HEALTH POLICY FOR CHILDREN
AND ADOLESCENTS, NO. 7

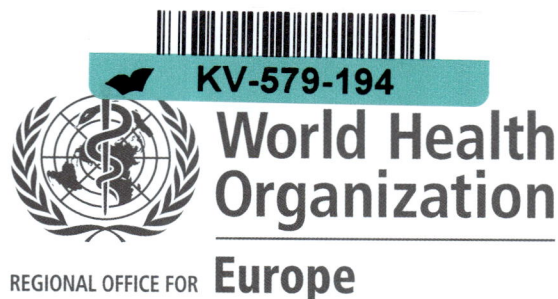

World Health Organization

REGIONAL OFFICE FOR **Europe**

Growing up unequal: gender and socioeconomic differences in young people's health and well-being

HEALTH BEHAVIOUR IN SCHOOL-AGED CHILDREN (HBSC) STUDY:
INTERNATIONAL REPORT FROM
THE 2013/2014 SURVEY

Edited by:
Jo Inchley, Dorothy Currie, Taryn Young,
Oddrun Samdal, Torbjørn Torsheim, Lise Augustson,
Frida Mathison, Aixa Aleman-Diaz, Michal Molcho,
Martin Weber and Vivian Barnekow

ABSTRACT

Health Behaviour in School-aged Children (HBSC), a WHO collaborative cross-national study, has provided information about the health, well-being, social environment and health behaviour of 11-, 13- and 15-year-old boys and girls for over 30 years. This latest international report from the study presents findings from the 2013/2014 survey, which collected data from almost 220 000 young people in 42 countries in Europe and North America. The data focus on social context (relations with family, peers and school), health outcomes (subjective health, injuries, obesity and mental health), health behaviours (patterns of eating, toothbrushing and physical activity) and risk behaviours (use of tobacco, alcohol and cannabis, sexual behaviour, fighting and bullying) relevant to young people's health and well-being. New items on family and peer support, migration, cyberbullying and serious injuries are also reflected in the report.

Keywords

HEALTH BEHAVIOR

HEALTH STATUS DISPARITIES

SOCIOECONOMIC FACTORS

GENDER IDENTITY

ADOLESCENT HEALTH

CHILD HEALTH

ADOLESCENT

CHILD

ISBN 978 92 890 5136 1

Data presented in this report can be accessed at the WHO Regional Office for Europe's health information gateway (http://portal.euro.who.int/en/) and via the WHO European health statistics mobile application (http://www.euro.who.int/en/data-and-evidence/the-european-health-statistics-app).

Address requests about publications of the WHO Regional Office for Europe to:

Publications

WHO Regional Office for Europe

UN City, Marmorvej 51

DK-2100 Copenhagen Ø, Denmark

Alternatively, complete an online request form for documentation, health information, or for permission to quote or translate, on the Regional Office web site (http://www.euro.who.int/pubrequest).

CONTENTS

CONTRIBUTORS

EDITORIAL BOARD

Jo Inchley	HBSC International Coordinator, Child and Adolescent Health Research Unit (CAHRU), School of Medicine, University of St Andrews, United Kingdom (Scotland)
Dorothy Currie	Deputy International Coordinator, CAHRU, School of Medicine, University of St Andrews, United Kingdom (Scotland)
Taryn Young	Assistant International Network Coordinator, CAHRU, School of Medicine, University of St Andrews, United Kingdom (Scotland)
Oddrun Samdal	HBSC Databank Manager, HBSC Data Management Centre, Department of Health Promotion and Development, University of Bergen, Norway
Torbjørn Torsheim	Professor, Department of Psychosocial Science, University of Bergen, Norway
Lise Augustson	Higher Executive Officer, Department of Health Promotion and Development, University of Bergen, Norway
Frida Mathisen	Researcher, Department of Health Promotion and Development, University of Bergen, Norway
Aixa Aleman-Diaz	Policy Officer, WHO Collaborating Centre for International Child and Adolescent Health Policy, School of Medicine, University of St Andrews, United Kingdom (Scotland)
Michal Molcho	Lecturer in Health Promotion, National University of Ireland, Galway, Ireland
Martin Weber	Programme Manager, Child and Adolescent Health, Noncommunicable Diseases and Health Promotion, WHO Regional Office for Europe
Vivian Barnekow	Consultant, WHO Regional Office for Europe

EDITORIAL AND PRODUCTION TEAM

Alex Mathieson	Freelance Writer and Editor, Edinburgh, United Kingdom (Scotland)
Damian Mullan	Designer, So it begins…, Edinburgh, United Kingdom (Scotland)
Jill Calder	Illustration and Calligraphy, Cellardyke, United Kingdom (Scotland)

Quotations were supplied by the HBSC Youth Engagement Group and collected by: Emmanuelle Godeau (France), Margarida Gaspar de Matos (Portugal), Zuzana Novakova (Slovakia), Colette Kelly (Ireland), Aixa Aleman-Diaz (United Kingdom (Scotland)) and Fiona Brooks (United Kingdom (England)).

WRITERS AND CONTRIBUTORS

Part/chapter	Writers
PART 1. INTRODUCTION	
HEALTH BEHAVIOUR IN SCHOOL-AGED CHILDREN (HBSC) STUDY	Jo Inchley (United Kingdom (Scotland)), Aixa Aleman-Diaz (United Kingdom (Scotland)), Colette Kelly (Ireland), Sophie Walsh (Israel), Gonneke Stevens (Netherlands)
PART 2. KEY DATA	
CHAPTER 1. UNDERSTANDING THIS REPORT	Dorothy Currie (United Kingdom (Scotland)), Frank Elgar (Canada), Lise Augustson (Norway), Torbjørn Torsheim (Norway)
CHAPTER 2. SOCIAL CONTEXT	
Family	Fiona Brooks (United Kingdom (England))
Peers	Michela Lenzi (Italy), Rob Gommans (Netherlands)
School	Mette Rasmussen (Denmark), John Freeman (Canada), Don Klinger (Canada), Kristiine Liiv (Estonia), Oddrun Samdal (Norway), Friedrich Teutsch (Austria), Jana Vasickova (Czech Republic)
CHAPTER 3. HEALTH OUTCOMES	
Positive health	Veronika Ottova-Jordan (Germany), Inese Gobina (Latvia), Joanna Mazur (Poland)
Medically attended injuries	Sophie Walsh (Israel), Alina Cosma (United Kingdom (Scotland))
Body weight	Giacomo Lazzeri (Italy), Kristiina Ojala (Finland), Arsaell Arnarsson (Iceland), Ágnes Németh (Hungary)
CHAPTER 4. HEALTH BEHAVIOURS	
Eating behaviour	Colette Kelly (Ireland), Giacomo Lazzeri (Italy), Anna Dzielska (Poland)
Oral health	Sisko Honkala (Finland)
Energy expenditure	Jens Bucksch (Germany), Zdenek Hamrik (Czech Republic), Hania Nalecz (Poland)
CHAPTER 5. RISK BEHAVIOURS	
Tobacco use	Anne Hublet (Belgium (Flemish))
Alcohol use	Margreet de Looze (Netherlands), Tibor Baska (Slovakia), Alessio Vieno (Italy), Daria Pavlova (Ukraine)
Cannabis use	Yossi Harel-Fisch (Israel), Anne Hublet (Belgium (Flemish))
Sexual behaviour	András Költő (Hungary), Josefine Magnusson (United Kingdom (England))
Fighting	Sophie Walsh (Israel), Alina Cosma (United Kingdom (Scotland))
Bullying	Sophie Walsh (Israel), Alina Cosma (United Kingdom (Scotland))

Part/chapter	Writers
PART 3. DISCUSSION	
CHAPTER 6. AGE	Oddrun Samdal (Norway)
CHAPTER 7. GENDER	Margreet De Looze (Netherlands)
CHAPTER 8. FAMILY AFFLUENCE	Frank Elgar (Canada)
CHAPTER 9. CONCLUSION	
Scientific conclusions	Jo Inchley (United Kingdom (Scotland)), Alina Cosma (United Kingdom (Scotland))
Policy conclusions	Michal Molcho (Ireland), Aixa Aleman-Diaz (United Kingdom (Scotland)), Wendy Craig (Canada)
ANNEX	Torbjørn Torsheim (Norway), Dorothy Currie (United Kingdom (Scotland)), Lise Augustson (Norway), Oddrun Samdal (Norway)

Function/organization	Contributors
DATA ANALYSIS	Torbjørn Torsheim (Norway), Lise Augustson (Norway), Frida Mathisen (Norway), Dorothy Currie (United Kingdom (Scotland))
INTERNATIONAL REPORT MANAGEMENT GROUP	Aixa Aleman-Diaz (United Kingdom (Scotland)), Lise Augustson (Norway), Vivian Barnekow (WHO Regional Office for Europe), Alina Cosma (United Kingdom (Scotland)), Dorothy Currie (United Kingdom (Scotland)), Inese Gobina (Latvia), Joseph Hancock (HBSC International Coordinating Centre), Jo Inchley (HBSC International Coordinator), Colette Kelly (Ireland), Tina Kiaer (WHO Regional Office for Europe), Frida Mathisen (Norway), Michal Molcho (Ireland), Oddrun Samdal (HBSC International Databank Manager), Torbjørn Torsheim (Norway), Martin Weber (WHO Regional Office for Europe), Taryn Young (HBSC International Coordinating Centre), Felicity Wild (HBSC International Coordinating Centre)
WHO REGIONAL OFFICE FOR EUROPE	Martin Weber (Programme Manager, Child and Adolescent Health), Vivian Barnekow (Consultant), Joao Joaquim Rodrigues da Silva Breda (Programme Manager, Nutrition, Physical Activity and Obesity), Lars Fodgaard Møller (Programme Manager, Alcohol, Illicit Drugs and Prison Health), Gunta Lazdane (Programme Manager, Sexual and Reproductive Health), Kristina Mauer-Stender (Programme Manager, Tobacco Control), Dinesh Sethi (Programme Manager, Violence and Injury Prevention), Isabel Yordi Aguirre (Technical Officer, Gender and Health)

HBSC PRINCIPAL INVESTIGATORS

HBSC international coordination for the 2013/2014 survey	Candace Currie (International Coordinator to June 2015), Jo Inchley (International Coordinator from June 2015), Aixa Aleman-Diaz, Dorothy Currie, Joseph Hancock, Felicity Wild, Taryn Young	HBSC International Coordinating Centre, CAHRU, School of Medicine, University of St Andrews, (United Kingdom (Scotland))
HBSC databank management for the 2013/2014 survey	Oddrun Samdal (International Databank Manager), Lise Augustson, Frida Mathisen, Torbjørn Torsheim	HBSC Data Management Centre, Department of Health Promotion and Development, University of Bergen, Norway

Country or region	Principal investigators	Institutions
Albania	Gentiana Qirjako	Faculty of Public Health, University of Medicine, Tirana
Armenia	Sergey Sargsyan	Arabkir Medical Centre – Institute of Child and Adolescent Health, Yerevan
Austria	Rosemarie Felder-Puig	Ludwig Boltzmann Institute for Health Promotion Research, University of Vienna
Belgium (Flemish)	Carine Vereecken (to 2012) Anne Hublet (from 2012)	Department of Public Health, University of Ghent
Belgium (French)	Danielle Piette	School of Public Health, Université Libre de Bruxelles
Bulgaria	Lidiya Vasileva	Institute for Population and Human Studies, Bulgarian Academy of Sciences, Sofia
Canada	John Freeman	Faculty of Education, Queen's University, Kingston
	Will Pickett	Faculty of Health Sciences, Queen's University, Kingston
Croatia	Marina Kuzman (to 2013) Ivana Pavic Simetin (from 2013)	Croatian Institute of Public Health, Zagreb
Czech Republic	Michal Kalman	Palacky University, Olomouc
Denmark	Pernille Due (to 2012) Mette Rasmussen (from 2012)	National Institute of Public Health, University of Southern Denmark, Copenhagen
Estonia	Katrin Aasvee	National Institute for Health Development, Tallinn
Finland	Jorma Tynjälä	Department of Health Sciences, University of Jyväskylä
France	Emmanuelle Godeau	Service Médical du Rectorat de Toulouse, Université Paul Sabatier, Toulouse

Country or region	Principal investigators	Institutions
Germany	Petra Kolip (to 2015) Matthias Richter (from 2015)	School of Public Health, University of Bielefeld Institute of Medical Sociology, Martin Luther University, Halle-Wittenberg
Greece	Anna Kokkevi	University Mental Health Research Institute, Athens
Greenland	Birgit Niclasen	Department of Health, Government of Greenland, Nuuk
Hungary	Ágnes Németh	National Institute for Health Promotion, Budapest
Iceland	Arsaell Arnarsson	University of Akureyri
Ireland	Saoirse Nic Gabhainn Michal Molcho	Health Promotion Research Centre, National University of Ireland, Galway (WHO Collaborating Centre for Health Promotion Research)
Israel	Yossi Harel-Fisch	International Research Programme on Adolescent Well-being and Health, School of Education, Bar-Ilan University, Ramat Gan
Italy	Franco Cavallo	Department of Public Health and Paediatrics, School of Medicine, University of Turin
Latvia	Iveta Pudule	Centre for Disease Prevention and Control, Riga
Lithuania	Apolinaras Zaborskis	Lithuanian University of Health Sciences
Luxembourg	Yolande Wagener	Directorate of Health/Division for School Health, Children and Adolescents, Ministry of Health, Luxembourg
Malta	Charmaine Gauci	Health Promotion Directorate, Msida
Netherlands	Wilma Vollebergh Tom ter Bogt	Department of Interdisciplinary Social Science, Faculty of Social and Behavioural Sciences, University of Utrecht
Norway	Oddrun Samdal	Department of Health Promotion and Development, University of Bergen
Poland	Joanna Mazur	Department of Child and Adolescent Health, Institute of Mother and Child, Warsaw
Portugal	Margarida Gaspar de Matos	Faculty of Human Kinetics, University of Lisbon
Republic of Moldova	Galina Lesco	National Resource Centre, youth-friendly health service NEOVITA, Chisinau

Country or region	Principal investigators	Institutions
Romania	Adriana Baban	Department of Psychology, Babes Bolyai University, Cluj-Napoca
Russian Federation	Oleg Churganov	Scientific-Research Institute of Physical Culture, St Petersburg
Slovakia	Andrea Madarasová Gecková	Department of Health Psychology, Faculty of Medicine, Pavol Jozef Šafárik University, Kosice
Slovenia	Helena Jericek	Institute of Public Health of the Republic of Slovenia, Ljubljana
Spain	Carmen Moreno Rodriguez	Department of Developmental and Educational Psychology, University of Seville
Sweden	Lilly Augustine (to 2015) Petra Lofstedt (from 2015)	Public Health Agency of Sweden
Switzerland	Emmanuel Kuntsche	Addiction Switzerland, Research Institute, Lausanne
The former Yugoslav Republic of Macedonia	Lina Kostarova Unkovska	Centre for Psychosocial and Crisis Action, Skopje
Turkey	Oya Ercan	Cerrahpasa Medical Faculty, Department of Paediatrics, Istanbul University
Ukraine	Olga Balakireva	Institute for Economy and Forecasting, National Academy of Sciences of Ukraine, Kiev
United Kingdom (England)	Antony Morgan (to 2015) Fiona Brooks	Centre for Research in Primary and Community Care, University of Hertfordshire, Hatfield
United Kingdom (Scotland)	Candace Currie (to 2015) Jo Inchley (from 2015)	CAHRU, School of Medicine, University of St Andrews
United Kingdom (Wales)	Chris Roberts	Health and Social Services Analytical Team, Social Research and Information Division, Welsh Government, Cardiff
United States of America	Ronald Iannotti	The CDM Group, Maryland

A list of all country teams and members can be found on the HBSC website.

ACKNOWLEDGEMENTS

Health Behaviour in School-aged Children (HBSC), a WHO collaborative cross-national study, involves a wide network of researchers from all participating countries and regions.

The data collection in each country or region was funded at national level. The editorial board is grateful for the financial support and guidance offered by government ministries, research foundations and other funding bodies in the participating countries and regions. We particularly thank NHS (National Health Service) Health Scotland (WHO Collaborating Centre for Health Promotion), which contributed funding to the HBSC International Coordinating Centre (until 2013) and to support printing of this report, and the Norwegian Directorate of Health, which contributed funding to the HBSC Data Management Centre. The report's production was supported by a generous contribution from the WHO Regional Office for Europe.

We are grateful for support from staff at the Norwegian Social Science Data Services, Bergen, for their assistance in preparing the international data file.

We would like to thank: our valued partners, particularly WHO Regional Office for Europe, for their continuing support; the young people who were willing to share their experiences with us and those who kindly allowed us to include some of their comments in this report; schools and education authorities in each participating country and region for making the survey possible; and all members of national HBSC teams involved in the research.

We are also grateful to Dr Peter Donnelly, President and Chief Executive Officer, Public Health Ontario, and Professor Bjorn Holstein, University of Southern Denmark, for providing very helpful feedback on an earlier draft.

Jo Inchley, Dorothy Currie, Taryn Young, Oddrun Samdal, Torbjørn Torsheim, Lise Augustson, Frida Mathison, Aixa Aleman-Diaz, Michal Molcho, Martin Weber and Vivian Barnekow

PREFACE

The Health Behaviour in School-aged Children (HBSC) study is now in its 33rd year. It continues to grow not only as a source of reliable and valid data on the health behaviours of 11-, 13- and 15-year-olds, but also in its membership – 44 countries and regions across Europe and North America are now included.

The European strategy for child and adolescent health, much of which is based on data from HBSC surveys, sets out a vision, guiding principles and priorities for countries to work across sectors and with partners to protect and promote the health and well-being of children and adolescents throughout the WHO European Region. It emphasizes how the health of children and adolescents is important for every society, now and for the future. It is within this context that HBSC sits, and to which it makes such an important contribution.

HBSC focuses on a wide range of health, education, social and family measures that affect young people's health and well-being. Previous reports from the study have highlighted age, geographic and family-affluence factors, and social determinants of health. This sixth international report, which presents data from the 2013/2014 survey, focuses on the effect of gender and socioeconomic differences on the way young people grow and develop.

But while gender issues are central to the report, they are not its only focus. As is the case with previous HBSC reports, the effects of age and socioeconomic status are also reviewed, building on the latest HBSC data and other scientific evidence to offer recommendations to policy-makers in countries and regions. The report adds to the growing body of evidence for effective interventions to tackle the pervasive effects of social and health inequalities, which are widening between and within countries.

In particular, it provides a lens on two areas that present threats to children and young people's health and well-being, one very old – migration – and the other very new – cyberbullying. At a time when Europe is witnessing unprecedented patterns of migration, we must remain alert to the health and well-being risks all immigrants, but perhaps particularly children and young people, face when leaving what was once home and moving to a new country. And while technological developments offer children and young people wonderful opportunities for personal development and growth, to stay in close touch with friends and families, and to have fun, they also present challenges that can lead to severe and lasting effects on health and well-being. Technology is unquestionably a positive presence in all our lives, but we must remain vigilant to the threats it poses to children and young people.

Once again, HBSC provides us with strong evidence to support positive policy action in countries and regions. It offers data that are of value to sectors beyond health as governments and their partners seek to develop and refine policies to promote and protect the health and well-being of children and young people.

HBSC supports the achievement of one of the main tenets of the European strategy for child and adolescent health – that children and adolescents have a right to be seen and heard. It is their voices that speak through the HBSC data. We all must listen.

Jo Inchley
HBSC International Coordinator

Dorothy Currie
HBSC Deputy International Coordinator

FOREWORD

The Health Behaviour in School-aged Children (HBSC) study demonstrates unequivocally the importance of adolescence to the short-, medium- and long-term health and well-being potential of girls, boys, women and men. That is why HBSC is such a valuable resource. It explains how social determinants and health behaviours in childhood and adolescence lead to ongoing physical and mental health problems in adulthood and, more important, points us to interventions that support the development of positive health behaviours and well-being in children and young people that can become lifelong.

Despite the considerable advances made in the WHO European Region over the decades in improving the health and well-being of young people and recent actions to reduce the health inequalities many of them face, some remain disadvantaged from birth by virtue of their gender. That disadvantage, which spreads across the life-course of girls and women in social, educational, employment and welfare spheres, has an early and lasting impact on health and well-being.

A recent report from the WHO Regional Office for Europe looking at women's health in Europe across the life-course shows that opportunities are present during childhood and adolescence for evidence-based actions to prevent future ill health and fully realize girls' health and well-being potential. But inequalities in health linked to gender and social factors, such as place of residence, maternal/family socioeconomic status, ethnicity and migrant status, persist for girls across the Region.

Gender issues arising in childhood and adolescence also affect the long-term health and well-being prospects of boys. Many of the health behaviours and habits that lead to illness, disability and premature death in adult men – cardiovascular disease, diabetes, cancer and mental health problems – have their roots in the adolescent period. Evidence from throughout the Region shows us that men die earlier and live considerable portions of their lives in poor health: HBSC helps us to understand why.

Addressing child and adolescent health and well-being requires whole-of-government and whole-of society approaches that reach far into the fabric of communities and societies to change entrenched attitudes and behaviours. The European policy for health and well-being, Health 2020, lays the foundations for intersectoral action that can serve to promote improvement across all the areas that affect the health and well-being of children and young people – education, welfare, transport, leisure and social protection, to name but a few.

The HBSC study takes its place among a rich trove of resources developed through the Regional Office, which includes Health 2020, the review of social determinants and the health divide in Europe, and the European strategy for child and adolescent health. The strategy for child and adolescent health in particular offers countries an invaluable tool to promote and nurture the positive health behaviours in childhood and adolescence that lay the foundations for healthy adulthoods.

Growing up unequal, the title of this sixth international report from the HBSC study, serves as a call to action to all of us involved in protecting and promoting the health and well-being of children and young people in Europe. HBSC invites children and young people to tell it like it is and highlight the issues that are important to them. Those issues must also be important to us.

Zsuzsanna Jakab
WHO Regional Director for Europe

ABBREVIATIONS

BMI	body mass index
EMC	electronic media communication
FAS	(HBSC) Family Affluence Scale
HBSC	Health Behaviour in School-aged Children (study/survey)
HiAP	health in all policies
IOTF	International Obesity Task Force
MSPSS	Multidimensional Scale of Perceived Social Support
MVPA	moderate-to-vigorous physical activity
SES	socioeconomic status
STIs	sexually transmitted infections
UNICEF	United Nations Children's Fund

INTRODUCTION

PART 1

HEALTH BEHAVIOUR IN SCHOOL-AGED CHILDREN (HBSC) STUDY

HBSC, a WHO collaborative cross-national study, asks 11-, 13- and 15-year-old boys and girls about their health and well-being, social environments and health behaviours every four years using a self-report survey. Full contact details for the international survey and national teams can be found on the HBSC website *(1)*.

HBSC uses findings at national and international levels to:
- gain new insight into young people's[1] health and well-being
- understand the social determinants of health
- inform policy and practice to improve young people's lives.

The first HBSC survey was conducted in 1983/1984 in five countries. The study has now grown to include 44 countries and regions across Europe and North America. The table shows the growth in the international network over the nine survey rounds.

RESEARCH APPROACH

HBSC focuses on understanding young people's health in their social context – at home, school, and with family and friends. Researchers in the HBSC network are interested in understanding how these factors, individually and collectively, influence young people's health as they move into young adulthood. Data are collected in all participating countries and regions through school-based surveys using a standard methodology detailed in the HBSC 2013/2014 international study protocol *(2)*.

Each country or region uses random sampling to select a proportion of young people aged 11, 13 and 15 years, ensuring that the sample is representative of all in the age range. Around 1500 students in each HBSC country or region were selected from each age group in the 2013/2014 survey, totalling almost 220 000 (see the Annex for further details).

Of the 44 countries and regions that are HBSC network members, 42 completed the 2013/2014 survey and met the guidelines for publication of data in this report. Those not included were unable to conduct the survey. Fieldwork took place mainly between September 2013 and June 2014, except in four countries, where an extended fieldwork period was necessary to reach the required sample size. Further information on the survey design, consent and fieldwork is given in the Annex, and a more detailed description of the research approach is set out in the HBSC 2013/2014 international study protocol *(2)*. Methodological development of the study since its inception is described by Roberts et al. *(3)*.

IMPORTANCE OF RESEARCH ON YOUNG PEOPLE'S HEALTH

Young people aged between 11 and 15 years face many pressures and challenges, including growing academic expectations, changing social relationships with family and peers, and the physical and emotional changes associated with maturation. These years mark a period of increased autonomy in which independent decision-making that may influence their health and health-related behaviour develops.

Behaviours established during this transition period can continue into adulthood, affecting issues such as mental health, the development of health complaints, alcohol and tobacco use, physical activity levels and diet. HBSC's findings show the changes in young people's health as they move from childhood through adolescence and into adulthood. They can be used to monitor young people's health and determine the effectiveness of health improvement interventions.

HBSC RESEARCH NETWORK

The number of researchers working on HBSC across the 44 countries and regions now exceeds 340. Information on each national team is available on the HBSC website *(1)*. The study is supported by two specialist centres: the International Coordinating Centre, based at the Child and Adolescent Health Research Unit, School of Medicine, University of St Andrews, United Kingdom (Scotland);

---

[1] This report uses the terms young people and adolescents interchangeably to describe respondents to the survey.

HBSC SURVEYS: COUNTRIES AND REGIONS INCLUDED IN THE INTERNATIONAL DATA FILES

#	1983/1984	1985/1986	1989/1990	1993/1994	1997/1998	2001/2002	2005/2006	2009/2010	2013/2014
1	England	Finland	Finland	Finland	Finland	Finland	Finland	Finland	Finland
2	Finland	Norway	Norway	Norway	Norway	Norway	Norway	Norway	Norway
3	Norway	Austria	Austria	Austria	Austria	Austria	Austria	Austria	Austria
4	Austria	Belgium (French)	Belgium[b]	Belgium (French)	Belgium (French)	Belgium (French)	Belgium (French)	Belgium (French)	Belgium (French)
5	Denmark[a]	Hungary	Hungary	Hungary	Hungary	Hungary	Hungary	Hungary	Hungary
6		Israel	Scotland	Israel	Israel	Israel	Israel	Israel	Israel
7		Scotland	Spain	Scotland	Scotland	Scotland	Scotland	Scotland	Scotland
8		Spain	Sweden	Spain	Spain	Spain	Spain	Spain	Spain
9		Sweden	Switzerland	Sweden	Sweden	Sweden	Sweden	Sweden	Sweden
10		Switzerland	Wales	Switzerland	Switzerland	Switzerland	Switzerland	Switzerland	Switzerland
11		Wales	Denmark[a]	Wales	Wales	Wales	Wales	Wales	Wales
12		Denmark[a]	Netherlands[a]	Denmark	Denmark	Denmark	Denmark	Denmark	Denmark
13		Netherlands[a]	Canada	Netherlands	Canada	Canada	Canada	Canada	Canada
14			Latvia[a]	Canada	Latvia	Latvia	Latvia	Latvia	Latvia
15			Northern Ireland[a]	Latvia	Northern Ireland	Poland	Poland	Poland	Poland
16			Poland	Northern Ireland	Poland	Belgium (Flemish)	Belgium (Flemish)	Belgium (Flemish)	Belgium (Flemish)
17				Poland	Belgium (Flemish)	Czech Republic	Czech Republic	Czech Republic	Czech Republic
18				Belgium (Flemish)	Czech Republic	Estonia	Estonia	Estonia	Estonia
19				Czech Republic	Estonia	France	France	France	France
20				Estonia	France	Germany	Germany	Germany	Germany
21				France	Germany	Greenland	Greenland	Greenland	Greenland
22				Germany	Greenland	Lithuania	Lithuania	Lithuania	Lithuania
23				Greenland	Lithuania	Russian Federation	Russian Federation	Russian Federation	Russian Federation
24				Lithuania	Russian Federation	Slovakia	Slovakia	Slovakia	Slovakia
25				Russian Federation	Slovakia	England	England	England	England
26				Slovakia	England	Greece	Greece	Greece	Greece
27					Greece	Portugal	Portugal	Portugal	Portugal
28					Portugal	Ireland	Ireland	Ireland	Ireland
29					Ireland	United States	United States	United States	MKD[c]
30					United States	MKD[c]	MKD[c]	MKD[c]	Netherlands
31						Netherlands	Netherlands	Netherlands	Italy
32						Italy	Italy	Italy	Croatia
33						Croatia	Croatia	Croatia	Malta
34						Malta	Malta	Malta	Slovenia
35						Slovenia	Slovenia	Slovenia	Ukraine
36						Ukraine	Ukraine	Ukraine	Iceland
37							Bulgaria	Iceland	Luxembourg
38							Iceland	Luxembourg	Romania
39							Luxembourg	Romania	Armenia
40							Romania	Turkey	Bulgaria
41							Turkey	Armenia	Albania
42									Republic of Moldova

[a] Carried out survey after scheduled fieldwork dates. [b] National data file. [c] The former Yugoslav Republic of Macedonia (MKD is an abbreviation of the International Organization for Standardization (ISO)).
Note: although Albania and Bulgaria participated in the 2009/2010 survey, they are not listed because the national data were not submitted to the international data centre by the deadline.

and the Data Management Centre, based at the Department of Health Promotion and Development, University of Bergen, Norway. It is led by the International Coordinator, Dr Jo Inchley, and the Databank Manager is Professor Oddrun Samdal. The study is funded at national level in each of its member countries and regions.

ENGAGING WITH YOUNG PEOPLE

The vision is to involve young people in all aspects of the HBSC study beyond completing questionnaires in the classroom, from identifying domains of inquiry to the dissemination of results. Youth engagement consequently has become a core and integral part of the work undertaken in the HBSC network. It represents a meaningful way of recognizing and including young people as critical stakeholders in the production of science and policy.

Fundamental to the work is Article 12 of the United Nations Convention on the Rights of the Child (4), which enshrines the rights of children to have their views and opinions heard, respected and taken into account. Young people have a right to participate in issues that concern their lives and in the determination of decisions that are relevant to them. Their role in research has traditionally been as a resource, but participatory research engages them to do more than provide responses to research instruments designed by adults. Given that children and young people are experts in their own lives, their active engagement in research that is relevant to them is essential.

The HBSC network has developed a range of methodologies to facilitate young people's active engagement in the research process. The approach explicitly concerns power within the research cycle and the requirement for research to be both empowering and health-promoting. Participatory research approaches with young people have been employed in the HBSC study in relation to data generation, devising new research areas and related questions, and data analysis, interpretation and dissemination.

There are countless examples of teams in the network embracing such approaches in their national projects, including those in Canada, Czech Republic, France, Ireland, Poland, Portugal, Scotland, Slovakia and United Kingdom (England) (5–7). Others aim to document the scientific evidence base on the benefits of involving young people in the development, implementation and evaluation of health-related programmes.

While there is still much to do in terms of streamlining practice at international level, the HBSC work will drive the case for youth engagement as an international standard in adolescent health research. The aim is to capture data that are meaningful to young people and which reflect their current lifestyles, while also being of significant value to programme and policy design.

Quotations supplied by the HBSC Youth Engagement Group appear throughout this report, highlighting issues young people have identified as being important to them.

ENGAGING WITH POLICY-MAKERS

Data such as those presented in this report provide an essential, but not sufficient, basis for policy action to improve young people's well-being. The HBSC network therefore works closely with external partners to maximize the impact of its findings and the reach of its experts.

Through its long-standing partnership with WHO, the study has become an integral part of efforts to invest in young people's health, such as the European child and adolescent health strategy for 2015 to 2020 (8), major publications on adolescent health (9), global adolescent health indicator coordination and the development of WHO collaborating centres[2] specifically aimed at increasing the knowledge base on adolescent health (10).

---

[2] Current centres include: the WHO Collaborating Centre for International Child and Adolescent Health Policy (Scotland); the WHO Collaborating Centre for Health Promotion and Education (Norway); the WHO Collaborating Centre for Health Promotion Research (Ireland); and the WHO Collaborating Centre for Health Promotion and Public Health Development (Scotland).

HBSC experts and data have been integral to the development, implementation and monitoring of strategies. This latest HBSC report, which is part of the WHO Health Policy for Children and Adolescents series established in 1999, represents an additional effort to raise the profile of children and young people's health for policy-makers.

One of the main aims of the HBSC network is to create and maintain active collaboration with health and education ministries, and other government entities responsible for the well-being of young people. The study has been at the forefront of making research relevant to policy and practice, while also engaging with policy-makers in identifying themes that should be included in the study.

The WHO/HBSC Forum series (11–13) convened researchers, policy-makers and practitioners to analyse data, review policies and interventions and formulate lessons learnt about priority public health issues from the perspective of social determinants of health. HBSC members work nationally to encourage the inclusion and use of adolescent health indicators in relevant policy and implementation documents.

The study has also built strong relationships with national and international stakeholders, such as other adolescent health surveys, lobbyists, and professional groups and networks, including the United Nations Children's Fund (UNICEF), the European Commission, the Organisation for Economic Co-operation and Development, Eurochild, the Excellence in Pediatrics Institute and the Schools for Health in Europe Network. These organizations work strategically and practically to advance the rights and well-being of young people and benefit from the use and dissemination of HBSC data. HBSC data and experts have featured, for example, in a number of UNICEF report cards, including the forthcoming Report Card 13 that will be published in 2016. HBSC continues to explore innovative ways to engage with stakeholders interested in improving young people's health and is willing to work with organizations and individuals seeking to advance this goal.

SOCIAL DETERMINANTS OF HEALTH AND WELL-BEING AMONG YOUNG PEOPLE

Evidence gathered over the last few decades shows that disadvantaged social circumstances are associated with increased health risks (14–16). As a result, health inequalities are now embedded in contemporary international policy development. The WHO Commission on Social Determinants of Health claims that the vast majority of inequalities in health within and between countries are avoidable (17), yet they continue to be experienced by young people across Europe and North America.

Young people are often neglected as a population group in health statistics, being either aggregated with younger children or with young adults. Less attention has been paid to inequalities related to socioeconomic status (SES), age and gender among this group. This report seeks to identify and discuss the extent of these inequalities and highlight the need for preventive action to, as UNICEF puts it (18), "turn this vulnerable age into an age of opportunity".

In general, young people in the WHO European Region enjoy better health and development than ever before, but are failing to achieve their full potential. This results in significant social, economic and human costs and wide variations in health. Health experience during the adolescent period has short- and long-term implications for individuals and society. Within a life-course approach (19), adolescence is critical in determining adult behaviour in relation to issues such as tobacco and alcohol use, dietary behaviour and physical activity. Health inequalities in adult life are partly determined by early life circumstances.

Findings presented in this report can contribute to WHO's European policy for health and well-being, Health 2020 (20), which aims to ensure an evidence-based and coherent policy framework capable of addressing present and future challenges to population health. It provides a clear common vision and roadmap for pursuing health and health equity across the European Region, strengthening the promotion of population health and reducing health inequities by addressing the social determinants of health. The data can also support implementation of the European child and adolescent health strategy (8), which calls for targeted action to break negative cycles in childhood and adolescence and give every child the opportunity to live a healthy and meaningful life.

Attempts to address health inequalities must include examination of differences in health status and their causes. The HBSC study has collected data on the health and health behaviours of young people since 1983, enabling it to describe how health varies across countries and regions and increase understanding of inequalities due to age, gender and SES. HBSC recognizes the importance of the relationships that comprise the immediate social context of young people's lives and shows how family, peers and school can provide supportive environments for healthy development. Importantly, the study has shown that it is not only health outcomes that are differentiated by age, gender and SES, but also the social circumstances in which young people grow up.

DIMENSIONS OF INEQUALITIES

Social inequalities in health are traditionally measured by examining differences in SES as defined by individuals' (or, in the case of young people, their parents') position in the labour market, education status or income. Gender, ethnicity, age, place of residence and disability are also important dimensions of social difference but have been insufficiently researched in relation to young people's health outcomes.

It has been argued that these determinants need to be researched in their own right to enable fully developed explanations of health inequalities to emerge (21). This is very important in policy terms, as evidence suggests that segments of the population respond differently to identical public health interventions. Researchers can therefore play an important role in advancing understanding of the individual influences of each of the dimensions of health inequalities and how they interact to affect health.

This report contributes to developing a better understanding of determinants of, and inequalities in, young people's health by presenting data from the HBSC 2013/2014 survey analysed in four dimensions: age, gender, country/region of residence and family affluence. First, however, it describes what is known about the relationship between social determinants and young people's health and well-being.

OVERVIEW OF PREVIOUS HBSC FINDINGS

A review of HBSC evidence presented through academic journals and reports which has produced key findings influenced by these dimensions of health provides a platform for the presentation of new data in this report.

Age differences

Young people's health choices change during adolescence. Health inequalities emerge or worsen and translate into continuing health problems and inequalities in the adult years (22,23). These findings have important implications for the timing of health interventions and reinforce the idea that investment in young people must be sustained to consolidate the achievements of early childhood interventions (18). This is vital for individuals as they grow, but is also important as a means of maximizing return on programmes focused on increasing investment in the early years and reducing the economic effects of health problems.

Gender differences

Previous HBSC reports have presented findings for boys and girls separately, providing clear evidence of gender differences in health that have persisted or changed over time. Boys in general engage more in externalizing or expressive forms of health behaviours, such as drinking or fighting, while girls tend to deal with health issues in a more emotional or internalizing way, often manifesting as psychosomatic symptoms or mental health problems (24).

Gender differences for some health behaviours and indicators, such as current attempts to lose weight (25) and psychosomatic complaints (24,26–31), tend to increase during adolescence, indicating that this is a crucial period for the development of health differentials that may track into adulthood. Targeting young people's health from a gender perspective has considerable potential to reduce health differentials based on gender in adulthood.

The magnitude of gender differences varies considerably cross-nationally. Gender difference in psychological and physical symptoms, for example, is stronger in countries with a low gender development index score (26). Similarly, the gender difference in drunkenness is greater in eastern European countries (31). These findings underscore the need to incorporate macro-level sociocontextual factors in the study of gender health inequalities among young people (27).

Socioeconomic differences

The HBSC study has found family affluence to be an important predictor of young people's health. In general, cost may restrict families' opportunities to adopt healthy behaviours, such as eating fruit and vegetables (32–34) and participating in fee-based physical activity (35,36). Young people living in low-affluence households are less likely to have adequate access to health resources (37) and more likely to be exposed to psychosocial stress, which underpin health inequalities in self-rated health and well-being (38). Many of these inequalities have persisted or increased over time (39,40). A better understanding of the effects may enable the identification of the origins of socioeconomic differences in adult health and offer opportunities to define possible pathways through which adult health inequalities are produced and reproduced.

The distribution of wealth within countries also significantly affects young people's health. In general, young people in countries and regions with large differences in wealth distribution are more vulnerable to poorer health outcomes, independent of their individual family wealth (27,30,40–44).

Country differences in health

Variations between countries and regions in patterns of health and its social determinants are seen. Over the 30 years of the HBSC study, it has been possible to monitor how young people's health and lifestyle patterns have developed in the context of political and economic change. Between the 1997/1998 and 2005/2006 HBSC surveys, for instance, the frequency of drunkenness increased by an average of 40% in all participating eastern European countries; at the same time, drunkenness declined by an average of 25% in 13 of 16 western European and North American countries. These trends may be attributed to policies that, respectively, either liberalized or restricted the alcohol industry (45) and to changes in social norms and economic factors.

The findings underline the importance of the wider societal context and the effect –positive and negative – it can have on young people's health. While geographic patterns are not analysed in this report, the maps featured in Chapters 2–5 allow comparison between countries and regions. Future HBSC publications may investigate these cross-national differences.

SOCIAL CONTEXT OF YOUNG PEOPLE'S HEALTH

There is some evidence to suggest that protective mechanisms and assets offered in the immediate social context of young people's lives can offset the effect of some structural determinants of health inequalities, including poverty and deprivation (46–48). Understanding how these social environments act as protective and risk factors can therefore support efforts to address health inequalities.

Research confirms that young people can accumulate protective factors, increasing the likelihood of coping with adverse situations even in poorer life circumstances (12). The HBSC study highlights a range of factors associated with these broad social environments that can create opportunities to improve young people's health.

Family

Communication with parents is key in establishing the family as a protective factor. Support from family equips young people to deal with stressful situations, buffering them against the adverse consequences of several negative influences (49). Young people who report ease of communication with their parents are also more likely to experience a range of positive health outcomes, such as higher self-rated health, higher life satisfaction (31) and fewer physical and psychological complaints (23). HBSC data show that ease of communication with mothers and fathers has increased in many countries in recent years (50).

The accumulation of support from parents, siblings and peers leads to an even stronger predictor of positive health: the higher the number of sources of support, the more likely it is that children will experience positive health (51). This suggests that professionals working in young people's health should not only address health problems directly, but also consider families' influence in supporting the development of health-promoting behaviours.

Peer relations

Developing positive peer relationships and friendships is crucial in helping adolescents deal with developmental tasks such as forming identity, developing social skills and self-esteem, and establishing autonomy. The HBSC study has identified areas across countries and regions in which having high-quality peer relationships serves as a protective factor, with the positive effects on adolescent health including fewer psychological complaints (52).

Adolescents who participate in social networks are found to have better perceived health and sense of well-being and take part in more healthy behaviours (31). Peers are therefore valuable social contacts who contribute to young people's health and well-being, but can also be negative influences in relation to risk behaviours such as smoking and drinking: this is a complex area (53,54).

School environment

Experiences in school can be crucial to the development of self-esteem, self-perception and health behaviour. HBSC findings show that those who perceive their school as supportive are more likely to engage in positive health behaviours and have better health outcomes, including good self-rated health, high levels of life satisfaction, few health complaints (55–59) and low smoking prevalence (60). These associations suggest that schools have an important role in supporting young people's well-being and in acting as buffers against negative health behaviours and outcomes.

Neighbourhood

Neighbourhoods that engender high levels of social capital create better mental health, more health-promoting behaviours, fewer risk-taking behaviours, better overall perceptions of health (12,61) and greater likelihood of physical activity (62). Building neighbourhood social capital is therefore a means of tackling health inequalities.

This review of research findings stemming from the HBSC study provides an introduction to the latest empirical findings and sets the scene in terms of understanding their importance and relevance to current debates on adolescent health.

NEW TOPICS INCLUDED IN THE 2013/2014 REPORT

The HBSC study has a continuous process of item review and development to address current issues affecting young people's health and well-being, and several new topics were introduced in the 2013/2014 survey. New topics presented here include peer and family support, serious injury, migration and cyberbullying. Data are included in the main chapters and/or the Annex.

Peer and family support

Social support from peers and parents is an important protective asset and is critical for adolescent psychosocial well-being. New items from the Multidimensional Scale of Perceived Social Support (MSPSS) (63) measuring perceived social support from parents and friends were added to existing items on family and peer relationships to provide insights into the role they play in young people's lives.

Serious injury

Three items on serious injury were included in the 2013/2014 survey: in the past 12 months, has the young person undergone a serious injury that needed medical treatment, such as stitches, a cast, surgery or overnight hospitalization; where were they when this happened; and what activity were they doing?

Serious injuries have important mortality and morbidity implications. Unintentional injuries (including traffic injuries, drowning, burns and falls) are the leading cause of death for children aged 10–19 years. Road traffic injuries alone are the leading cause of death among 15–19-year-olds and the second leading cause among those aged 10–14 (18,64). Severe injuries can require hospital treatment and cause lost school days, disabilities and physical and psychological wounds, with long-term consequences for the young person and substantial financial costs to the family and society. Consequently, monitoring and understanding serious injuries has been prioritized (65). Surveillance can allow the identification of more distinct patterns of occurrence of burdensome events and their potential causes, which can help to focus prevention strategies.

Migration

Recent years have seen growth in understanding of the vulnerability of immigrant adolescents and their susceptibility to reduced well-being and greater involvement in risk behaviours (66–69). Global migration and the increasing numbers of young people with immigrant roots (70) make the subject a critical public health issue. A mandatory question asking young people where they and each of their parents were born was introduced in the 2013/2014 survey: a summary table of results can be found in the Annex.

Cyberbullying

Two new mandatory questions on cyberbullying victimization were included, asking young people: if they had experienced being sent mean messages, emails, texts or wall-postings, or someone had created a website that made fun of them; or someone had taken unflattering or inappropriate photographs of them without permission and posted them online.

Constant access to internet and media devices has changed the way young people interact with and connect to each other. While this offers a wide range of benefits, it may also present the context for negative outcomes (71).

Cyberbullying is typically defined as aggression that is intentionally and repeatedly carried out in an electronic context (through, for example, email, blogs, instant messages and text messages) against a person who cannot easily defend him- or herself (72). Exposure to cyberbullying has been related to a wide range of negative outcomes, including anxiety, depression, substance abuse, increased physical symptoms, dropping out of school and decline in school performance (73,74). The new questions allow monitoring of the prevalence of this new, relevant and worrying phenomenon and understanding of its relationship to other facets of adolescent lives such as well-being, social relationships, academic performance and risk behaviours.

Accessing data

Data presented in this report can be accessed at the WHO Regional Office for Europe's health information gateway (75) and via the WHO European health statistics mobile application (76).

REFERENCES

1. HBSC [website]. St Andrews: Child and Adolescent Health Research Unit, University of St Andrews; 2015 (http://www.hbsc.org/, accessed 17 November 2015).

2. Currie C, Inchley J, Molcho M, Lenzi M, Veselska Z, Wild F, editors. Health Behaviour in School-Aged Children (HBSC) study protocol: background, methodology and mandatory items for the 2013/14 survey. St Andrews: Child and Adolescent Health Research Unit, University of St Andrews; 2014 (http://www.hbsc.org/news/index.aspx?ni=2418, accessed 17 November 2015).

3. Roberts C, Freeman J, Samdal O, Schnohr CW, de Looze ME, Nic Gabhainn S et al. The Health Behaviour in School-aged Children (HBSC) study: methodological developments and current tensions. Int J Public Health 2009;54:S140–50.

4. Convention on the Rights of the Child. Adopted and opened for signature, ratification and accession by General Assembly resolution 44/25 of 20 November 1989 entry into force 2 September 1990, in accordance with Article 49. New York (NY): United Nations; 1989 (http://www.ohchr.org/EN/ProfessionalInterest/Pages/CRC.aspx, accessed 17 November 2015).

5. Daniels N, Burke L, O'Donnell A, McGovern O, Kelly C, D'Eath M et al. Expanding the role of young people in research: towards a better understanding of their lives. Zdrowie Publiczne i Zarządzanie [Public Health and Management] 2014;12(1):36–44.

6. Gaspar de Matos M, Simones C, Gaspar T, Camacho I, Tome G, Reis M et al. Adolescentes, navegação segura poráguas desconhecidas [Adolescents in safe navigation through unknown waters]. Lisbon: Coisas de Ler; 2015.

7. Dzielska A, Salonna F, Małkowska-Szkutnik A, Mazur J, Tabak I, Vorlíček M et al. Are we growing up healthy? Social norms approach to promote healthy adolescent lifestyle in Visegrad as an example of e-health intervention. In: ESRII 3rd Conference, 17th–18th September 2015, Warsaw, Poland [website]. Warsaw: University of Social Sciences and Humanities; 2015 (http://www.esrii2015.org/?page_id=708, accessed 17 November 2015).

8. Investing in children: the European child and adolescent health strategy 2015–2020. Copenhagen: WHO Regional Office for Europe; 2014 (http://www.pnsd.msssi.gob.es/novedades/pdf/Investing_in_children_European_strategy.pdf, accessed 24 August 2015).

9. Health for the world's adolescents. A second chance in the second decade. Geneva: World Health Organization; 2014 (http://apps.who.int/adolescent/second-decade/, accessed 24 August 2015).

10. WHO collaborating centres global database [online database]. Geneva: World Health Organization; undated (http://apps.who.int/whocc//, accessed 17 November 2015).

11. Addressing the socioeconomic determinants of healthy eating habits and physical activity levels among adolescents: report from the 2006 HBSC/WHO Forum. Copenhagen: WHO Regional Office for Europe; 2006 (http://www.euro.who.int/__data/assets/pdf_file/0005/98231/e89375.pdf, accessed 24 August 2015).

12. Social cohesion for mental well-being among adolescents. Copenhagen: WHO Regional Office for Europe; 2008 (http://www.euro.who.int/__data/assets/pdf_file/0005/84623/E91921.pdf, accessed 16 November 2015).

13. Socio-environmentally determined health inequities among children and adolescents. Copenhagen: WHO Regional Office for Europe; 2010 (http://www.euro.who.int/__data/assets/pdf_file/0009/135891/e94866.pdf, accessed 16 November 2015).

14. Acheson D. Independent inquiry into inequalities in health report. London: The Stationery Office; 1998 (https://www.gov.uk/government/uploads/system/uploads/attachment_data/file/265503/ih.pdf, accessed 16 November 2015).

15. Mackenbach J, Bakker M, editors. Reducing inequalities in health: a European perspective. London: Routledge; 2002.

16. Equity in health and health care: a WHO/SIDA initiative. Geneva: World Health Organization; 1996 (https://extranet.who.int/iris/restricted/handle/10665/63119, accessed 16 November 2015).

17. Commission on Social Determinants of Health. Closing the gap in a generation – health equity through action on the social determinants of health. Final report of the Commission on Social Determinants of Health. Geneva: World Health Organization; 2008 (http://apps.who.int/iris/bitstream/10665/43943/1/9789241563703_eng.pdf, accessed 16 November 2015).

18. The state of the world's children 2011. Adolescence: an age of opportunity. New York (NY): UNICEF; 2011 (http://www.unicef.org/adolescence/files/SOWC_2011_Main_Report_EN_02092011.pdf, accessed 16 November 2015).

19. Graham H, Power C. Childhood disadvantage and adult health: a lifecourse framework. London: Health Development Agency; 2004 (https://www.nice.org.uk/proxy/?sourceUrl=http%3A%2F%2Fwww.nice.org.uk%2Fnicemedia%2Fdocuments%2Fchildhood_disadvantage.pdf, accessed 16 November 2015).

20. Health 2020: a European policy framework supporting action across government and society for health and well-being. Copenhagen: WHO Regional Office for Europe; 2012 (EUR/RC62/9; http://www.euro.who.int/en/who-we-are/governance/regional-committeefor- europe/sixty-second-session/working-documents/eurrc629-health-2020-a-europeanpolicy- framework-supporting-action-across-government-and-society-for-health-and-wellbeing, accessed 17 November 2015).

21. Kelly M, Morgan A, Bonnefoy J, Butt J, Bergman V. The social determinants of health: developing an evidence base for political action. Final report to the WHO Commission on the Social Determinants of Health. London: National Institute for Health and Clinical Excellence, United Kingdom, Universidad del Desarrollo, Chile; 2007 (http://www.who.int/social_determinants/resources/mekn_report_10oct07.pdf, accessed 16 November 2015).

22. Brener ND, Kann L, Garcia D, MacDonald G, Ramsey F, Honeycutt S et al. Youth risk behavior surveillance – selected steps communities, 2005. MMWR Surveill Summ. 2007;56(2):1–16.

23. Woodward M, Oliphant J, Lowe G, Tunstall-Pedoe H. Contribution of contemporaneous risk factors to social inequality in coronary heart disease and all causes mortality. Prev Med. 2003;36(5):561–8.

24. Hurrelmann K, Richter M. Risk behaviour in adolescence: the relationship between developmental and health problems. J Public Health 2006;14:20–8.

25. Ojala K, Vereecken C, Välimaa R, Currie C, Villberg J, Tynjälä J et al. Attempts to lose weight among overweight and non-overweight adolescents: a cross-national survey. Int J Behav Nutr Phys Act. 2007;4(1):50–60.

26. Haugland S, Wold B, Stevenson J, Aaroe LE, Woynarowska B. Subjective health complaints in adolescence. A cross-national comparison of prevalence and dimensionality. Eur J Public Health 2001;11(1):4–10.

27. Torsheim T, Ravens-Sieberer U, Hetland J, Välimaa R, Danielson M, Overpeck M. Cross-national variation of gender differences in adolescent subjective health in Europe and North America. Soc Sci Med. 2006;62(4):815–27.

28. Cavallo F, Zambon A, Borraccino A, Raven-Sieberer U, Torsheim T, Lemma P. Girls growing through adolescence have a higher risk of poor health. Qual Life Res. 2006;15(10):1577–85.

29. Ravens-Sieberer U, Torsheim T, Hetland J, Vollebergh W, Cavallo F, Jericek H et al. Subjective health, symptom load and quality of life of children and adolescents in Europe. Int J Public Health 2009;54(Suppl. 2):151–9.

30. Holstein BE, Currie C, Boyce W, Damsgaard MT, Gobina I, Kökönyei G et al. Socio-economic inequality in multiple health complaints among adolescents: international comparative study in 37 countries. Int J Public Health 2009;54(Suppl. 2):260–70.

31. Moreno C, Sánchez-Queija I, Muñoz-Tinoco V, de Matos MG, Dallago L, Bogt TT et al. Cross-national associations between parent and peer communication and psychological complaints. Int J Public Health 2009;54(Suppl. 2):235–42.

32. Richter M, Vereecken CA, Boyce W, Maes L, Nic Gabhainn S, Currie CE. Parental occupation, family affluence and adolescent health behaviour in 28 countries. Int J Public Health 2009;54(4):203–12.

33. Vereecken CA, Inchley J, Subramanian SV, Hublet A, Maes L. The relative influence of individual and contextual socio-economic status on consumption of fruit and soft drinks among adolescents in Europe. Eur J Public Health 2005;15(3):224–32.

34. Vereecken C, Dupuy M, Rasmussen M, Kelly C, Nansel TR, Al Sabbah H et al. Breakfast consumption and its socio-demographic and lifestyle correlates in schoolchildren in 41 countries participating in the HBSC study. Int J Public Health 2009;54(Suppl. 2):180–90.

35. Borraccino A, Lemma P, Iannotti RJ, Zambon A, Dalmasso P, Lazzeri G et al. Socio-economic effects on meeting PA guidelines: comparisons among 32 countries. Med Sci Sports Exerc. 2009;41(4):749–56.

36. Zambon A, Boyce W, Cois E, Currie C, Lemma P, Dalmasso P et al. Do welfare regimes mediate the effect of socioeconomic position on health in adolescence? A cross-national comparison in Europe, North America, and Israel. Int J Health Serv. 2006;36(2):309–29.

37. Nic Gabhainn S, Baban A, Boyce W, Godeau E, HBSC Sexual Health Focus Group. How well protected are sexually active 15-year-olds? Cross-national patterns in condom and contraceptive pill use 2002–2006. Int J Public Health 2009:54(Suppl. 2):209–15.

38. Kuusela S, Kannas L, Tynjälä J, Honkala E, Tudor-Smith C. Frequent use of sugar products by schoolchildren in 20 European countries, Israel and Canada in 1993/1994. Int Dent J. 1999;49(2):105–14.

39. Moor I, Richter M, Ravens-Sieberer U, Ottova-Jordan V, Elgar FJ, Pfortner T-K. Trends in social inequalities in adolescent health complaints from 1994 to 2010 in Europe, North America and Israel: the HBSC study. Eur J Public Health 2015;25:S57–60.

40. Elgar FJ, Pförtner T-K, Moor I, de Clercq B, Stevens GWJM, Currie C. Socioeconomic inequalities in adolescent health 2002–2010: a time-series analysis of 34 countries participating in the Health Behaviour in School-aged Children study. Lancet 2015;385(9982):2088–95.

41. Elgar FJ, Roberts C, Parry-Langdon N, Boyce W. Income inequality and alcohol use: a multilevel analysis of drinking and drunkenness in adolescents in 34 countries. Eur J Public Health 2005;15(3):245–50.

42. Torsheim T, Currie C, Boyce W, Kalnins I, Overpeck M, Haugland S. Material deprivation and self-rated health: a multilevel study of adolescents from 22 European and North American countries. Soc Sci Med. 2004;59(1):1–12.

43. Due P, Damsgaard MT, Rasmussen M, Holstein BE, Wardle J, Merlo J et al. Socioeconomic position, macroeconomic environment and overweight among adolescents in 35 countries. Int J Obes. 2009;33(10):1084–93.

44. Elgar FJ, Craig W, Boyce W, Morgan A, Vella-Zarb R. Income inequality and school bullying: multilevel study of adolescents in 37 countries. J Adolesc Health 2009;45(4):351–9.

45. Kuntsche E, Kuntsche S, Knibbe R, Simons-Morton B, Farhat T, Hublet A et al. Cultural and gender convergence in adolescent drunkenness: evidence from 23 European and North American countries. Arch Pediatr Adolesc Med. 2011;165(2):152–8.

46. Blum RW, McNeely C, Nonnemaker J. Vulnerability, risk, and protection. J Adolesc Health 2002;31(1):S28–39.

47. Morgan A. Social capital as a health asset for young people's health and wellbeing. J Child Adolesc Psychol. 2010;Suppl. 2:19–42.

48. Scales P. Reducing risks and building development assets: essential actions for promoting adolescent health. J Sch Health 1999;69(3):13–9.

49. Waylen A, Stallard N, Stewart-Brown S. Parenting and health in mid-childhood: a longitudinal study. Eur J Public Health 2008;18(3):300–5.

50. Brooks F, Zaborskis A, Tabak I, del Carmen Granado Alcon M, Zemaitiene N, de Roos S et al. Trends in adolescents' perceived parental communication across 32 countries in Europe and North America from 2002 to 2010. Eur J Public Health 2015;25(Suppl. 2):46–50.

51. Molcho M, Nic Gabhainn S, Kelleher C. Interpersonal relationships as predictors of positive health among Irish youth: the more the merrier. Ir Med J. 2007;100(8):33–6.

52. Zambon A, Morgan A, Vereecken C, Colombini S, Boyce W, Mazur J et al. The contribution of club participation to adolescent health: evidence from six countries. J Epidemiol Community Health 2010;64(1):89–95.

53. Kuntsche E. Decrease in adolescent cannabis use from 2002 to 2006 and links to evenings out with friends in 31 European and North American countries and regions. Arch Pediatr Adolesc Med. 2009;163(2):119–25.

54. Simons-Morton B, Chen RS. Over time relationships between early adolescent and peer substance use. Addict Behav. 2006;31(7):1211–23.

55. Ravens-Sieberer U, Kokonyet G, Thonmas C. School and health. In: Currie C, Roberts C, Morgan A, Smith R, Settertobulte W, Samdal O et al., editors. Young people's health in context. Health Behaviour in School-aged Children (HBSC) study: international report from the 2001/2002 survey. Copenhagen: WHO Regional Office for Europe; 2004 (Health Policy for Children and Adolescents, No.4; http://www.euro.who.int/__data/assets/pdf_file/0008/110231/e82923.pdf, accessed 17 November 2015).

56. Due P, Lynch J, Holstein B, Modvig J. Socioeconomic health inequalities among a nationally representative sample of Danish adolescents: the role of different types of social relations. J Epidemiol Community Health 2003;57(9):692–8.

57. Vieno A, Santinello M, Pastore M, Perkins DD. Social support, sense of community in school, and self-efficacy as resources during early adolescence: an integrative model. Am J Community Psychol. 2007;39:177–90.

58. Vieno A, Santinello M, Galbiati E, Mirandola M. School climate and well being in early adolescence: a comprehensive model. Eur J Soc Psychol. 2004;2:219–37.

59. Freeman JG, Samdal O, Klinger DA, Dur W, Griebler R, Currie D et al. The relationship of schools to emotional health and bullying. Int J Public Health 2009;54(Suppl. 2):251–59.

60. Rasmussen M, Damsgaard MT, Holstein BE, Poulsen LH, Due P. School connectedness and daily smoking among boys and girls: the influence of parental smoking norms. Eur J Public Health 2005;15(6):607–12.

61. Boyce WF, Davies D, Gallupe O, Shelley D. Adolescent risk taking, neighborhood social capital, and health. J Adolesc Health 2008;43(3):246–52.

62. Nichol M, Janssen I, Pickett W. Associations between neighborhood safety, availability of recreational facilities, and adolescent physical activity among Canadian youth. J Phys Act Health 2010;7(4):442–50.

63. Zimet GD, Dahlem NW, Zimet SG, Farley GK. The Multidimensional Scale of Perceived Social Support. J Pers Assess. 1988;52(1):30–41.

64. Peden M, Oyegbite K, Ozanne-Smith J, Hyder AA, Branche C, Rhaman AKMF et al., editors. World report on child injury prevention. Geneva: World Health Organization; 2008 (http://apps.who.int/iris/bitstream/10665/43851/1/9789241563574_eng.pdf, accessed 24 August 2015).

65. Sethi D, Racioppi F, Baumgarten I, Vida P. Injuries and violence in Europe: why they matter and what can be done. Copenhagen: WHO Regional Office for Europe; 2006 (http://www.euro.who.int/__data/assets/pdf_file/0005/98762/E88037.pdf, accessed 24 August 2015).

66. Stevens GWJM, Vollebergh WAM. Mental health in migrant children. J Child Psychol Psychiatry 2008;49:276–94.

67. Molcho M, Cristini F, Nic Gabhainn S, Santinello M, Moreno C, Gaspar de Matos M et al. Health and well-being among child immigrants in Europe. Eurohealth 2010;16:20–3.

68. Sam DL, Vedder P, Liebkind K, Netod F, Virtae E. Immigration, acculturation and the paradox of adaptation in Europe. Eur J Dev Psychol. 2008;5:138–58.

69. Walsh SD, Djalovski A, Boniel-Nissim M, Harel-Fisch Y. Parental, peer and school experiences as predictors of alcohol drinking among first and second generation immigrant adolescents in Israel. Drug Alcohol Depend. 2014;138:39–47.

70. Strohmeier D, Schmitt-Rodermund E. Immigrant youth in European countries: the manifold challenges of adaptation. Eur J Dev Psychol. 2008;5(2):129–37.

71. Holfeld B, Grabe M. Middle school students' perceptions of and responses to cyber bullying. J Educ Comput Res. 2012;46(4):395–413.

72. Kowalski RM, Limber SP, Agatston PW. Cyberbullying: bullying in the digital age. Chichester: John Wiley & Sons Ltd; 2012.

73. Kowalski RM, Giumetti GW, Schroeder AN, Lattanner MR. Bullying in the digital age: a critical review and meta-analysis of cyberbullying research among youth. Psychol Bull. 2014;140(4):1073.

74. Mitchell KJ, Ybarra M, Finkelhor D. The relative importance of online victimization in understanding depression, delinquency, and substance use. Child Maltreat. 2007;12(4):314–24.

75. European health information gateway [website]. Copenhagen: WHO Regional Office for Europe; 2015 (http://portal.euro.who.int/en/, accessed 30 November 2015).

76. The European health statistics app [website]. Copenhagen: WHO Regional Office for Europe; 2015 (http://www.euro.who.int/en/data-and-evidence/the-european-health-statistics-app, accessed 30 November 2015).

GROWING UP UNEQUAL: GENDER AND SOCIOECONOMIC
DIFFERENCES IN YOUNG PEOPLE'S HEALTH AND WELL-BEING

KEY DATA

GROWING UP UNEQUAL: GENDER AND SOCIOECONOMIC
DIFFERENCES IN YOUNG PEOPLE'S HEALTH AND WELL-BEING
PART 2. KEY DATA | CHAPTER 1. UNDERSTANDING THIS REPORT

1

UNDERSTANDING THIS REPORT

UNDERSTANDING THIS REPORT

The report presents findings from the HBSC 2013/2014 survey across 42 countries and regions. Data are drawn from the mandatory component of the HBSC survey questionnaire, which was used in all countries and regions.

In addition to presenting individual country/region prevalence for a range of health and health-related indicators, the report also describes cross-national patterns in magnitude and direction of differences in prevalence between subgroups. Statistical analyses are used to systematically identify meaningful differences in the prevalence of health and social indicators by levels of age, gender and family affluence. Findings are presented in Chapters 2–5, with further details on analyses performed provided in the Annex.

Data for some indicators were not available from specific countries and regions. Some, including Greenland and Norway, excluded items on sensitive topics such as sexual health.

TYPES OF INDICATOR REPORTED

Chapters 2–5 consider four types of indicator:
- social context, relating to family, peers and school, which often serve as protective factors
- health outcomes, describing current levels of health and well-being
- health behaviour, relating to behaviours and activities seen as potentially health-sustaining
- risk behaviours, relating to those seen as potentially health-damaging.

Each chapter includes the following subsections:
- a brief overview of the importance of the topic and a summary of what is known about it based on scientific literature;
- descriptions of how the indicators have been measured;
- bar charts showing the relationship between family affluence and each of the indicators;
- bar charts showing country/region-specific prevalence by age and gender;
- maps illustrating cross-national differences among 15-year-olds;
- a short summary of the cross-national associations with age, gender and family affluence for each indicator and a brief presentation of results;
- scientific discussion, interpreting the findings based on relevant scientific literature; and
- policy reflections, outlining where and how policy-makers could take action.

AGE AND GENDER

The rapid changes in physical and mental development that occur across adolescence mean that differences in reporting of health and well-being between age groups and boys and girls are to be expected. Bar charts present data for boys and girls in each age group (11-, 13- and 15-year-olds) separately for each country and region in descending order of prevalence (for boys and girls combined). The HBSC average presented in the charts is based on equal weighting of each country or region, regardless of differences in achieved sample size or population. Percentages in the charts are rounded to the nearest whole number.

Interpretation of differences is also based on rounded numbers, as they appear in the charts. A real difference of 10.3 will count as a 10 percentage-point difference and a difference of 10.6 as an 11 percentage-point difference. This affects the interpretation of differences: to have a difference of more than 10%, the rounded difference must be at least 11.

It is important to avoid overinterpretation of the rankings. Frequently, few percentage points separate adjacent countries and regions and prevalence differences may not be statistically significant. Countries highlighted in bold in the charts are those in which there was a statistically significant gender difference in prevalence.

GROWING UP UNEQUAL: GENDER AND SOCIOECONOMIC
DIFFERENCES IN YOUNG PEOPLE'S HEALTH AND WELL-BEING
PART 2. KEY DATA | CHAPTER 1. UNDERSTANDING THIS REPORT

1

FAMILY AFFLUENCE

Family affluence is a robust determinant of adolescent health. A socioeconomic gradient in health in which health and well-being improve as affluence rises is found in many cultures throughout the life-course (1). This social pattern emerges early in life and shapes future inequalities in social development, education, employment and adult health. Though the so-called healthy years of adolescence are not often a focus of health policy, a robust body of evidence shows that health and social inequalities in health track strongly from childhood and adolescence through to late adulthood.

Investigating social inequalities in young people's health requires age-appropriate measures of socioeconomic conditions. The HBSC 2013/2014 survey used a six-item assessment of common material assets or activities:

- Does your family own a car, van or truck? (Responses: no, one, two or more);
- Do you have your own bedroom for yourself? (No, yes);
- How many times did you and your family travel out of [insert country/region name] for a holiday/vacation last year? (Not at all, once, twice, more than twice);
- How many computers do your family own? (None, one, two, more than two);
- Does your family have a dishwasher at home? (No, yes); and
- How many bathrooms (rooms with a bath/shower or both) are in your home? (None, one, two, more than two).

Responses are scored and summed to form a HBSC Family Affluence Scale (FAS) summary score (2–4).

Responses to these items are used in the report to estimate relative socioeconomic position in society by comparing the individual's summary score from the FAS to all other scores in the respective country/region. The ridit-based relative affluence score is then used to identify groups of young people in the lowest 20% (low affluence), middle 60% (medium affluence) and highest 20% (high affluence) in each country and region.

This approach to measuring health inequalities differs from previous HBSC survey cycles and international reports, in which uniform cut-point criteria were used to create groups of low, medium and high affluence. Due to the vast heterogeneity in country wealth in the HBSC network (in 2013, per capita gross domestic product ranged from US$ 2244 (the Republic of Moldova) to US$ 110 665 (Luxembourg) (5)), these absolute affluence groupings are unevenly distributed and therefore complicate the interpretation of health inequalities. By equalizing the distribution of low, medium and high relative family affluence, this report effectively disregards country/region differences in absolute poverty and material standards of living. Although percentages of young people in low-, medium- and high-affluence groups are equivalent across countries and regions, the distribution of material assets is not. The same summary score on the FAS may therefore correspond to medium affluence in a high-income country and high affluence in a low-income country.

Interpretation of FAS bar charts

Bar charts illustrate the relationship between family affluence and various indicators throughout Chapters 2–5. The charts show whether the prevalence of an indicator increases or decreases with higher family affluence, the extent of any difference corresponding to high and low family affluence, and whether there is a statistically significant linear trend in prevalence across low-, medium- and high-affluence groups.

A sample bar chart including only six countries is presented below. It shows that the proportion of young people taking soft drinks daily in Armenia is higher among those from families with higher affluence, as denoted by the bars being above the 0% line (that is, being positive). This positive linear trend is statistically significant in boys and girls, as shown by the bars being shaded blue for boys and red for girls. The height of the bars shows the extent of the difference between high- and low-affluence groups only, but statistical significance is based on linear trend across all three family affluence groups. In this case, the proportion of boys taking soft drinks daily in high-affluence families is almost 15 percentage points higher than in those of low affluence.

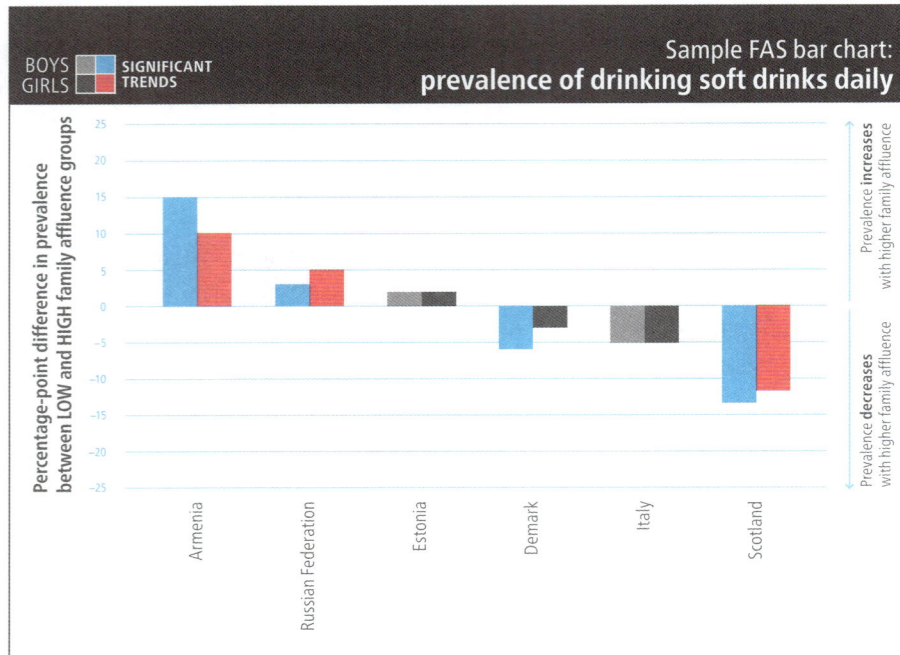

Sample FAS bar chart: prevalence of drinking soft drinks daily

BOYS / GIRLS — SIGNIFICANT TRENDS

Source: Currie et al. *(6). Note:* low- and high-affluence groups represent the lowest 20% and highest 20% in each country and region.

Prevalence is also higher among those from high-affluence families in Estonia and the Russian Federation, but the differences in Estonia are small and there is no statistically significant linear trend. The increase in prevalence of taking soft drinks with family affluence in the Russian Federation is statistically significant only among girls. Bars shaded grey denote that there is no statistically significant linear trend across family affluence groups for the indicator (dark grey for boys, light grey for girls).

The relationship is in the opposite direction in Denmark, Italy and Scotland, where prevalence of taking soft drinks daily is lower among young people from higher-affluence families, denoted by the bars lying below the 0% line (that is, being negative). The extent of the decline in prevalence with higher affluence in Scotland is particularly strong, with a decrease of more than 10 percentage points between those from low- and high-affluence families. This difference is reflected in a statistically significant linear trend (the bars are red and blue). Although Denmark and Italy show the same pattern, it is statistically significant only among boys in Denmark.

GEOGRAPHIC PATTERNS

Maps of prevalence are presented for most health indicators. These show broad patterns of prevalence across Europe and North America and are useful in highlighting cross-national differences and patterning between genders. As with age and gender differences, care must be taken not to overinterpret small differences in prevalence. The cut-off points between colour bands are fixed: there may be only a few percentage points between two regions falling within different colour shades.

REFERENCES

1.   Viner RM, Ozer EM, Denny S, Marmot M, Resnick M, Fatusi A et al. Adolescence and the social determinants of health. Lancet 2012;379(9826):1641–52.

2.   Elgar FJ, McKinnon B, Torsheim T, Schnohr CW, Mazur J, Cavallo F, Currie C. Patterns of socioeconomic inequality in adolescent health differ according to the measure of socioeconomic position. Soc Indic Res. 2015;doi:10.1007/s11205-015-0994-6.

3.   Hartley JEK, Leven K, Currie C. A new version of the HBSC Family Affluence Scale – FAS III: Scottish qualitative findings from the international FAS Development Study. Child Indic Res. 2015;doi:10.1007/s12187-015-9325-3.

GROWING UP UNEQUAL: GENDER AND SOCIOECONOMIC
DIFFERENCES IN YOUNG PEOPLE'S HEALTH AND WELL-BEING
PART 2. KEY DATA | CHAPTER 1. UNDERSTANDING THIS REPORT

1

4.   Torsheim T, Cavallo F, Levin KA, Schnohr C, Mazur J, Niclasen B, et al. Psychometric validation of the revised Family Affluence Scale: a latent variable approach. Child Indic Res. 2015;doi:10.1007/s12187-015-9339-x.

5.   Data. GDP per capita (current US$) [online database]. Washington (DC): The World Bank; 2015 (http://data.worldbank.org/indicator/NY.GDP.PCAP. CD, accessed 13 November 2015).

6.   Currie C, Zanotti C, Morgan A, Currie D, de Looze M, Roberts C et al., editors. Social determinants of health and well-being among young people. Health Behaviour in School-aged Children (HBSC) study: international report from the 2009/2010 survey. Copenhagen: WHO Regional Office for Europe; 2012 (Health Policy for Children and Adolescents, No. 6; http://www.euro.who.int/en/what-we-publish/abstracts/socialdeterminants-of-health-and-well-being-among-young-people.-health-behaviour-in-schoolaged-children-hbsc-study, accessed 24 August 2015).

GROWING UP UNEQUAL: GENDER AND SOCIOECONOMIC
DIFFERENCES IN YOUNG PEOPLE'S HEALTH AND WELL-BEING
PART 2. KEY DATA | CHAPTER 2. SOCIAL CONTEXT

2

SOCIAL CONTEXT

**FAMILY
PEERS
SCHOOL**

"Having a friend makes everything better."

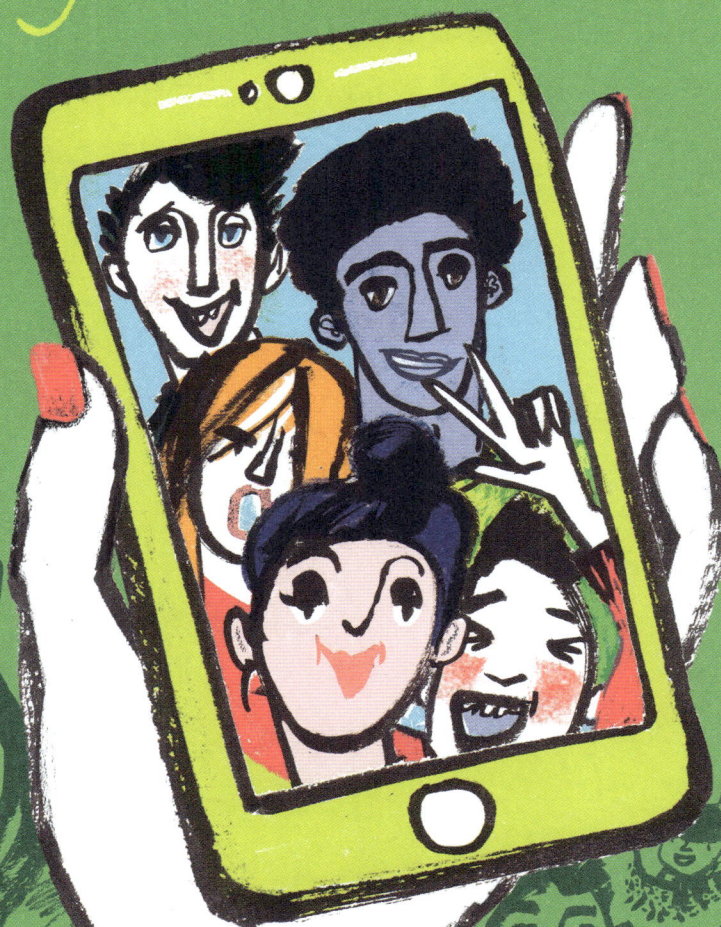

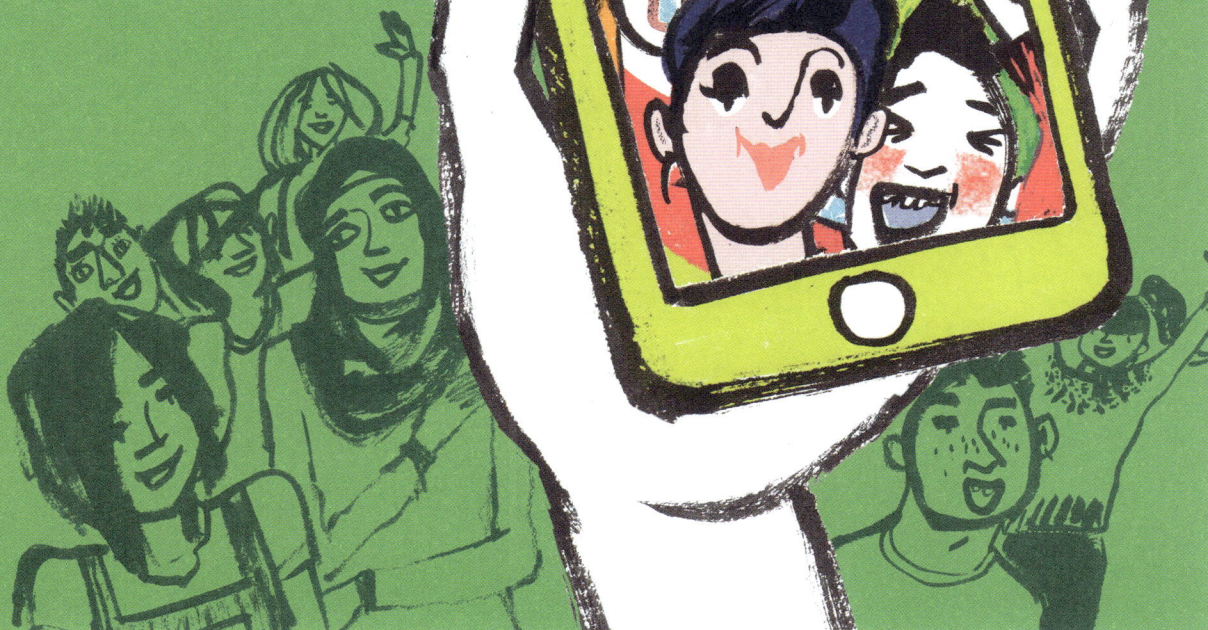

QUOTES FROM YOUNG PEOPLE ON SOCIAL CONTEXT

"It's important that there is someone you can talk to in case you have some problems such as being stressed or bullying/friendship problems."

"I think it is very important that you can talk to your friends about your problems because that is what they are there for and once you tell them your problem, they can help you to deal with it. Sometimes, also, you don't think your parents really understand you with some of your problems so it's great to have someone there who knows and understands you."

"It is essential to have a good peer group that we can trust when life is tough."

GROWING UP UNEQUAL: GENDER AND SOCIOECONOMIC
DIFFERENCES IN YOUNG PEOPLE'S HEALTH AND WELL-BEING
PART 2. KEY DATA | CHAPTER 2. SOCIAL CONTEXT

2

FAMILY:
COMMUNICATION WITH MOTHER

Parental communication is one of the key portals through which the family functions as a protective health asset, equipping young people to deal with stressful situations and buffering them against adverse influences. Ease of communication between adolescents and their mother is particularly important for life satisfaction (1). Supportive communication with parents also moderates the negative effects of electronic media use on life satisfaction during adolescence (2).

Adolescents who report ease of communication with their mothers are less likely to be current smokers (3), frequent alcohol drinkers (4) or sexually active (5). Communication with parents also has protective effects on their dietary and physical activity behaviours (6).

Communication in the family is an indicator of social support and of the family's connectedness (7). Easy communication with parents can facilitate self-disclosure, which can be a predictor of the most effective forms of parental monitoring (parents' knowledge of the child's whereabouts, activities and associations) and can prevent young people from participating in health-risk behaviours (8).

HBSC survey 2013/2014

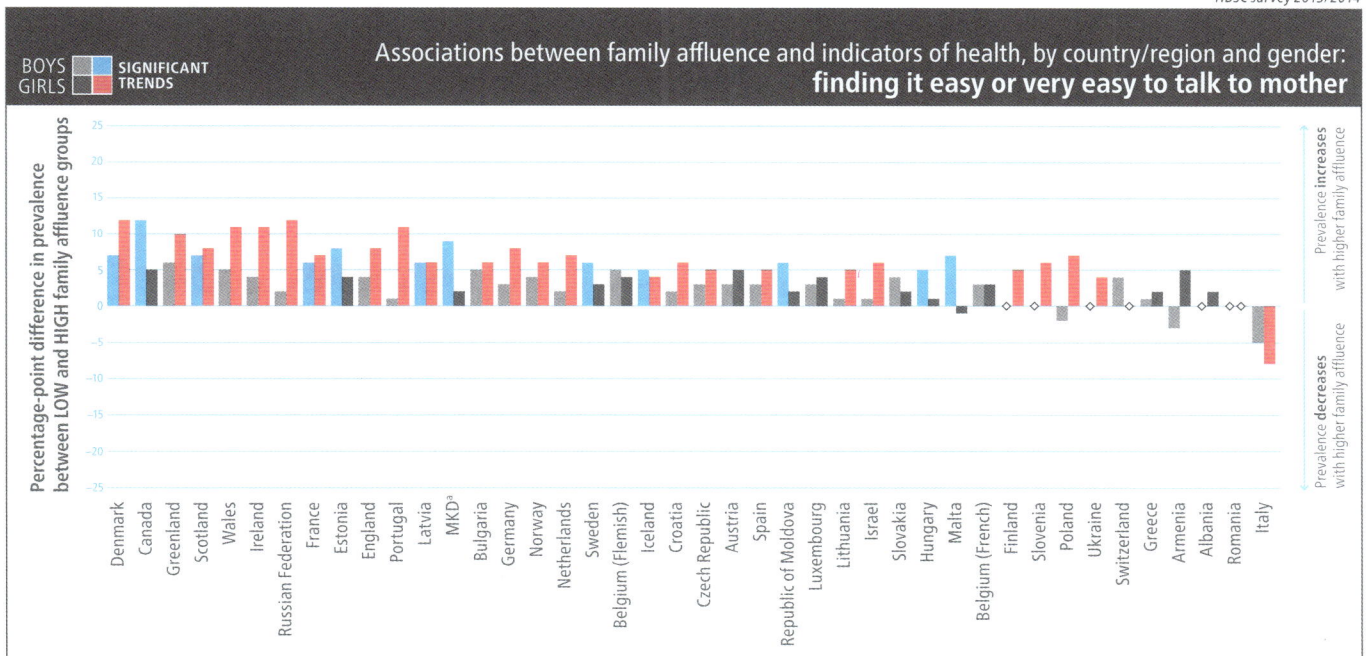

Associations between family affluence and indicators of health, by country/region and gender: **finding it easy or very easy to talk to mother**

ᵃThe former Yugoslav Republic of Macedonia. *Note:* low- and high-affluence groups represent the lowest 20% and highest 20% in each country. ◇ means less than +/-0.5%.

MEASURE

Young people were asked how easy it is for them to talk to their mother about things that really bother them. Response options ranged from very easy to very difficult.

Supplementary data on the quality of family communication are provided in the Annex.

RESULTS

Findings presented here show the proportions who reported finding it easy and very easy to talk to their mothers.

Age

A significant decline among boys and girls between ages 11 and 15 was found in almost all countries and regions. The biggest negative differences in percentages of boys was detected in England and Lithuania (between 11- and 13-year-olds) and in France, Greece and Scotland (13- and 15-year-olds). Very high negative differences were found in girls between 11 and 13 and 13 and 15 in Belgium (Flemish), England and France. Two exceptions were found: a small increase was identified between 11- and 13-year-old boys in Ireland and between girls of 13 and 15 in Greenland.

Gender

Differences in prevalence were small and no clear patterns were found. Although some differences were significant, none was greater than 10 percentage points.

Family affluence

Comparable percentages of boys reported easy communication with their mother across affluence groups in most countries and regions. There was a positive relationship with family affluence in 12, with boys from high-affluence families being most likely to report easy communication. In girls, associations were found in over half of the countries and regions. As with boys, girls from high-affluence families were most likely to report easy communication with their mother. Italy was a notable exception, with easy communication being higher among girls from low-affluence families.

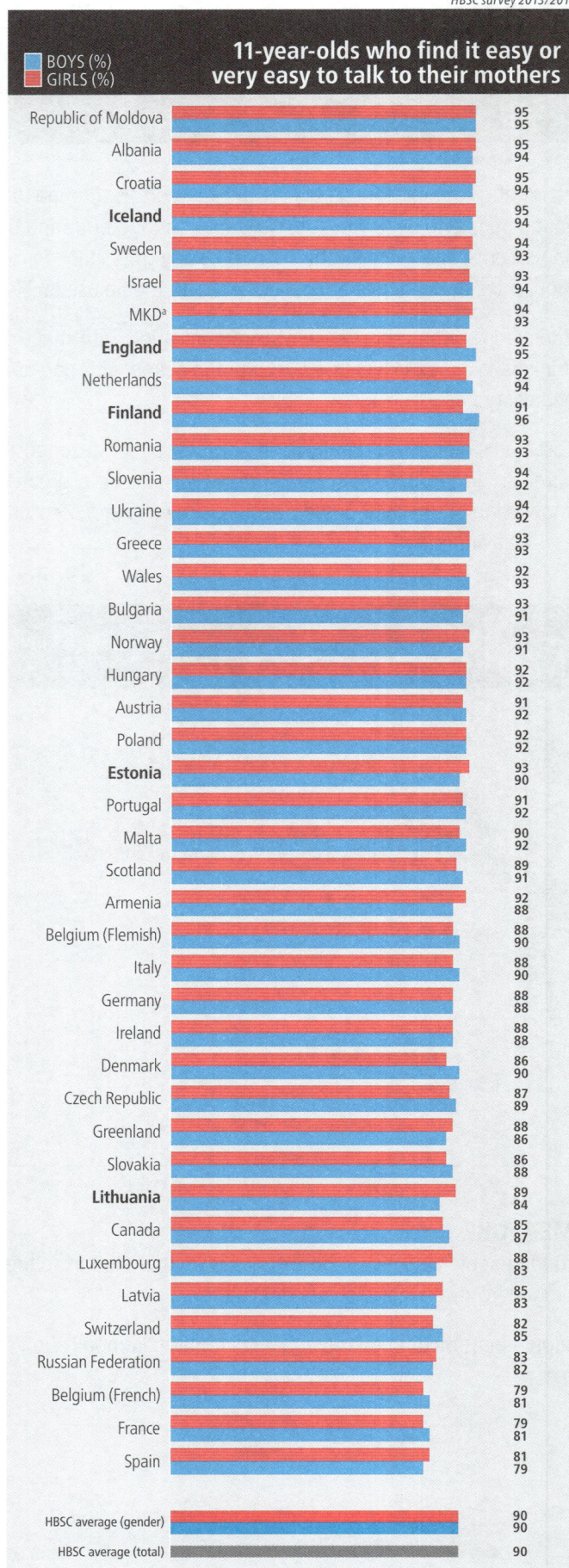

HBSC survey 2013/2014

	11-year-olds who find it easy or very easy to talk to their mothers	BOYS (%)	GIRLS (%)
Republic of Moldova		95	95
Albania		95	94
Croatia		95	94
Iceland		95	94
Sweden		94	93
Israel		93	94
MKD[a]		94	93
England		92	95
Netherlands		92	94
Finland		91	96
Romania		93	93
Slovenia		94	92
Ukraine		94	92
Greece		93	93
Wales		92	93
Bulgaria		93	91
Norway		93	91
Hungary		92	92
Austria		91	92
Poland		92	92
Estonia		93	90
Portugal		91	92
Malta		90	92
Scotland		89	91
Armenia		92	88
Belgium (Flemish)		88	90
Italy		88	90
Germany		88	88
Ireland		88	88
Denmark		86	90
Czech Republic		87	89
Greenland		88	86
Slovakia		86	88
Lithuania		89	84
Canada		85	87
Luxembourg		88	83
Latvia		85	83
Switzerland		82	85
Russian Federation		83	82
Belgium (French)		79	81
France		79	81
Spain		81	79
HBSC average (gender)		90	90
HBSC average (total)		90	

a The former Yugoslav Republic of Macedonia.

GROWING UP UNEQUAL: GENDER AND SOCIOECONOMIC
DIFFERENCES IN YOUNG PEOPLE'S HEALTH AND WELL-BEING
PART 2. KEY DATA | CHAPTER 2. SOCIAL CONTEXT
FAMILY: COMMUNICATION WITH MOTHER

2

13-year-olds who find it easy or very easy to talk to their mothers

HBSC survey 2013/2014

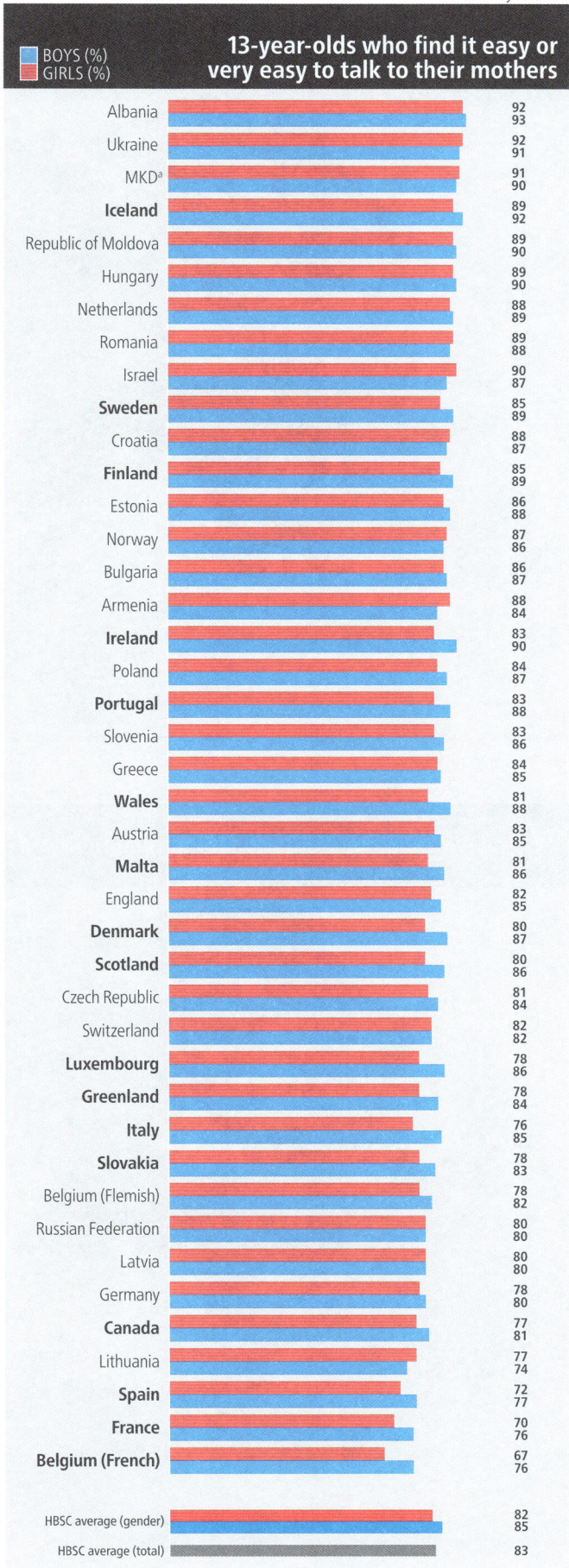

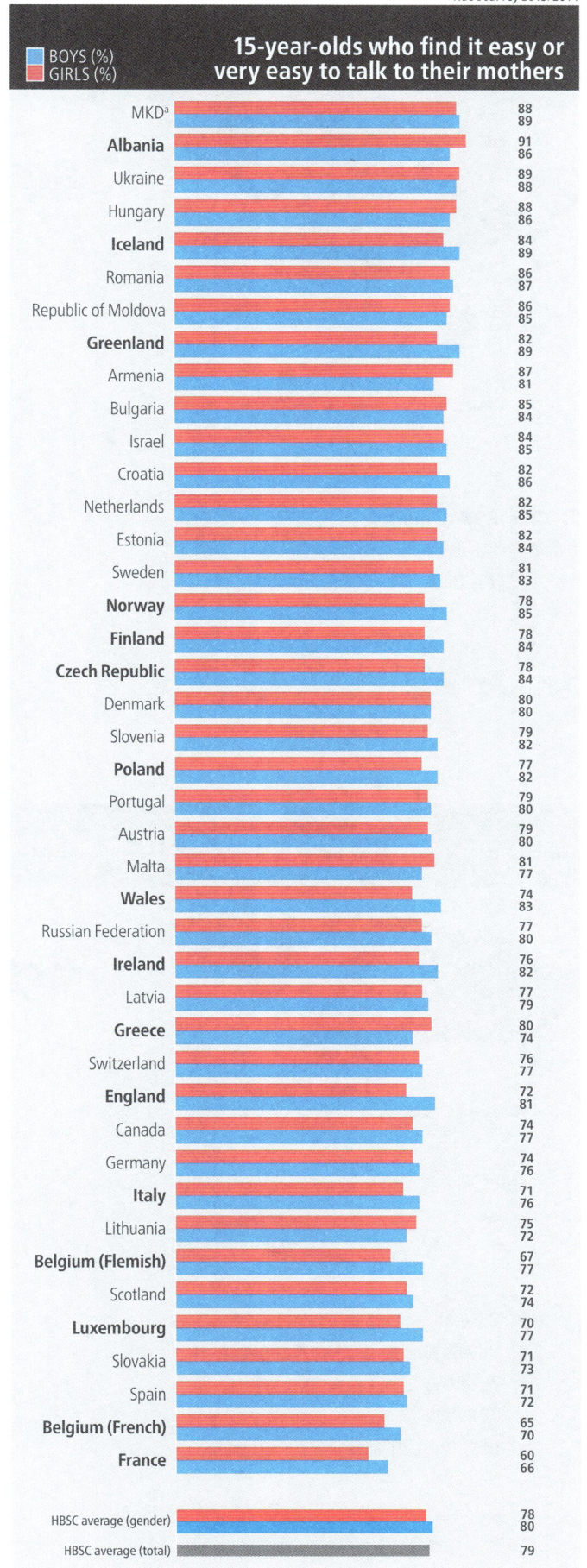

Legend: BOYS (%) · GIRLS (%)

Country	Girls (%)	Boys (%)
Albania	92	93
Ukraine	92	91
MKD[a]	91	90
Iceland	89	92
Republic of Moldova	89	90
Hungary	89	90
Netherlands	88	89
Romania	89	88
Israel	90	87
Sweden	85	89
Croatia	88	87
Finland	85	89
Estonia	86	88
Norway	87	86
Bulgaria	86	87
Armenia	88	84
Ireland	83	90
Poland	84	87
Portugal	83	88
Slovenia	83	86
Greece	84	85
Wales	81	88
Austria	83	85
Malta	81	86
England	82	85
Denmark	80	87
Scotland	80	86
Czech Republic	81	84
Switzerland	82	82
Luxembourg	78	86
Greenland	78	84
Italy	76	85
Slovakia	78	83
Belgium (Flemish)	78	82
Russian Federation	80	80
Latvia	80	80
Germany	78	80
Canada	77	81
Lithuania	77	74
Spain	72	77
France	70	76
Belgium (French)	67	76
HBSC average (gender)	82	85
HBSC average (total)		83

15-year-olds who find it easy or very easy to talk to their mothers

HBSC survey 2013/2014

Legend: BOYS (%) · GIRLS (%)

Country	Girls (%)	Boys (%)
MKD[a]	88	89
Albania	91	86
Ukraine	89	88
Hungary	88	86
Iceland	84	89
Romania	86	87
Republic of Moldova	86	85
Greenland	82	89
Armenia	87	81
Bulgaria	85	84
Israel	84	85
Croatia	82	86
Netherlands	82	85
Estonia	82	84
Sweden	81	83
Norway	78	85
Finland	78	84
Czech Republic	78	84
Denmark	80	80
Slovenia	79	82
Poland	77	82
Portugal	79	80
Austria	79	80
Malta	81	77
Wales	74	83
Russian Federation	77	80
Ireland	76	82
Latvia	77	79
Greece	80	74
Switzerland	76	77
England	72	81
Canada	74	77
Germany	74	76
Italy	71	76
Lithuania	75	72
Belgium (Flemish)	67	77
Scotland	72	74
Luxembourg	70	77
Slovakia	71	73
Spain	71	72
Belgium (French)	65	70
France	60	66
HBSC average (gender)	78	80
HBSC average (total)		79

Note: **indicates** significant gender difference (at p<0.05).

HBSC survey 2013/2014

15-year-old girls who find it easy or very easy to talk to their mothers

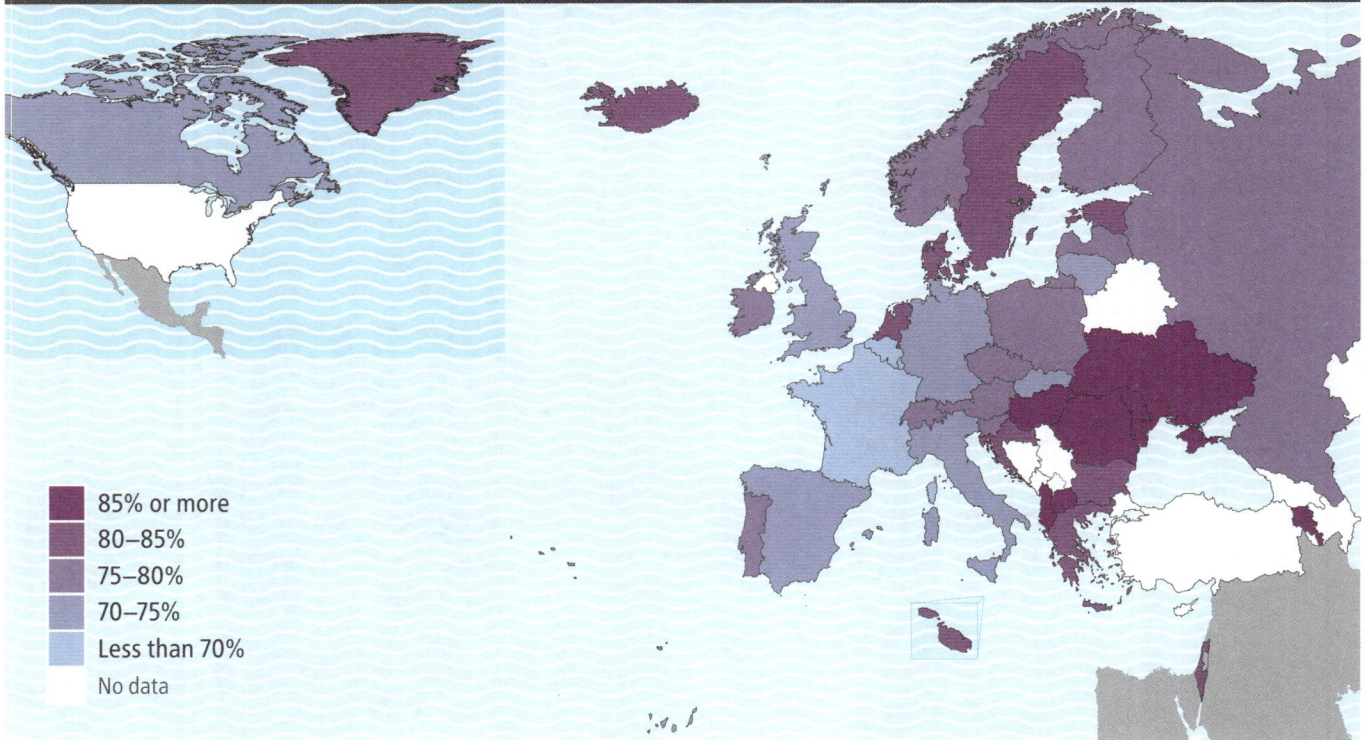

- 85% or more
- 80–85%
- 75–80%
- 70–75%
- Less than 70%
- No data

Note: HBSC teams provided disaggregated data for Belgium and the United Kingdom; these data appear in the map above.

HBSC survey 2013/2014

15-year-old boys who find it easy or very easy to talk to their mothers

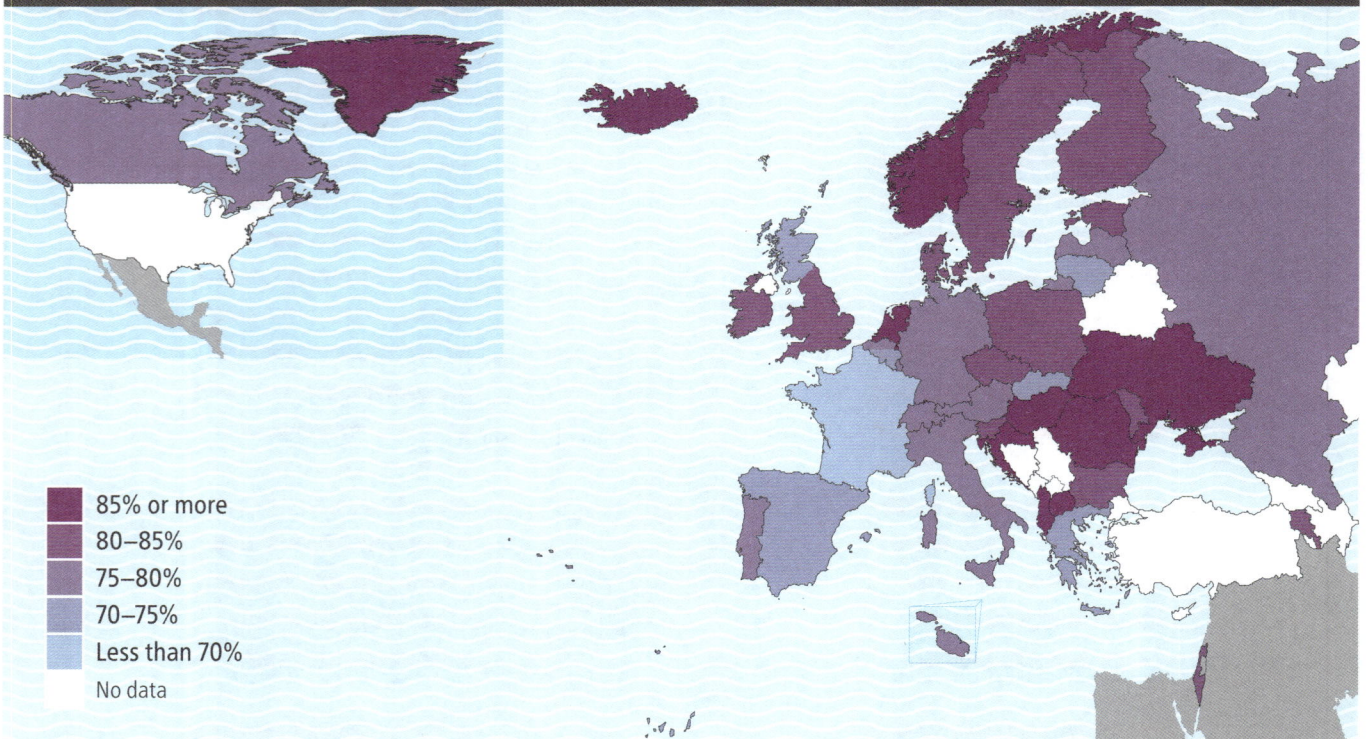

- 85% or more
- 80–85%
- 75–80%
- 70–75%
- Less than 70%
- No data

Note: HBSC teams provided disaggregated data for Belgium and the United Kingdom; these data appear in the map above.

GROWING UP UNEQUAL: GENDER AND SOCIOECONOMIC
DIFFERENCES IN YOUNG PEOPLE'S HEALTH AND WELL-BEING
PART 2. KEY DATA | CHAPTER 2. SOCIAL CONTEXT

2

FAMILY:
COMMUNICATION WITH FATHER

A positive father–child relationship is associated with child well-being. Ease of communication with their father has a protective role in maintaining young people's emotional well-being, self-esteem and positive body image, particularly for girls (9–13).

Communication with a father-figure appears to influence and affect boys and girls in distinct ways (14). Communication difficulties with fathers are associated with internalizing problems, especially in girls (15), but perceived closeness, paternal attachment and open communication reduces girls' engagement with health-risk behaviours (16).

The quality of the relationship with a father-figure has been found to be predictive of the development of negative emotions such as aggression in boys and emotional difficulties in girls (12,17).

HBSC survey 2013/2014

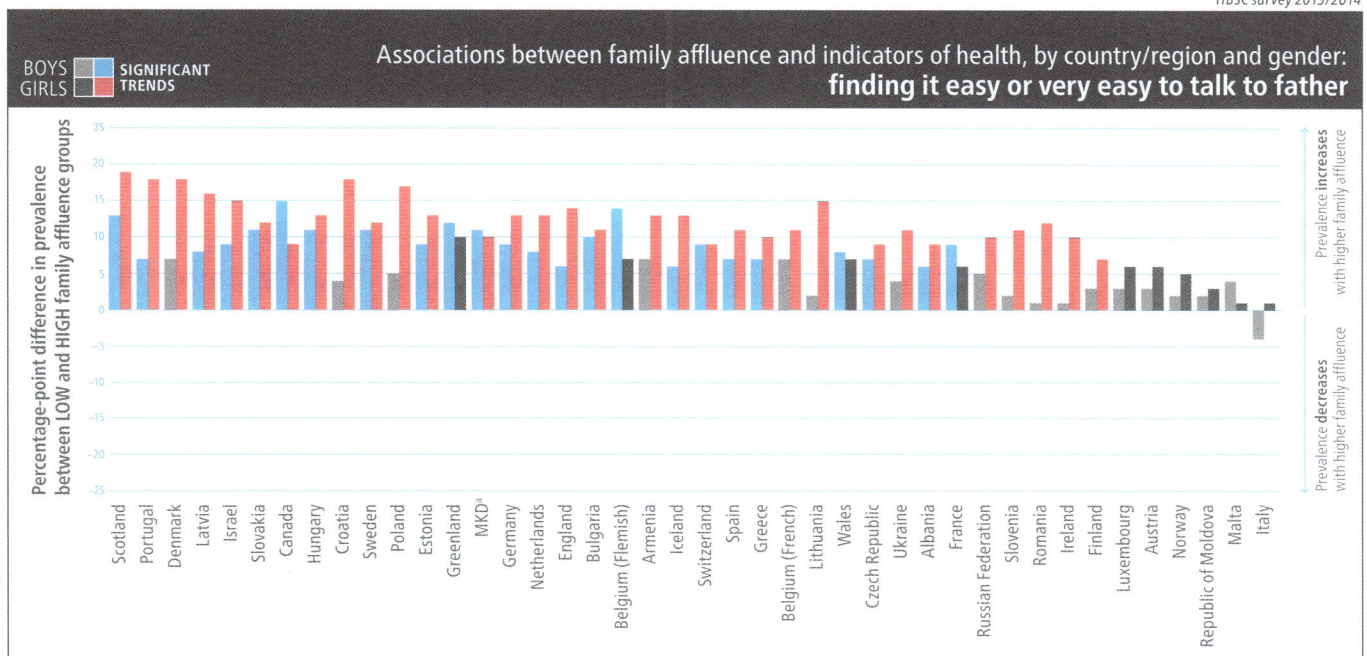

Associations between family affluence and indicators of health, by country/region and gender: **finding it easy or very easy to talk to father**

ᵃ The former Yugoslav Republic of Macedonia. *Note:* low- and high-affluence groups represent the lowest 20% and highest 20% in each country.

MEASURE

Young people were asked how easy it is for them to talk to their father about things that really bother them. Response options ranged from very easy to very difficult.

Supplementary data on the quality of family communication are provided in the Annex.

RESULTS

Findings presented here show the proportions who reported finding it easy and very easy to talk to their fathers.

Age

Ease of communication with father declined with age for girls in all countries and regions and around 80% for boys. The change with age was more than 10 percentage points in around half for boys and almost all for girls.

Gender

Boys at all ages in all countries and regions were more likely to report ease of communication with their fathers. The gender difference was greater than 15 percentage points in almost all at ages 13 and 15. Between 70% and 90% of 13-year-old boys in almost all reported easy communication, but this percentage was reached in only a few for girls.

Family affluence

Easy communication with fathers was associated with higher family affluence in three quarters of countries and regions for girls and one half for boys. The difference in prevalence was more than 10 percentage points in most for girls but in less than a quarter for boys.

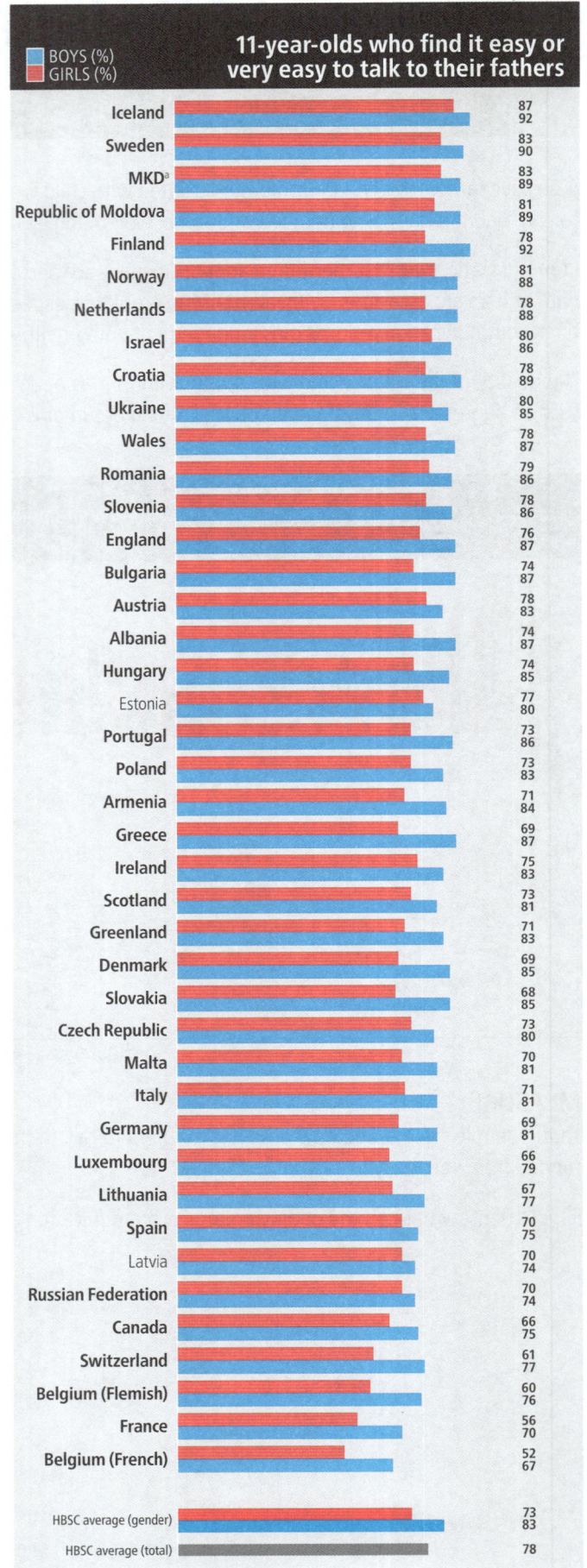

HBSC survey 2013/2014

BOYS (%)
GIRLS (%)

11-year-olds who find it easy or very easy to talk to their fathers

Country	Girls (%)	Boys (%)
Iceland	87	92
Sweden	83	90
MKD[a]	83	89
Republic of Moldova	81	89
Finland	78	92
Norway	81	88
Netherlands	78	88
Israel	80	86
Croatia	78	89
Ukraine	80	85
Wales	78	87
Romania	79	86
Slovenia	78	86
England	76	87
Bulgaria	74	87
Austria	78	83
Albania	74	87
Hungary	74	85
Estonia	77	80
Portugal	73	86
Poland	73	83
Armenia	71	84
Greece	69	87
Ireland	75	83
Scotland	73	81
Greenland	71	83
Denmark	69	85
Slovakia	68	85
Czech Republic	73	80
Malta	70	81
Italy	71	81
Germany	69	81
Luxembourg	66	79
Lithuania	67	77
Spain	70	75
Latvia	70	74
Russian Federation	70	74
Canada	66	75
Switzerland	61	77
Belgium (Flemish)	60	76
France	56	70
Belgium (French)	52	67
HBSC average (gender)	73	83
HBSC average (total)		78

[a] The former Yugoslav Republic of Macedonia.

GROWING UP UNEQUAL: GENDER AND SOCIOECONOMIC
DIFFERENCES IN YOUNG PEOPLE'S HEALTH AND WELL-BEING
PART 2. KEY DATA | CHAPTER 2. SOCIAL CONTEXT
FAMILY: COMMUNICATION WITH FATHER

2

13-year-olds who find it easy or very easy to talk to their fathers

HBSC survey 2013/2014

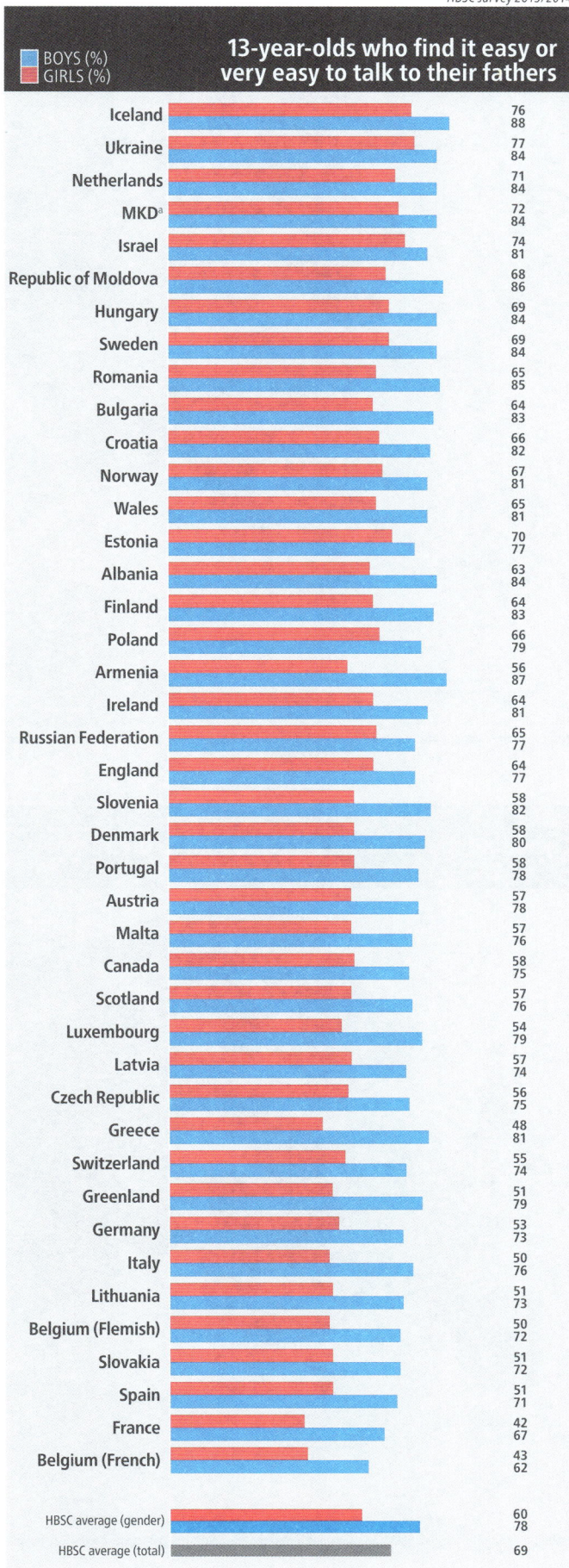

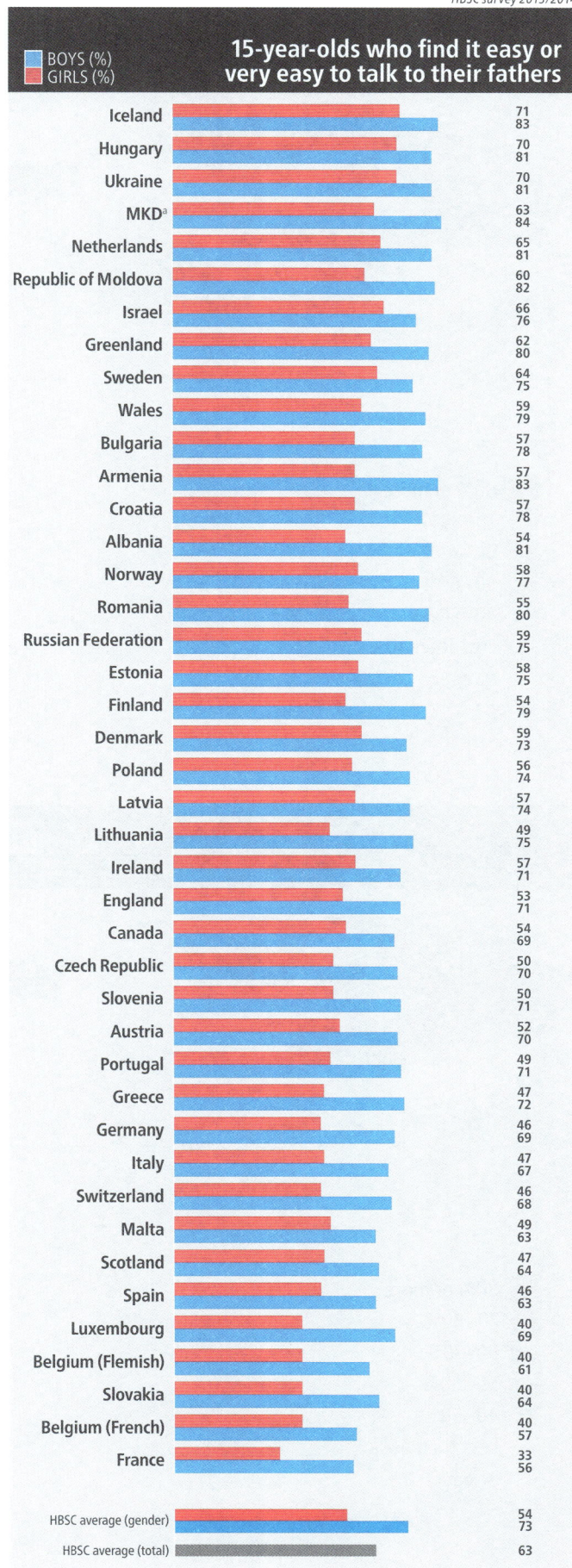

BOYS (%)
GIRLS (%)

Country	Girls (%)	Boys (%)
Iceland	76	88
Ukraine	77	84
Netherlands	71	84
MKD[a]	72	84
Israel	74	81
Republic of Moldova	68	86
Hungary	69	84
Sweden	69	84
Romania	65	85
Bulgaria	64	83
Croatia	66	82
Norway	67	81
Wales	65	81
Estonia	70	77
Albania	63	84
Finland	64	83
Poland	66	79
Armenia	56	87
Ireland	64	81
Russian Federation	65	77
England	64	77
Slovenia	58	82
Denmark	58	80
Portugal	58	78
Austria	57	78
Malta	57	76
Canada	58	75
Scotland	57	76
Luxembourg	54	79
Latvia	57	74
Czech Republic	56	75
Greece	48	81
Switzerland	55	74
Greenland	51	79
Germany	53	73
Italy	50	76
Lithuania	51	73
Belgium (Flemish)	50	72
Slovakia	51	72
Spain	51	71
France	42	67
Belgium (French)	43	62
HBSC average (gender)	60	78
HBSC average (total)		69

15-year-olds who find it easy or very easy to talk to their fathers

HBSC survey 2013/2014

BOYS (%)
GIRLS (%)

Country	Girls (%)	Boys (%)
Iceland	71	83
Hungary	70	81
Ukraine	70	81
MKD[a]	63	84
Netherlands	65	81
Republic of Moldova	60	82
Israel	66	76
Greenland	62	80
Sweden	64	75
Wales	59	79
Bulgaria	57	78
Armenia	57	83
Croatia	57	78
Albania	54	81
Norway	58	77
Romania	55	80
Russian Federation	59	75
Estonia	58	75
Finland	54	79
Denmark	59	73
Poland	56	74
Latvia	57	74
Lithuania	49	75
Ireland	57	71
England	53	71
Canada	54	69
Czech Republic	50	70
Slovenia	50	71
Austria	52	70
Portugal	49	71
Greece	47	72
Germany	46	69
Italy	47	67
Switzerland	46	68
Malta	49	63
Scotland	47	64
Spain	46	63
Luxembourg	40	69
Belgium (Flemish)	40	61
Slovakia	40	64
Belgium (French)	40	57
France	33	56
HBSC average (gender)	54	73
HBSC average (total)		63

Note: **indicates** significant gender difference (at p<0.05).

HBSC survey 2013/2014

15-year-old girls who find it easy or very easy to talk to their fathers

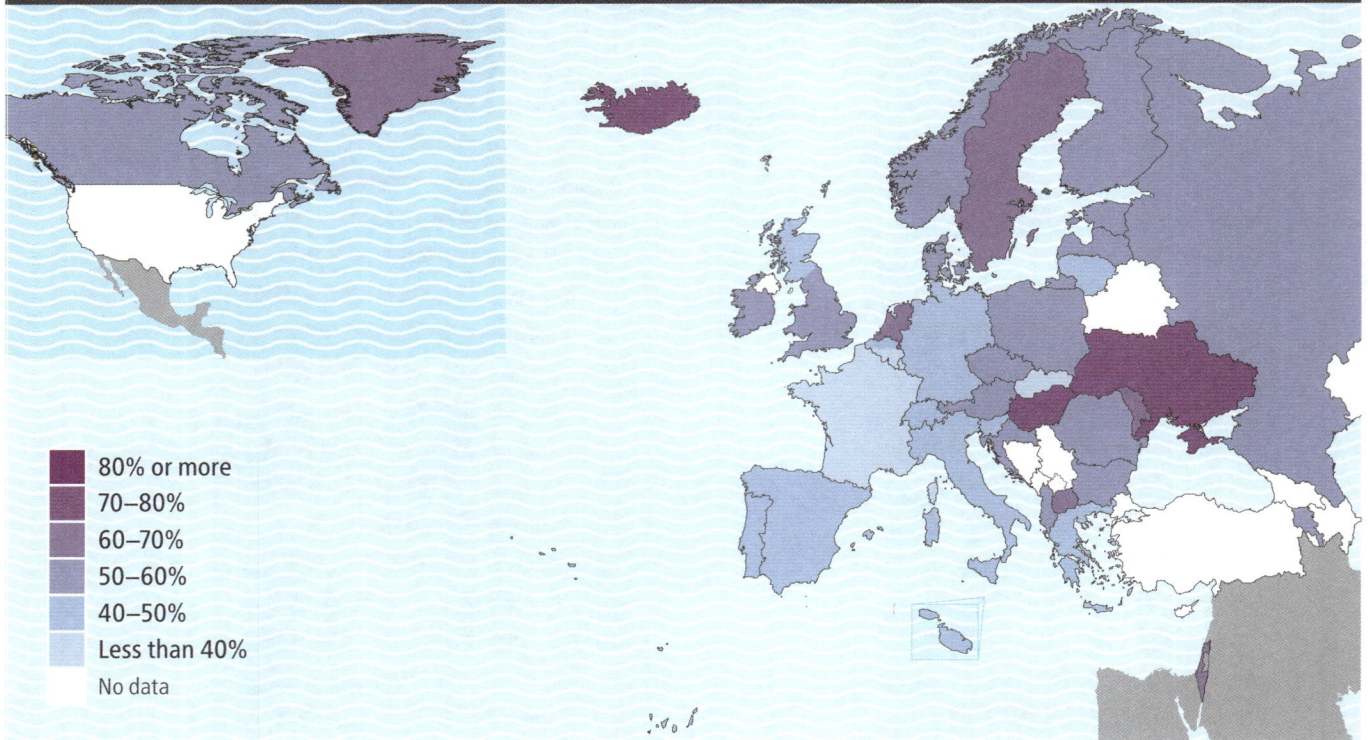

- 80% or more
- 70–80%
- 60–70%
- 50–60%
- 40–50%
- Less than 40%
- No data

Note: HBSC teams provided disaggregated data for Belgium and the United Kingdom; these data appear in the map above.

HBSC survey 2013/2014

15-year-old boys who find it easy or very easy to talk to their fathers

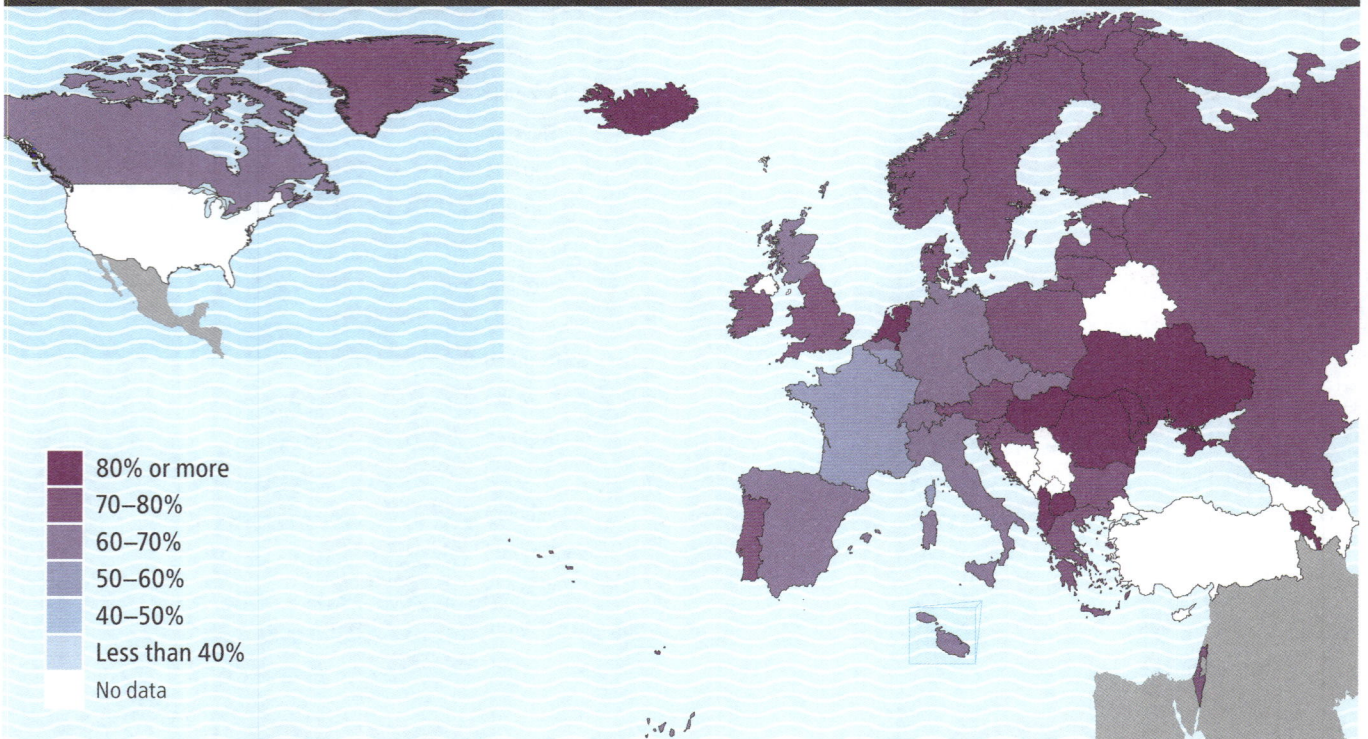

- 80% or more
- 70–80%
- 60–70%
- 50–60%
- 40–50%
- Less than 40%
- No data

Note: HBSC teams provided disaggregated data for Belgium and the United Kingdom; these data appear in the map above.

GROWING UP UNEQUAL: GENDER AND SOCIOECONOMIC
DIFFERENCES IN YOUNG PEOPLE'S HEALTH AND WELL-BEING
PART 2. KEY DATA | CHAPTER 2. SOCIAL CONTEXT

2

FAMILY:
PERCEIVED FAMILY SUPPORT

Supportive family relationships play a fundamental role in adolescent development, socialization, health and well-being *(18,19)*. A high level of perceived family support is related to better mental health *(20)* and lower levels of risk behaviours *(21,22)*. Parental support is also a protective factor for children in adverse environments *(23)*.

HBSC survey 2013/2014

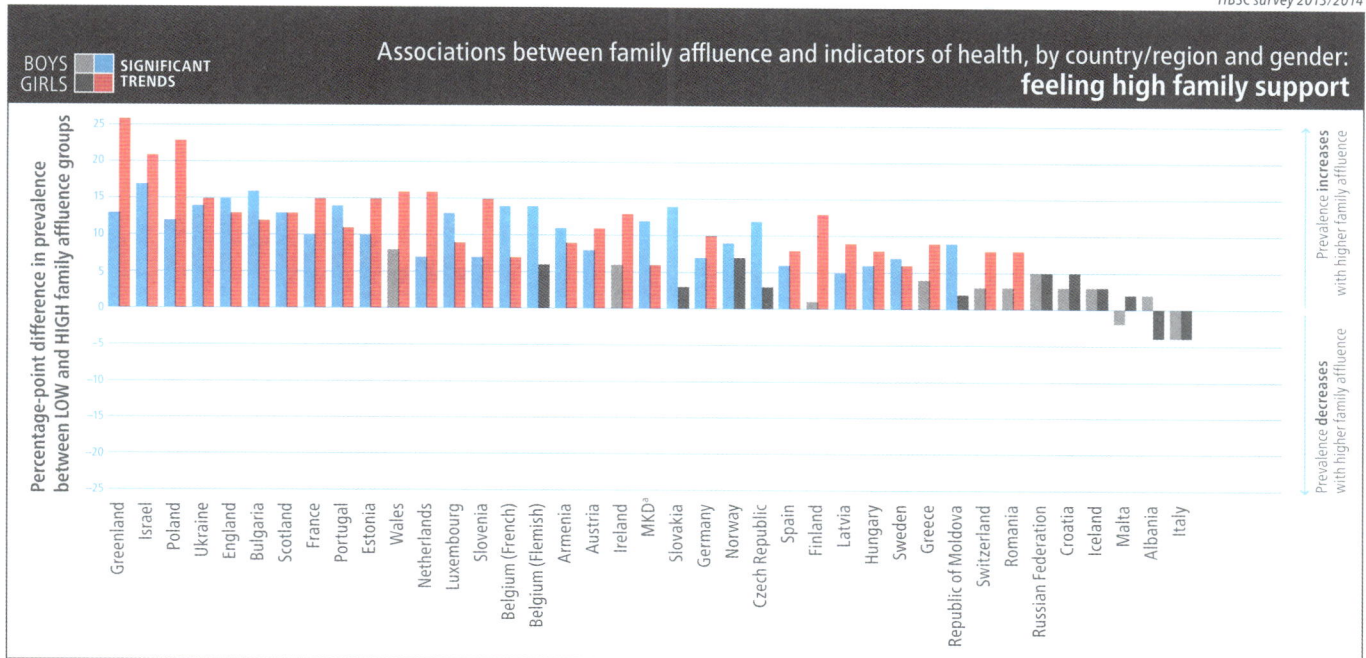

Associations between family affluence and indicators of health, by country/region and gender: **feeling high family support**

BOYS / GIRLS — SIGNIFICANT TRENDS

Percentage-point difference in prevalence between LOW and HIGH family affluence groups

Prevalence **increases** with higher family affluence

Prevalence **decreases** with higher family affluence

ᵃ The former Yugoslav Republic of Macedonia. *Note:* low- and high-affluence groups represent the lowest 20% and highest 20% in each country. No data were received from Canada, Denmark and Lithuania.

MEASURE

Family support was measured using the MSPSS *(24)*. Young people were asked if they feel that their family really tries to help them, that they can get emotional support from them when they need it, they can talk to their family about problems, and if the family is prepared to help them make decisions. Response options ranged from very strongly disagree to very strongly agree.

RESULTS

Findings presented here show the proportions who scored 5.5 or more on the MSPSS, categorized as high perceived family support (25,26).

Age

A significant age difference was found among boys and girls in almost all countries and regions (except Armenia and Bulgaria for both genders and Estonia and Romania for boys). Generally, the percentage who perceived their families as highly supportive decreased with age, but a different age pattern was detected in some countries and regions.

Gender

Significant gender differences in the youngest age group were found in only nine countries and regions, with higher proportions of girls reporting high family support in six. A reverse relationship was found in three (Belgium (Flemish), Greece and Greenland). Gender differences were more pronounced among 13- and 15-year-olds, with significant differences in 20 for 13-year-olds and 14 for those aged 15. Boys were more likely to report high family support in most but a reverse relationship was found in Albania, the Republic of Moldova and Ukraine in 13-year-olds and in Bulgaria for those who were 15.

Family affluence

Family affluence was associated with perceived family support in around two thirds of the countries and regions among boys and girls. Prevalence was higher for girls and boys from more affluent families. Differences between high- and low-affluence groups were more than 10 percentage points in around one third for both genders.

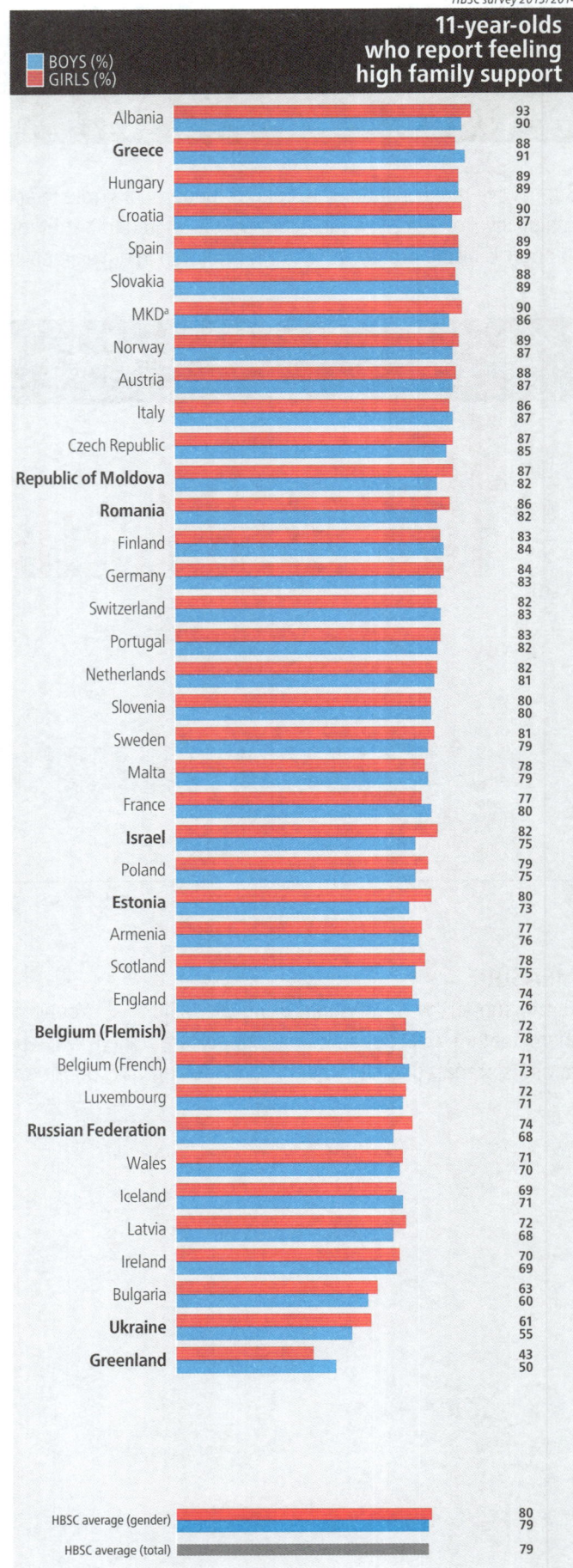

HBSC survey 2013/2014

11-year-olds who report feeling high family support

BOYS (%)
GIRLS (%)

Country	Girls (%)	Boys (%)
Albania	93	90
Greece	88	91
Hungary	89	89
Croatia	90	87
Spain	89	89
Slovakia	88	89
MKD[a]	90	86
Norway	89	87
Austria	88	87
Italy	86	87
Czech Republic	87	85
Republic of Moldova	87	82
Romania	86	82
Finland	83	84
Germany	84	83
Switzerland	82	83
Portugal	83	82
Netherlands	82	81
Slovenia	80	80
Sweden	81	79
Malta	78	79
France	77	80
Israel	82	75
Poland	79	75
Estonia	80	73
Armenia	77	76
Scotland	78	75
England	74	76
Belgium (Flemish)	72	78
Belgium (French)	71	73
Luxembourg	72	71
Russian Federation	74	68
Wales	71	70
Iceland	69	71
Latvia	72	68
Ireland	70	69
Bulgaria	63	60
Ukraine	61	55
Greenland	43	50
HBSC average (gender)	80	79
HBSC average (total)	79	

[a] The former Yugoslav Republic of Macedonia.

GROWING UP UNEQUAL: GENDER AND SOCIOECONOMIC
DIFFERENCES IN YOUNG PEOPLE'S HEALTH AND WELL-BEING
PART 2. KEY DATA | CHAPTER 2. SOCIAL CONTEXT
FAMILY: PERCEIVED FAMILY SUPPORT

2

13-year-olds who report feeling high family support

HBSC survey 2013/2014

- BOYS (%)
- GIRLS (%)

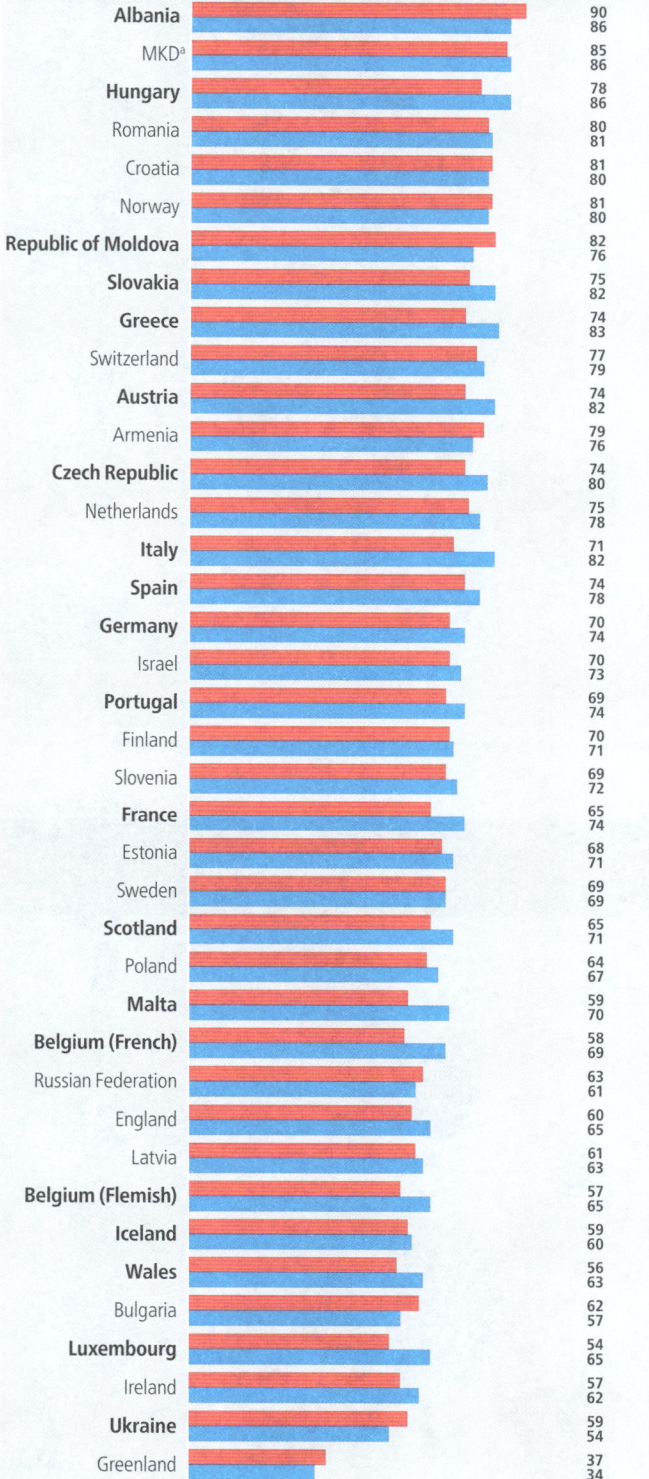

Country	Girls	Boys
Albania	90	86
MKD[a]	85	86
Hungary	78	86
Romania	80	81
Croatia	81	80
Norway	81	80
Republic of Moldova	82	76
Slovakia	75	82
Greece	74	83
Switzerland	77	79
Austria	74	82
Armenia	79	76
Czech Republic	74	80
Netherlands	75	78
Italy	71	82
Spain	74	78
Germany	70	74
Israel	70	73
Portugal	69	74
Finland	70	71
Slovenia	69	72
France	65	74
Estonia	68	71
Sweden	69	69
Scotland	65	71
Poland	64	67
Malta	59	70
Belgium (French)	58	69
Russian Federation	63	61
England	60	65
Latvia	61	63
Belgium (Flemish)	57	65
Iceland	59	60
Wales	56	63
Bulgaria	62	57
Luxembourg	54	65
Ireland	57	62
Ukraine	59	54
Greenland	37	34
HBSC average (gender)	69	72
HBSC average (total)		71

15-year-olds who report feeling high family support

HBSC survey 2013/2014

- BOYS (%)
- GIRLS (%)

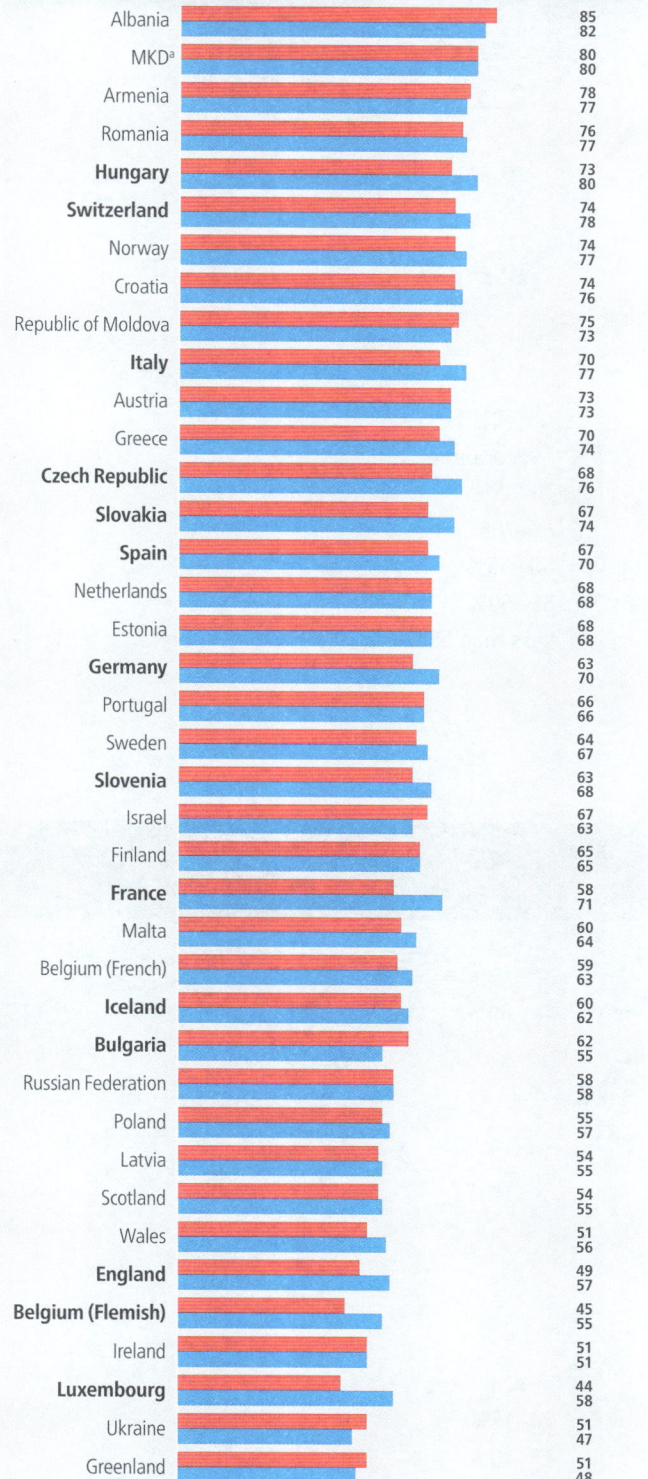

Country	Girls	Boys
Albania	85	82
MKD[a]	80	80
Armenia	78	77
Romania	76	77
Hungary	73	80
Switzerland	74	78
Norway	74	77
Croatia	74	76
Republic of Moldova	75	73
Italy	70	77
Austria	73	73
Greece	70	74
Czech Republic	68	76
Slovakia	67	74
Spain	67	70
Netherlands	68	68
Estonia	68	68
Germany	63	70
Portugal	66	66
Sweden	64	67
Slovenia	63	68
Israel	67	63
Finland	65	65
France	58	71
Malta	60	64
Belgium (French)	59	63
Iceland	60	62
Bulgaria	62	55
Russian Federation	58	58
Poland	55	57
Latvia	54	55
Scotland	54	55
Wales	51	56
England	49	57
Belgium (Flemish)	45	55
Ireland	51	51
Luxembourg	44	58
Ukraine	51	47
Greenland	51	48
HBSC average (gender)	64	67
HBSC average (total)		65

Note: **indicates** significant gender difference (at p<0.05).
No data were received from Canada, Denmark and Lithuania.

HBSC survey 2013/2014

15-year-old girls who report feeling high family support

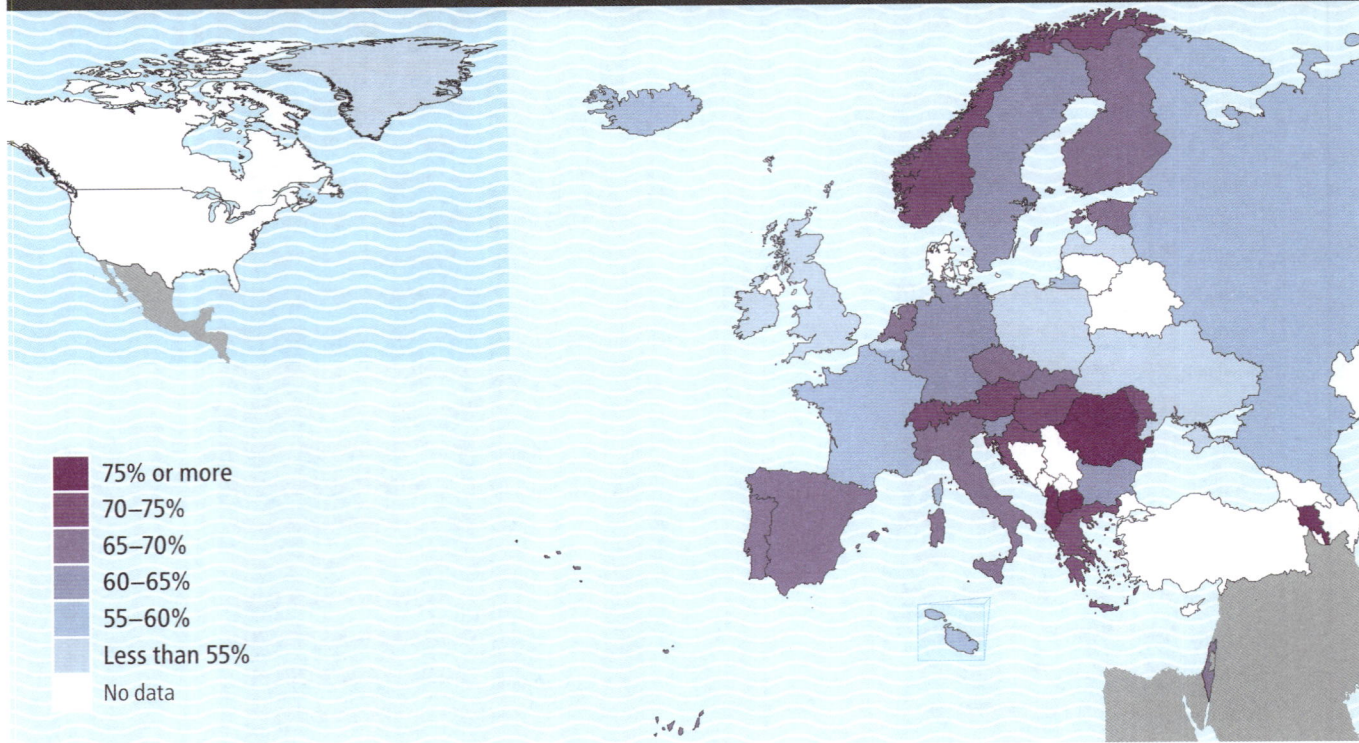

75% or more
70–75%
65–70%
60–65%
55–60%
Less than 55%
No data

Note: HBSC teams provided disaggregated data for Belgium and the United Kingdom; these data appear in the map above.

HBSC survey 2013/2014

15-year-old boys who report feeling high family support

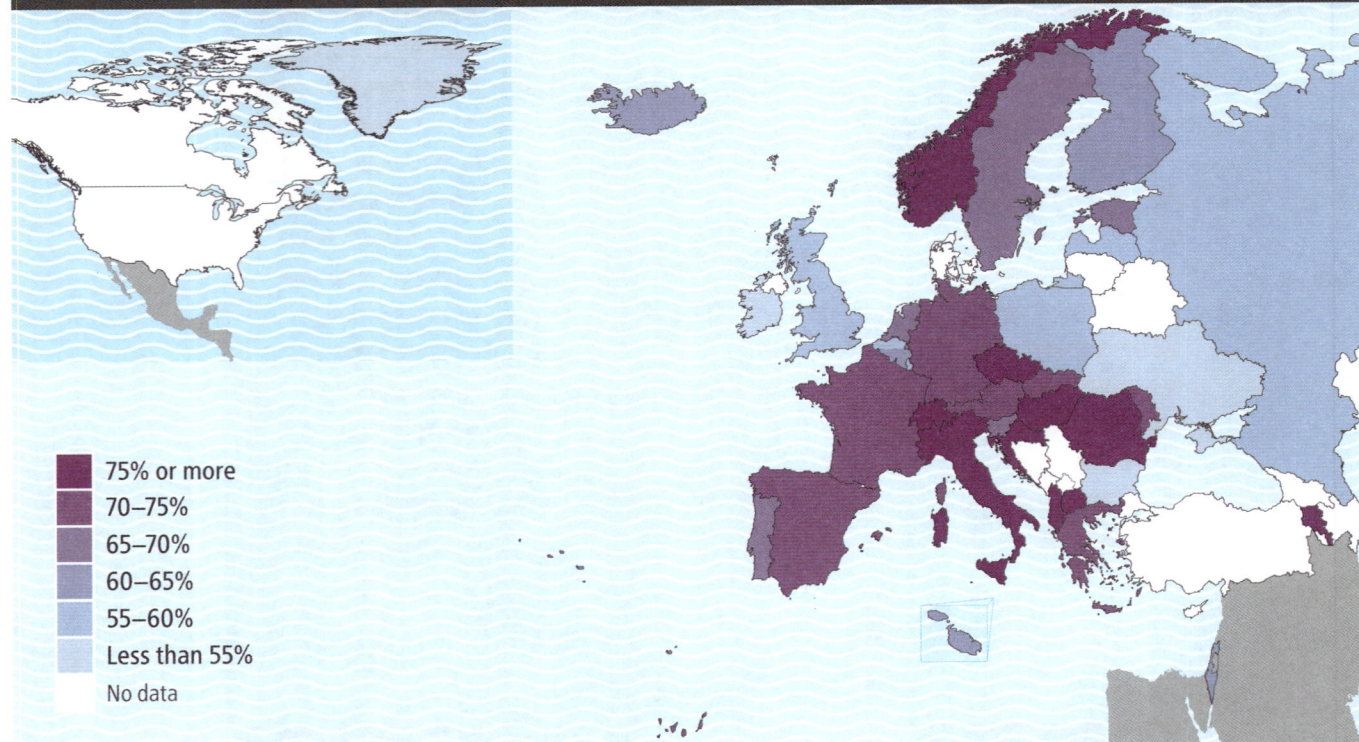

75% or more
70–75%
65–70%
60–65%
55–60%
Less than 55%
No data

Note: HBSC teams provided disaggregated data for Belgium and the United Kingdom; these data appear in the map above.

GROWING UP UNEQUAL: GENDER AND SOCIOECONOMIC
DIFFERENCES IN YOUNG PEOPLE'S HEALTH AND WELL-BEING
PART 2. KEY DATA | CHAPTER 2. SOCIAL CONTEXT
FAMILY

2

FAMILY:
SCIENTIFIC DISCUSSION AND POLICY REFLECTIONS

SCIENTIFIC DISCUSSION

The findings suggest that most young people feel their parents are interested and engaged with them, although parental engagement and support are significantly related to family affluence. Gender and age are strongly associated with effective parental communication and support.

The quality of parental communication can be influential in the development of pro-social values, provides young people with an important resource for managing stressful situations (27,28) and helps them navigate adverse influences that lead to health-risk behaviours such as smoking, substance use and aggressive behaviours (29,30). Open family communication on sexual issues corresponds with less high-risk sexual behaviours in adolescence (31). Findings relating to lower levels of reported ease of communication with parents for many young people traversing adolescence consequently have important implications for their health and well-being and actions to address health-risk behaviours.

Subjective life satisfaction is an important indicator of overall well-being. Young people during late childhood to mid-adolescence who report good communication with their parents or guardians have higher overall life satisfaction and report fewer physical or psychological complaints (32). Girls who find it easy to talk to their fathers, for example, report higher life satisfaction and a more positive body image (33). Findings raise particular concerns about the way older girls and young people with lower family affluence experience parental communication.

Parental support and strong family bonds are linked to positive emotional well-being in adolescence and reduced prevalence of engagement in health-risk behaviours. Findings in relation to family affluence highlight the significance of a social-determinants approach to understanding how disadvantage and inequality is constructed in adolescence (34).

POLICY REFLECTIONS

Consideration of how parenting influences child development has tended to give primacy to the early years. The effects of family dynamics on life chances and the nature of external relationships during adolescence have recently been highlighted by research, particularly the family's role in maintaining emotional well-being and health behaviours during mid-childhood and early adolescence (34): stability and sense of belonging within a family, for example, has been linked with young people's life satisfaction (28). How best to support families during adolescence, particularly those from disadvantaged backgrounds, represents a key challenge for policy-makers, as intervention in family life often cuts to the heart of ideological tensions concerning the role of government in the private lives and domains of its citizens.

Research has brought into question the displacement theory, which suggests that parents' influence on adolescents' lives wanes over time and peers and communities assume greater importance. Parents clearly have a key role as a protective health asset for young people in the successful navigation of adolescence and into early adulthood.

WHO's Early Years, Family and Education Task Group has highlighted the importance of all sectors and professionals working together to support young people to develop self-efficacy and agency (35). Its report stresses the importance of schools working directly with children and other services to provide parents with support and advice on parenting strategies during the later years of childhood.

REFERENCES

1. Levin KA, Currie C. Family structure, mother–child communication, father–child communication, and adolescent life satisfaction: a cross-sectional multilevel analysis. Health Educ. 2010;110(3):152–68.

2. Boniel-Nissim M, Tabak I, Mazur J, Borraccino A, Brooks F, Gommans R et al. Supportive communication with parents moderates the negative effects of electronic media use on life satisfaction during adolescence. Int J Public Health 2015;60(2):189–98.

3. Luk JW, Farhat T, Iannotti RJ, Simons-Morton BG. Parent–child communication and substance use among adolescents: do father and mother communication play a different role for sons and daughters? Addict Behav. 2010;35(5):426–31.

4. Zambon A, Lemma P, Borraccino A, Dalmasso P, Cavallo F. Socioeconomic position and adolescents' health in Italy: the role of the quality of social relations. Eur J Public Health 2006;16:627–32.

5. Lenciauskiene I, Zaborskis A. The effects of family structure, parent–child relationship and parental monitoring on early sexual behaviour among adolescents in nine European countries. Scand J Public Health 2008;36(6):607–18.

6. Small ML, Morgan N, Bailey-Davis L, Maggs JL. The protective effects of parent–college student communication on dietary and physical activity behaviors. J Adolesc Health 2013;53(2):300–2.

7. Le Poire BA. Family communication. Nurturing and control in a changing world. Thousand Oaks (CA): Sage; 2006.

8. Stattin H, Kerr M. Parental monitoring: a reinterpretation. Child Dev. 2000;71(4):1072–85.

9. Bulanda RE, Majumdar D. Perceived parent–child relations and adolescent self-esteem. J Child Fam Stud. 2009;18(2):203–12.

10. Cava M-J, Buelga S, Musitu G. Parental communication and life satisfaction in adolescence. Span J Psychol. 2014;17:E98.

11. Fenton C, Brooks F, Spencer NH, Morgan A. Sustaining a positive body image in adolescence: an assets-based analysis. Health Soc Care Community 2010;18(2):189–98.

12. Jafari M, Baharudin, R, Archer M. Fathers' parenting behaviors and Malaysian adolescents' anxiety: family income as a moderator. J Fam Issues 2013; doi:10.1177/0192513X13513580.

13. Clair A. The relationship between parents' subjective well-being and the life satisfaction of their children in Britain. Child Indic Res. 2012;5(4):631–50.

14. Levin KA, Dallago L, Currie C. The association between adolescent life satisfaction, family structure, family affluence and gender differences in parent–child communication. Soc Indic Res. 2012;106(2):287–305.

15. Demidenko N, Manion I, Lee CM. Father–daughter attachment and communication in depressed and nondepressed adolescent girls. J Child Fam Stud. 2015;24:1727–34.

16. Rostad WL. The influence of Dad: an investigation of adolescent females' perceived closeness with fathers and risky behaviors. Missoula (MT): University of Montana; 2012 (Theses, Dissertations, Professional Papers: Paper 1027; http://scholarworks.umt.edu/cgi/viewcontent.cgi?article=2046&context=etd, accessed 18 August 2015).

17. Gallarin M, Alonso-Arbiol I. Parenting practices, parental attachment and aggressiveness in adolescence: a predictive model. J Adolesc. 2012;35(6):1601–10.

18. Collins WA, Laursen B. Changing relationships, changing youth interpersonal contexts of adolescent development. J Early Adolesc. 2004;24(1):55–62.

19. Collins WA, Steinberg L. Adolescent development in interpersonal context. In: Eisenberg N, Damon W, Lerner RM, editors. Handbook of child psychology. Vol. 3. Hoboken (NJ): John Wiley & Sons Inc.; 2006:1003–67.

20. Rothon C, Goodwin L, Stansfeld S. Family social support, community "social capital" and adolescents' mental health and educational outcomes: a longitudinal study in England. Soc Psychiatry Psychiatr Epidemiol. 2012;47(5):697–709.

21. White R, Renk K. Externalizing behavior problems during adolescence: an ecological perspective. J Child Fam Stud. 2012;21(1):158–71.

22. Dunn MS, Kitts C, Lewis S, Goodrow B, Scherzer GD. Effects of youth assets on adolescent alcohol, tobacco, marijuana use, and sexual behavior. J Alcohol Drug Educ. 2011;55(3):23–40.

23. Stadler C, Feifel J, Rohrmann S, Vermeiren R, Poustka F. Peer-victimization and mental health problems in adolescents: are parental and school support protective? Child Psychiatry Hum Dev. 2010;41(4):371–86.

24. Zimet GD, Dahlem NW, Zimet SG, Farley GK. The Multidimensional Scale of Perceived Social Support. J Pers Assess. 1988;52(1):30–41.

25. Zimet GD, Powell SS, Farley GK, Werkman S, Berkoff KA. Psychometric characteristics of the Multidimensional Scale of Perceived Social Support. J Pers Assess. 1990;55(3–4):610–7.

26. Canty-Mitchell J, Zimet GD. Psychometric properties of the Multidimensional Scale of Perceived Social Support in urban adolescents. Am J Community Psychol. 2000;28(3):391–400.

27. Duncan P, Garcia A, Frankowski B, Carey P, Kallock E, Dixon R et al. Inspiring healthy adolescent choices: a rationale for and guide to strength promotion in primary care. J Adolesc Health 2007;41:525–35.

28. Ward P, Zabriskie R. Positive youth development within a family leisure context: youth perspectives of family outcomes. New Dir Youth Dev. 2011;130:29–42.

29. Lambert S, Cashwell C. Preteens talking to parents: perceived communication and school-based aggression. The Family Journal 2004;12(2):22–128.

30. Pedersen M, Carmen Granado Alcon M, Moreno C. Family and health. In: Currie C, Roberts C, Morgan A, Smith R, Settertobulte W, Samdal O et al., editors. Young people's health in context. Health Behaviour in School-aged Children (HBSC) study: international report from the 2001/2002 survey. Copenhagen: WHO Regional Office for Europe; 2004 (Health Policy for Children and Adolescents, No. 4; http://www.euro.who.int/__data/assets/pdf_file/0008/110231/e82923.pdf, accessed 18 August 2015).

31. Whitaker DJ, Miller KS. Parent–adolescent discussions about sex and condoms: impact on peer influences of sexual risk behavior. J Adolesc Res. 2000;15(2):251–73.

32. Moreno C, Sanchez-Queija I, Munoz-Tinoco V, de Matos MG, Dallago L, Ter Bogt T et al. Cross-national associations between parent and peer communication and psychological complaints. Int J Public Health 2009;54:235–42.

33. Fenton C, Brooks F, Spencer N, Morgan A. Sustaining a positive body image in adolescence: an assets-based analysis. Health Soc Care Community 2010;18(2):189–98.

34. Bell NJ, Forthun LF, Sun SW. Attachment, adolescent competencies and substance use: developmental consideration in the study of risk behaviours. Subst Use Misuse 2000;35:1177–206.

35. Jensen BB, Currie C, Dyson A, Eisenstadt N, Melhuish E. Early Years, Family and Education Task Group: report. European review of social determinants of health and the health divide in the WHO European Region. Copenhagen: WHO Regional Office for Europe; 2013 (http://www.euro.who.int/__data/assets/pdf_file/0006/236193/Early-years,-family-and-education-task-group-report.pdf, accessed 18 August 2015).

GROWING UP UNEQUAL: GENDER AND SOCIOECONOMIC
DIFFERENCES IN YOUNG PEOPLE'S HEALTH AND WELL-BEING
PART 2. KEY DATA | CHAPTER 2. SOCIAL CONTEXT

2

PEERS:
PERCEIVED PEER SUPPORT

Perceived peer support has a critical impact on adolescents' physical and mental health *(1)*. Adolescents who perceive their friends as supportive experience higher levels of psychological well-being and have better social competences and fewer emotional and behavioural problems *(2,3)*. Peer support can be protective in the face of stressors and has a direct positive association with well-being *(4,5)*. It is therefore critical to understand how peer relationships (and other socializing agents) influence adolescents' well-being and identify factors that promote peer support *(6)*.

HBSC survey 2013/2014

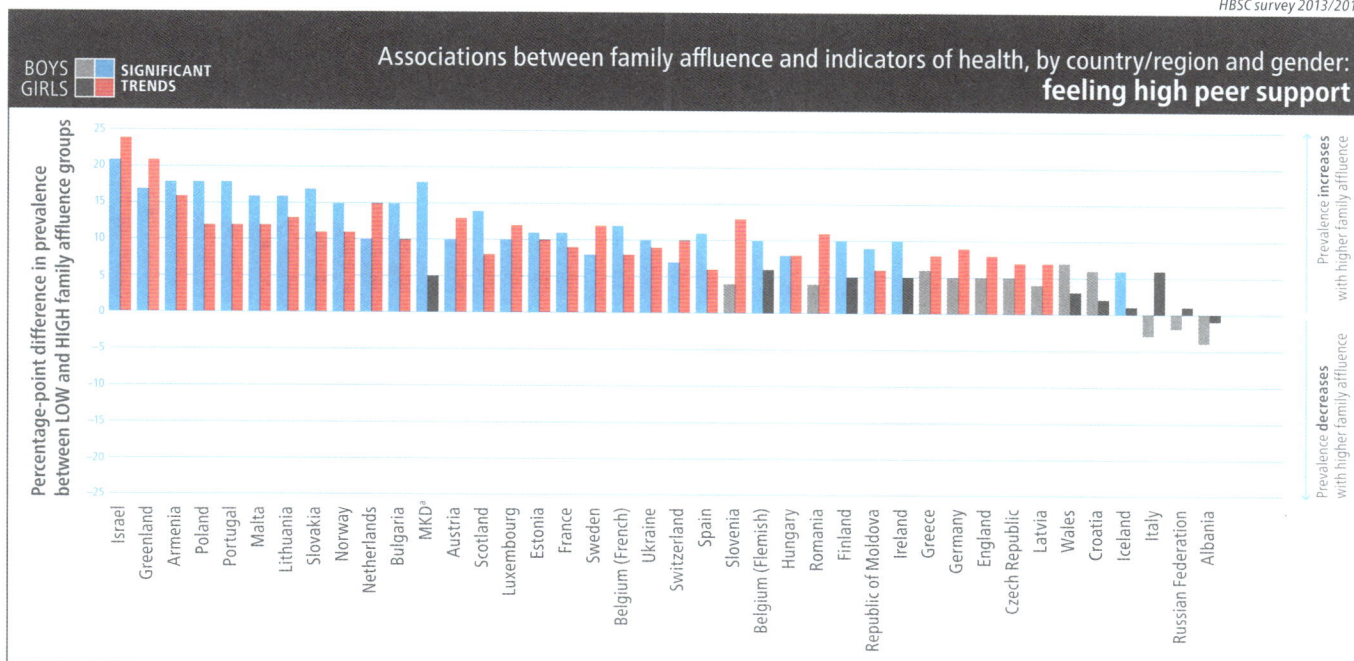

Associations between family affluence and indicators of health, by country/region and gender: **feeling high peer support**

ª The former Yugoslav Republic of Macedonia. *Note*: low- and high-affluence groups represent the lowest 20% and highest 20% in each country. No data were received from Canada and Denmark.

MEASURE

Peer support was measured using the MSPSS *(7)*. Young people were asked if they perceive that their friends really try to help them, that they can count on them when things go wrong, if they have friends with whom they can share their sorrows and joys, and if they can talk to them about their problems. Response options ranged from very strongly disagree to very strongly agree.

RESULTS

Findings presented here show the proportions reporting an average score of 5.5 or more (high peer support) on the MSPSS *(7)*.

Age

Comparable percentages of boys reported high levels of peer support across ages in most countries and regions, but there was a decreasing trend by age in 10, with smaller percentages of older boys reporting it: the most pronounced differences were between 11- and 13-year-olds. An opposite trend was detected in five countries and regions, with older boys more likely to report high levels of support.

Similar patterns were identified for girls, with no significant age differences in most countries and regions. Peer support decreased with age in 10 and the opposite trend was observed in five.

Gender

Reporting high levels of social support from peers was more common among girls in almost all countries and regions and at every age. Gender differences tended to be most pronounced among 13-year-olds.

Family affluence

Affluence levels were positively associated with perceived peer support in most countries and regions. Girls and boys from high-affluence families were more likely to report high levels of support. Differences between high- and low-affluence groups exceeded 20 percentage points in Israel (girls and boys) and Greenland (girls only).

HBSC survey 2013/2014

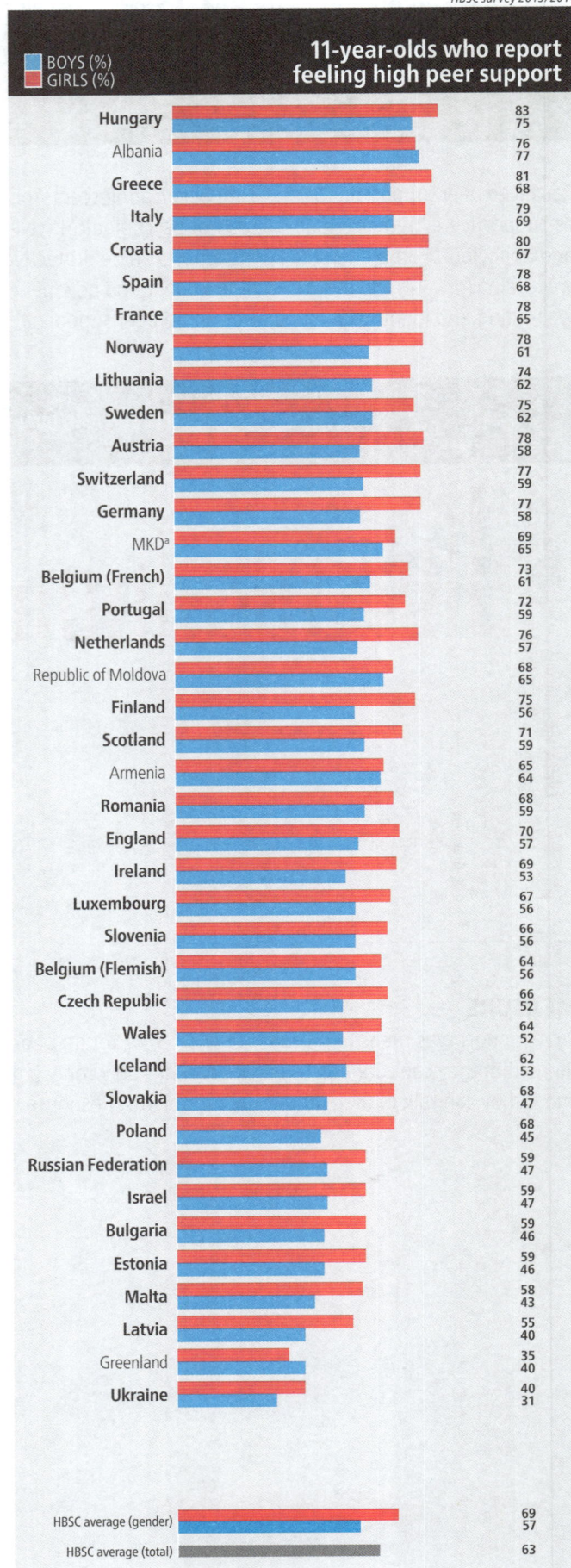

11-year-olds who report feeling high peer support

BOYS (%)
GIRLS (%)

Country	Girls	Boys
Hungary	83	75
Albania	76	77
Greece	81	68
Italy	79	69
Croatia	80	67
Spain	78	68
France	78	65
Norway	78	61
Lithuania	74	62
Sweden	75	62
Austria	78	58
Switzerland	77	59
Germany	77	58
MKD[a]	69	65
Belgium (French)	73	61
Portugal	72	59
Netherlands	76	57
Republic of Moldova	68	65
Finland	75	56
Scotland	71	59
Armenia	65	64
Romania	68	59
England	70	57
Ireland	69	53
Luxembourg	67	56
Slovenia	66	56
Belgium (Flemish)	64	56
Czech Republic	66	52
Wales	64	52
Iceland	62	53
Slovakia	68	47
Poland	68	45
Russian Federation	59	47
Israel	59	47
Bulgaria	59	46
Estonia	59	46
Malta	58	43
Latvia	55	40
Greenland	35	40
Ukraine	40	31
HBSC average (gender)	69	57
HBSC average (total)	63	

[a] The former Yugoslav Republic of Macedonia.

GROWING UP UNEQUAL: GENDER AND SOCIOECONOMIC
DIFFERENCES IN YOUNG PEOPLE'S HEALTH AND WELL-BEING
PART 2. KEY DATA | CHAPTER 2. SOCIAL CONTEXT
PEERS: PERCEIVED PEER SUPPORT

2

HBSC survey 2013/2014

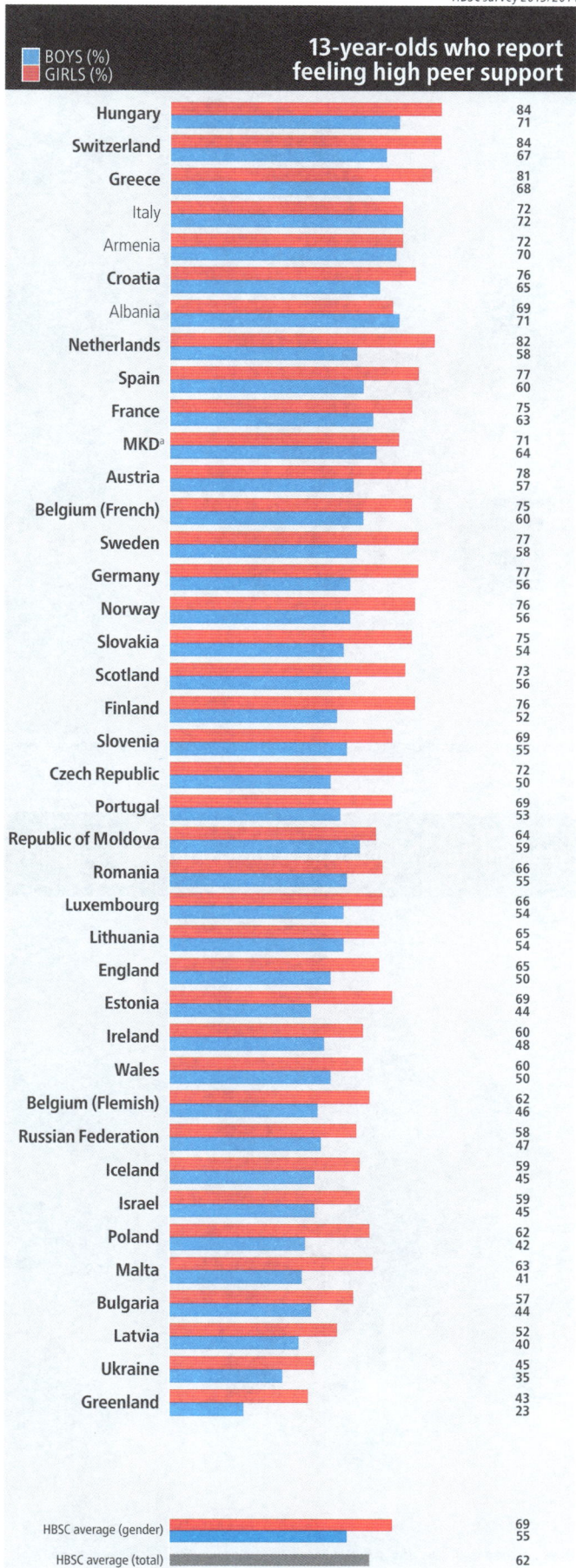

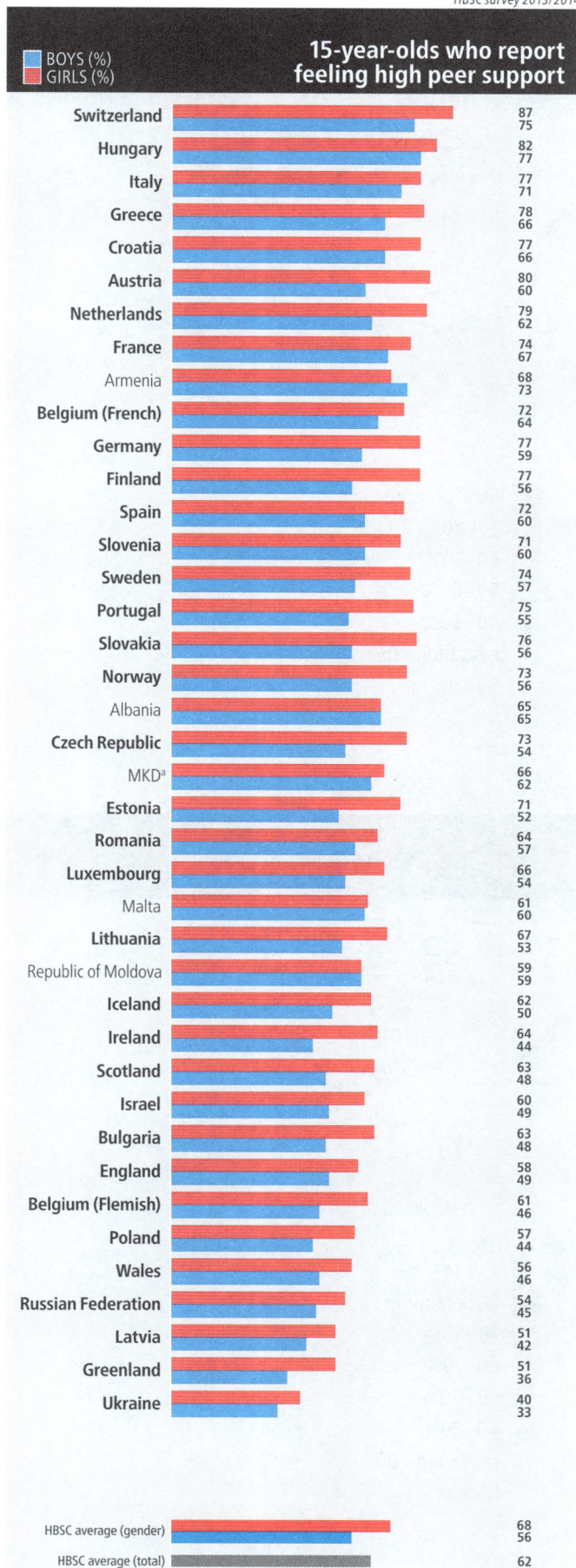

13-year-olds who report feeling high peer support

- BOYS (%)
- GIRLS (%)

Country	Girls	Boys
Hungary	84	71
Switzerland	84	67
Greece	81	68
Italy	72	72
Armenia	72	70
Croatia	76	65
Albania	69	71
Netherlands	82	58
Spain	77	60
France	75	63
MKD[a]	71	64
Austria	78	57
Belgium (French)	75	60
Sweden	77	58
Germany	77	56
Norway	76	56
Slovakia	75	54
Scotland	73	56
Finland	76	52
Slovenia	69	55
Czech Republic	72	50
Portugal	69	53
Republic of Moldova	64	59
Romania	66	55
Luxembourg	66	54
Lithuania	65	54
England	65	50
Estonia	69	44
Ireland	60	48
Wales	60	50
Belgium (Flemish)	62	46
Russian Federation	58	47
Iceland	59	45
Israel	59	45
Poland	62	42
Malta	63	41
Bulgaria	57	44
Latvia	52	40
Ukraine	45	35
Greenland	43	23
HBSC average (gender)	69	55
HBSC average (total)		62

HBSC survey 2013/2014

15-year-olds who report feeling high peer support

- BOYS (%)
- GIRLS (%)

Country	Girls	Boys
Switzerland	87	75
Hungary	82	77
Italy	77	71
Greece	78	66
Croatia	77	66
Austria	80	60
Netherlands	79	62
France	74	67
Armenia	68	73
Belgium (French)	72	64
Germany	77	59
Finland	77	56
Spain	72	60
Slovenia	71	60
Sweden	74	57
Portugal	75	55
Slovakia	76	56
Norway	73	56
Albania	65	65
Czech Republic	73	54
MKD[a]	66	62
Estonia	71	52
Romania	64	57
Luxembourg	66	54
Malta	61	60
Lithuania	67	53
Republic of Moldova	59	59
Iceland	62	50
Ireland	64	44
Scotland	63	48
Israel	60	49
Bulgaria	63	48
England	58	49
Belgium (Flemish)	61	46
Poland	57	44
Wales	56	46
Russian Federation	54	45
Latvia	51	42
Greenland	51	36
Ukraine	40	33
HBSC average (gender)	68	56
HBSC average (total)		62

Note: **indicates** significant gender difference (at p<0.05). No data were received from Canada and Denmark.

HBSC survey 2013/2014

15-year-old girls who report feeling high peer support

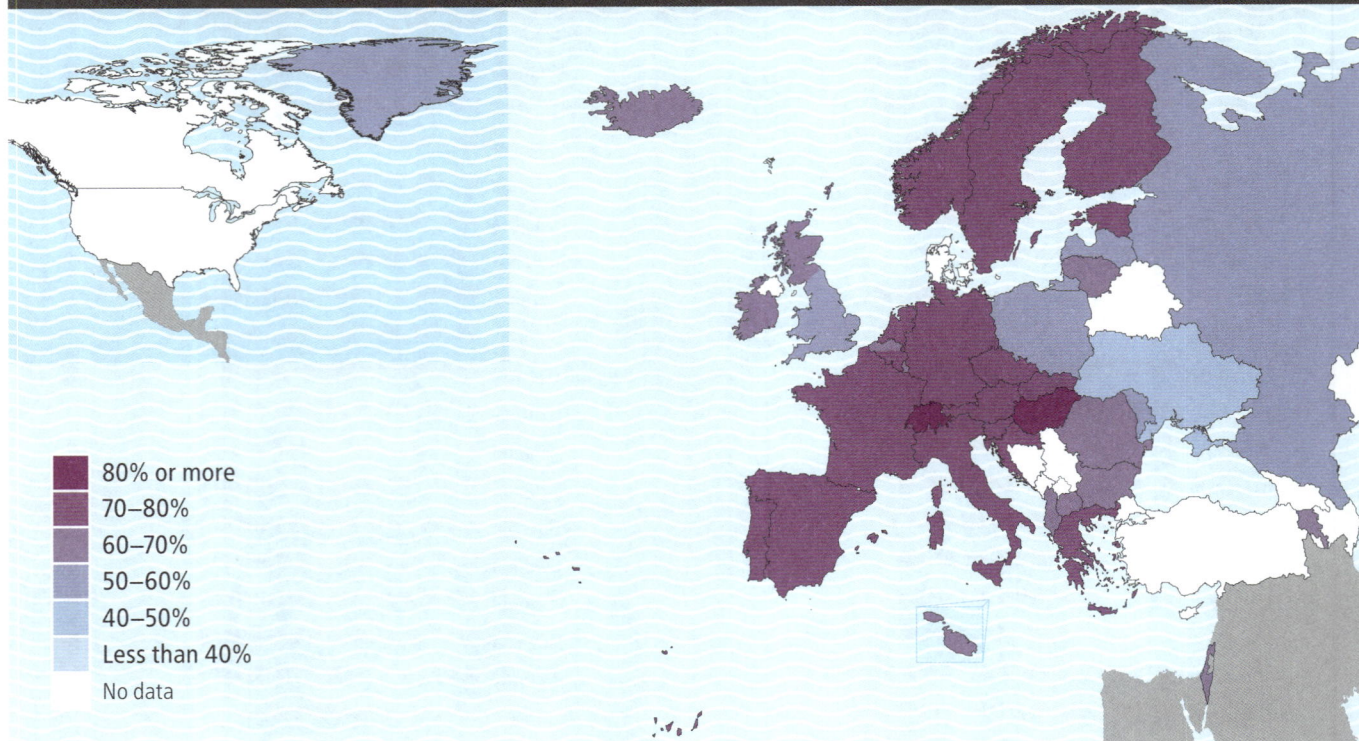

80% or more
70–80%
60–70%
50–60%
40–50%
Less than 40%
No data

Note: HBSC teams provided disaggregated data for Belgium and the United Kingdom; these data appear in the map above.

HBSC survey 2013/2014

15-year-old boys who report feeling high peer support

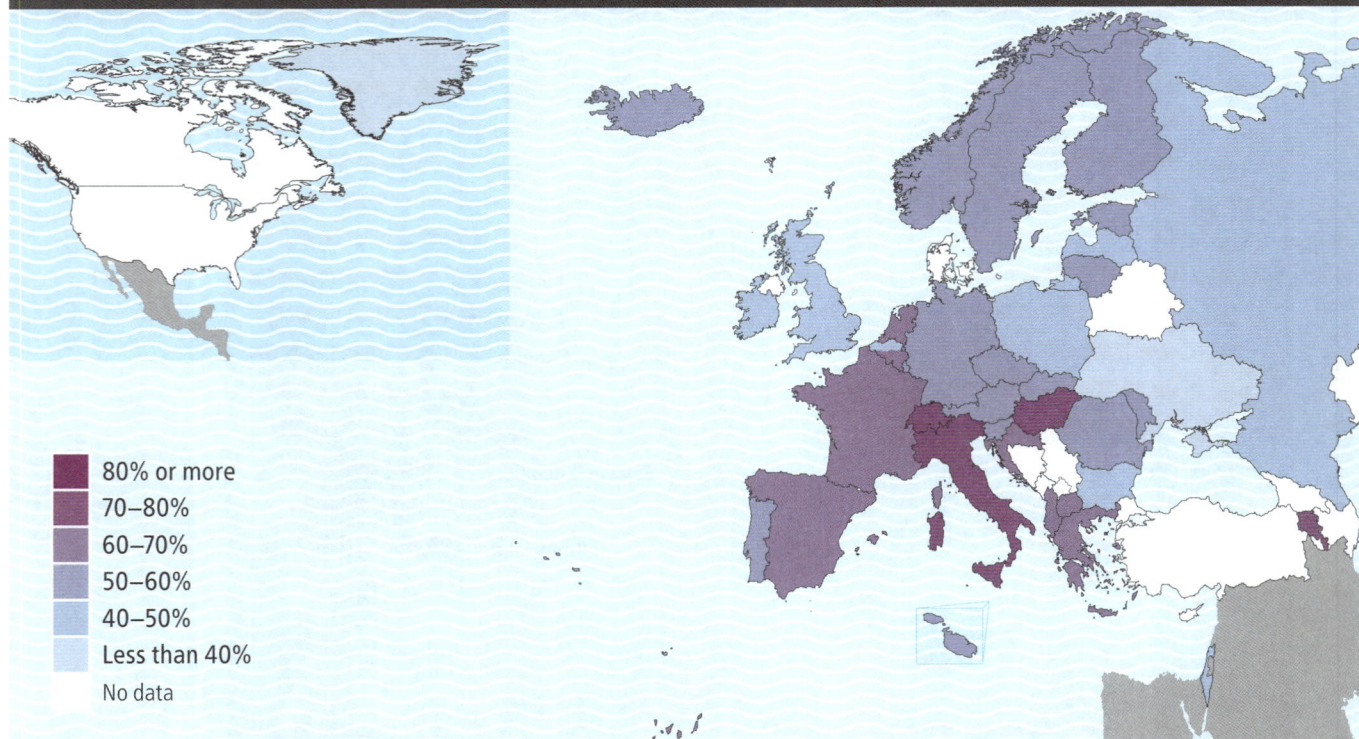

80% or more
70–80%
60–70%
50–60%
40–50%
Less than 40%
No data

Note: HBSC teams provided disaggregated data for Belgium and the United Kingdom; these data appear in the map above.

GROWING UP UNEQUAL: GENDER AND SOCIOECONOMIC
DIFFERENCES IN YOUNG PEOPLE'S HEALTH AND WELL-BEING
PART 2. KEY DATA | CHAPTER 2. SOCIAL CONTEXT

2

PEERS:
TIME WITH FRIENDS (BEFORE 8 PM (20:00))

Adolescence is a significant period of social transition. As family relationships change, adolescents begin to spend less time with parents and more with peers (8), either through direct or online relationships (9). Spending time with friends is therefore very important for adolescents, who turn to them in times of need (10) to access emotional support and a safe environment in which to explore their identities. At the same time, however, several studies have found a positive association between time spent with friends and risk behaviours such as (binge) drinking and risky sexual behaviours (9,11).

HBSC survey 2013/2014

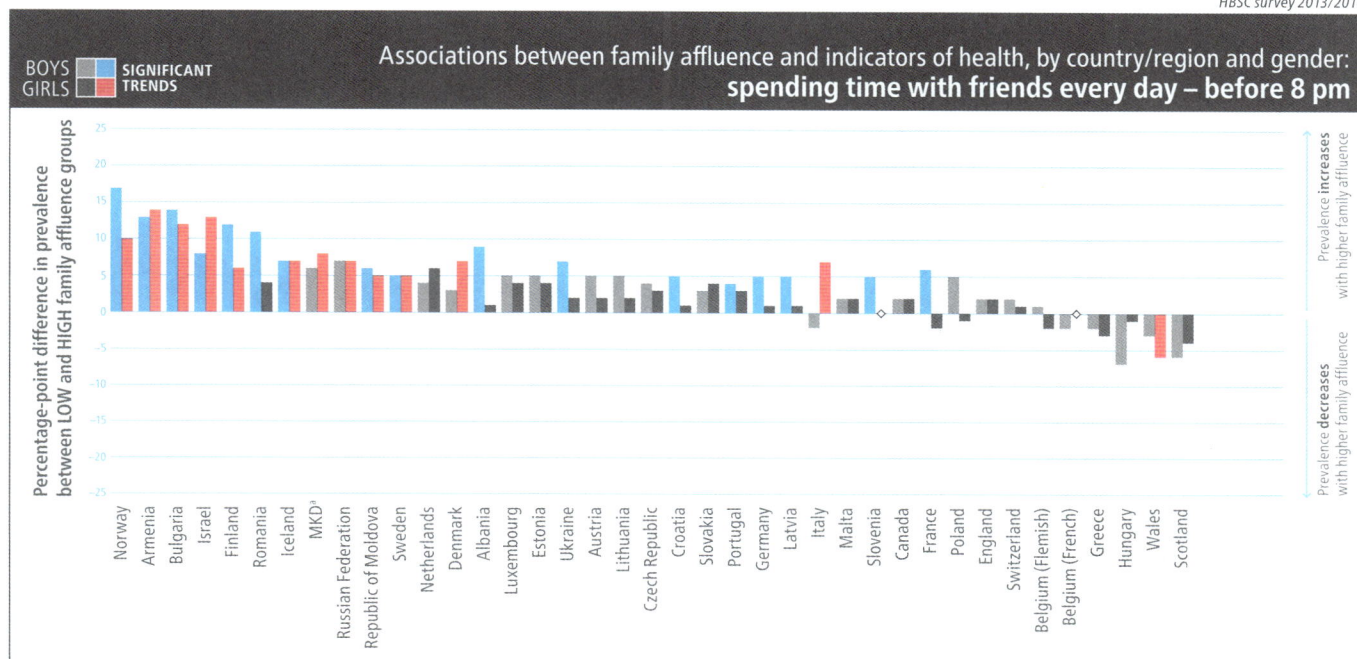

BOYS
GIRLS
SIGNIFICANT TRENDS

Associations between family affluence and indicators of health, by country/region and gender:
spending time with friends every day – before 8 pm

Percentage-point difference in prevalence between LOW and HIGH family affluence groups

Prevalence **increases** with higher family affluence

Prevalence **decreases** with higher family affluence

Norway, Armenia, Bulgaria, Israel, Finland, Romania, Iceland, MKD^a, Russian Federation, Republic of Moldova, Sweden, Netherlands, Denmark, Albania, Luxembourg, Estonia, Ukraine, Austria, Lithuania, Czech Republic, Croatia, Slovakia, Portugal, Germany, Latvia, Italy, Malta, Slovenia, Canada, France, Poland, England, Switzerland, Belgium (Flemish), Belgium (French), Greece, Hungary, Wales, Scotland

^aThe former Yugoslav Republic of Macedonia. *Note:* low- and high-affluence groups represent the lowest 20% and highest 20% in each country. ◇ means less than +/-0.5%.
No data were received from Greenland, Ireland and Spain.

MEASURE

Young people were asked how often they meet friends outside of school time before 8 o'clock in the evening. Response options ranged from hardly ever or never to daily.

Supplementary data on meeting friends after 8 o'clock in the evening are provided in the Annex.

RESULTS

Findings presented here show the proportions who reported meeting friends daily.

Age

Comparable percentages of boys and girls across all ages reported meeting with friends before 8 o'clock in the evening every day in approximately half of the countries and regions. Prevalence increased with age in 13 for boys and 16 for girls, but the opposite trend was observed in a few, particularly in northern Europe.

Gender

Meeting friends every day was more common among boys in most countries and regions and at all ages. Girls were more likely to report it in Iceland (11- and 13-year-olds), Latvia and the Russian Federation (13-year-olds only). The biggest differences across age groups were observed in Albania, Austria and Malta, where the percentages for boys were around double those for girls.

Family affluence

Affluence was positively associated with spending time with friends in around half of countries and regions, with the highest prevalence among high-affluence groups. Associations were statistically significant in 17 countries and regions for boys and 12 for girls. Girls in one country (United Kingdom (Wales)) showed the opposite relationship.

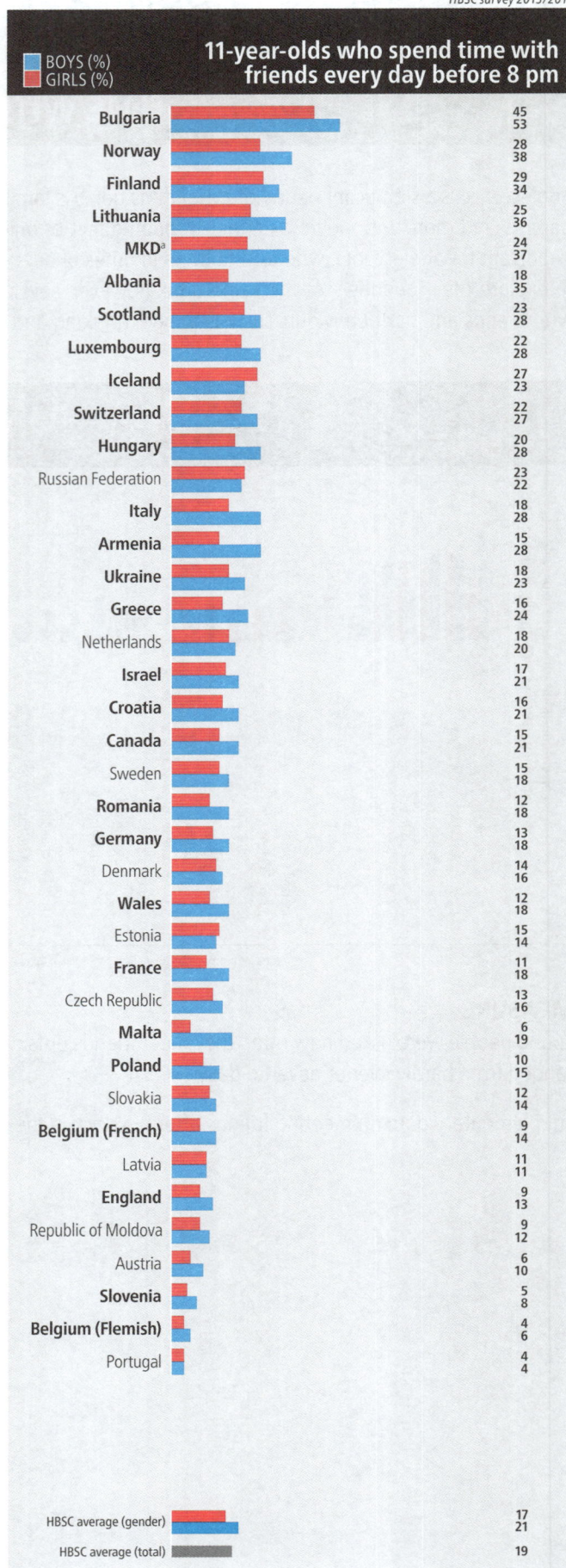

HBSC survey 2013/2014

BOYS (%)
GIRLS (%)

11-year-olds who spend time with friends every day before 8 pm

Country	Girls (%)	Boys (%)
Bulgaria	45	53
Norway	28	38
Finland	29	34
Lithuania	25	36
MKD[a]	24	37
Albania	18	35
Scotland	23	28
Luxembourg	22	28
Iceland	27	23
Switzerland	22	27
Hungary	20	28
Russian Federation	23	22
Italy	18	28
Armenia	15	28
Ukraine	18	23
Greece	16	24
Netherlands	18	20
Israel	17	21
Croatia	16	21
Canada	15	21
Sweden	15	18
Romania	12	18
Germany	13	18
Denmark	14	16
Wales	12	18
Estonia	15	14
France	11	18
Czech Republic	13	16
Malta	6	19
Poland	10	15
Slovakia	12	14
Belgium (French)	9	14
Latvia	11	11
England	9	13
Republic of Moldova	9	12
Austria	6	10
Slovenia	5	8
Belgium (Flemish)	4	6
Portugal	4	4
HBSC average (gender)	17	21
HBSC average (total)		19

[a] The former Yugoslav Republic of Macedonia.

GROWING UP UNEQUAL: GENDER AND SOCIOECONOMIC
DIFFERENCES IN YOUNG PEOPLE'S HEALTH AND WELL-BEING
PART 2. KEY DATA | CHAPTER 2. SOCIAL CONTEXT
PEERS: TIME WITH FRIENDS (BEFORE 8 PM (20:00))

2

13-year-olds who spend time with friends every day before 8 pm

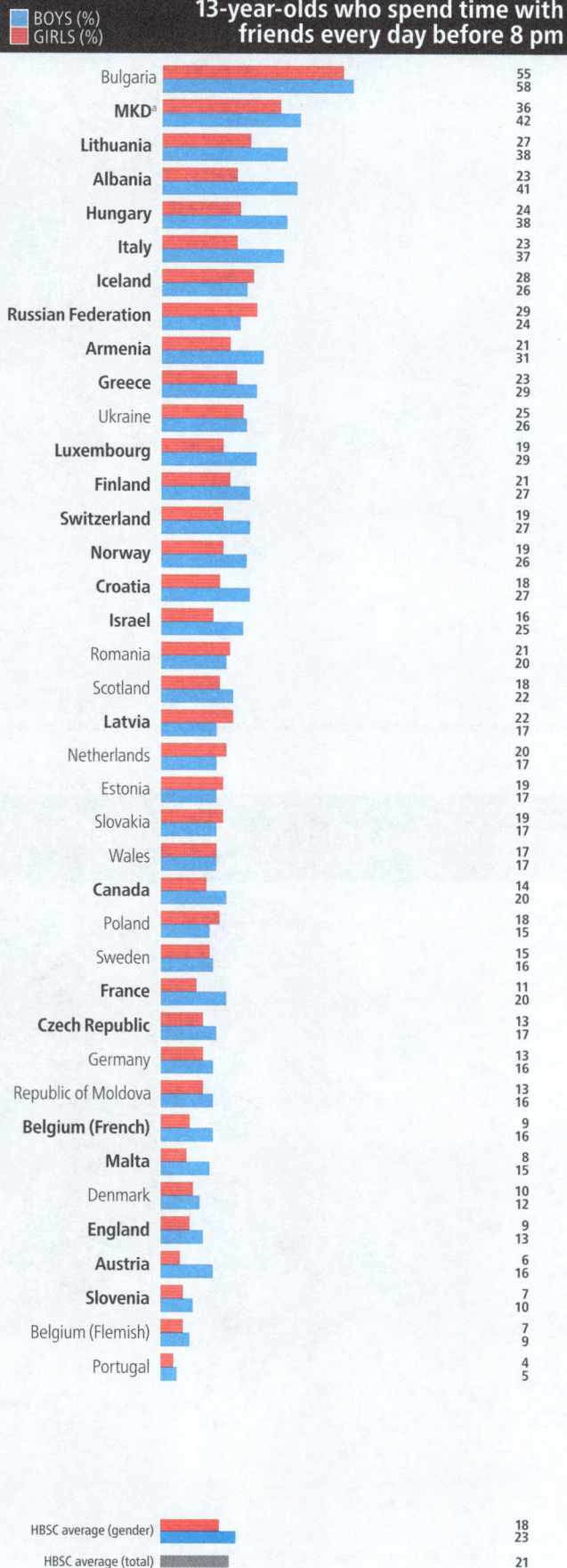

HBSC survey 2013/2014

- BOYS (%)
- GIRLS (%)

Country	Girls	Boys
Bulgaria	55	58
MKD[a]	36	42
Lithuania	27	38
Albania	23	41
Hungary	24	38
Italy	23	37
Iceland	28	26
Russian Federation	29	24
Armenia	21	31
Greece	23	29
Ukraine	25	26
Luxembourg	19	29
Finland	21	27
Switzerland	19	27
Norway	19	26
Croatia	18	27
Israel	16	25
Romania	21	20
Scotland	18	22
Latvia	22	17
Netherlands	20	17
Estonia	19	17
Slovakia	19	17
Wales	17	17
Canada	14	20
Poland	18	15
Sweden	15	16
France	11	20
Czech Republic	13	17
Germany	13	16
Republic of Moldova	13	16
Belgium (French)	9	16
Malta	8	15
Denmark	10	12
England	9	13
Austria	6	16
Slovenia	7	10
Belgium (Flemish)	7	9
Portugal	4	5
HBSC average (gender)	18	23
HBSC average (total)		21

15-year-olds who spend time with friends every day before 8 pm

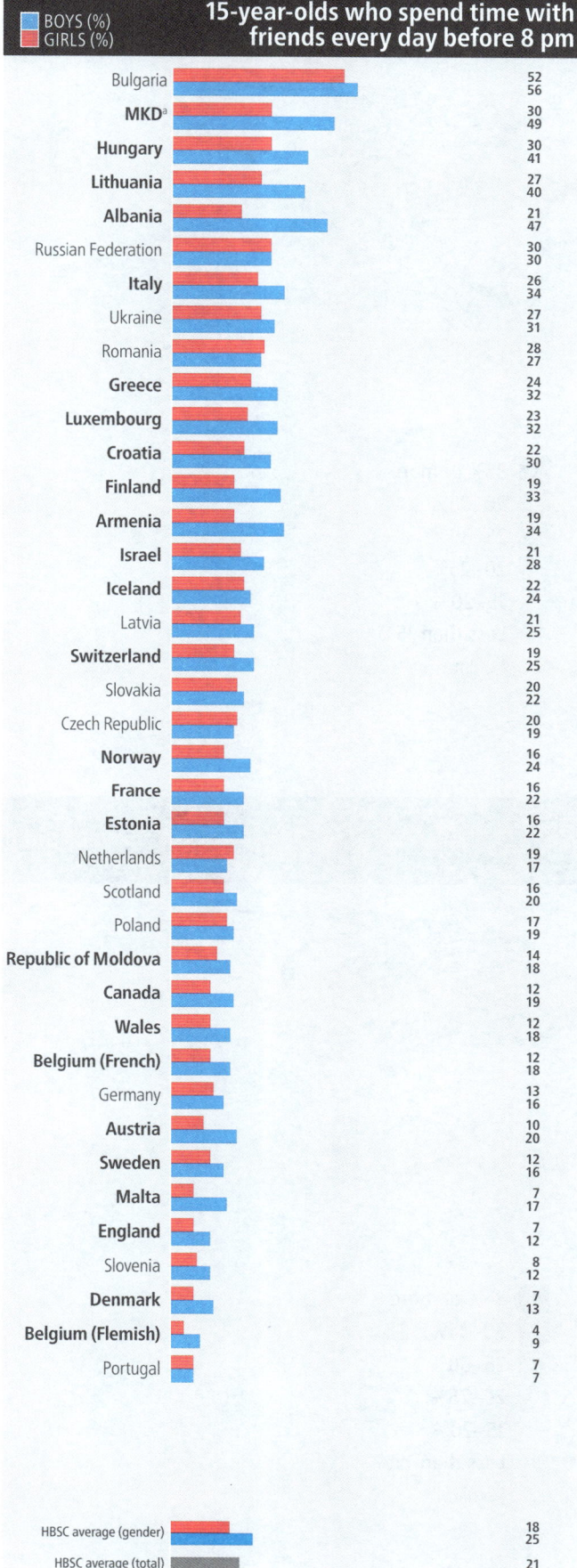

HBSC survey 2013/2014

- BOYS (%)
- GIRLS (%)

Country	Girls	Boys
Bulgaria	52	56
MKD[a]	30	49
Hungary	30	41
Lithuania	27	40
Albania	21	47
Russian Federation	30	30
Italy	26	34
Ukraine	27	31
Romania	28	27
Greece	24	32
Luxembourg	23	32
Croatia	22	30
Finland	19	33
Armenia	19	34
Israel	21	28
Iceland	22	24
Latvia	21	25
Switzerland	19	25
Slovakia	20	22
Czech Republic	20	19
Norway	16	24
France	16	22
Estonia	16	22
Netherlands	19	17
Scotland	16	20
Poland	17	19
Republic of Moldova	14	18
Canada	12	19
Wales	12	18
Belgium (French)	12	18
Germany	13	16
Austria	10	20
Sweden	12	16
Malta	7	12
England	7	12
Slovenia	8	12
Denmark	7	13
Belgium (Flemish)	4	9
Portugal	7	7
HBSC average (gender)	18	25
HBSC average (total)		21

Note: **indicates** significant gender difference (at p<0.05).
No data were received from Greenland, Ireland and Spain.

HBSC survey 2013/2014

15-year-old girls who spend time with friends every day before 8 pm

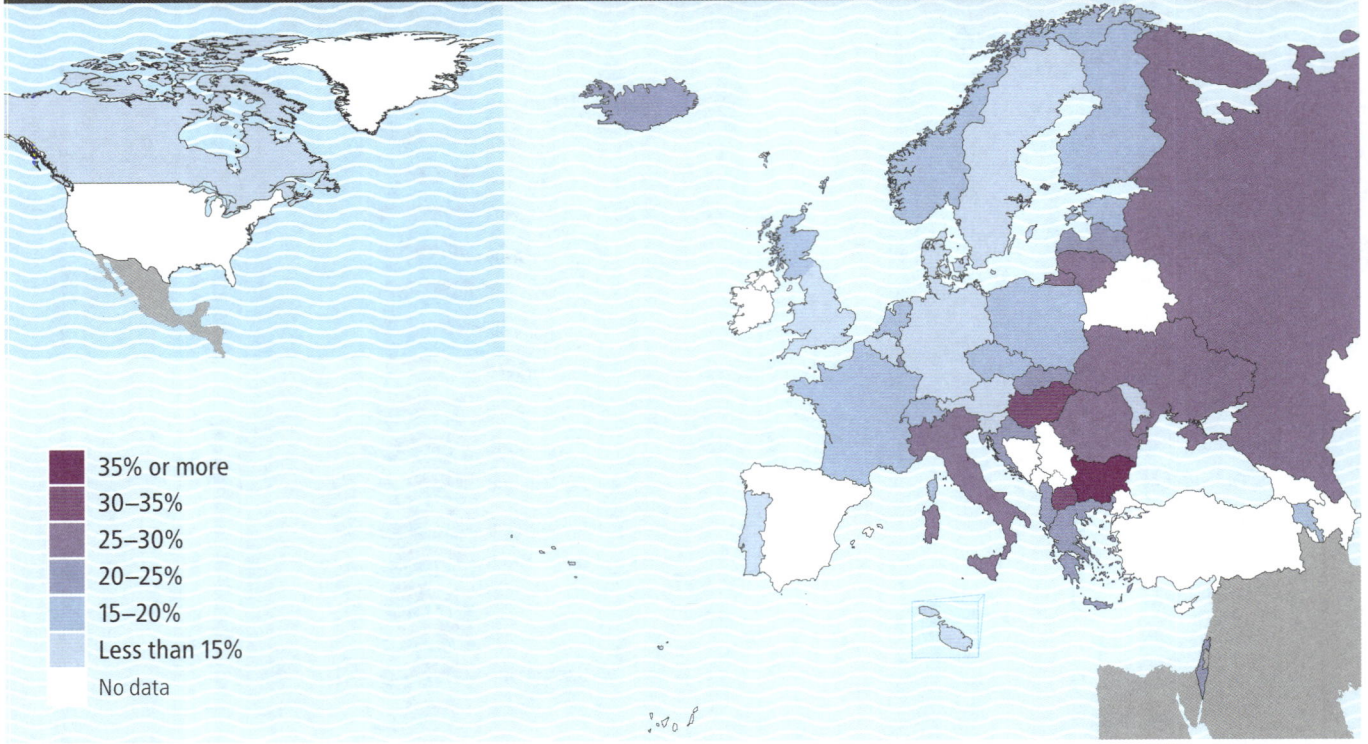

35% or more
30–35%
25–30%
20–25%
15–20%
Less than 15%
No data

Note: HBSC teams provided disaggregated data for Belgium and the United Kingdom; these data appear in the map above.

HBSC survey 2013/2014

15-year-old boys who spend time with friends every day before 8 pm

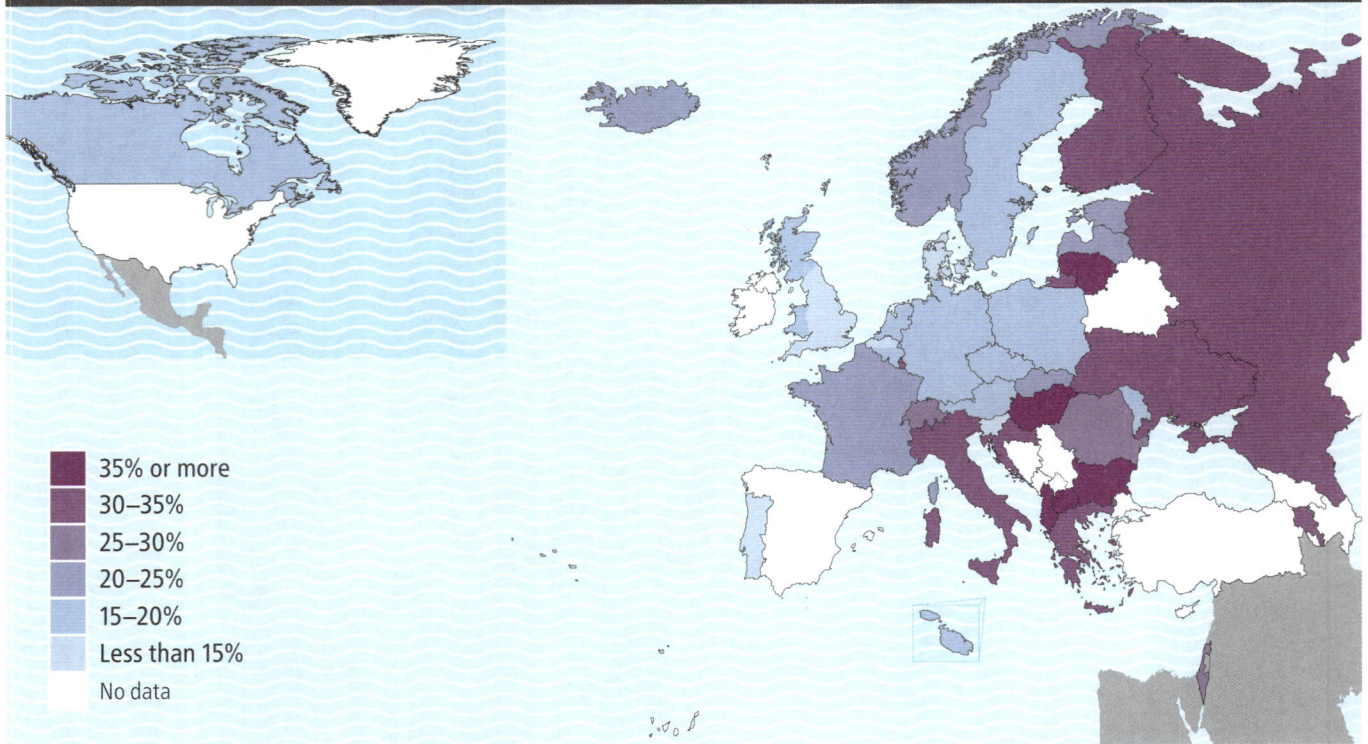

35% or more
30–35%
25–30%
20–25%
15–20%
Less than 15%
No data

Note: HBSC teams provided disaggregated data for Belgium and the United Kingdom; these data appear in the map above.

GROWING UP UNEQUAL: GENDER AND SOCIOECONOMIC
DIFFERENCES IN YOUNG PEOPLE'S HEALTH AND WELL-BEING
PART 2. KEY DATA | CHAPTER 2. SOCIAL CONTEXT

2

PEERS:
ELECTRONIC MEDIA COMMUNICATION – SOCIAL MEDIA

Electronic media communication (EMC) has become an integral part of adolescent life and is an important predictor of adolescent health and well-being.

Increases in EMC *(12)* mean that the contexts of adolescents' interactions with peers have expanded from the physical (offline) to the virtual (online) world *(13,14)*. EMC has become a central component of young people's lives and how they communicate with one another. It also plays an important role in learning, entertainment and socialization *(15)*.

A substantial body of research suggests the emergence of positive (social competence and well-being) and negative (substance use, sleeping habits, dietary behaviour) effects on teenagers' lives *(12,16–20)* over and above those associated with face-to-face interactions with friends *(9,19)*. Similar results have been found for screen-based media use, which is to some extent related to EMC *(21,22)*.

EMC is associated with general life satisfaction but shows a distinctive pattern in which adolescents who report very low or very high levels also report the lowest life-satisfaction scores. The frequency of EMC associated with the highest life-satisfaction score differs by country/region, gender and age group *(23)*.

HBSC survey 2013/2014

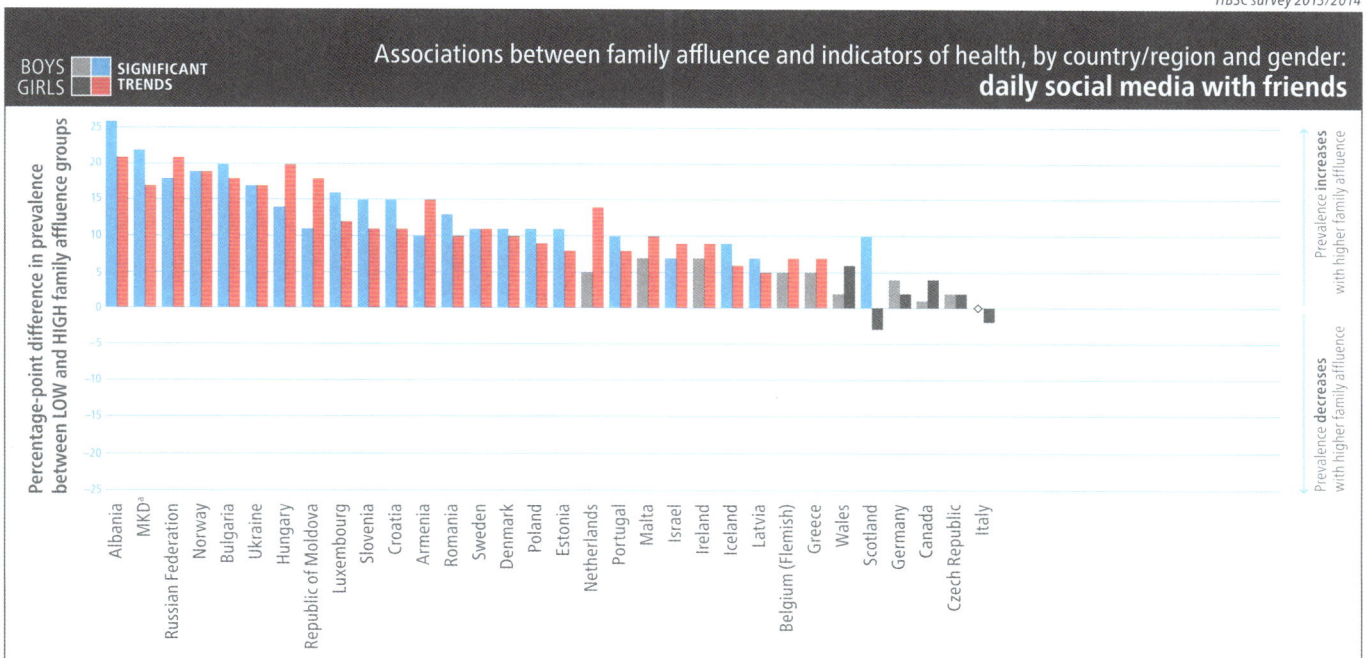

Associations between family affluence and indicators of health, by country/region and gender: **daily social media with friends**

BOYS / GIRLS — SIGNIFICANT TRENDS

ᵃ The former Yugoslav Republic of Macedonia. Note: low- and high-affluence groups represent the lowest 20% and highest 20% in each country. ◇ means less than +/-0.5%. No data were received from Austria, Belgium (French), England, Finland, France, Greenland, Lithuania, Slovakia, Spain and Switzerland.

MEASURE
Young people were asked how often they contact their friends using various social media outlets. Response options ranged from hardly ever or never to daily.

Supplementary data on daily contact via texting/SMS are provided in the Annex.

RESULTS

Findings presented here show the proportion who reported daily EMC contact via social media.

Age

A significant age effect was found in most countries and regions, with older adolescents using social media more frequently. A significant increase between age 11 and 15 was seen in 26 countries and regions for boys and 29 for girls. The largest age differences were in Luxembourg (boys) and Greece and Ukraine (girls), where prevalence increased by over 30 percentage points.

Gender

Significant differences between boys and girls were found in around half of countries and regions and across all age groups. There was no clear trend at age 11, with boys being more frequent users in some countries and regions and girls in others. In contrast, where a significant difference was found at ages 13 and 15, girls generally reported more frequent use.

Family affluence

In general, a positive association was observed between family affluence and daily social media contact. This was significant in 22 countries and regions for boys and 26 for girls.

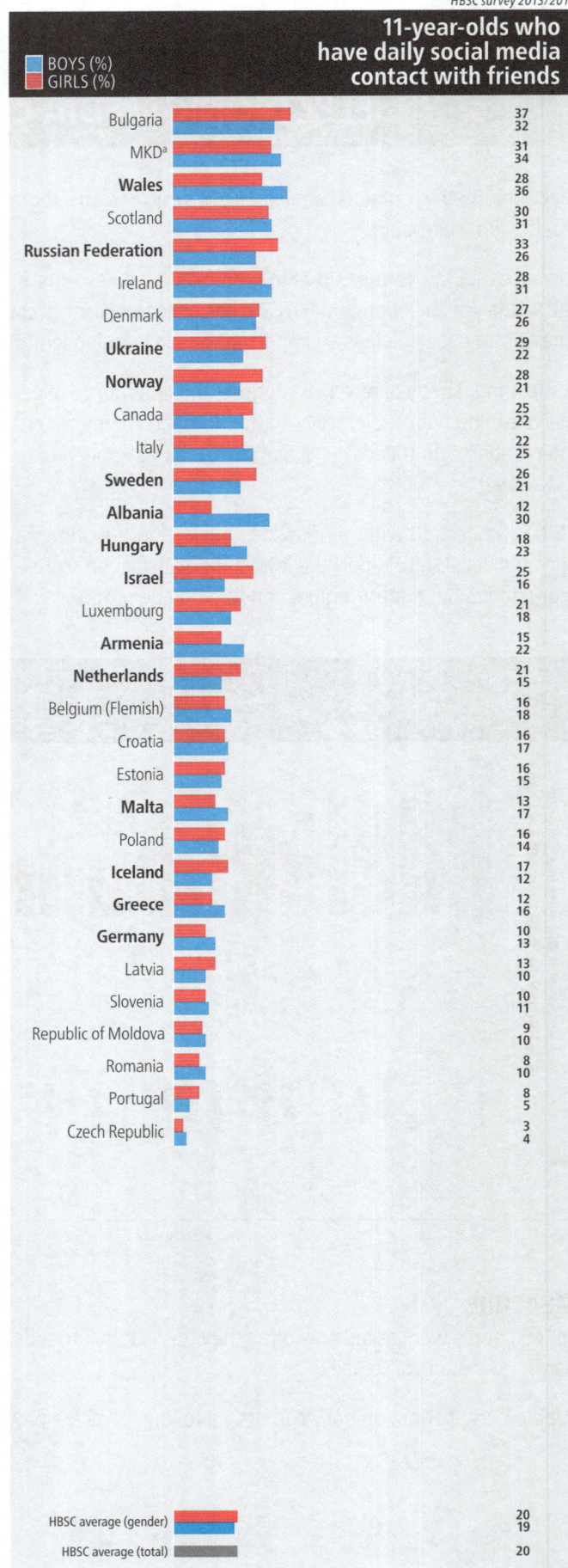

HBSC survey 2013/2014

11-year-olds who have daily social media contact with friends

BOYS (%)
GIRLS (%)

Country	Boys	Girls
Bulgaria	37	32
MKD[a]	31	34
Wales	28	36
Scotland	30	31
Russian Federation	33	26
Ireland	28	31
Denmark	27	26
Ukraine	29	22
Norway	28	21
Canada	25	22
Italy	22	25
Sweden	26	21
Albania	12	30
Hungary	18	23
Israel	25	16
Luxembourg	21	18
Armenia	15	22
Netherlands	21	15
Belgium (Flemish)	16	18
Croatia	16	17
Estonia	16	15
Malta	13	17
Poland	16	14
Iceland	17	12
Greece	12	16
Germany	10	13
Latvia	13	10
Slovenia	10	11
Republic of Moldova	9	10
Romania	8	10
Portugal	8	5
Czech Republic	3	4
HBSC average (gender)	20	19
HBSC average (total)	20	

[a] The former Yugoslav Republic of Macedonia.

GROWING UP UNEQUAL: GENDER AND SOCIOECONOMIC
DIFFERENCES IN YOUNG PEOPLE'S HEALTH AND WELL-BEING
PART 2. KEY DATA | CHAPTER 2. SOCIAL CONTEXT
PEERS: ELECTRONIC MEDIA COMMUNICATION – SOCIAL MEDIA

2

13-year-olds who have daily social media contact with friends

HBSC survey 2013/2014

- **■ BOYS (%)**
- **■ GIRLS (%)**

Country	Girls	Boys
MKD[a]	45	48
Bulgaria	48	40
Ukraine	52	35
Russian Federation	50	35
Ireland	44	40
Luxembourg	41	38
Wales	34	40
Norway	36	37
Greece	36	37
Italy	35	36
Scotland	34	36
Belgium (Flemish)	39	31
Croatia	33	34
Finland	34	31
Canada	36	28
Netherlands	36	28
Albania	24	39
Sweden	36	27
Belgium (French)	31	30
Hungary	29	31
Poland	32	25
Estonia	32	25
Denmark	29	28
Malta	27	27
Armenia	24	25
Latvia	31	17
Germany	22	24
Iceland	24	22
Slovenia	25	18
Israel	25	17
Republic of Moldova	15	11
Portugal	15	11
Romania	14	10
Czech Republic	4	4

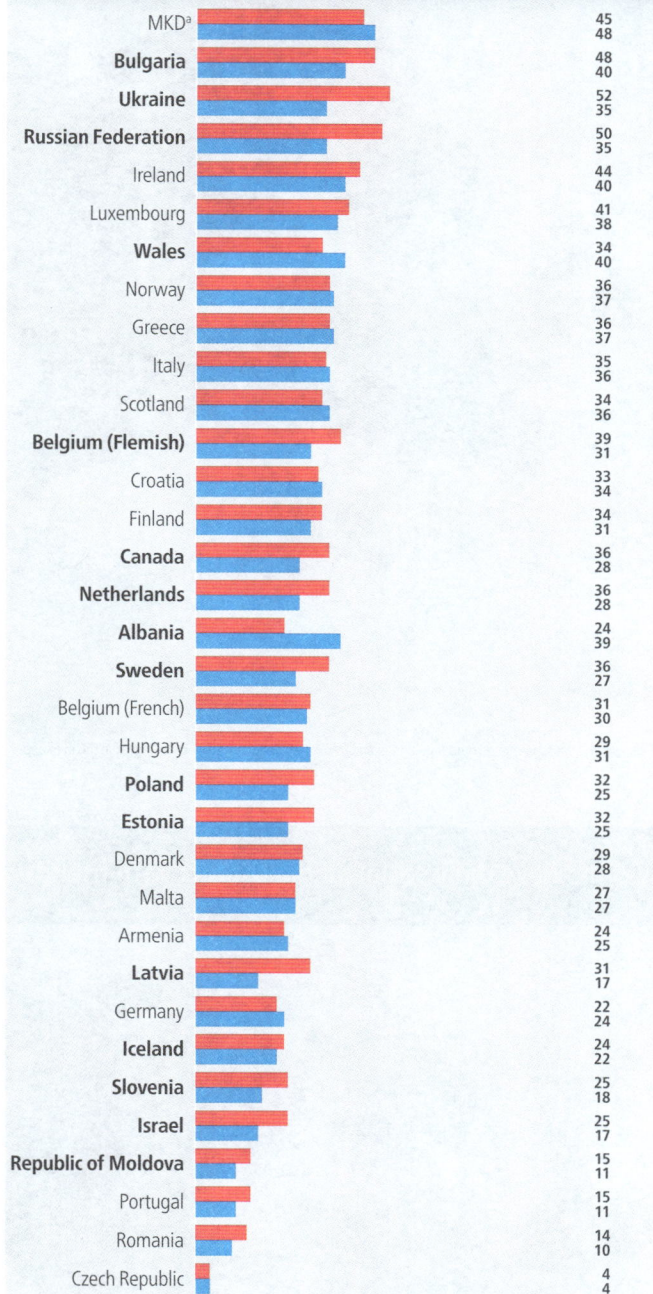

	Girls	Boys
HBSC average (gender)	32	28
HBSC average (total)		30

15-year-olds who have daily social media contact with friends

HBSC survey 2013/2014

- **■ BOYS (%)**
- **■ GIRLS (%)**

Country	Girls	Boys
Austria	63	53
Ukraine	61	48
Russian Federation	57	45
Luxembourg	48	55
MKD[a]	49	52
Ireland	48	38
Bulgaria	47	39
Wales	41	42
Hungary	41	41
Greece	43	39
Belgium (Flemish)	39	38
Norway	37	38
Croatia	40	35
Scotland	39	35
Albania	29	45
Canada	40	32
Malta	34	37
England	35	36
Belgium (French)	37	32
Netherlands	36	32
Estonia	36	30
Finland	34	31
Denmark	31	34
Poland	37	27
Italy	32	32
Latvia	36	23
Sweden	32	27
France	30	26
Armenia	25	28
Slovenia	28	23
Iceland	27	25
Switzerland	24	25
Israel	24	21
Germany	20	25
Portugal	21	15
Republic of Moldova	19	16
Romania	19	14
Czech Republic	4	3

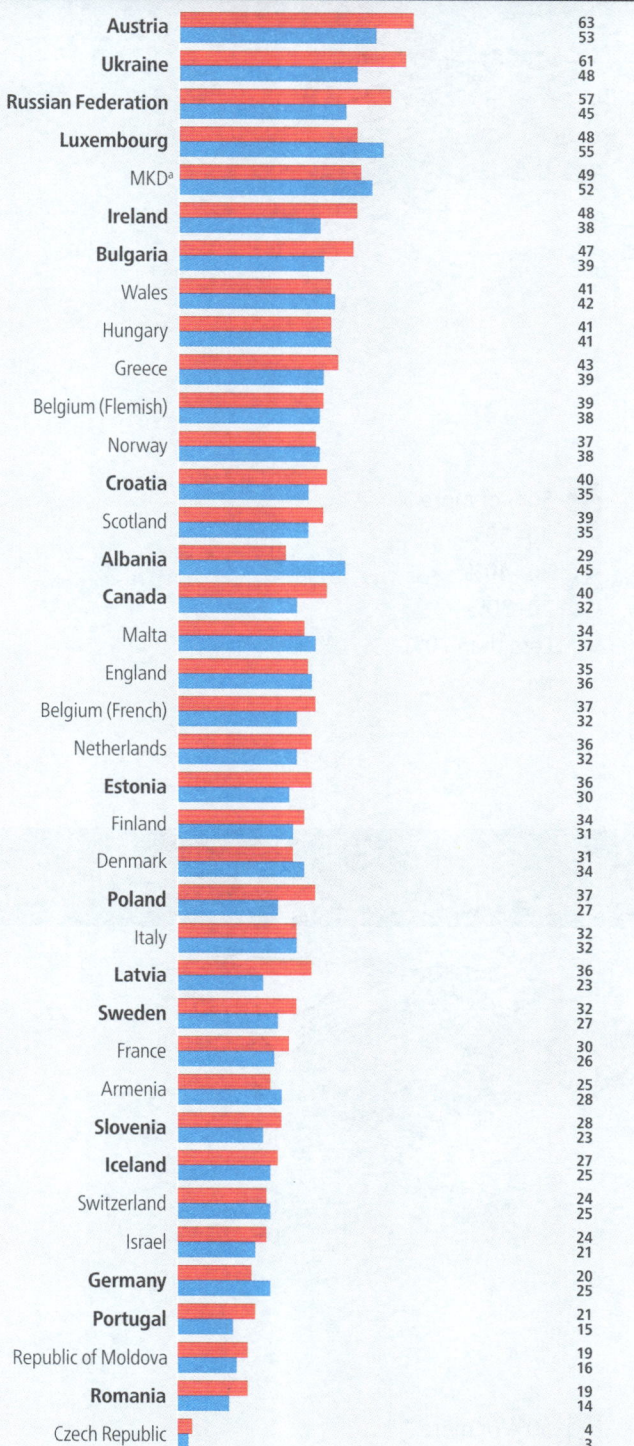

	Girls	Boys
HBSC average (gender)	35	32
HBSC average (total)		33

Note: **indicates** significant gender difference (at p<0.05). No data were received from: Greenland, Lithuania, Slovakia and Spain (all ages); Belgium (French), Finland and France (11-year-olds); and Austria, England and Switzerland (11- and 13-year-olds).

HBSC survey 2013/2014

15-year-old girls who have daily social media contact with friends

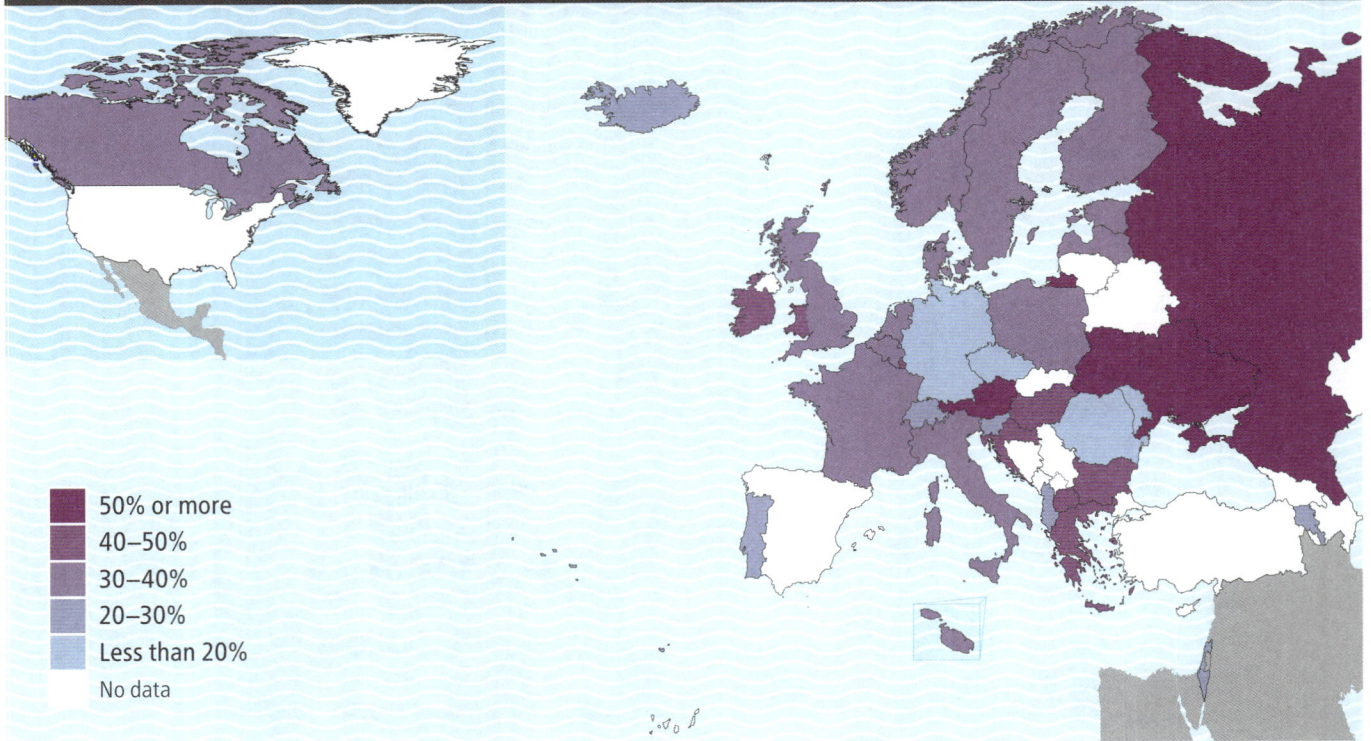

- 50% or more
- 40–50%
- 30–40%
- 20–30%
- Less than 20%
- No data

Note: HBSC teams provided disaggregated data for Belgium and the United Kingdom; these data appear in the map above.

HBSC survey 2013/2014

15-year-old boys who have daily social media contact with friends

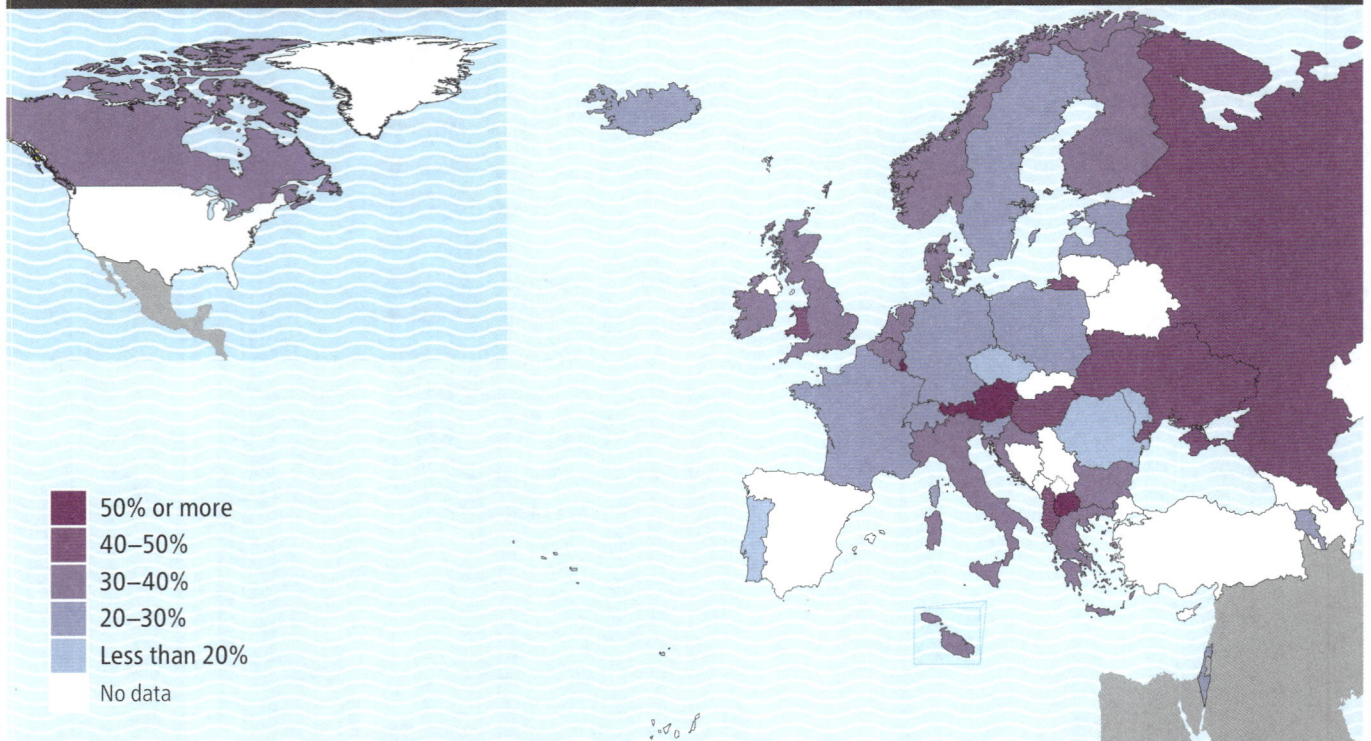

- 50% or more
- 40–50%
- 30–40%
- 20–30%
- Less than 20%
- No data

Note: HBSC teams provided disaggregated data for Belgium and the United Kingdom; these data appear in the map above.

GROWING UP UNEQUAL: GENDER AND SOCIOECONOMIC
DIFFERENCES IN YOUNG PEOPLE'S HEALTH AND WELL-BEING
PART 2. KEY DATA | CHAPTER 2. SOCIAL CONTEXT
PEERS

2

PEERS:
SCIENTIFIC DISCUSSION AND POLICY REFLECTIONS

SCIENTIFIC DISCUSSION

Findings are in line with the literature on perceived social support in adolescence: girls and adolescents from high-affluence families tend to report higher levels of social support *(24)*. Gender differences in social support are generally interpreted as deriving from gender role socialization. The feminine role is widely considered to be warm, supportive, nurturing, sensitive to the feelings of others and emotionally expressive *(24)*, although it is constantly changing and varies across cultures. In relation to SES, economic hardship can hinder the creation of supportive ties by reducing access to social events and time to nurture social relationships.

Results on time with friends are also in line with the literature, showing that boys tend to spend more time in this pursuit. Girls' parents might set more restrictions on their independence during adolescence and exert a higher level of parental monitoring.

Although observed in only around a quarter of countries and regions, findings show a positive association between age and time spent with friends. Adolescents become more independent as they grow older and begin to spend less time with parents and more with peers *(8)*. The association between family affluence and time spent with friends was observed in only a minority, underlining that economic factors might not be the primary driver.

Findings on EMC are in line with the literature *(15,25)*. Older and high-affluence adolescents use EMC more frequently. Older adolescents have higher levels of autonomy, greater opportunities (with more frequent access to EMC devices) and increased levels of unsupervised time, so are able to explore a broader social context more freely. Those with high affluence tend to have more opportunities to use EMC through, for example, access to a smartphone *(25)*.

Girls are more frequent users of social media among older age groups. Again, this is in line with the literature *(25)* and can be associated with a commonly described gender difference *(26,27)*. Girls tend to be more verbal and network- and connection-oriented; their friendships are associated with stronger interpersonal engagement, extended dyadic (one-to-one) interactions, greater disclosure and more effective and emotional exchanges. Boys tend to focus more on agentic (self-directed actions aimed at personally chosen goals) and status-oriented goals; their friendships are characterized by being together in larger groups doing something of similar interest, such as organized play.

POLICY REFLECTIONS

Reflecting the importance of peer support to adolescents' well-being, programmes that foster the creation of supportive ties should be promoted. Boys and young people from low-affluence families, who tend to experience lower levels of support from friends, require particular attention. Collaborative teaching methods, for example, should be adopted in schools and opportunities for interactions in local communities that might promote supportive ties with friends encouraged. Ecological programmes that include local neighbourhoods among the contexts of interventions (such as local events and common spaces) can increase opportunities for young people to get to know and interact with peers and develop more supportive networks.

Policies should aim to promote the establishment and maintenance of supportive friendships among adolescents by, for instance, providing them with adequate opportunities to interact with peers in safe, (semi-)supervised and structured settings. Parents and educators should be informed about the false and misleading notion that time spent solely with peers may lead to risk-taking and offending: it very much depends on the conditions under which these interactions take place *(28)*.

Young people commonly communicate through electronic means, so teaching them about healthy and responsible interactions with peers online is important in preventing problems such as addiction and cyberbullying *(15)*. It is useful to include in adolescent prevention programmes the negative consequences of online activities (such as the unlimited retention of information posted online) and the potential inaccuracy and one-sidedness of peers' online activities (perhaps presenting a rose-tinted picture of their lives). Such programmes will help adolescents and parents to become informed users of the internet.

REFERENCES

1. Kerr M, Stattin H, Biesecker G, Ferrer-Wreder L. Relationships with parents and peers in adolescence. In Lerner R, Easterbrooks MA, Mistry J, editors. Developmental psychology. Vol. 6. New York (NY): John Wiley & Sons Inc.; 2003:395–419.

2. Colaros LG, Eccles JS. Differential effects of support providers on adolescents' mental health. Soc Work Res. 2003;27:19–30.

3. Lenzi M, Vieno A, Perkins DD, Santinello M, Pastor M, Mazzardis S. Perceived neighborhood social resources as determinants of prosocial behavior in early adolescence. Am J Community Psychol. 2012;50(1–2):37–49.

4. Cohen S, Wills TA. Stress, social support, and the buffering hypothesis. Psychol Bull. 1985;98:310–57.

5. Wilkinson RB. The role of parental and peer attachment in the psychological health and self-esteem of adolescents. J Youth Adolesc. 2004;33:479–93.

6. Bronfenbrenner U. The ecology of human development: experiments by nature and design. Cambridge (MA): Harvard University Press; 1979.

7. Zimet GD, Dahlem NW, Zimet SG, Farley GK. The Multidimensional Scale of Perceived Social Support. J Pers Assess. 1988;52:30–41.

8. Nickerson A, Nagle RJ. Parent and peer attachment in late childhood and early adolescence. J Early Adolesc. 2005;25:223–49.

9. Gommans R, Stevens GWJM, Finne E, Cillessen AHN, Boniel-Nissim M, ter Bogt TFM. Frequent electronic media communication with friends is associated with higher substance use. Int J Public Health 2015;60:167–77.

10. Buhrmester D. Intimacy of friendship, interpersonal competence, and adjustment during preadolescence and adolescence. Child Dev. 1990;61(4):1101–11.

11. Jaccard J, Blanton H, Dodge T. Peer influences on risk behavior: an analysis of the effects of a close friend. Dev Psychol. 2005;41(1):135–47.

12. Valkenburg PM, Peter J. Online communication among adolescents: an integrated model of its attraction, opportunities, and risks. J Adolesc Health 2010;48:121–7.

13. Brechwald WA, Prinstein MJ. Beyond homophily: a decade of advances in understanding peer influence processes. J Res Adolesc. 2011;21:166–79.

14. Brown BB, Larson J. Peer relationships in adolescence. In: Lerner R, Steinberg L, editors. Handbook of adolescent psychology, third edition. Hoboken (NJ): John Wiley & Sons Inc.; 2009:74–103.

15. Matos MG, Ferreira M. Nascidos digitais: novas linguagens, lazer e dependências [Born digital: new languages, leisure and addiction]. Lisbon: Coisas de Ler; 2013.

16. Li S, Jin X, Wu S, Jiang F, Yan C, Shen X. The impact of media use on sleep patterns and sleep disorders among school-aged children in China. Sleep 2007;30:361–7.

17. Jackson LA, von Eye A, Fitzgerald HE, Witt EA, Zhao Y. Internet use, videogame playing and cell phone use as predictors of children's body mass index (BMI), body weight, academic performance, and social and overall self-esteem. Computers in Human Behavior 2011;27:599–604.

18. Leena K, Tomi L, Arja R. Intensity of mobile phone use and health compromising behaviours. How is information and communication technology connected to health-related lifestyle in adolescence? J Adolesc. 2005;28:35–47.

19. Huang GC, Unger JB, Soto D, Fujimoto K, Pentz MA, Jordan-Marsh M et al. Peer influences: the impact of online and offline friendship networks on adolescent smoking and alcohol use. J Adolesc Health 2014;54:508–14.

20. Stoddard SA, Bauermeister JA, Gordon-Messer D, Johns M, Zimmerman MA. Permissive norms and young adults' alcohol and marijuana use: the role of online communities. J Stud Alcohol Drugs 2012;73:968–75.

21. Iannotti RJ, Janssen I, Haug E, Kololo H, Annaheim B, Borraccino A et al. Interrelationships of adolescent physical activity, screen-based sedentary behaviour, and social and psychological health. Int J Public Health 2009;54:191–8.

22. Iannotti RJ, Kogan MD, Janssen I, Boyce WF. Patterns of adolescent physical activity, screen-based media use, and positive and negative health indicators in the US and Canada. J Adolesc Health 2009;44:493–9.

23. Boniel-Nissim M, Tabak I, Mazur J, Borraccino A, Brooks F, Gommans R et al. Supportive communication with parents moderates the negative effects of electronic media use on life satisfaction during adolescence. Int J Public Health 2015;60:189–98.

24. Reevy GM, Maslach C. Use of social support: gender and personality differences. Sex Roles 2001;44:437–59.

25. Lenhart A. Teens, smartphones, and texting. Washington (DC): Pew Research Center's Internet & American Life Project; 2012 (http://pewinternet.org/Reports/2012/Teens-and-smartphones.aspx, accessed 18 August 2015).

26. Rose AJ, Rudolph KD. A review of sex differences in peer relationship processes: potential trade-offs for the emotional and behavioral development of girls and boys. Psychol Bull. 2006;132:98–131.

27. Rose AJ, Smith RL. Sex differences in peer relationships. In: Rubin KH, Bukowski WM, Laursen B, editors. Handbook of peer interactions, relationships, and groups. New York (NY): Guilford Press; 2009:379–93.

28. Hoeben E, Weerman F. Situational conditions and adolescent offending: does the impact of unstructured socializing depend on its location? Eur J Criminol. 2014;11:481–99.

GROWING UP UNEQUAL: GENDER AND SOCIOECONOMIC
DIFFERENCES IN YOUNG PEOPLE'S HEALTH AND WELL-BEING
PART 2. KEY DATA | CHAPTER 2. SOCIAL CONTEXT

2

SCHOOL:
LIKING SCHOOL

Children and adolescents spend a substantial amount of time in the school setting. School therefore constitutes a significant influence on children's cognitive, social and emotional development *(1,2)*.

A positive school experience is considered a resource for health and well-being, while a negative one may constitute a risk factor, affecting mental and physical health. Liking school consequently has been identified as a protective factor against health-compromising behaviours, and not liking – or not feeling connected to – school is associated with health-risk behaviours, low self-rated health and increased somatic and psychological symptoms *(3)*.

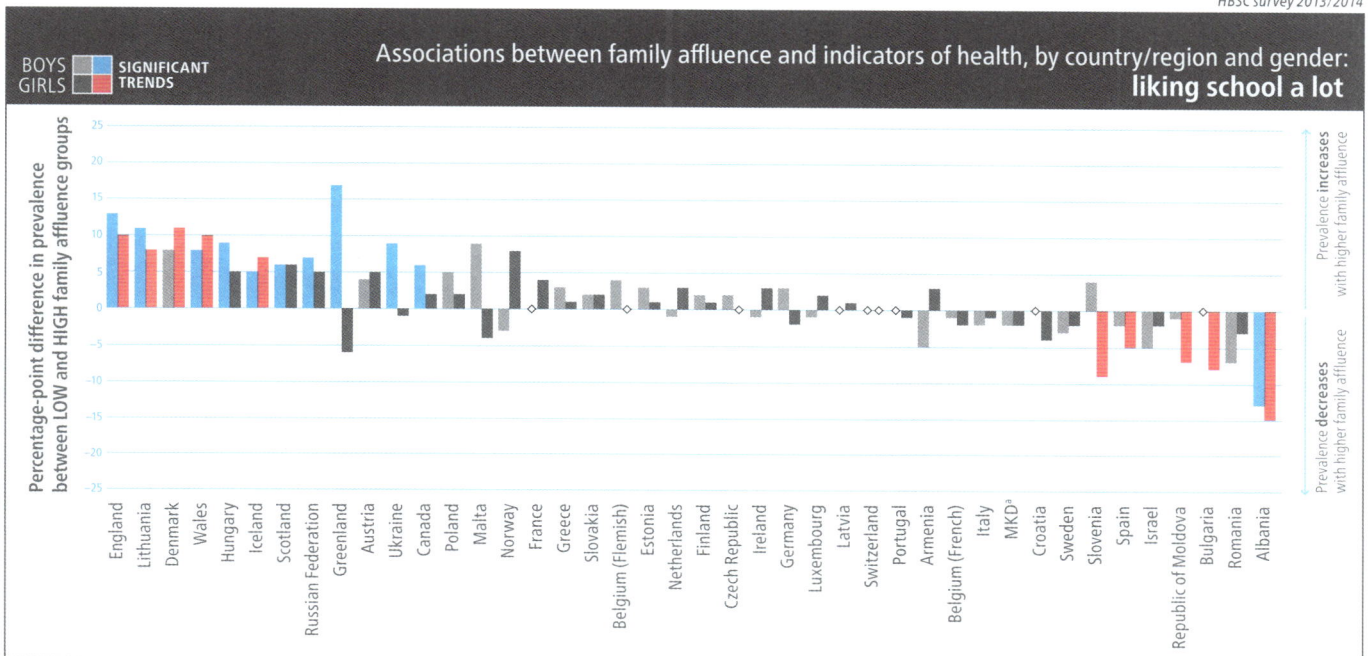

HBSC survey 2013/2014

Associations between family affluence and indicators of health, by country/region and gender: **liking school a lot**

ª The former Yugoslav Republic of Macedonia. *Note*: low- and high-affluence groups represent the lowest 20% and highest 20% in each country. ◇ means less than +/-0.5%.

MEASURE
Young people were asked how they feel about school at present. Response options ranged from liking it a lot to not liking it at all.

RESULTS

Findings presented here show the proportions who reported liking school a lot.

Age

The highest proportion was found among 11-year-olds, with a decrease by increasing age.

Boys in 36 countries and regions showed a significant decrease with age. A difference of 10 or more percentage points between ages 11 and 15 was seen in 29, with the difference being greater than 20 in 13.

For girls, 39 countries and regions showed a significant decrease with age. The difference between 11 and 15 years was 10 or more percentage points in 36 and greater than 20 in 22. Liking school increased with age in two countries (Hungary and Slovenia).

Gender

Overall, girls were more likely to report liking school a lot at all three ages, but especially at age 11. The difference between boys and girls was less than 10 percentage points in most cases and decreased with age. Two countries (England and Sweden) had higher prevalence among boys at age 15.

Family affluence

No general pattern was seen for boys or girls. Only a few countries and regions showed significant associations with family affluence.

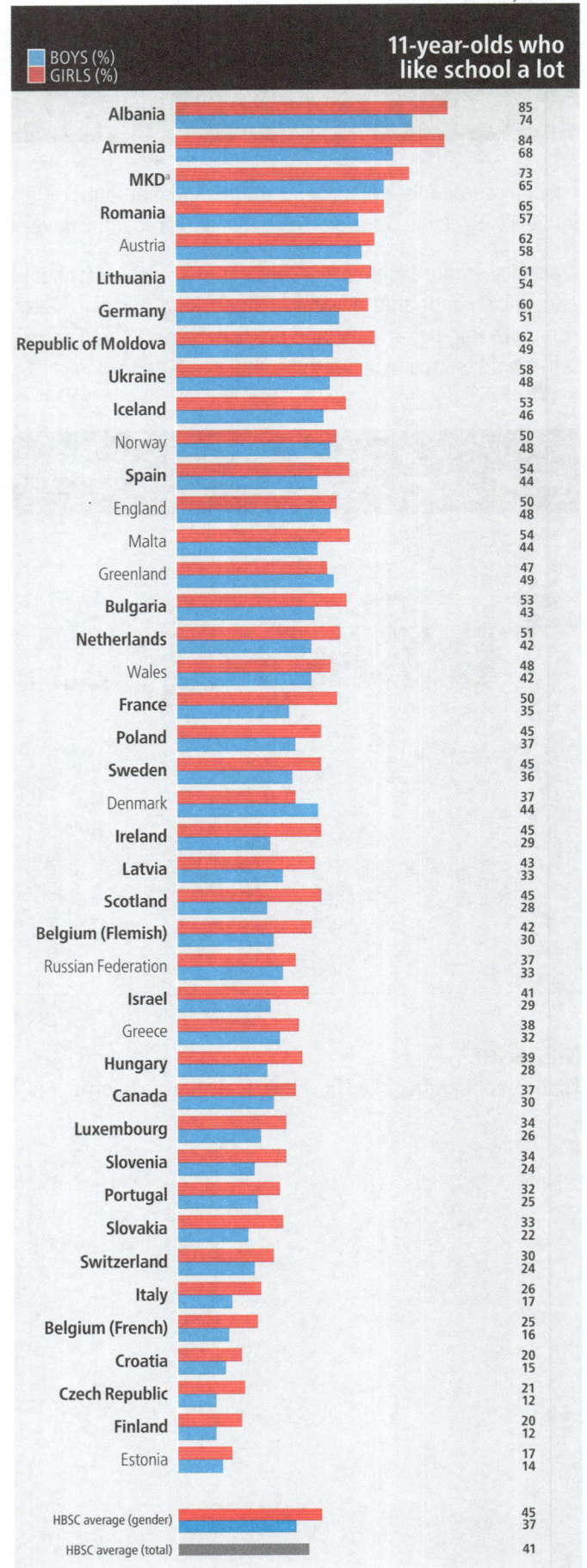

HBSC survey 2013/2014

11-year-olds who like school a lot

BOYS (%)
GIRLS (%)

Country	Boys (%)	Girls (%)
Albania	74	85
Armenia	68	84
MKD[a]	65	73
Romania	57	65
Austria	58	62
Lithuania	54	61
Germany	51	60
Republic of Moldova	49	62
Ukraine	48	58
Iceland	46	53
Norway	48	50
Spain	44	54
England	48	50
Malta	44	54
Greenland	49	47
Bulgaria	43	53
Netherlands	42	51
Wales	42	48
France	35	50
Poland	37	45
Sweden	36	45
Denmark	44	37
Ireland	29	45
Latvia	33	43
Scotland	28	45
Belgium (Flemish)	30	42
Russian Federation	33	37
Israel	29	41
Greece	32	38
Hungary	28	39
Canada	30	37
Luxembourg	26	34
Slovenia	24	34
Portugal	25	32
Slovakia	22	33
Switzerland	24	30
Italy	17	26
Belgium (French)	16	25
Croatia	15	20
Czech Republic	12	21
Finland	12	20
Estonia	14	17
HBSC average (gender)	37	45
HBSC average (total)		41

[a] The former Yugoslav Republic of Macedonia.

GROWING UP UNEQUAL: GENDER AND SOCIOECONOMIC
DIFFERENCES IN YOUNG PEOPLE'S HEALTH AND WELL-BEING
PART 2. KEY DATA | CHAPTER 2, SOCIAL CONTEXT
SCHOOL: LIKING SCHOOL

2

HBSC survey 2013/2014

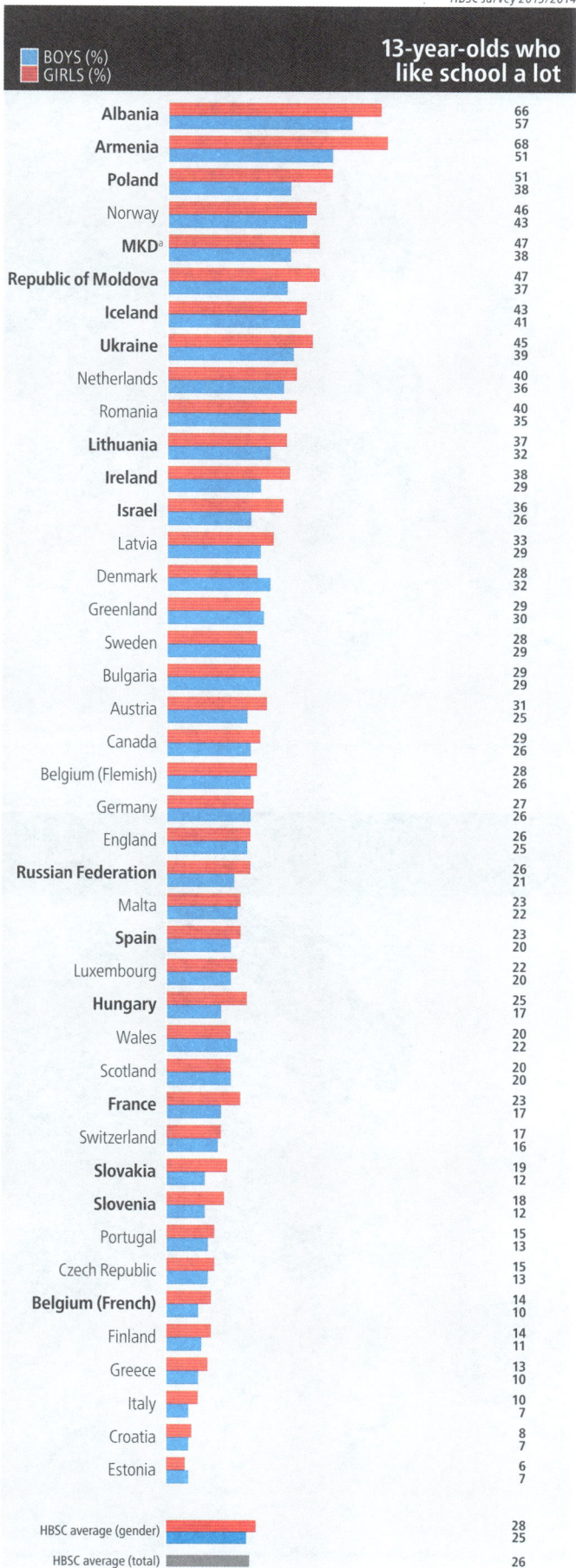

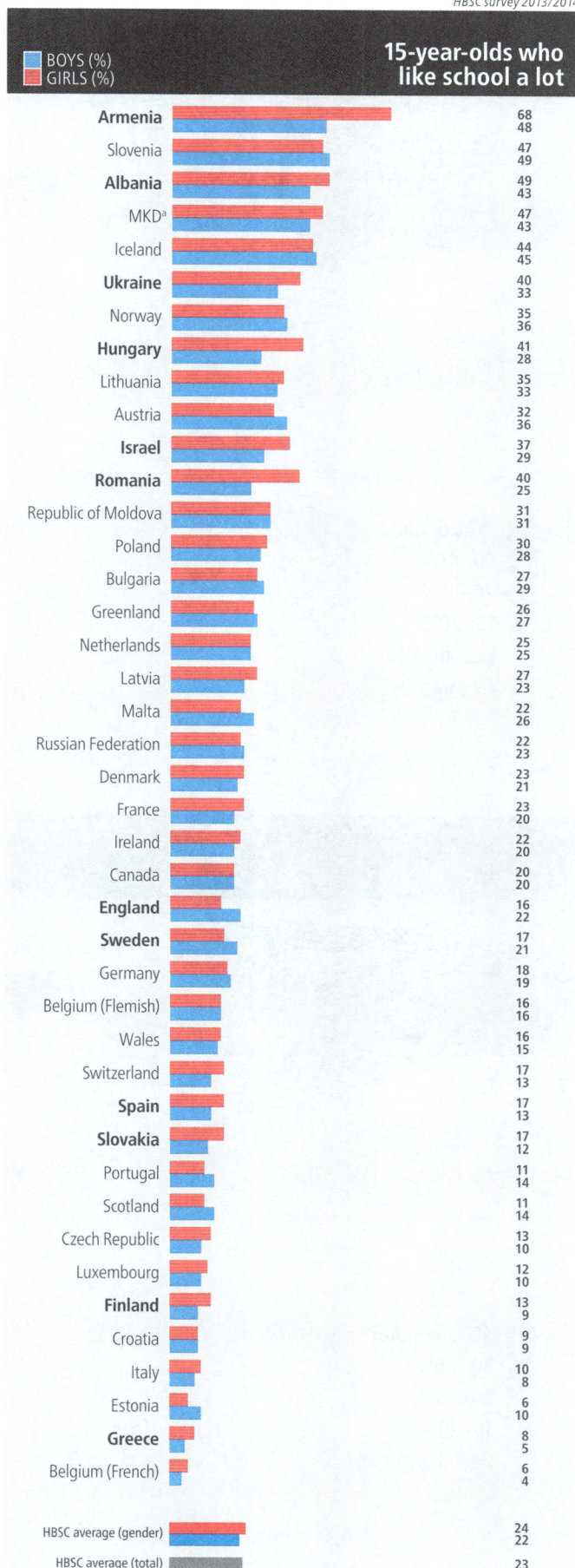

13-year-olds who like school a lot

- BOYS (%)
- GIRLS (%)

Country	Girls (%)	Boys (%)
Albania	66	57
Armenia	68	51
Poland	51	38
Norway	46	43
MKD[a]	47	38
Republic of Moldova	47	37
Iceland	43	41
Ukraine	45	39
Netherlands	40	36
Romania	40	35
Lithuania	37	32
Ireland	38	29
Israel	36	26
Latvia	33	29
Denmark	28	32
Greenland	29	30
Sweden	28	29
Bulgaria	29	29
Austria	31	25
Canada	29	26
Belgium (Flemish)	28	26
Germany	27	26
England	26	25
Russian Federation	26	21
Malta	23	22
Spain	23	20
Luxembourg	22	20
Hungary	25	17
Wales	20	22
Scotland	20	20
France	23	17
Switzerland	17	16
Slovakia	19	12
Slovenia	18	12
Portugal	15	13
Czech Republic	15	13
Belgium (French)	14	10
Finland	14	11
Greece	13	10
Italy	10	7
Croatia	8	7
Estonia	6	7
HBSC average (gender)	28	25
HBSC average (total)	26	

HBSC survey 2013/2014

15-year-olds who like school a lot

- BOYS (%)
- GIRLS (%)

Country	Girls (%)	Boys (%)
Armenia	68	48
Slovenia	47	49
Albania	49	43
MKD[a]	47	43
Iceland	44	45
Ukraine	40	33
Norway	35	36
Hungary	41	28
Lithuania	35	33
Austria	32	36
Israel	37	29
Romania	40	25
Republic of Moldova	31	31
Poland	30	28
Bulgaria	27	29
Greenland	26	27
Netherlands	25	25
Latvia	27	23
Malta	22	26
Russian Federation	22	23
Denmark	23	21
France	23	20
Ireland	22	20
Canada	20	20
England	16	22
Sweden	17	21
Germany	18	19
Belgium (Flemish)	16	16
Wales	16	15
Switzerland	17	13
Spain	17	13
Slovakia	17	12
Portugal	11	14
Scotland	11	14
Czech Republic	13	10
Luxembourg	12	10
Finland	13	9
Croatia	9	9
Italy	10	8
Estonia	6	10
Greece	8	5
Belgium (French)	6	4
HBSC average (gender)	24	22
HBSC average (total)	23	

Note: **indicates** significant gender difference (at p<0.05).

HBSC survey 2013/2014

15-year-old girls who like school a lot

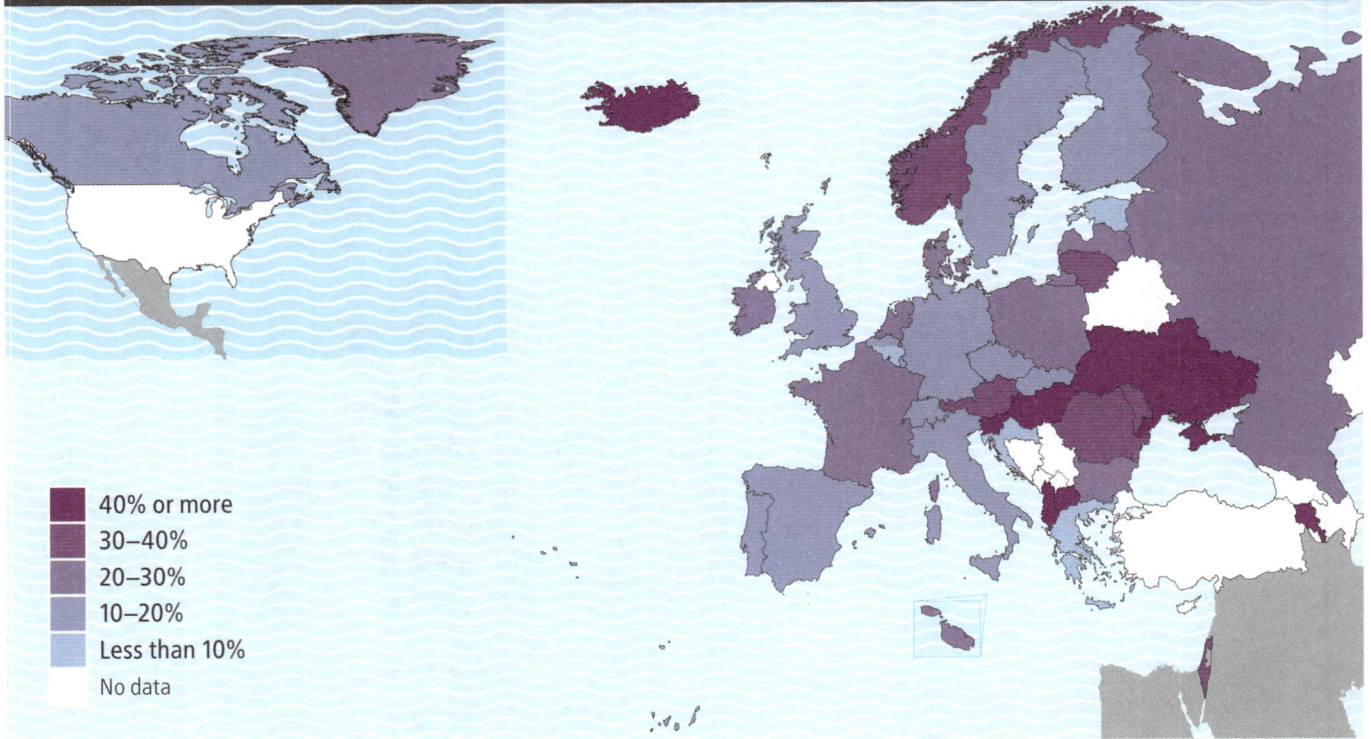

40% or more
30–40%
20–30%
10–20%
Less than 10%
No data

Note: HBSC teams provided disaggregated data for Belgium and the United Kingdom; these data appear in the map above.

HBSC survey 2013/2014

15-year-old boys who like school a lot

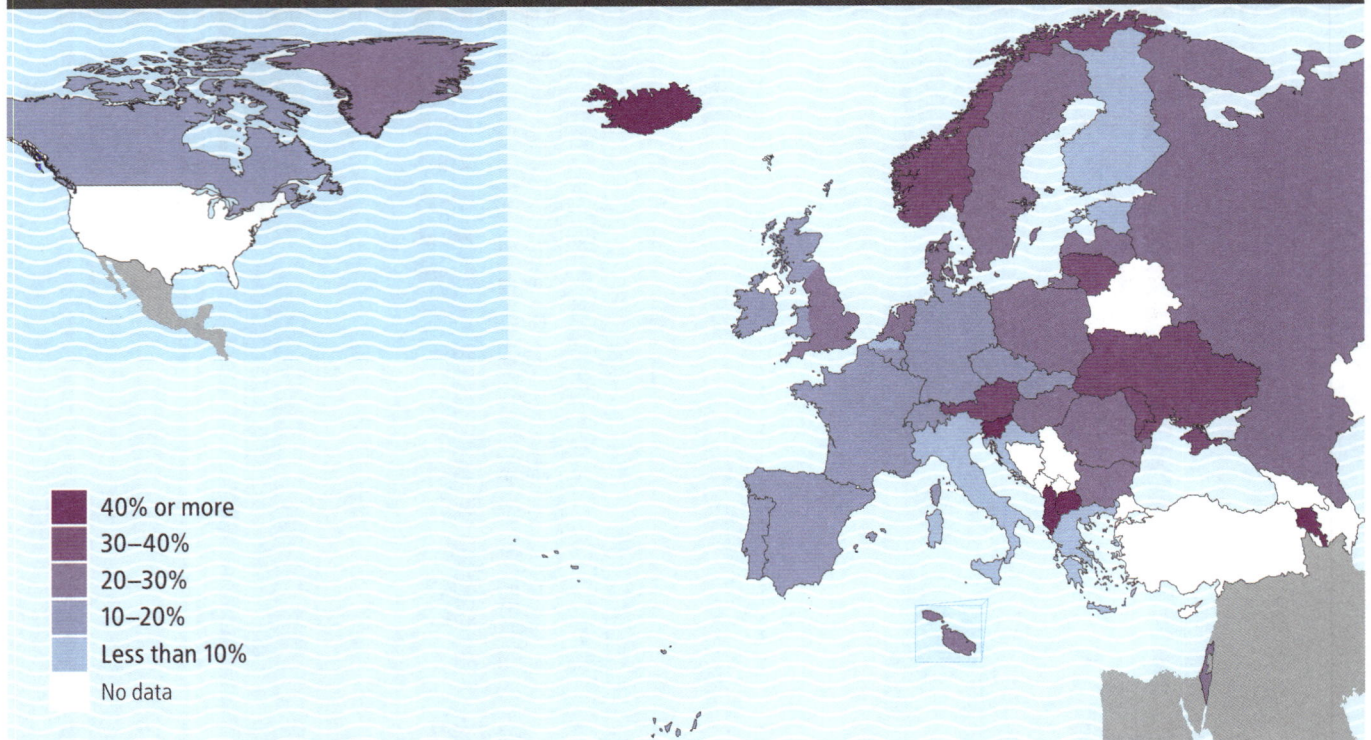

40% or more
30–40%
20–30%
10–20%
Less than 10%
No data

Note: HBSC teams provided disaggregated data for Belgium and the United Kingdom; these data appear in the map above.

GROWING UP UNEQUAL: GENDER AND SOCIOECONOMIC
DIFFERENCES IN YOUNG PEOPLE'S HEALTH AND WELL-BEING
PART 2. KEY DATA | CHAPTER 2. SOCIAL CONTEXT

2

SCHOOL:
PERCEIVED SCHOOL PERFORMANCE

Studies focusing on young people's academic achievement and health show significant links between low academic performance at school and low self-rated health and well-being (4,5). Some longitudinal studies have also found that academic achievement functions as a predictor of future health (6).

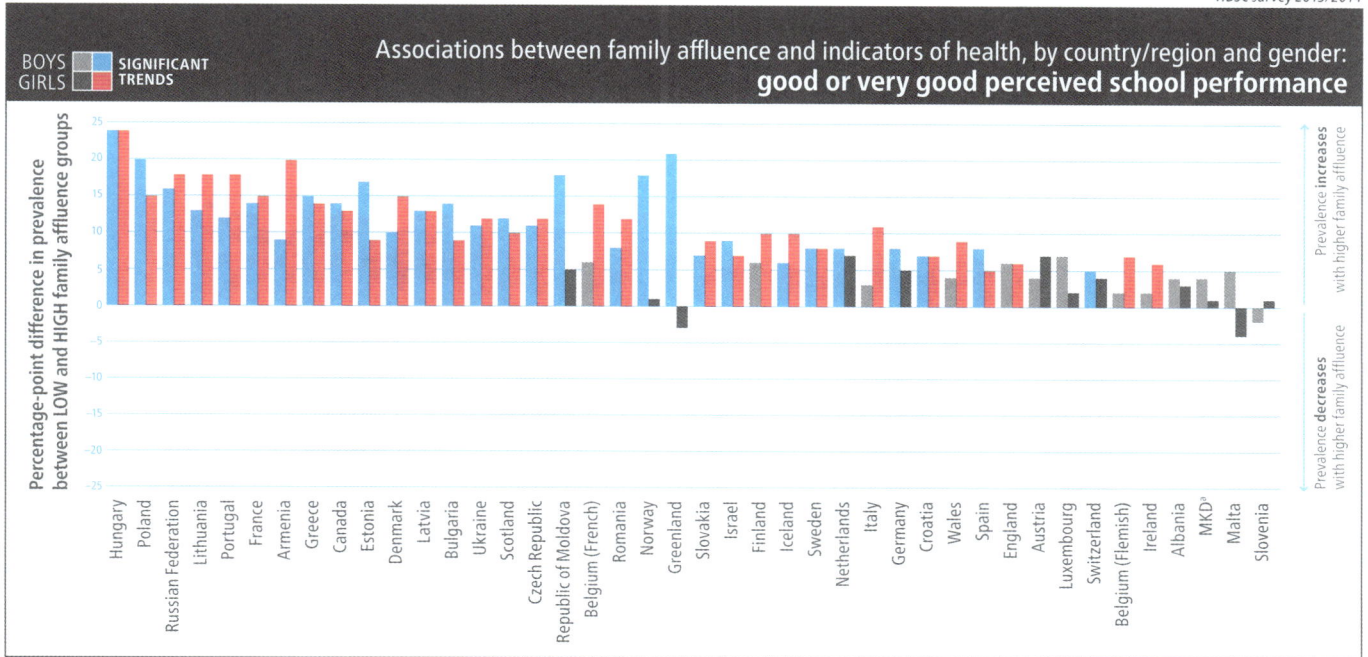

HBSC survey 2013/2014

Associations between family affluence and indicators of health, by country/region and gender:
good or very good perceived school performance

BOYS
GIRLS
**SIGNIFICANT
TRENDS**

ª The former Yugoslav Republic of Macedonia. *Note:* low- and high-affluence groups represent the lowest 20% and highest 20% in each country.

MEASURE

Young people were asked what, in their opinion, their class teacher(s) thinks about their school performance compared to their classmates. Response options ranged from below average to very good.

RESULTS

Findings presented here show the proportions who reported good or very good perceived school performance.

Age

Generally, the proportion decreased with increasing age, with a significant decrease in 40 countries and regions for boys and 39 for girls. The difference between 11- and 15-year-olds was 20 or more percentage points in around half.

Gender

Girls were more likely to report good or very good perceived school performance at all three ages. Most of the differences between boys and girls were less than 10 percentage points. A significant difference was seen among 11-year-olds in 26 countries and regions, 13-year-olds in 23 and 15-year-olds in 14. The opposite trend (in which prevalence was higher among boys) was observed in three countries: Belgium (French) and Greenland (13-year-olds only), and Portugal (13- and 15-year-olds).

Family affluence

Prevalence was generally highest in those from high-affluence backgrounds, a finding observed in 29 countries and regions for boys and 30 for girls.

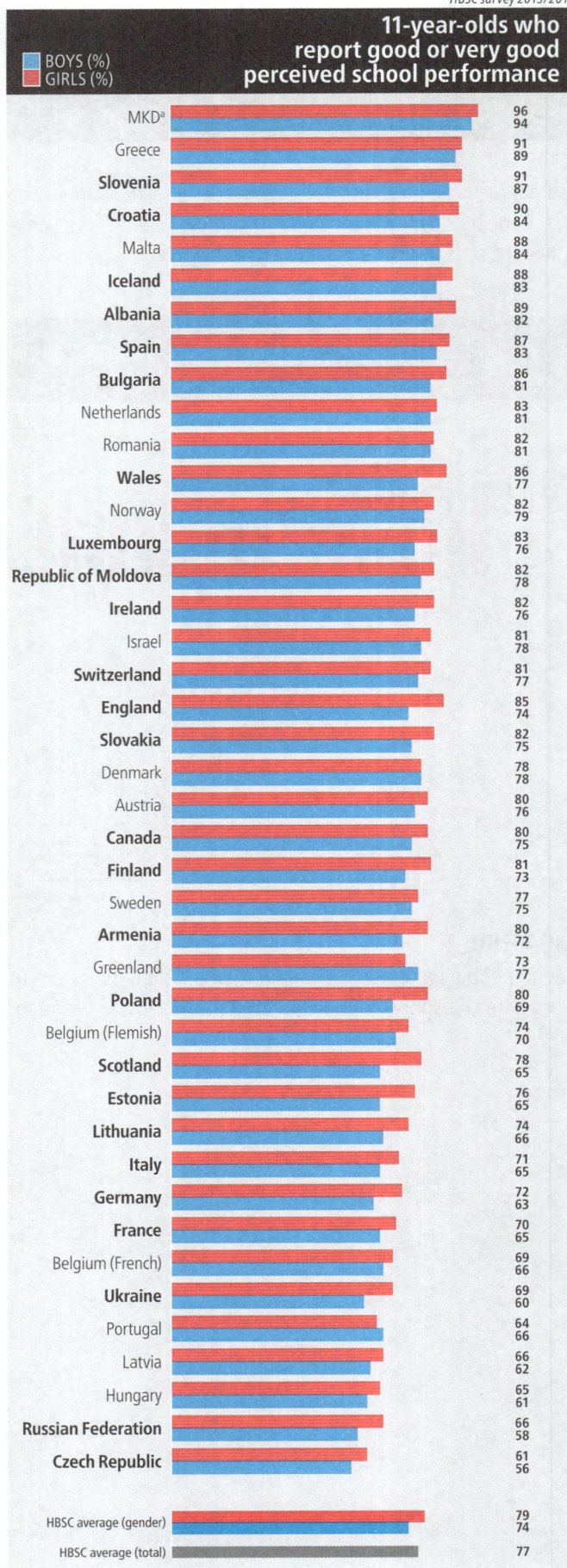

HBSC survey 2013/2014

11-year-olds who report good or very good perceived school performance

BOYS (%)
GIRLS (%)

Country	Girls (%)	Boys (%)
MKDª	96	94
Greece	91	89
Slovenia	91	87
Croatia	90	84
Malta	88	84
Iceland	88	83
Albania	89	82
Spain	87	83
Bulgaria	86	81
Netherlands	83	81
Romania	82	81
Wales	86	77
Norway	82	79
Luxembourg	83	76
Republic of Moldova	82	78
Ireland	82	76
Israel	81	78
Switzerland	81	77
England	85	74
Slovakia	82	75
Denmark	78	78
Austria	80	76
Canada	80	75
Finland	81	73
Sweden	77	75
Armenia	80	72
Greenland	73	77
Poland	80	69
Belgium (Flemish)	74	70
Scotland	78	65
Estonia	76	65
Lithuania	74	66
Italy	71	65
Germany	72	63
France	70	65
Belgium (French)	69	66
Ukraine	69	60
Portugal	64	66
Latvia	66	62
Hungary	65	61
Russian Federation	66	58
Czech Republic	61	56
HBSC average (gender)	79	74
HBSC average (total)	77	

ª The former Yugoslav Republic of Macedonia.

GROWING UP UNEQUAL: GENDER AND SOCIOECONOMIC
DIFFERENCES IN YOUNG PEOPLE'S HEALTH AND WELL-BEING
PART 2. KEY DATA | CHAPTER 2. SOCIAL CONTEXT
SCHOOL: PERCEIVED SCHOOL PERFORMANCE

2

HBSC survey 2013/2014

13-year-olds who report good or very good perceived school performance

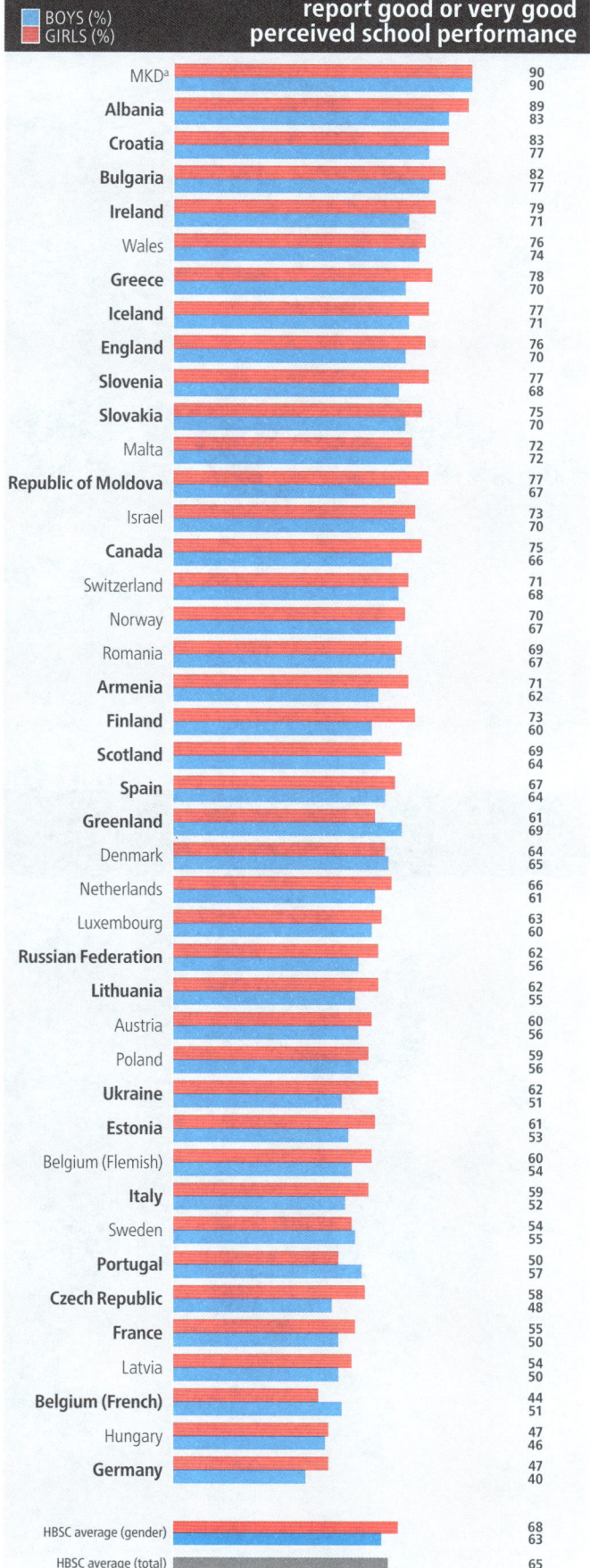

- BOYS (%)
- GIRLS (%)

Country	Girls (%)	Boys (%)
MKD[a]	90	90
Albania	89	83
Croatia	83	77
Bulgaria	82	77
Ireland	79	71
Wales	76	74
Greece	78	70
Iceland	77	71
England	76	70
Slovenia	77	68
Slovakia	75	70
Malta	72	72
Republic of Moldova	77	67
Israel	73	70
Canada	75	66
Switzerland	71	68
Norway	70	67
Romania	69	67
Armenia	71	62
Finland	73	60
Scotland	69	64
Spain	67	64
Greenland	61	69
Denmark	64	65
Netherlands	66	61
Luxembourg	63	60
Russian Federation	62	56
Lithuania	62	55
Austria	60	56
Poland	59	56
Ukraine	62	51
Estonia	61	53
Belgium (Flemish)	60	54
Italy	59	52
Sweden	54	55
Portugal	50	57
Czech Republic	58	48
France	55	50
Latvia	54	50
Belgium (French)	44	51
Hungary	47	46
Germany	47	40
HBSC average (gender)	68	63
HBSC average (total)	65	

HBSC survey 2013/2014

15-year-olds who report good or very good perceived school performance

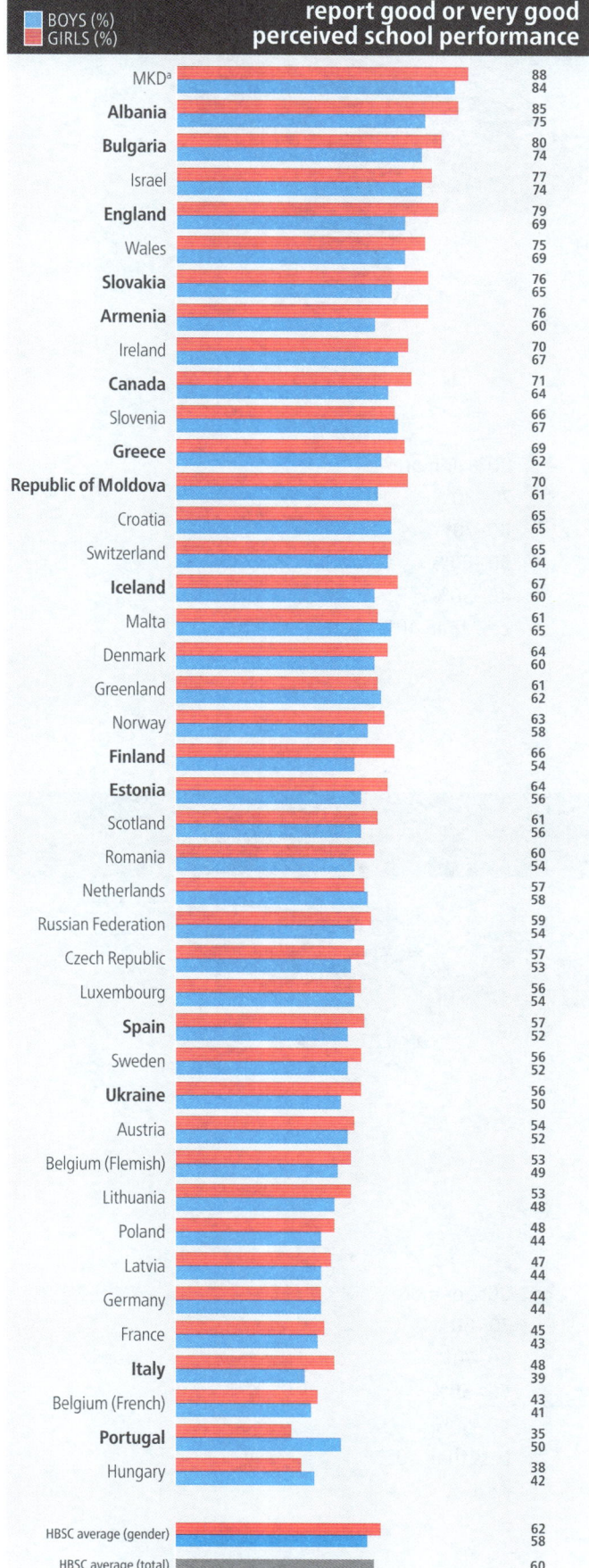

- BOYS (%)
- GIRLS (%)

Country	Girls (%)	Boys (%)
MKD[a]	88	84
Albania	85	75
Bulgaria	80	74
Israel	77	74
England	79	69
Wales	75	69
Slovakia	76	65
Armenia	76	60
Ireland	70	67
Canada	71	64
Slovenia	66	67
Greece	69	62
Republic of Moldova	70	61
Croatia	65	65
Switzerland	65	64
Iceland	67	60
Malta	61	65
Denmark	64	60
Greenland	61	62
Norway	63	58
Finland	66	54
Estonia	64	56
Scotland	61	56
Romania	60	54
Netherlands	57	58
Russian Federation	59	54
Czech Republic	57	53
Luxembourg	56	54
Spain	57	52
Sweden	56	52
Ukraine	56	50
Austria	54	52
Belgium (Flemish)	53	49
Lithuania	53	48
Poland	48	44
Latvia	47	44
Germany	44	44
France	45	43
Italy	48	39
Belgium (French)	43	41
Portugal	35	50
Hungary	38	42
HBSC average (gender)	62	58
HBSC average (total)	60	

*Note: **indicates** significant gender difference (at p<0.05).*

HBSC survey 2013/2014

15-year-old girls who report good or very good perceived school performance

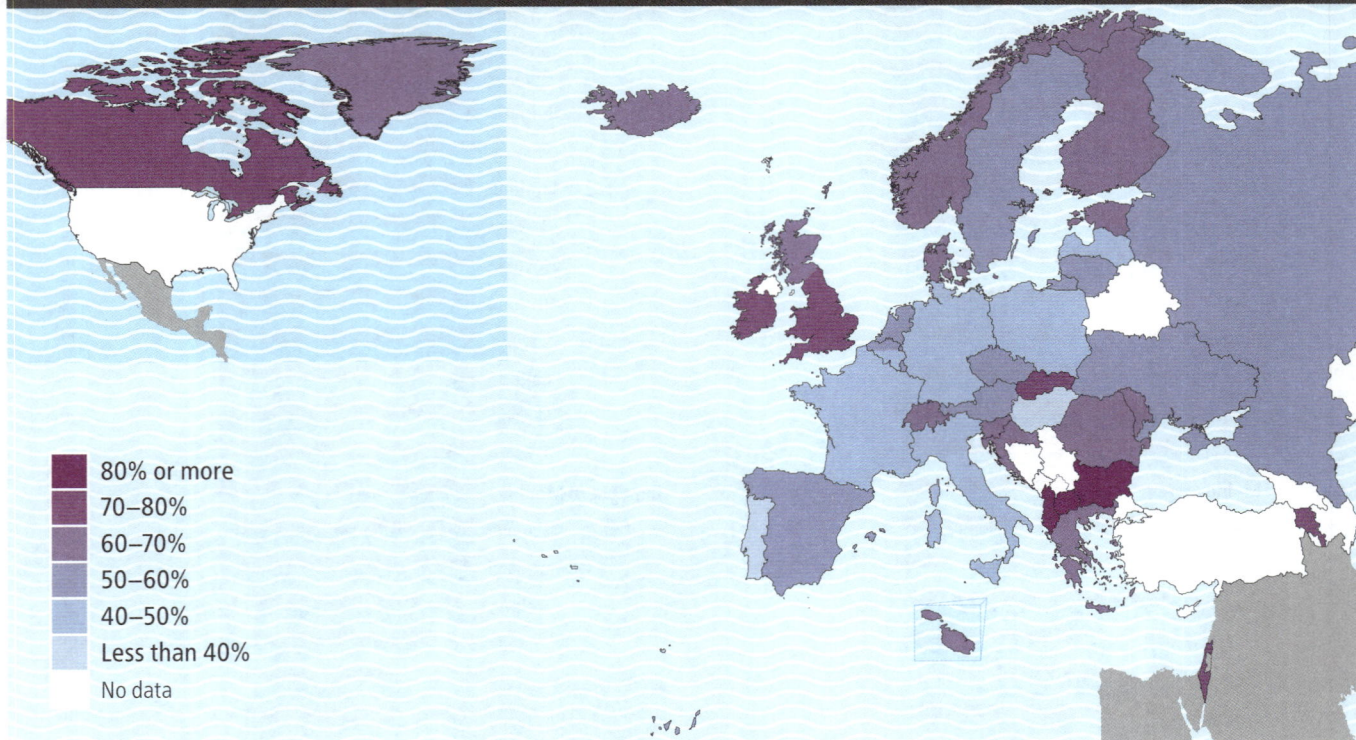

80% or more
70–80%
60–70%
50–60%
40–50%
Less than 40%
No data

Note: HBSC teams provided disaggregated data for Belgium and the United Kingdom; these data appear in the map above.

HBSC survey 2013/2014

15-year-old boys who report good or very good perceived school performance

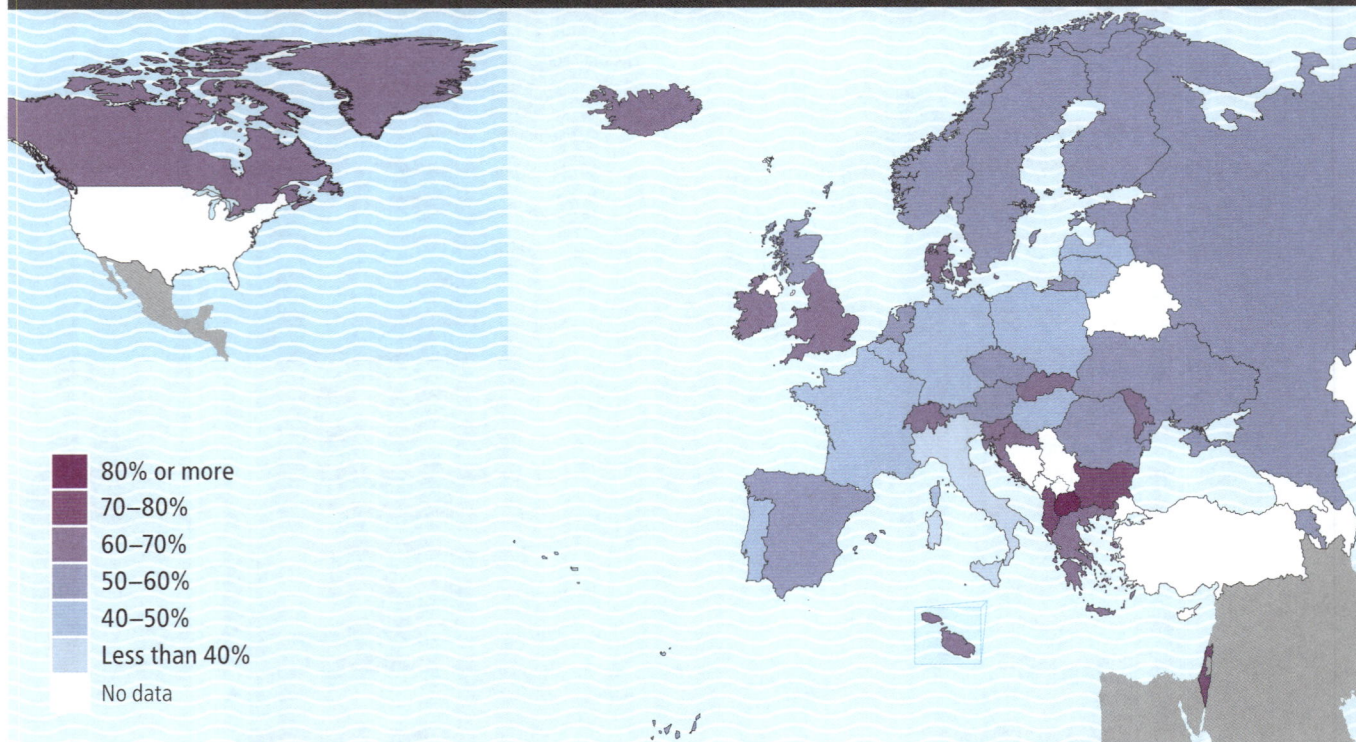

80% or more
70–80%
60–70%
50–60%
40–50%
Less than 40%
No data

Note: HBSC teams provided disaggregated data for Belgium and the United Kingdom; these data appear in the map above.

GROWING UP UNEQUAL: GENDER AND SOCIOECONOMIC
DIFFERENCES IN YOUNG PEOPLE'S HEALTH AND WELL-BEING
PART 2. KEY DATA | CHAPTER 2. SOCIAL CONTEXT

2

SCHOOL:
PRESSURED BY SCHOOLWORK

School-related stress tends to be experienced by young people with higher levels of pressure at school and is characterized by increased compromising health behaviours, more frequent health problems (headache, abdominal pain, backache and dizziness) and psychological complaints such as feeling sad, tense and nervous (7,8). High levels of school pressure are also associated with lower self-reported health, life satisfaction and levels of well-being.

HBSC survey 2013/2014

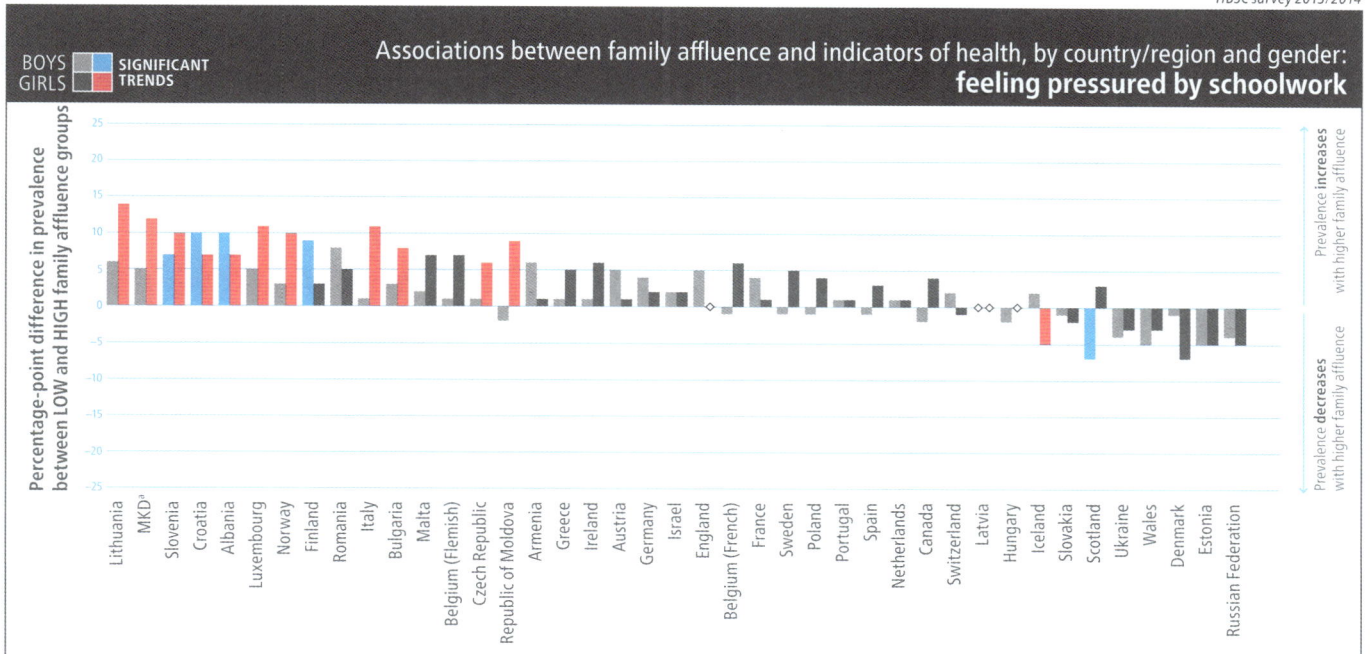

Associations between family affluence and indicators of health, by country/region and gender: **feeling pressured by schoolwork**

ᵃ The former Yugoslav Republic of Macedonia. *Note:* low- and high-affluence groups represent the lowest 20% and highest 20% in each country. ◇ means less than +/-0.5%. No data were received from Greenland.

MEASURE
Young people were asked how pressured they feel by the schoolwork they have to do. Response options ranged from not at all to a lot.

RESULTS

Findings presented here show the proportions who reported feeling pressured by schoolwork some or a lot.

Age

Proportions increased with increasing age, a pattern that was more apparent among girls. Compared with 11-year-olds, boys of 15 showed a higher prevalence in 33 countries and regions, with a difference of 20 or more percentage points being seen in 11. Among girls, there was an increase between 11 and 15 years in 39 countries and regions, with a difference of more than 20 percentage points in 28.

Gender

Gender differences changed with age. Boys were more likely to report being pressured by schoolwork at age 11 and girls at 15. Higher prevalence among 11-year-old girls was seen in three countries and regions and among boys in 13. Twenty countries and regions had higher prevalence among girls at age 13 and one among boys. Higher prevalence among 15-year-old girls was seen in 36 countries and regions, with a difference of 10 or more percentage points in 27.

Family affluence

No general pattern was seen for boys and girls. Only a few countries and regions showed significant patterns by family affluence.

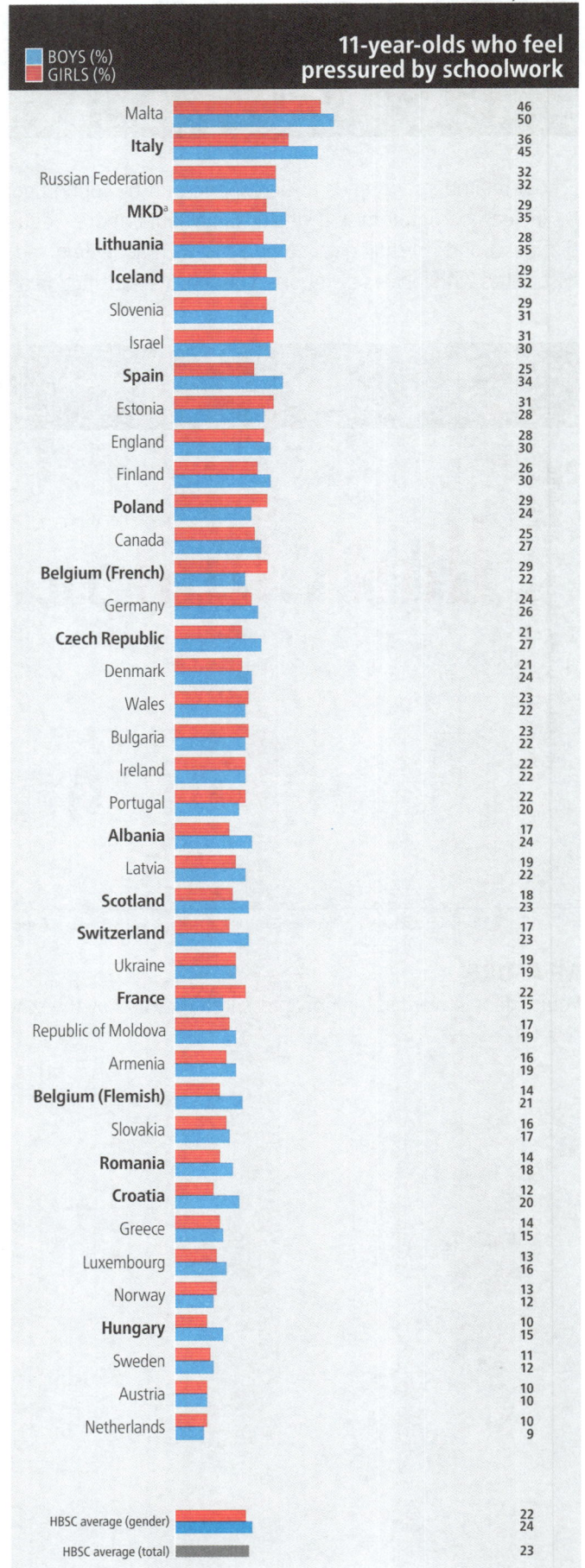

HBSC survey 2013/2014

11-year-olds who feel pressured by schoolwork

BOYS (%)
GIRLS (%)

Country	Girls	Boys
Malta	46	50
Italy	36	45
Russian Federation	32	32
MKD[a]	29	35
Lithuania	28	35
Iceland	29	32
Slovenia	29	31
Israel	31	30
Spain	25	34
Estonia	31	28
England	28	30
Finland	26	30
Poland	29	24
Canada	25	27
Belgium (French)	29	22
Germany	24	26
Czech Republic	21	27
Denmark	21	24
Wales	23	22
Bulgaria	23	22
Ireland	22	22
Portugal	22	20
Albania	17	24
Latvia	19	22
Scotland	18	23
Switzerland	17	23
Ukraine	19	19
France	22	15
Republic of Moldova	17	19
Armenia	16	19
Belgium (Flemish)	14	21
Slovakia	16	17
Romania	14	18
Croatia	12	20
Greece	14	15
Luxembourg	13	16
Norway	13	12
Hungary	10	15
Sweden	11	12
Austria	10	10
Netherlands	10	9
HBSC average (gender)	22	24
HBSC average (total)		23

[a] The former Yugoslav Republic of Macedonia.

GROWING UP UNEQUAL: GENDER AND SOCIOECONOMIC
DIFFERENCES IN YOUNG PEOPLE'S HEALTH AND WELL-BEING
PART 2. KEY DATA | CHAPTER 2. SOCIAL CONTEXT
SCHOOL: PRESSURED BY SCHOOLWORK

2

13-year-olds who feel pressured by schoolwork

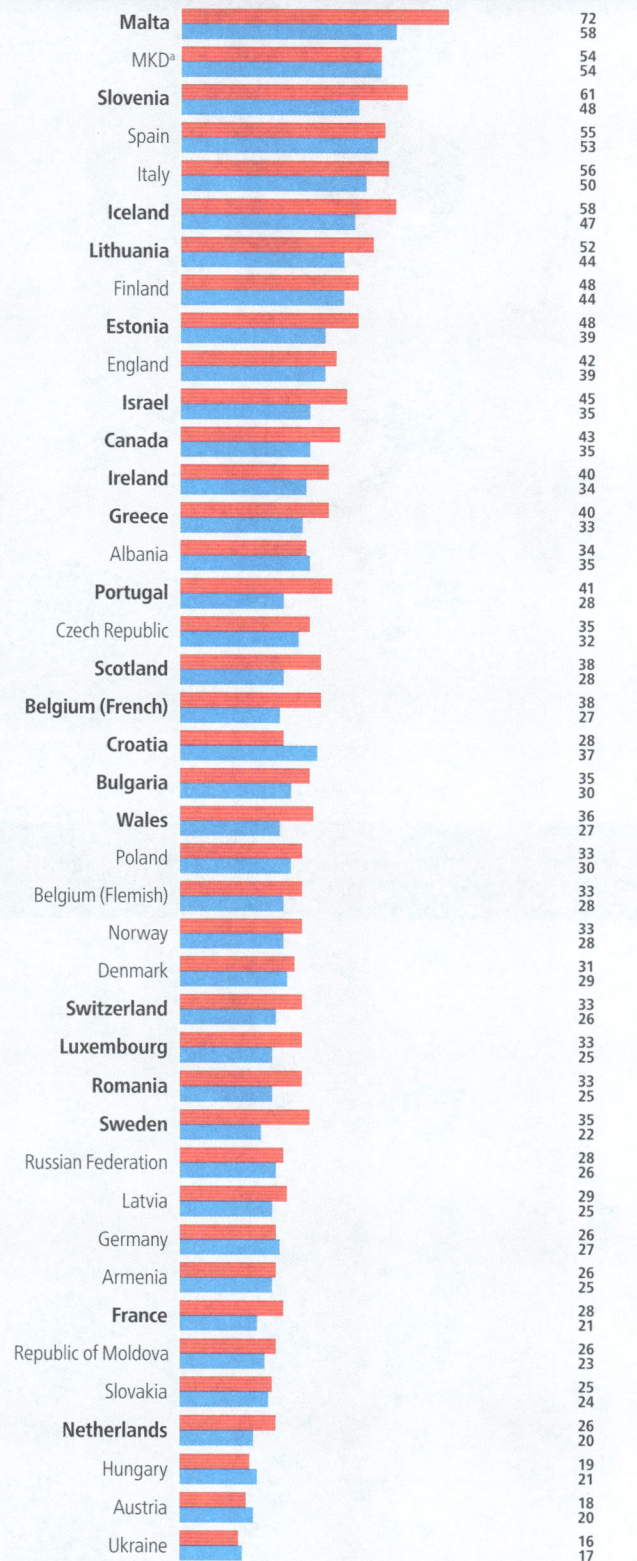

HBSC survey 2013/2014

- BOYS (%)
- GIRLS (%)

Country	Girls	Boys
Malta	72	58
MKD[a]	54	54
Slovenia	61	48
Spain	55	53
Italy	56	50
Iceland	58	47
Lithuania	52	44
Finland	48	44
Estonia	48	39
England	42	39
Israel	45	35
Canada	43	35
Ireland	40	34
Greece	40	33
Albania	34	35
Portugal	41	28
Czech Republic	35	32
Scotland	38	28
Belgium (French)	38	27
Croatia	28	37
Bulgaria	35	30
Wales	36	27
Poland	33	30
Belgium (Flemish)	33	28
Norway	33	28
Denmark	31	29
Switzerland	33	26
Luxembourg	33	25
Romania	33	25
Sweden	35	22
Russian Federation	28	26
Latvia	29	25
Germany	26	27
Armenia	26	25
France	28	21
Republic of Moldova	26	23
Slovakia	25	24
Netherlands	26	20
Hungary	19	21
Austria	18	20
Ukraine	16	17
HBSC average (gender)	38	33
HBSC average (total)	36	

15-year-olds who feel pressured by schoolwork

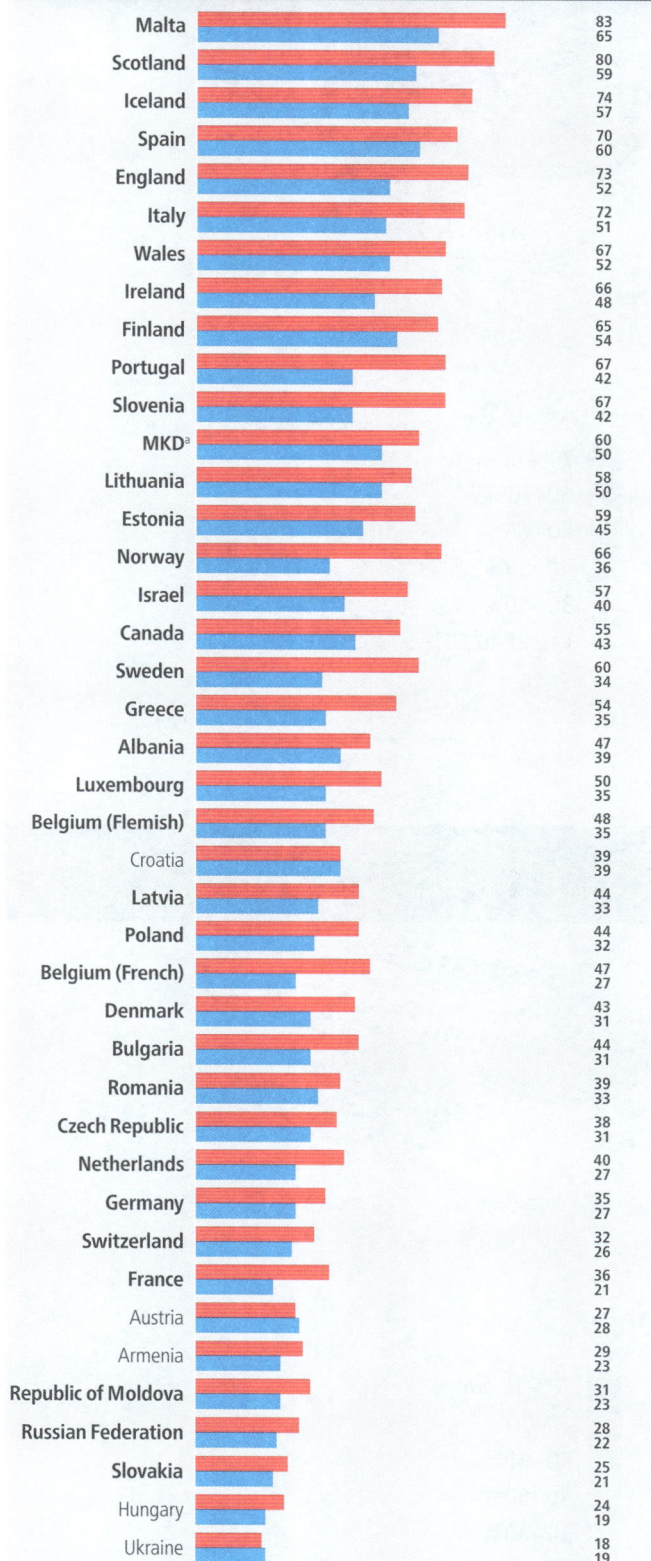

HBSC survey 2013/2014

- BOYS (%)
- GIRLS (%)

Country	Girls	Boys
Malta	83	65
Scotland	80	59
Iceland	74	57
Spain	70	60
England	73	52
Italy	72	51
Wales	67	52
Ireland	66	48
Finland	65	54
Portugal	67	42
Slovenia	67	42
MKD[a]	60	50
Lithuania	58	50
Estonia	59	45
Norway	66	36
Israel	57	40
Canada	55	43
Sweden	60	34
Greece	54	35
Albania	47	39
Luxembourg	50	35
Belgium (Flemish)	48	35
Croatia	39	39
Latvia	44	33
Poland	44	32
Belgium (French)	47	27
Denmark	43	31
Bulgaria	44	31
Romania	39	33
Czech Republic	38	31
Netherlands	40	27
Germany	35	27
Switzerland	32	26
France	36	21
Austria	27	28
Armenia	29	23
Republic of Moldova	31	23
Russian Federation	28	22
Slovakia	25	21
Hungary	24	19
Ukraine	18	19
HBSC average (gender)	51	39
HBSC average (total)	45	

*Note: **indicates** significant gender difference (at p<0.05). No data were received from Greenland.*

HBSC survey 2013/2014

15-year-old girls who feel pressured by school work

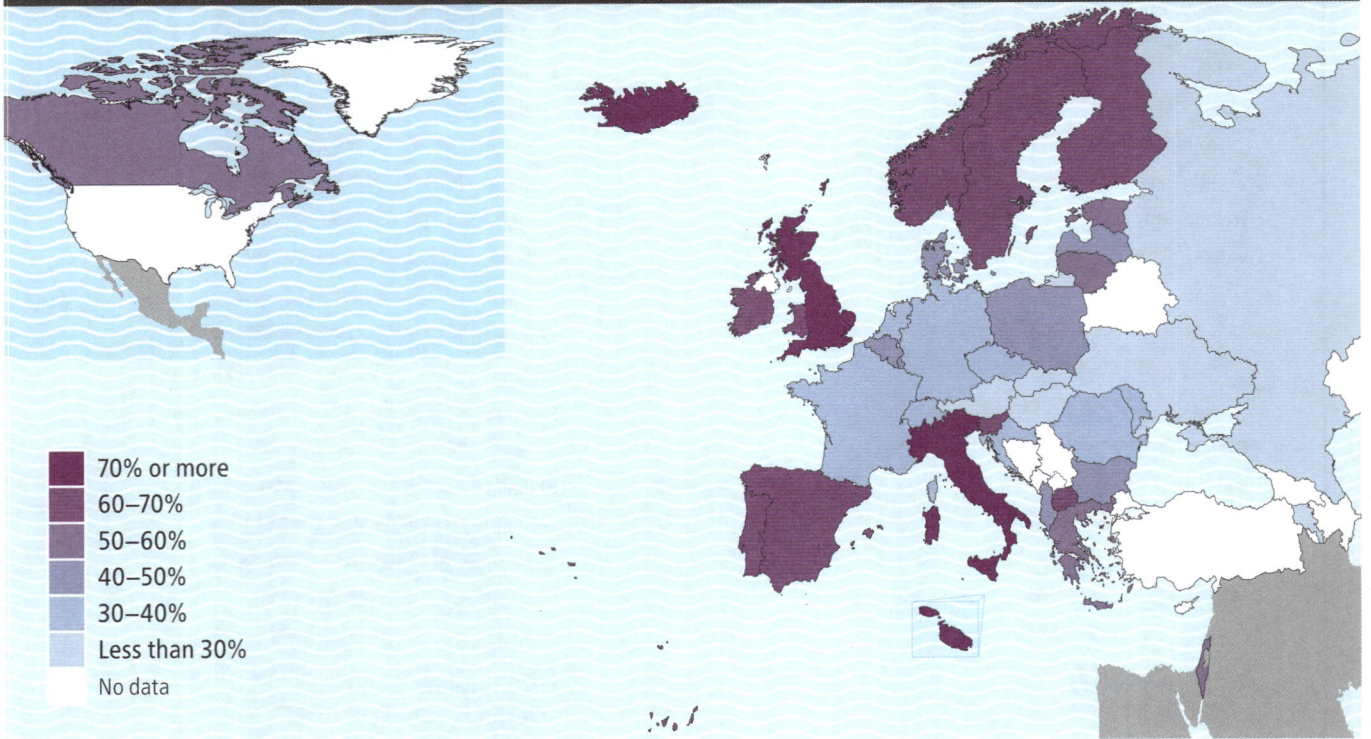

70% or more
60–70%
50–60%
40–50%
30–40%
Less than 30%
No data

Note: HBSC teams provided disaggregated data for Belgium and the United Kingdom; these data appear in the map above.

HBSC survey 2013/2014

15-year-old boys who feel pressured by school work

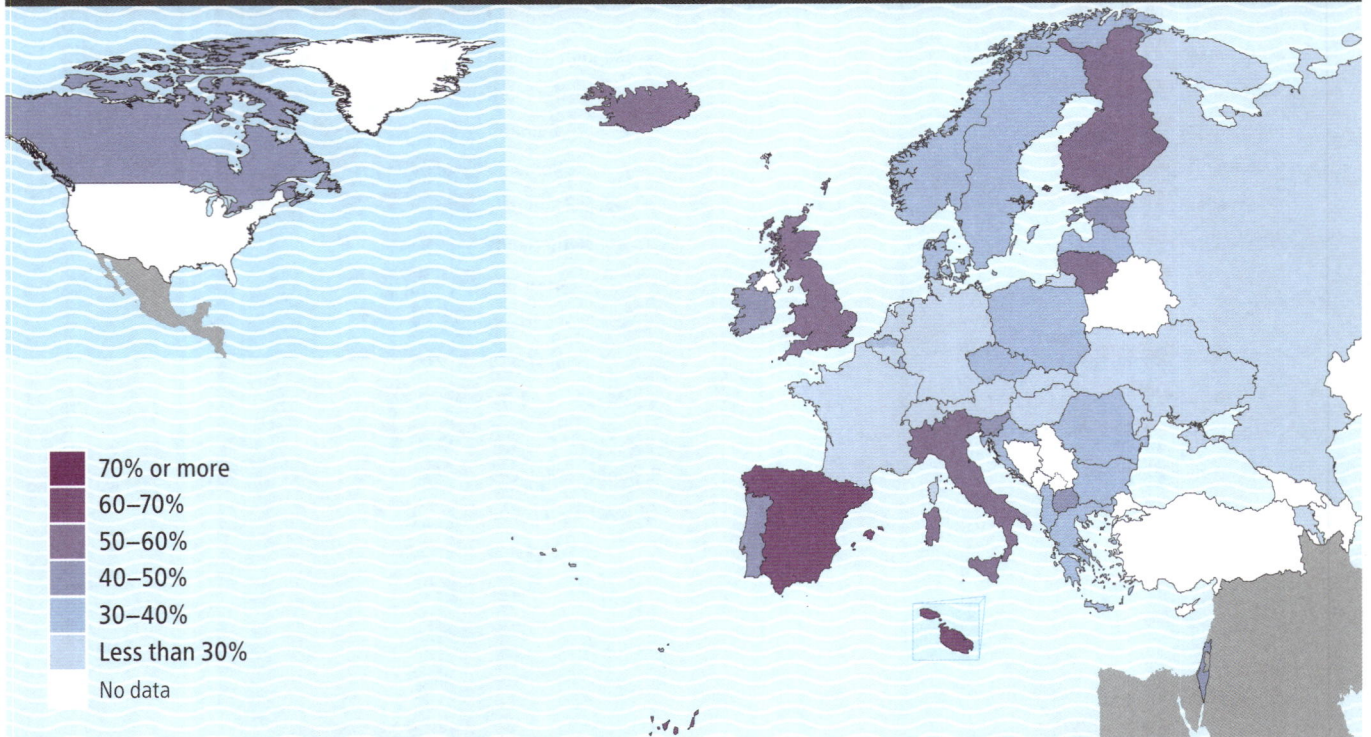

70% or more
60–70%
50–60%
40–50%
30–40%
Less than 30%
No data

Note: HBSC teams provided disaggregated data for Belgium and the United Kingdom; these data appear in the map above.

GROWING UP UNEQUAL: GENDER AND SOCIOECONOMIC
DIFFERENCES IN YOUNG PEOPLE'S HEALTH AND WELL-BEING
PART 2. KEY DATA | CHAPTER 2. SOCIAL CONTEXT

2

SCHOOL:
CLASSMATE SUPPORT

Experiencing social support is central to child and adolescent well-being *(9)*. Young people derive social support from a number of sources, such as parents and family, peers, classmates and teachers, with each source being associated with beneficial outcomes *(10)*. Peer support may improve psychological well-being, self-esteem, achievement of academic goals and social adjustment to school *(11)*, and support from classmates makes a significant contribution to realizing the basic need for relatedness.

HBSC survey 2013/2014

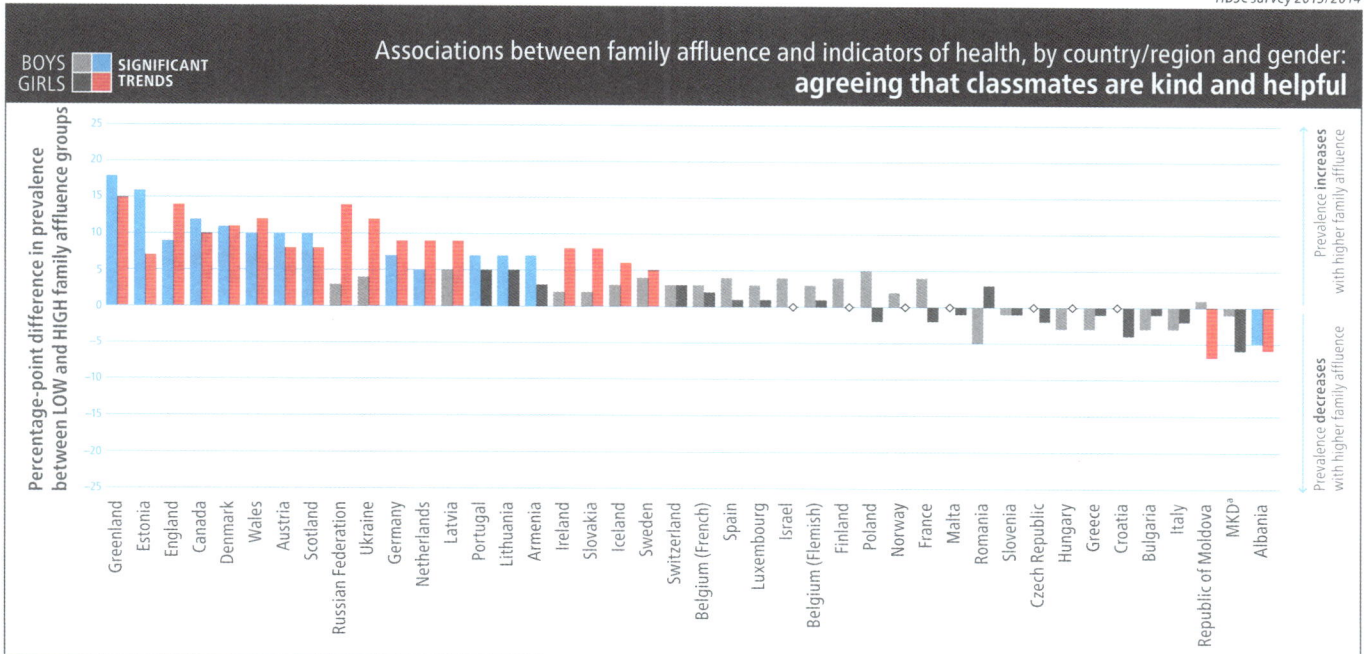

BOYS
GIRLS
SIGNIFICANT TRENDS

Associations between family affluence and indicators of health, by country/region and gender:
agreeing that classmates are kind and helpful

Percentage-point difference in prevalence between LOW and HIGH family affluence groups

Prevalence **increases** with higher family affluence

Prevalence **decreases** with higher family affluence

Greenland, Estonia, England, Canada, Denmark, Wales, Austria, Scotland, Russian Federation, Ukraine, Germany, Netherlands, Latvia, Portugal, Lithuania, Armenia, Ireland, Slovakia, Iceland, Sweden, Switzerland, Belgium (French), Spain, Luxembourg, Israel, Belgium (Flemish), Finland, Poland, Norway, France, Malta, Romania, Slovenia, Czech Republic, Hungary, Greece, Croatia, Bulgaria, Italy, Republic of Moldova, MKD[a], Albania

[a] The former Yugoslav Republic of Macedonia. *Note:* low- and high-affluence groups represent the lowest 20% and highest 20% in each country. ◇ means less than +/-0.5%.

MEASURE

Young people were asked to indicate their agreement or disagreement with the statement that most of the students in their class(es) are kind and helpful. Response options ranged from strongly disagree to strongly agree.

RESULTS

Findings presented here show the proportions who agreed or strongly agreed.

Age

The proportion was highest among 11-year-olds in most countries and regions. A significant decrease with age was seen among boys in 25 and an increase in two. For girls, there was a significant decrease in 30 and an increase in two.

Gender

Gender differences were evident in only a few countries and regions and changed with age. Where there was a significant difference, girls tended to report higher classmate support at age 11 and boys at 15. Relatively few differences, however, were statistically significant.

Family affluence

Around half of countries and regions showed significant patterns by family affluence in at least one gender. Of these, high classmate support was associated with high affluence in most.

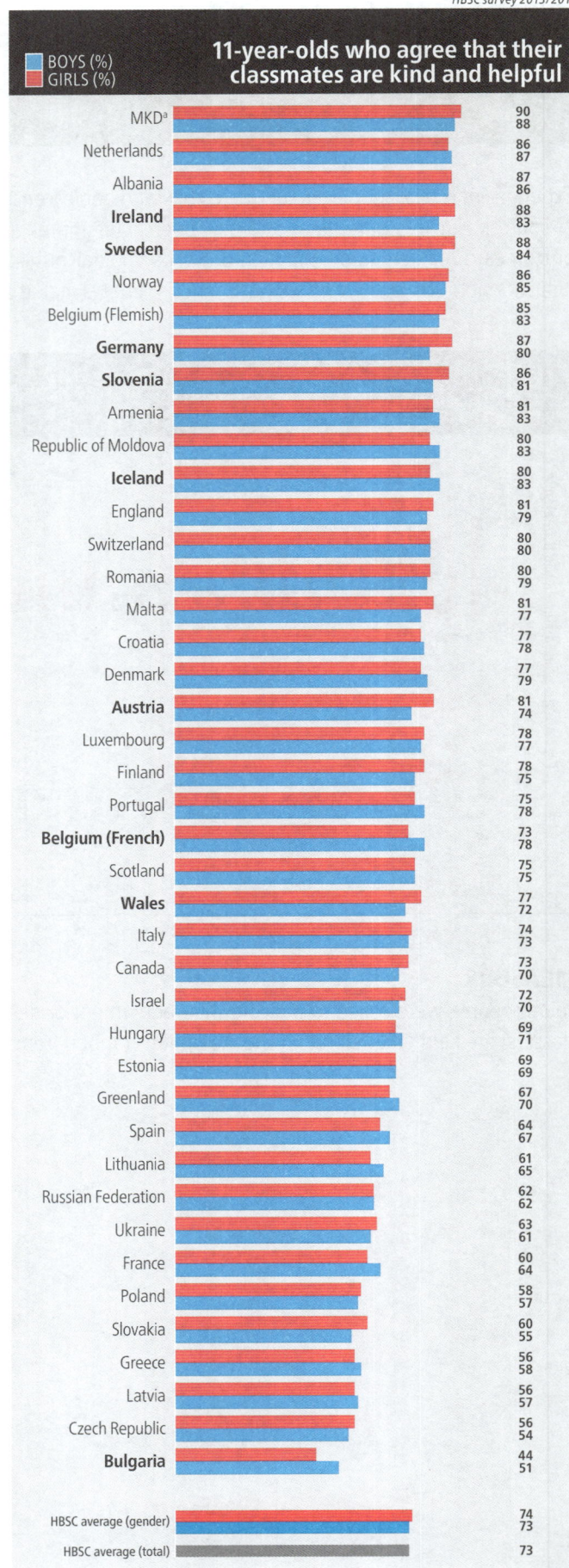

HBSC survey 2013/2014

11-year-olds who agree that their classmates are kind and helpful

BOYS (%)
GIRLS (%)

Country	Girls	Boys
MKDª	90	88
Netherlands	86	87
Albania	87	86
Ireland	88	83
Sweden	88	84
Norway	86	85
Belgium (Flemish)	85	83
Germany	87	80
Slovenia	86	81
Armenia	81	83
Republic of Moldova	80	83
Iceland	80	83
England	81	79
Switzerland	80	80
Romania	80	79
Malta	81	77
Croatia	77	78
Denmark	77	79
Austria	81	74
Luxembourg	78	77
Finland	78	75
Portugal	75	78
Belgium (French)	73	78
Scotland	75	75
Wales	77	72
Italy	74	73
Canada	73	70
Israel	72	70
Hungary	69	71
Estonia	69	69
Greenland	67	70
Spain	64	67
Lithuania	61	65
Russian Federation	62	62
Ukraine	63	61
France	60	64
Poland	58	57
Slovakia	60	55
Greece	56	58
Latvia	56	57
Czech Republic	56	54
Bulgaria	44	51
HBSC average (gender)	74	73
HBSC average (total)	73	

ª The former Yugoslav Republic of Macedonia.

GROWING UP UNEQUAL: GENDER AND SOCIOECONOMIC
DIFFERENCES IN YOUNG PEOPLE'S HEALTH AND WELL-BEING
PART 2. KEY DATA | CHAPTER 2. SOCIAL CONTEXT
SCHOOL: CLASSMATE SUPPORT

2

HBSC survey 2013/2014

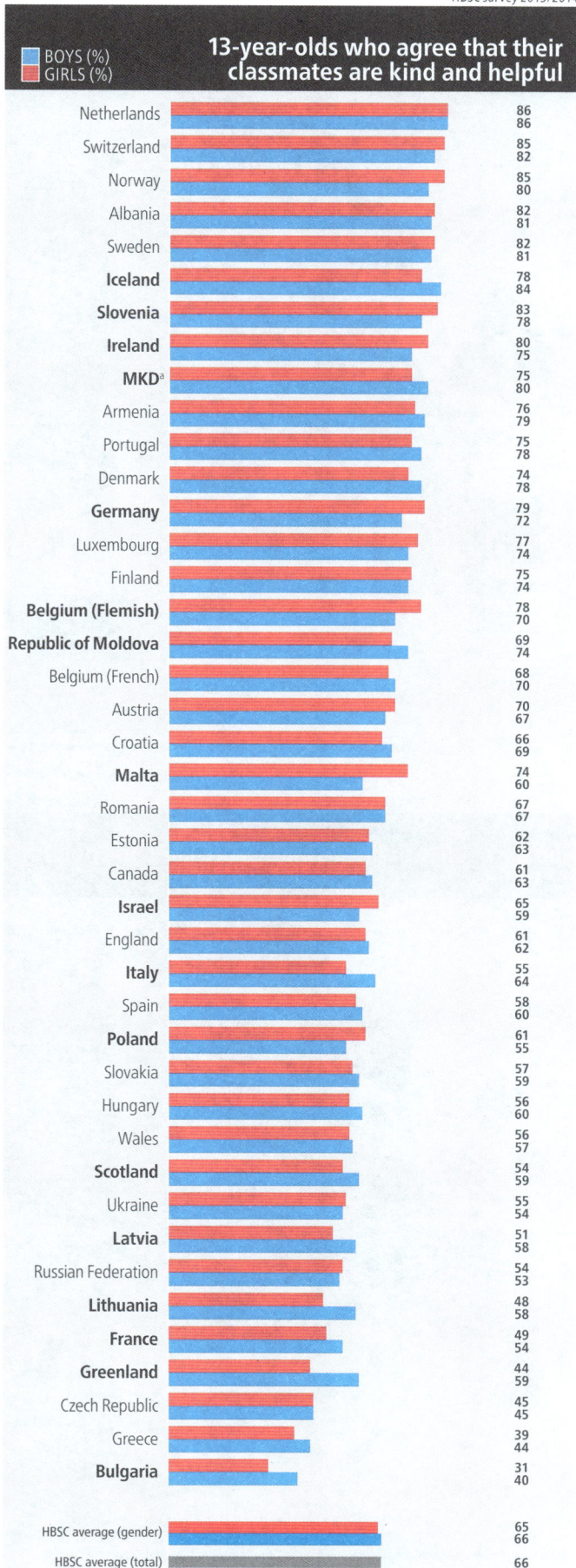

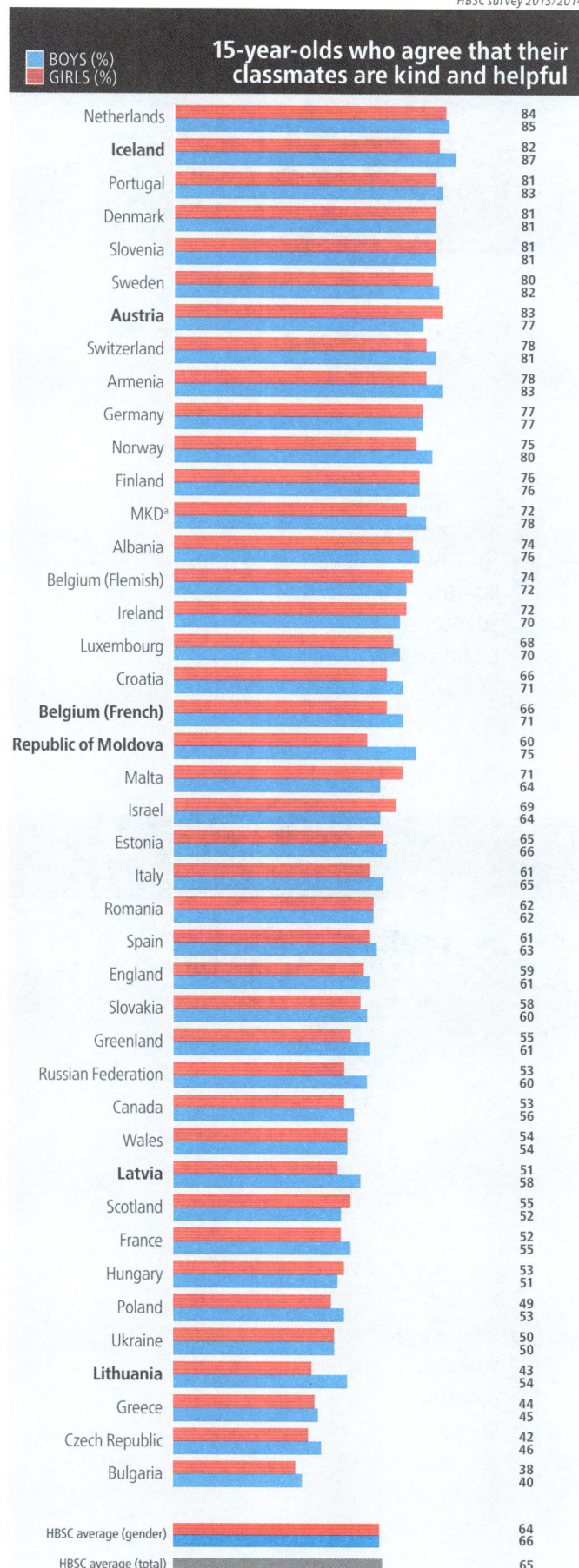

13-year-olds who agree that their classmates are kind and helpful

■ BOYS (%)
■ GIRLS (%)

Country	Girls (%)	Boys (%)
Netherlands	86	86
Switzerland	85	82
Norway	85	80
Albania	82	81
Sweden	82	81
Iceland	78	84
Slovenia	83	78
Ireland	80	75
MKD[a]	75	80
Armenia	76	79
Portugal	75	78
Denmark	74	78
Germany	79	72
Luxembourg	77	74
Finland	75	74
Belgium (Flemish)	78	70
Republic of Moldova	69	74
Belgium (French)	68	70
Austria	70	67
Croatia	66	69
Malta	74	60
Romania	67	67
Estonia	62	63
Canada	61	63
Israel	65	59
England	61	62
Italy	55	64
Spain	58	60
Poland	61	55
Slovakia	57	59
Hungary	56	60
Wales	56	57
Scotland	54	59
Ukraine	55	54
Latvia	51	58
Russian Federation	54	53
Lithuania	48	58
France	49	54
Greenland	44	59
Czech Republic	45	45
Greece	39	44
Bulgaria	31	40
HBSC average (gender)	65	66
HBSC average (total)		66

HBSC survey 2013/2014

15-year-olds who agree that their classmates are kind and helpful

■ BOYS (%)
■ GIRLS (%)

Country	Girls (%)	Boys (%)
Netherlands	84	85
Iceland	82	87
Portugal	81	83
Denmark	81	81
Slovenia	81	81
Sweden	80	82
Austria	83	77
Switzerland	78	81
Armenia	78	83
Germany	77	77
Norway	75	80
Finland	76	76
MKD[a]	72	78
Albania	74	76
Belgium (Flemish)	74	72
Ireland	72	70
Luxembourg	68	70
Croatia	66	71
Belgium (French)	66	71
Republic of Moldova	60	75
Malta	71	64
Israel	69	64
Estonia	65	66
Italy	61	65
Romania	62	62
Spain	61	63
England	59	61
Slovakia	58	60
Greenland	55	61
Russian Federation	53	60
Canada	53	56
Wales	54	54
Latvia	51	58
Scotland	55	52
France	52	55
Hungary	53	51
Poland	49	53
Ukraine	50	50
Lithuania	43	54
Greece	44	45
Czech Republic	42	46
Bulgaria	38	40
HBSC average (gender)	64	66
HBSC average (total)		65

Note: **indicates** significant gender difference (at p<0.05).

HBSC survey 2013/2014

15-year-old girls who agree that their classmates are kind and helpful

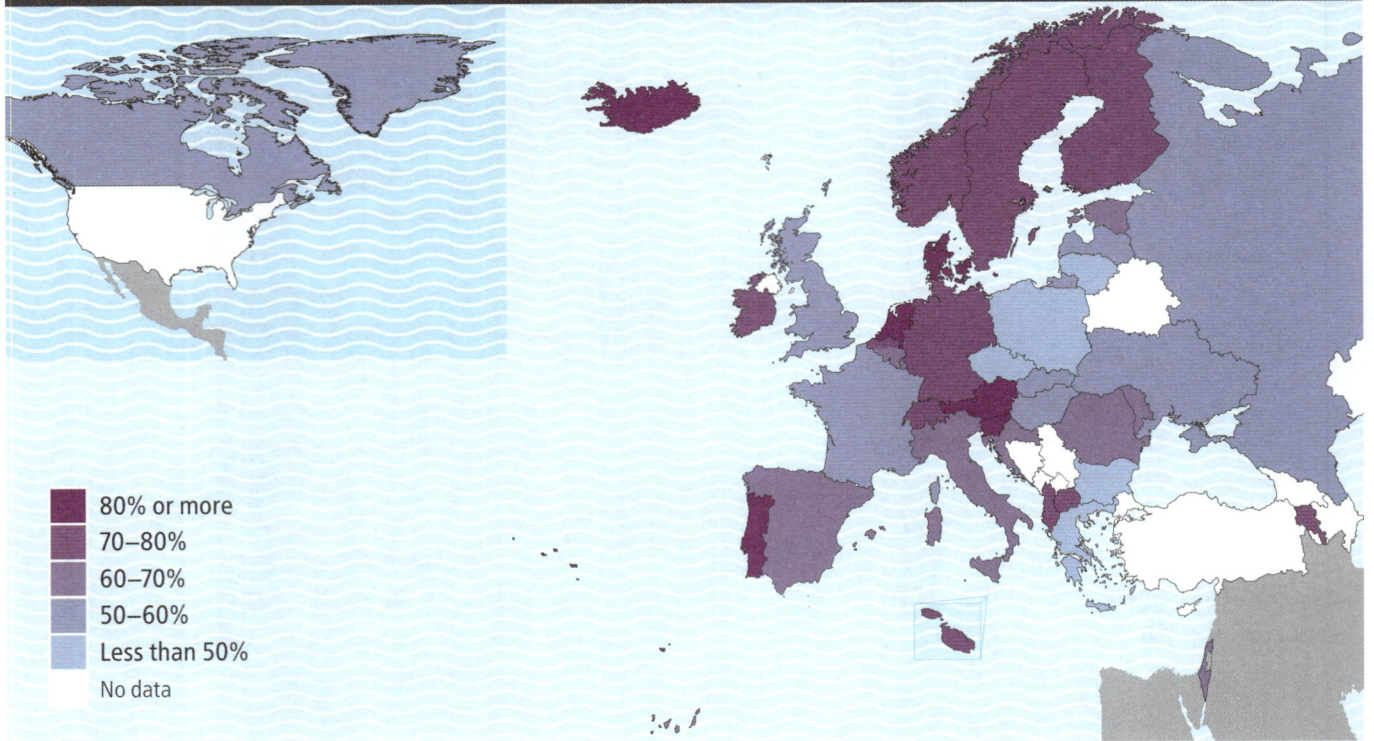

- 80% or more
- 70–80%
- 60–70%
- 50–60%
- Less than 50%
- No data

Note: HBSC teams provided disaggregated data for Belgium and the United Kingdom; these data appear in the map above.

HBSC survey 2013/2014

15-year-old boys who agree that their classmates are kind and helpful

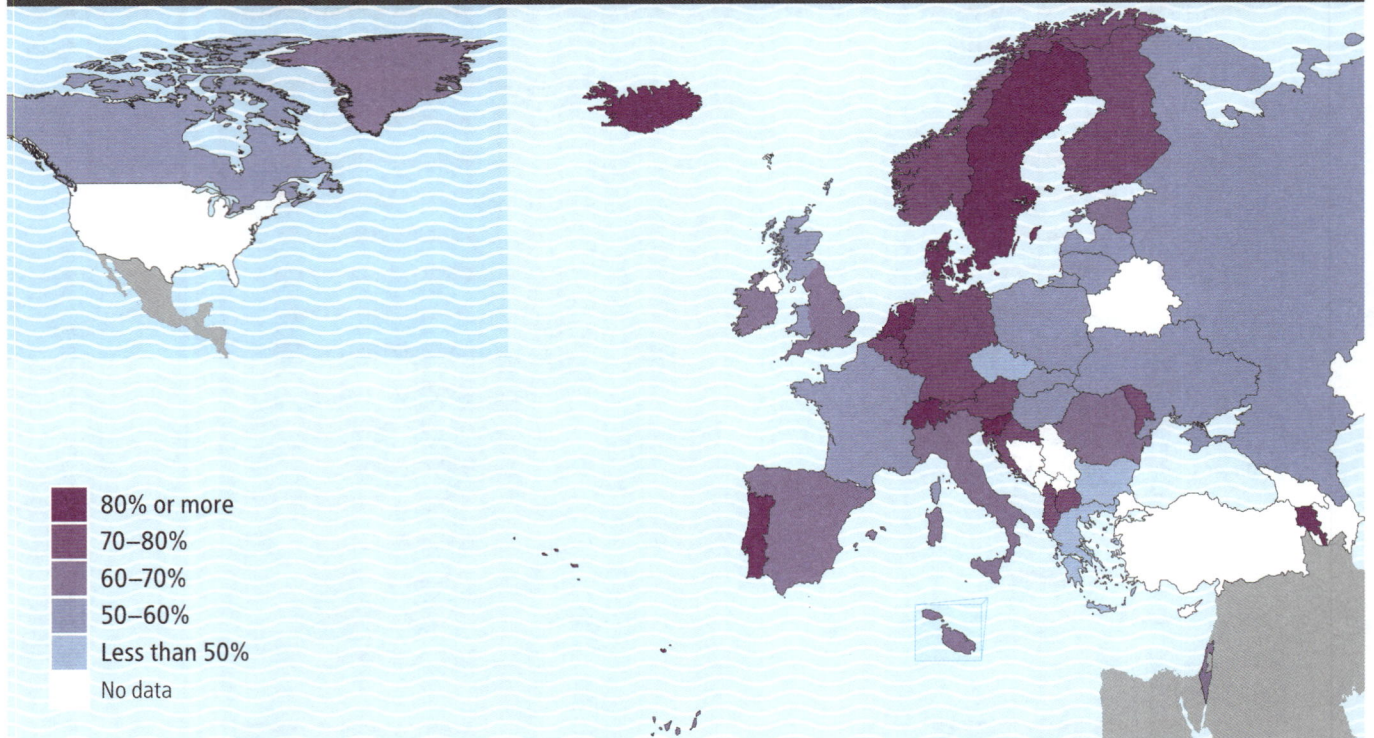

- 80% or more
- 70–80%
- 60–70%
- 50–60%
- Less than 50%
- No data

Note: HBSC teams provided disaggregated data for Belgium and the United Kingdom; these data appear in the map above.

GROWING UP UNEQUAL: GENDER AND SOCIOECONOMIC
DIFFERENCES IN YOUNG PEOPLE'S HEALTH AND WELL-BEING
PART 2. KEY DATA | CHAPTER 2. SOCIAL CONTEXT
SCHOOL

2

SCHOOL:
SCIENTIFIC DISCUSSION AND POLICY REFLECTIONS

SCIENTIFIC DISCUSSION

Older students generally seem to be more challenged by their school life, while younger age groups like school to a greater extent, feel less pressured by schoolwork and generally report better school performance. The perception of having kind and helpful classmates is also higher among younger students.

Girls tend to like school to a greater extent and generally report better school performance. The picture for school-related stress is more complex, however, as the gender patterns change with age. Boys in the younger group in some countries and regions are more challenged by school pressure and report lower classmate support, but the situation is reversed among older students.

School performance generally increases with increasing affluence, but no clear pattern by family affluence is seen for liking school, school pressure and classmate support. School should constitute a supportive environment irrespective of students' family background. It is therefore positive that no marked SES differences are observed across countries and regions.

POLICY REFLECTIONS

Children spend increasing time in school as they age. Positive perceptions of, and attitudes towards, school are therefore important to healthy child development. WHO continues to emphasize the significance of school as a setting in which to influence young people's health and health behaviour. Empirical evidence demonstrates that school-based health-promotion programmes are effective, not least those that achieve changes in the school environment *(12)*.

Certain programmes also increase the chances of academic achievement *(13)*. Evidence-based, professionally guided health-promotion activities are rare, however, with those advocating a whole-school approach even more so.

The findings suggest that gender-sensitive policies to bring boys' perceptions of school closer to those of girls should be encouraged from an early age.

REFERENCES

1. Wells J. Promoting emotional well-being in schools. In: Buchanan A, Hudson B, editors. Promoting children's emotional well-being. London: Oxford University Press; 2000:161–92.
2. Wang MT, Dishion TJ. The trajectories of adolescents' perceptions of school climate, deviant peer affiliation, and behavioural problems during the middle school years. J Res Adolesc. 2012;22:40–53.
3. Bond L, Butler H, Thomas L, Carlin J, Glover S, Bowes G et al. Social and school connectedness in early secondary school as predictors of late teenage substance use, mental health, and academic outcomes. J Adolesc Health 2007;40(4):357.
4. Van Ryzin MJ, Gravely AA, Roseth CJ. Autonomy, belongingness, and engagement in school as contributors to adolescent psychological well-being. J Youth Adolesc. 2009;38:1–12.
5. Bird JM, Markle RS. Subjective well-being in school environments: promoting positive youth development through evidence-based assessment and intervention. Am J Orthopsychiatry 2012;82:61–66.
6. Cole D, Jacquez F, Maschman T. Social origins of depressive cognitions: a longitudinal study of self-perceived competences in children. Cognit Ther Res. 2001;25(4):377–95.
7. Torsheim T, Aaro LE, Wold B. School-related stress, social support, and distress: prospective analysis of reciprocal and multilevel relationships. Scand J Psychol. 2003;44:153–9.
8. Ottová-Jordan W, Smith ORF, Augustine L, Gobina I, Rathmann K, Torsheim T et al. Trends in health complaints from 2002 to 2010 in 34 countries and their association with health behaviours and social context factors at individual and macro-level. Eur J Public Health 2015;25(2):83–9.
9. Shin R, Daly B, Vera E. The relationship of peer norms, ethnic identity, and peer support to school engagement in urban youth. Professional School Counselling 2007;10:379–88.
10. Malecki CK, Demaray MK. What type of support do they need? Investigating student adjustment as related to emotional, appraisal, information, and instrumental support. Sch Psychol Q. 2003;18(3):231–52.
11. Danielsen AG, Samdal O, Hetland J, Wold B. School-related social support and students' perceived life satisfaction. J Educ Res. 2009;102:303–18.

12. Stewart-Brown S. What is the evidence on school health promotion in improving health or preventing disease and, specifically, what is the effectiveness of the health promoting schools approach? Copenhagen: WHO Regional Office for Europe; 2006 (Health Evidence Network report; http://www.oru.se/ExternalWebsites/NCFF/Maten%20i%20skolan/L%C3%A4sf%C3%B6nster/rapporter/E88185.pdf, accessed 24 August 2015).

13. Murray NG, Low BJ, Hollis C, Cross AW, Davis SM. Coordinated school health programmes and academic achievement: a systematic review of the literature. J Sch Health 2007;77:589–600.

GROWING UP UNEQUAL: GENDER AND SOCIOECONOMIC
DIFFERENCES IN YOUNG PEOPLE'S HEALTH AND WELL-BEING
PART 2. KEY DATA | CHAPTER 3. HEALTH OUTCOMES

3

HEALTH OUTCOMES

POSITIVE HEALTH
MEDICALLY ATTENDED INJURIES
BODY WEIGHT

"When you are ill, it's dark, you are in a closed room. And when you are healthy you are outside and the sun is shining."

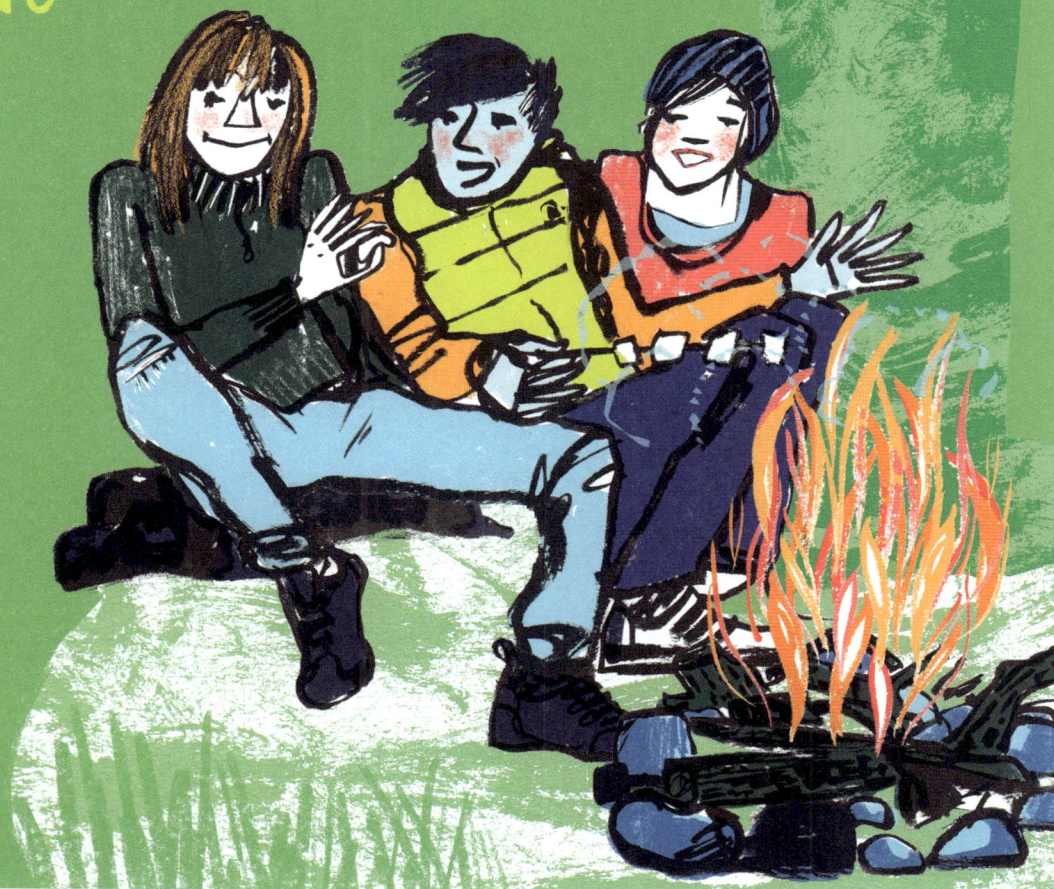

QUOTES FROM YOUNG PEOPLE ON HEALTH OUTCOMES

"The future is unknown and we all care about what is going to happen to us. The academic future is the worst and gives us the larger worries. We have doubts such as 'What can I study? Will I like it? Can I get a job in the end?'"

"It can be hard to find yourself, 'who you are'."

"As teenagers grow older, their problems grow much more complex, in school, homework, relationships and their perception of these."

GROWING UP UNEQUAL: GENDER AND SOCIOECONOMIC
DIFFERENCES IN YOUNG PEOPLE'S HEALTH AND WELL-BEING
PART 2. KEY DATA | CHAPTER 3. HEALTH OUTCOMES

3

POSITIVE HEALTH:
SELF-RATED HEALTH

Self-rated health is a subjective indicator of general health. In adolescence, it refers not only to the presence or absence of chronic disease or disability, but also to a more general understanding of self.

Empirical studies have shown that self-rated health is an independent predictor of future morbidity and mortality even after controlling for other factors *(1)*. Poor health in early childhood may result in long-term negative effects that can continue throughout adolescence into adulthood and may also influence use of health services *(2)*. Adolescent self-rated health is influenced by a broad range of health indicators, including medical, psychological, socioenvironmental and behavioural *(3,4)*, and wider social contextual factors such as family, peers, school and cultural status.

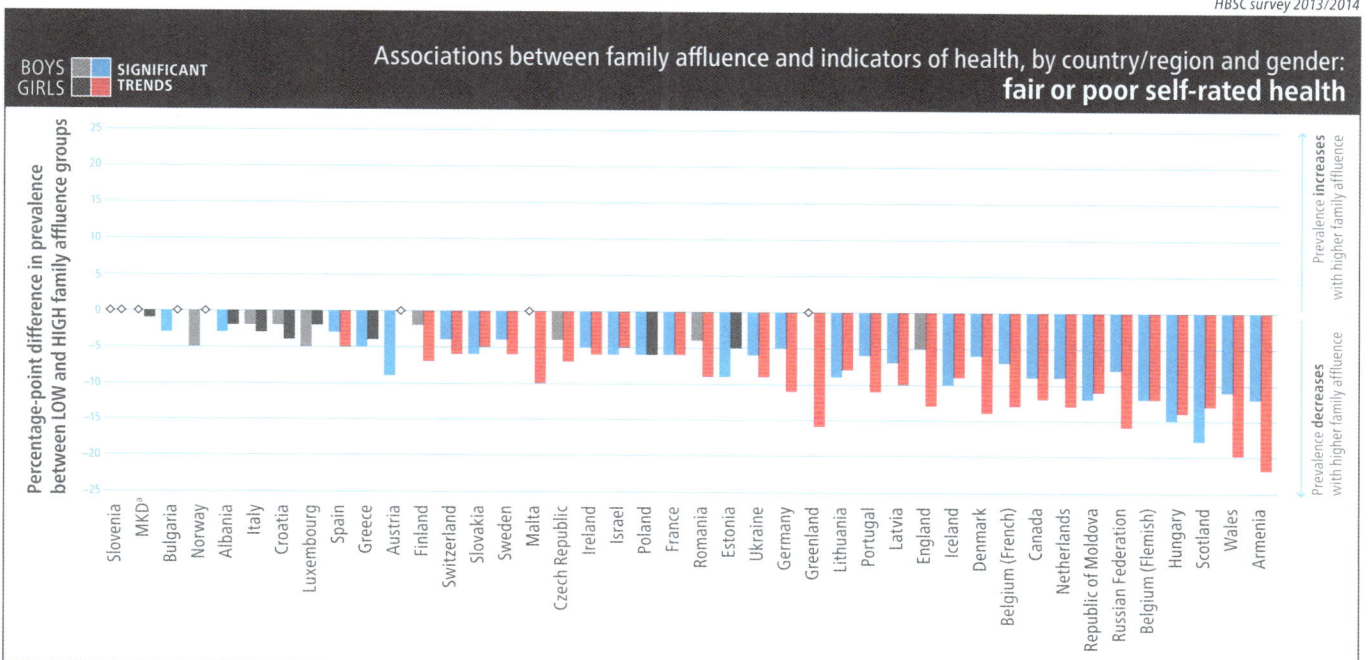

HBSC survey 2013/2014

Associations between family affluence and indicators of health, by country/region and gender: **fair or poor self-rated health**

BOYS
GIRLS | SIGNIFICANT TRENDS

Percentage-point difference in prevalence between LOW and HIGH family affluence groups

Prevalence **increases** with higher family affluence
Prevalence **decreases** with higher family affluence

Slovenia, MKDª, Bulgaria, Norway, Albania, Italy, Croatia, Luxembourg, Spain, Greece, Austria, Finland, Switzerland, Slovakia, Sweden, Malta, Czech Republic, Ireland, Israel, Poland, France, Romania, Estonia, Ukraine, Germany, Greenland, Lithuania, Portugal, Latvia, England, Iceland, Denmark, Belgium (French), Canada, Netherlands, Republic of Moldova, Russian Federation, Belgium (Flemish), Hungary, Scotland, Wales, Armenia

ª The former Yugoslav Republic of Macedonia. *Note*: low- and high-affluence groups represent the lowest 20% and highest 20% in each country. ◇ means less than +/-0.5%.

MEASURE

Young people were asked to describe their health (Would you say your health is …?). Response options were excellent, good, fair and poor.

RESULTS

Findings presented here show the proportions reporting their health as either fair or poor.

Age

Older adolescents tended to report poor or fair health more often, with the effect being stronger among girls. Three quarters of countries and regions saw an increase of 10 or more percentage points in girls between age 11 and 15, but this increase was seen in only two (Finland and Wales) for boys.

Gender

Girls reported fair or poor health more frequently across all age groups. Gender differences were significant at age 11 in only a few countries and regions, but were significant for nearly all at 15. Differences increased with increasing age.

Family affluence

A significant association with low affluence was found in most countries and regions. A difference of 10 or more percentage points between high- and low-affluence groups was observed in 17 countries and regions for girls and seven for boys.

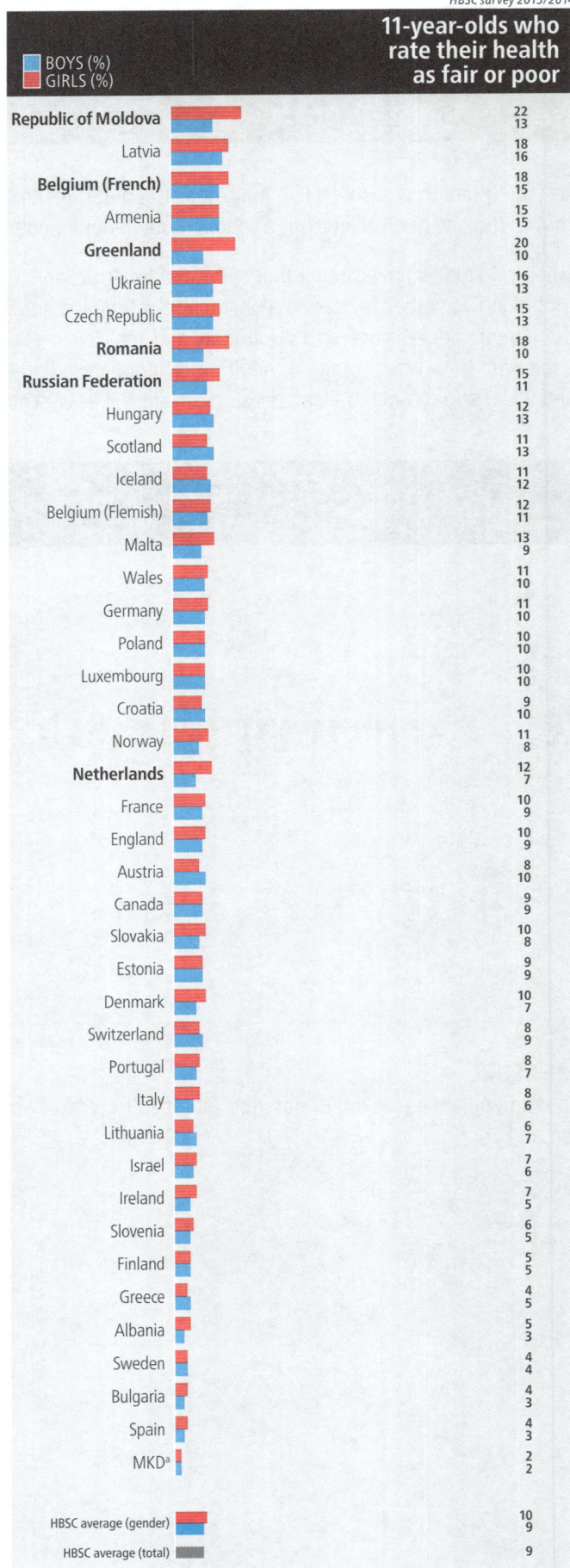

HBSC survey 2013/2014

11-year-olds who rate their health as fair or poor

BOYS (%)
GIRLS (%)

Country	Girls	Boys
Republic of Moldova	22	13
Latvia	18	16
Belgium (French)	18	15
Armenia	15	15
Greenland	20	10
Ukraine	16	13
Czech Republic	15	13
Romania	18	10
Russian Federation	15	11
Hungary	12	13
Scotland	11	13
Iceland	11	12
Belgium (Flemish)	12	11
Malta	13	9
Wales	11	10
Germany	11	10
Poland	10	10
Luxembourg	10	10
Croatia	9	10
Norway	11	8
Netherlands	12	7
France	10	9
England	10	9
Austria	8	10
Canada	9	9
Slovakia	10	8
Estonia	9	9
Denmark	10	7
Switzerland	8	9
Portugal	8	7
Italy	8	6
Lithuania	6	7
Israel	7	6
Ireland	7	5
Slovenia	6	5
Finland	5	5
Greece	4	5
Albania	5	3
Sweden	4	4
Bulgaria	4	3
Spain	4	3
MKD[a]	2	2
HBSC average (gender)	10	9
HBSC average (total)		9

[a] The former Yugoslav Republic of Macedonia.

GROWING UP UNEQUAL: GENDER AND SOCIOECONOMIC
DIFFERENCES IN YOUNG PEOPLE'S HEALTH AND WELL-BEING
PART 2. KEY DATA | CHAPTER 3. HEALTH OUTCOMES
POSITIVE HEALTH: SELF-RATED HEALTH

3

13-year-olds who rate their health as fair or poor

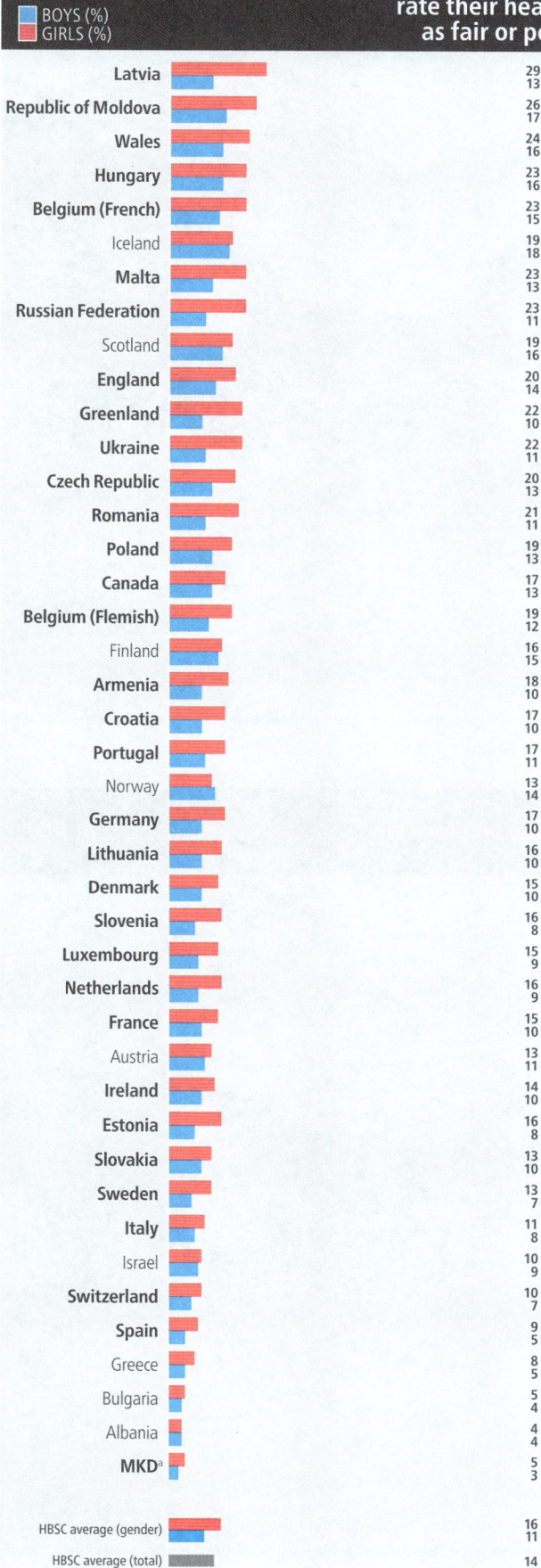

HBSC survey 2013/2014

■ BOYS (%)
■ GIRLS (%)

Country	Boys	Girls
Latvia	29	13
Republic of Moldova	26	17
Wales	24	16
Hungary	23	16
Belgium (French)	23	15
Iceland	19	18
Malta	23	13
Russian Federation	23	11
Scotland	19	16
England	20	14
Greenland	22	10
Ukraine	22	11
Czech Republic	20	13
Romania	21	11
Poland	19	13
Canada	17	13
Belgium (Flemish)	19	12
Finland	16	15
Armenia	18	10
Croatia	17	10
Portugal	17	11
Norway	13	14
Germany	17	10
Lithuania	16	10
Denmark	15	10
Slovenia	16	8
Luxembourg	15	9
Netherlands	16	9
France	15	10
Austria	13	11
Ireland	14	10
Estonia	16	8
Slovakia	13	10
Sweden	13	7
Italy	11	8
Israel	10	9
Switzerland	10	7
Spain	9	5
Greece	8	5
Bulgaria	5	4
Albania	4	4
MKD[a]	5	3
HBSC average (gender)	16	11
HBSC average (total)	14	

15-year-olds who rate their health as fair or poor

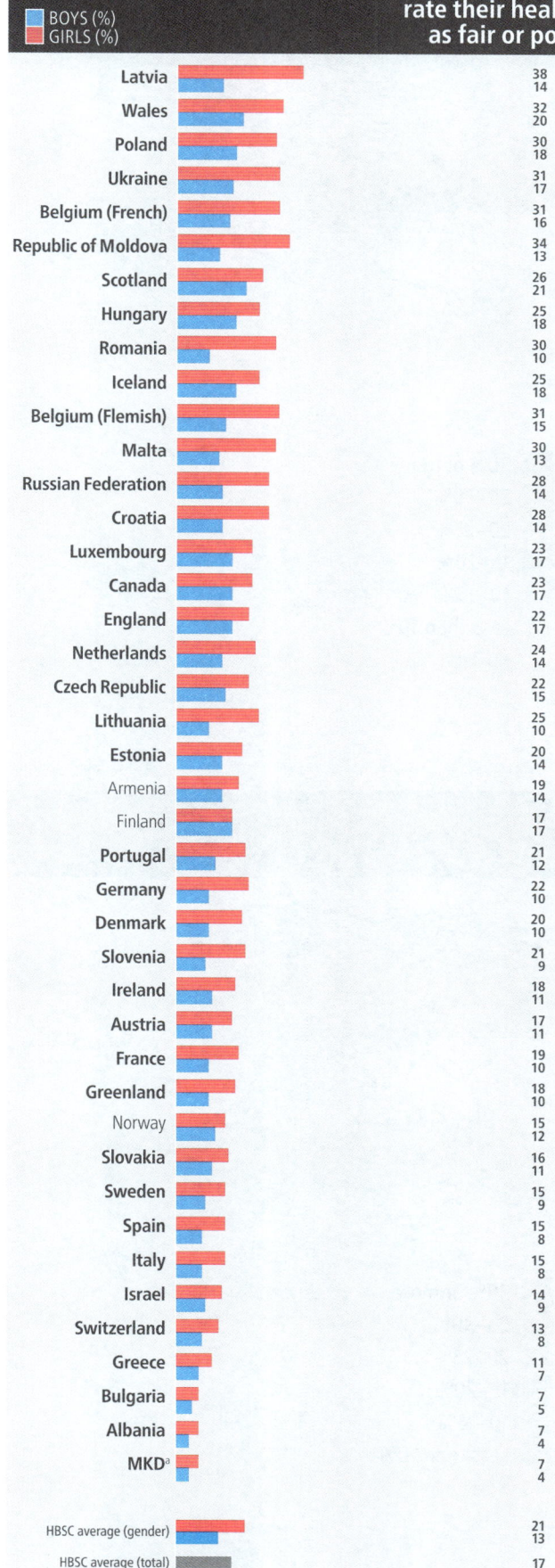

HBSC survey 2013/2014

■ BOYS (%)
■ GIRLS (%)

Country	Boys	Girls
Latvia	38	14
Wales	32	20
Poland	30	18
Ukraine	31	17
Belgium (French)	31	16
Republic of Moldova	34	13
Scotland	26	21
Hungary	25	18
Romania	30	10
Iceland	25	18
Belgium (Flemish)	31	15
Malta	30	13
Russian Federation	28	14
Croatia	28	14
Luxembourg	23	17
Canada	23	17
England	22	17
Netherlands	24	14
Czech Republic	22	15
Lithuania	25	10
Estonia	20	14
Armenia	19	14
Finland	17	17
Portugal	21	12
Germany	22	10
Denmark	20	10
Slovenia	21	9
Ireland	18	11
Austria	17	11
France	19	10
Greenland	18	10
Norway	15	12
Slovakia	16	11
Sweden	15	9
Spain	15	8
Italy	15	8
Israel	14	9
Switzerland	13	8
Greece	11	7
Bulgaria	7	5
Albania	7	4
MKD[a]	7	4
HBSC average (gender)	21	13
HBSC average (total)	17	

Note: **indicates** significant gender difference (at p<0.05).

HBSC survey 2013/2014

15-year-old girls who rate their health as fair or poor

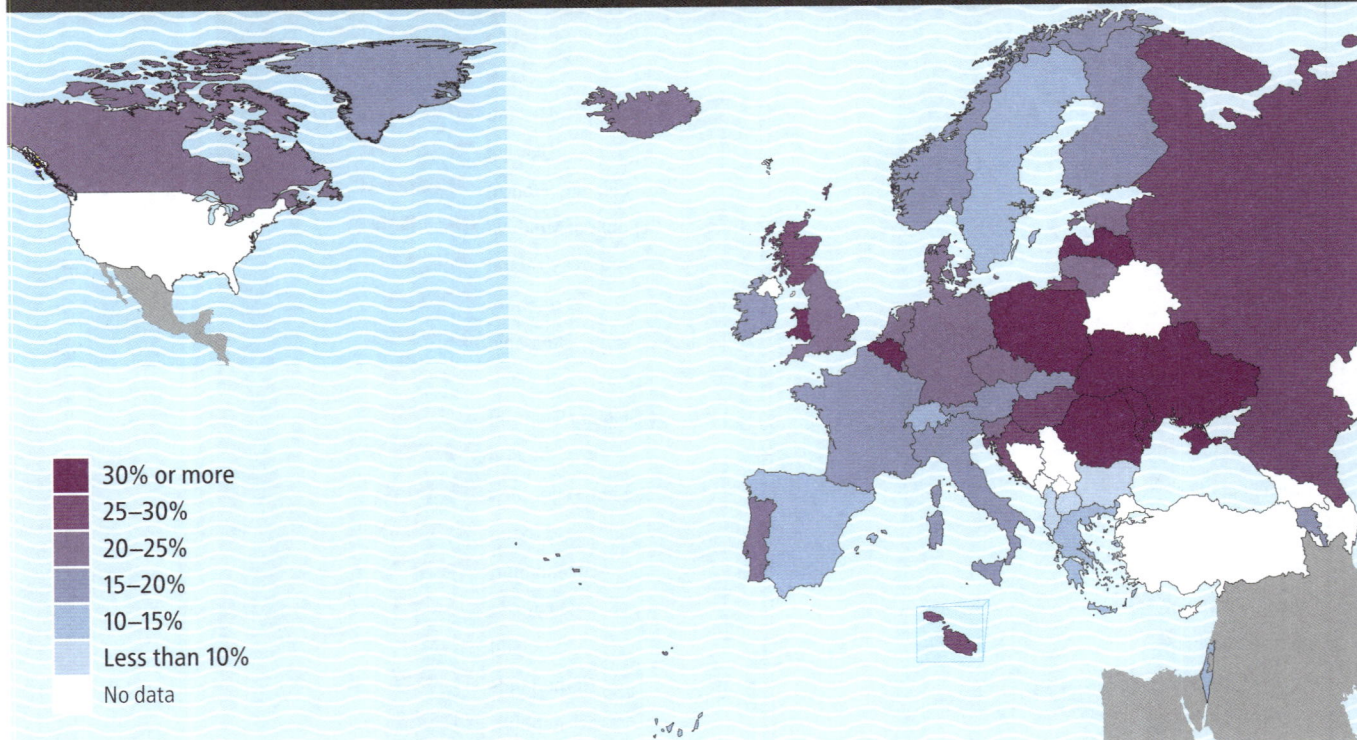

- 30% or more
- 25–30%
- 20–25%
- 15–20%
- 10–15%
- Less than 10%
- No data

Note: HBSC teams provided disaggregated data for Belgium and the United Kingdom; these data appear in the map above.

HBSC survey 2013/2014

15-year-old boys who rate their health as fair or poor

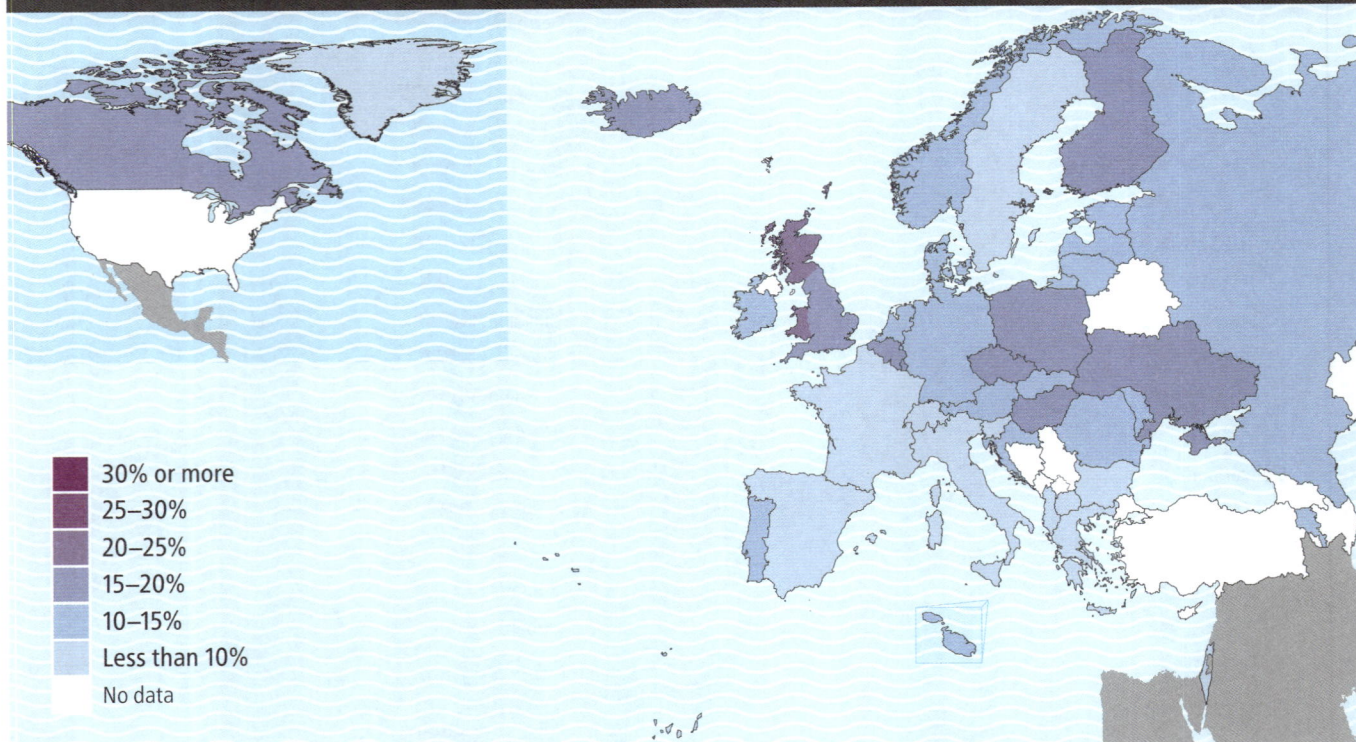

- 30% or more
- 25–30%
- 20–25%
- 15–20%
- 10–15%
- Less than 10%
- No data

Note: HBSC teams provided disaggregated data for Belgium and the United Kingdom; these data appear in the map above.

GROWING UP UNEQUAL: GENDER AND SOCIOECONOMIC
DIFFERENCES IN YOUNG PEOPLE'S HEALTH AND WELL-BEING
PART 2. KEY DATA | CHAPTER 3. HEALTH OUTCOMES

3

POSITIVE HEALTH:
LIFE SATISFACTION

Life satisfaction is closely associated with subjective health and well-being (5). It is considered to be relatively stable over time, in contrast to spontaneous feelings related to immediate experiences (6). During adolescence, it is strongly influenced by life experiences and relationships, particularly in the family environment (7–9) and with peers (10). Family structure and psychosocial factors play a role, especially in relation to self-perception and self-esteem (11–13).

The school environment is also important to adolescent life satisfaction. Acquiring academic competence constitutes one of the developmental goals of adolescence (14). Academic success has a strong positive effect on life satisfaction (15), while other factors, such as bullying, pose a risk and are associated with low life satisfaction and subjective health status (16–18). Better life satisfaction may act as a buffer against the negative effects of stress and the development of psychopathological behaviour (5).

HBSC survey 2013/2014

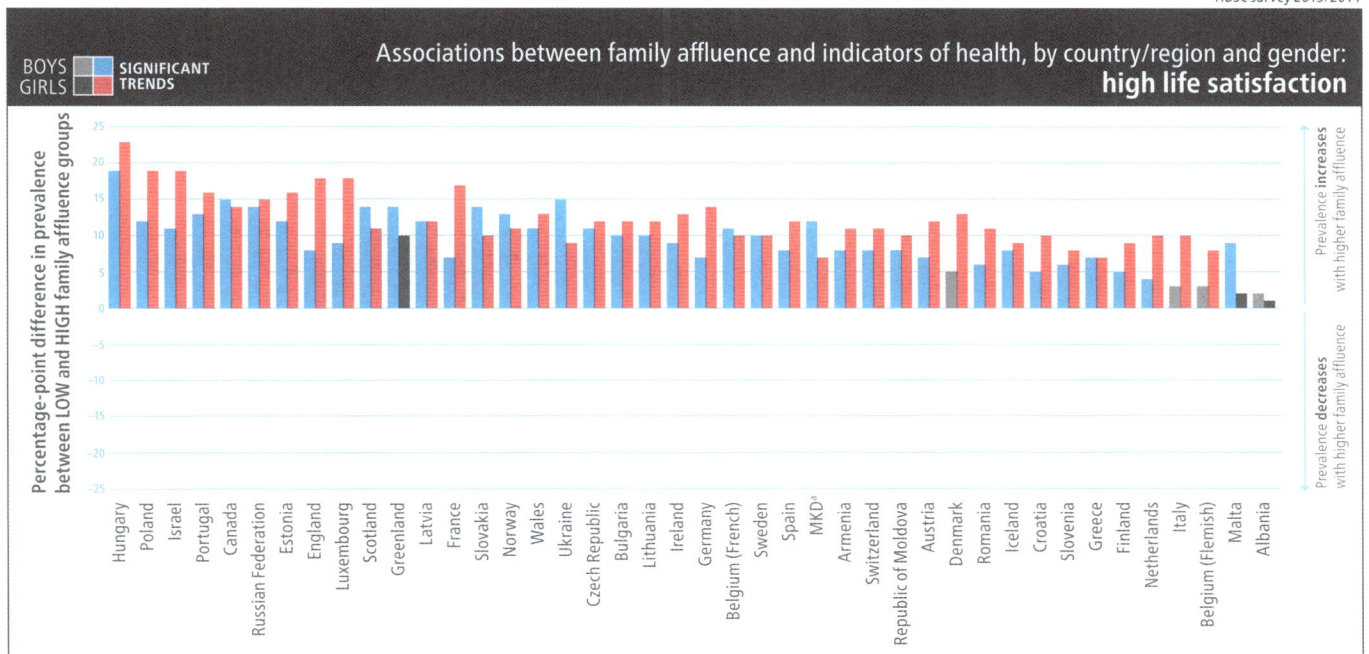

Associations between family affluence and indicators of health, by country/region and gender: **high life satisfaction**

BOYS
GIRLS

SIGNIFICANT TRENDS

Percentage-point difference in prevalence between LOW and HIGH family affluence groups

Prevalence **increases** with higher family affluence

Prevalence **decreases** with higher family affluence

[a] The former Yugoslav Republic of Macedonia. *Note:* low- and high-affluence groups represent the lowest 20% and highest 20% in each country.

MEASURE

Young people were asked to rate their life satisfaction using a visual analogue scale. The Cantril ladder has 11 steps: the top indicates the best possible life and the bottom the worst. Respondents were asked to indicate the ladder step at which they would place their lives at present (from zero to 10).

RESULTS

Findings presented here show the proportion reporting high life satisfaction, defined as a score of six or more on the Cantril ladder.

Age

Prevalence decreased with age in both genders. While the difference between age 11 and 15 was less than 10 percentage points for boys, it was 10 or more in 23 countries and regions for girls. Significant age differences were found for girls in 41 countries and regions, but in only 16 for boys.

Gender

Boys generally reported higher life satisfaction across all age groups. Gender differences increased significantly by age, emerging in only nine countries and regions for 11-year-olds but in 35 for those aged 15.

Family affluence

A significant positive association with high affluence was found for both genders in nearly all countries and regions. The social gradient in life satisfaction was significant in nearly all (38 for boys and 39 for girls).

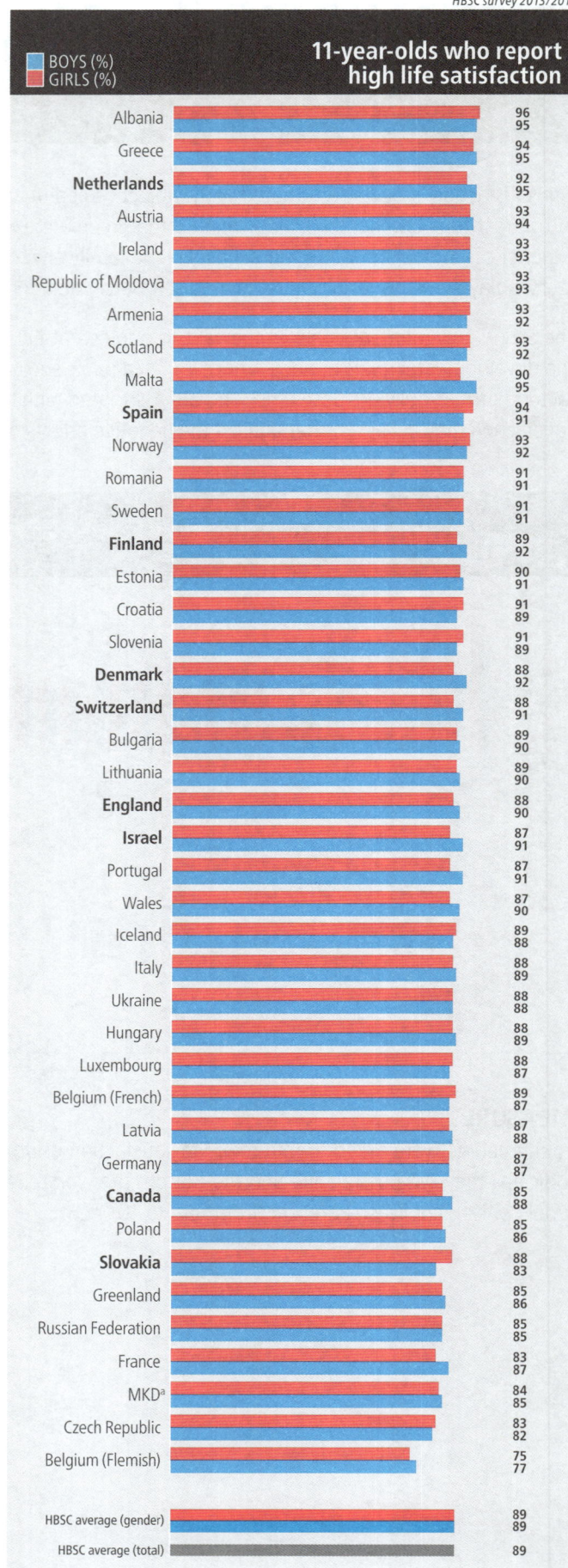

HBSC survey 2013/2014

11-year-olds who report high life satisfaction

BOYS (%)
GIRLS (%)

Country	Girls	Boys
Albania	96	95
Greece	94	95
Netherlands	92	95
Austria	93	94
Ireland	93	93
Republic of Moldova	93	93
Armenia	93	92
Scotland	93	92
Malta	90	95
Spain	94	91
Norway	93	92
Romania	91	91
Sweden	91	91
Finland	89	92
Estonia	90	91
Croatia	91	89
Slovenia	91	89
Denmark	88	92
Switzerland	88	91
Bulgaria	89	90
Lithuania	89	90
England	88	90
Israel	87	91
Portugal	87	91
Wales	87	90
Iceland	89	88
Italy	88	89
Ukraine	88	88
Hungary	88	89
Luxembourg	88	87
Belgium (French)	89	87
Latvia	87	88
Germany	87	87
Canada	85	88
Poland	85	86
Slovakia	88	83
Greenland	85	86
Russian Federation	85	85
France	83	87
MKD[a]	84	85
Czech Republic	83	82
Belgium (Flemish)	75	77
HBSC average (gender)	89	89
HBSC average (total)		89

[a] The former Yugoslav Republic of Macedonia.

GROWING UP UNEQUAL: GENDER AND SOCIOECONOMIC
DIFFERENCES IN YOUNG PEOPLE'S HEALTH AND WELL-BEING
PART 2. KEY DATA | CHAPTER 3. HEALTH OUTCOMES
POSITIVE HEALTH: LIFE SATISFACTION

3

13-year-olds who report high life satisfaction

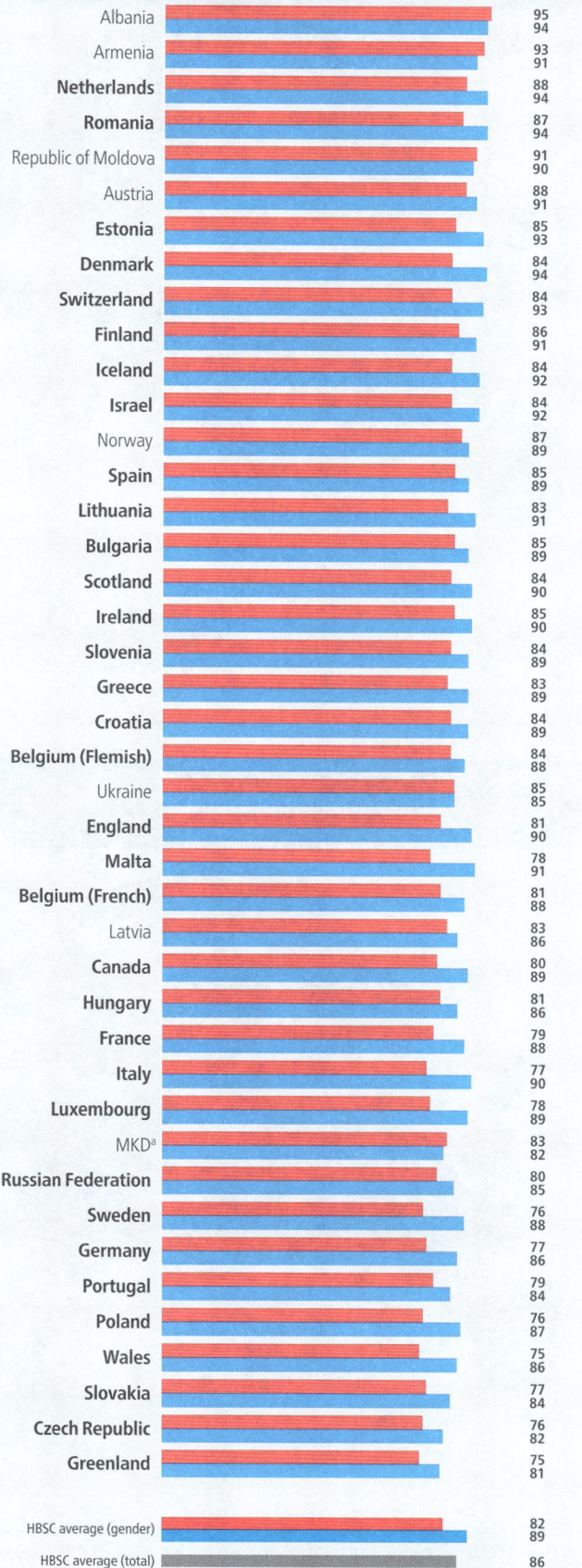

HBSC survey 2013/2014

BOYS (%) · GIRLS (%)

Country	Girls (%)	Boys (%)
Albania	95	94
Armenia	93	91
Netherlands	88	94
Romania	87	94
Republic of Moldova	91	90
Austria	88	91
Estonia	85	93
Denmark	84	94
Switzerland	84	93
Finland	86	91
Iceland	84	92
Israel	84	92
Norway	87	89
Spain	85	89
Lithuania	83	91
Bulgaria	85	89
Scotland	84	90
Ireland	85	90
Slovenia	84	89
Greece	83	89
Croatia	84	89
Belgium (Flemish)	84	88
Ukraine	85	85
England	81	90
Malta	78	91
Belgium (French)	81	88
Latvia	83	86
Canada	80	89
Hungary	81	86
France	79	88
Italy	77	90
Luxembourg	78	89
MKD[a]	83	82
Russian Federation	80	85
Sweden	76	88
Germany	77	86
Portugal	79	84
Poland	76	87
Wales	75	86
Slovakia	77	84
Czech Republic	76	82
Greenland	75	81
HBSC average (gender)	82	89
HBSC average (total)		86

15-year-olds who report high life satisfaction

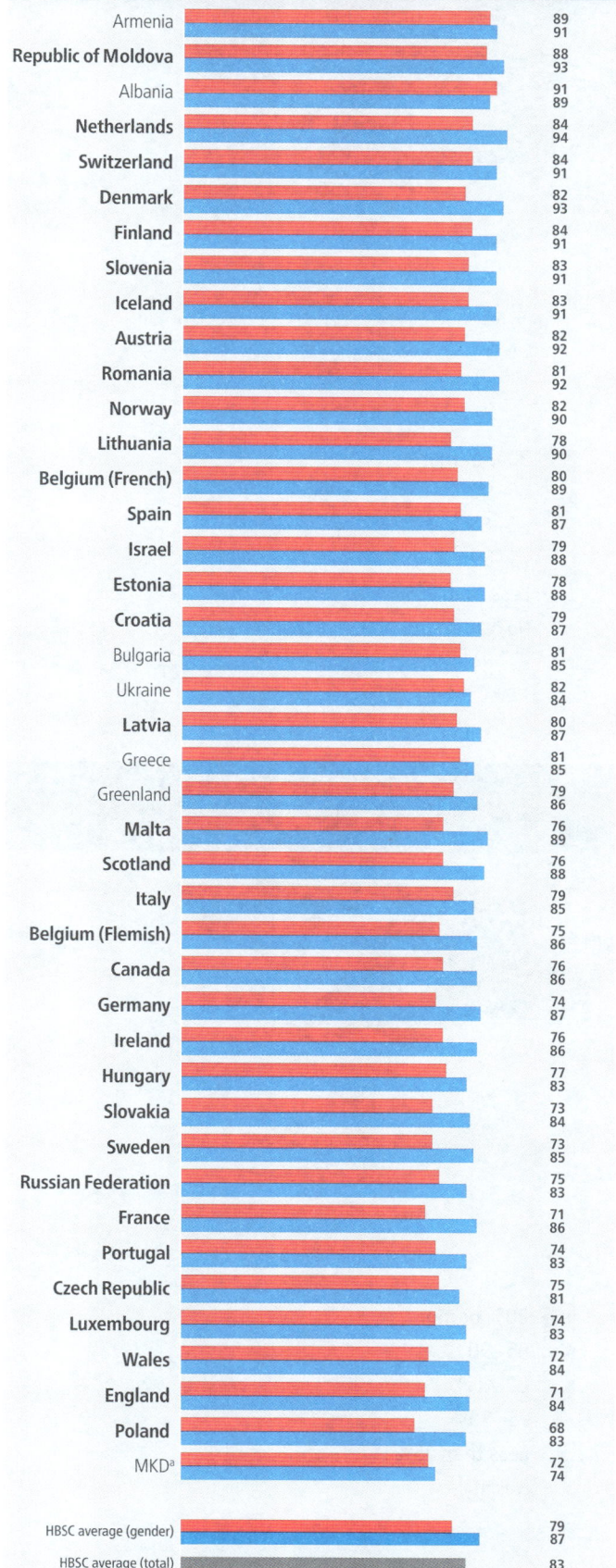

HBSC survey 2013/2014

BOYS (%) · GIRLS (%)

Country	Girls (%)	Boys (%)
Armenia	89	91
Republic of Moldova	88	93
Albania	91	89
Netherlands	84	94
Switzerland	84	91
Denmark	82	93
Finland	84	91
Slovenia	83	91
Iceland	83	91
Austria	82	92
Romania	81	92
Norway	82	90
Lithuania	78	90
Belgium (French)	80	89
Spain	81	87
Israel	79	88
Estonia	78	88
Croatia	79	87
Bulgaria	81	85
Ukraine	82	84
Latvia	80	87
Greece	81	85
Greenland	79	86
Malta	76	89
Scotland	76	88
Italy	79	85
Belgium (Flemish)	75	86
Canada	76	86
Germany	74	87
Ireland	76	86
Hungary	77	83
Slovakia	73	84
Sweden	73	85
Russian Federation	75	83
France	71	86
Portugal	74	83
Czech Republic	75	81
Luxembourg	74	83
Wales	72	84
England	71	84
Poland	68	83
MKD[a]	72	74
HBSC average (gender)	79	87
HBSC average (total)		83

Note: **indicates** significant gender difference (at p<0.05).

HBSC survey 2013/2014

15-year-old girls who report high life satisfaction

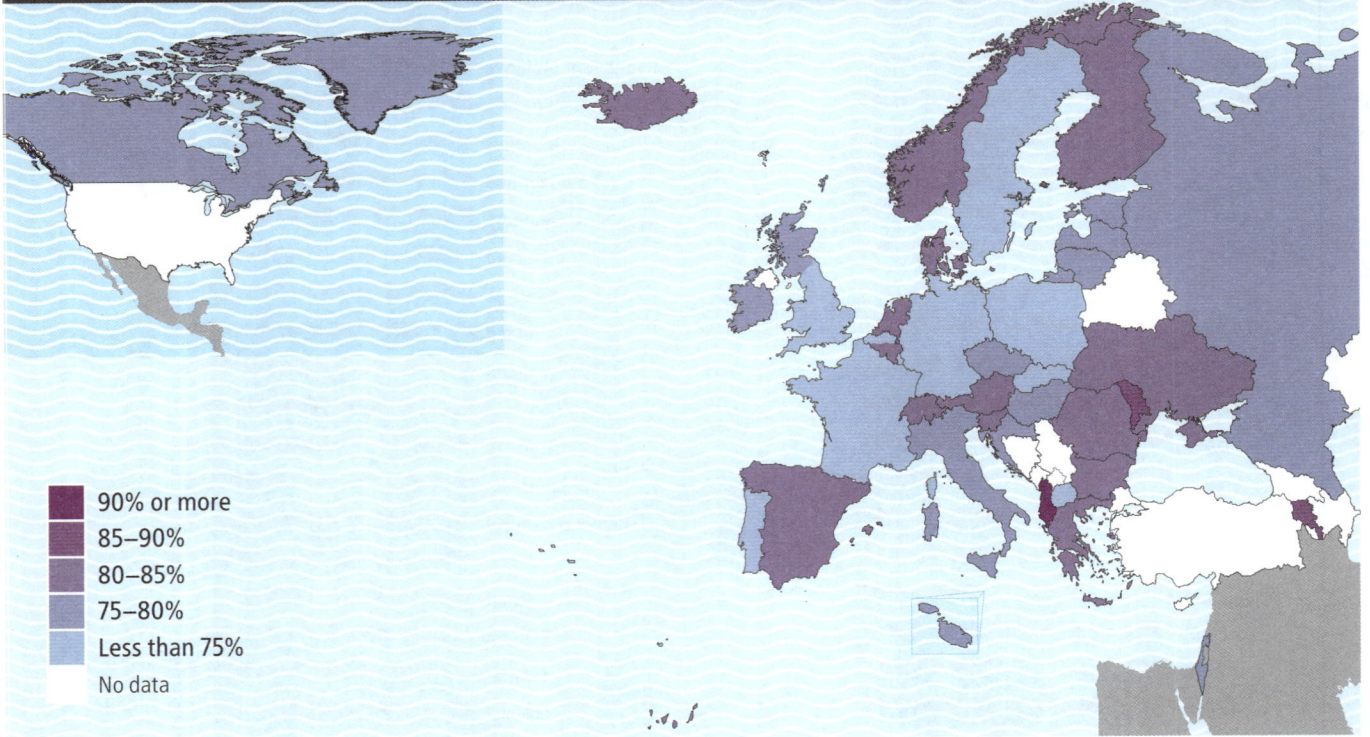

90% or more
85–90%
80–85%
75–80%
Less than 75%
No data

Note: HBSC teams provided disaggregated data for Belgium and the United Kingdom; these data appear in the map above.

HBSC survey 2013/2014

15-year-old boys who report high life satisfaction

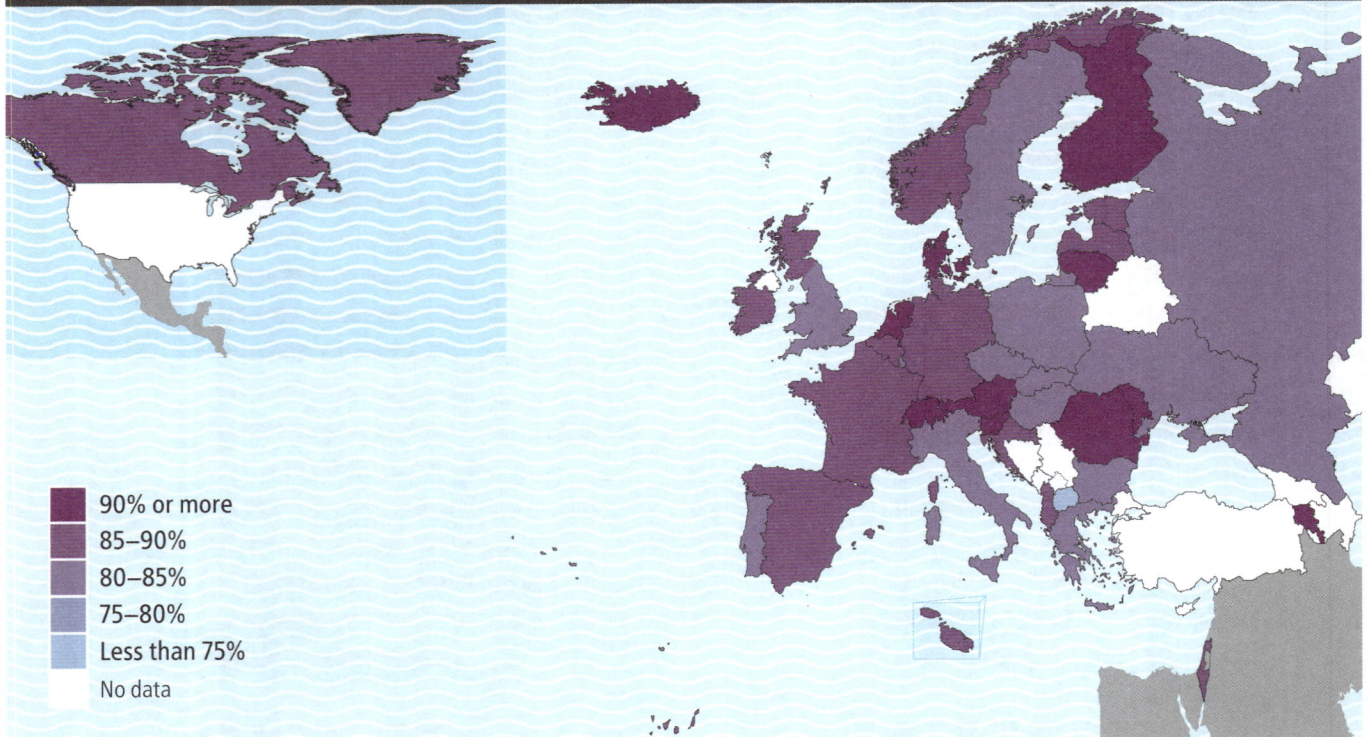

90% or more
85–90%
80–85%
75–80%
Less than 75%
No data

Note: HBSC teams provided disaggregated data for Belgium and the United Kingdom; these data appear in the map above.

GROWING UP UNEQUAL: GENDER AND SOCIOECONOMIC
DIFFERENCES IN YOUNG PEOPLE'S HEALTH AND WELL-BEING
PART 2. KEY DATA | CHAPTER 3. HEALTH OUTCOMES

3

POSITIVE HEALTH:
MULTIPLE HEALTH COMPLAINTS

Having multiple health complaints is an important indicator for measuring subjective well-being, as it reflects individual burden and personal experience related to negative life events in the social context of family, school and peers (18–23). Multiple health complaints are highly prevalent among adolescents cross-nationally (24–27).

Age and gender differences and socioeconomic inequality in multiple health complaints have been recognized (23,28–32). Their recurrence negatively affects adolescents' everyday functioning and general well-being (33–39).

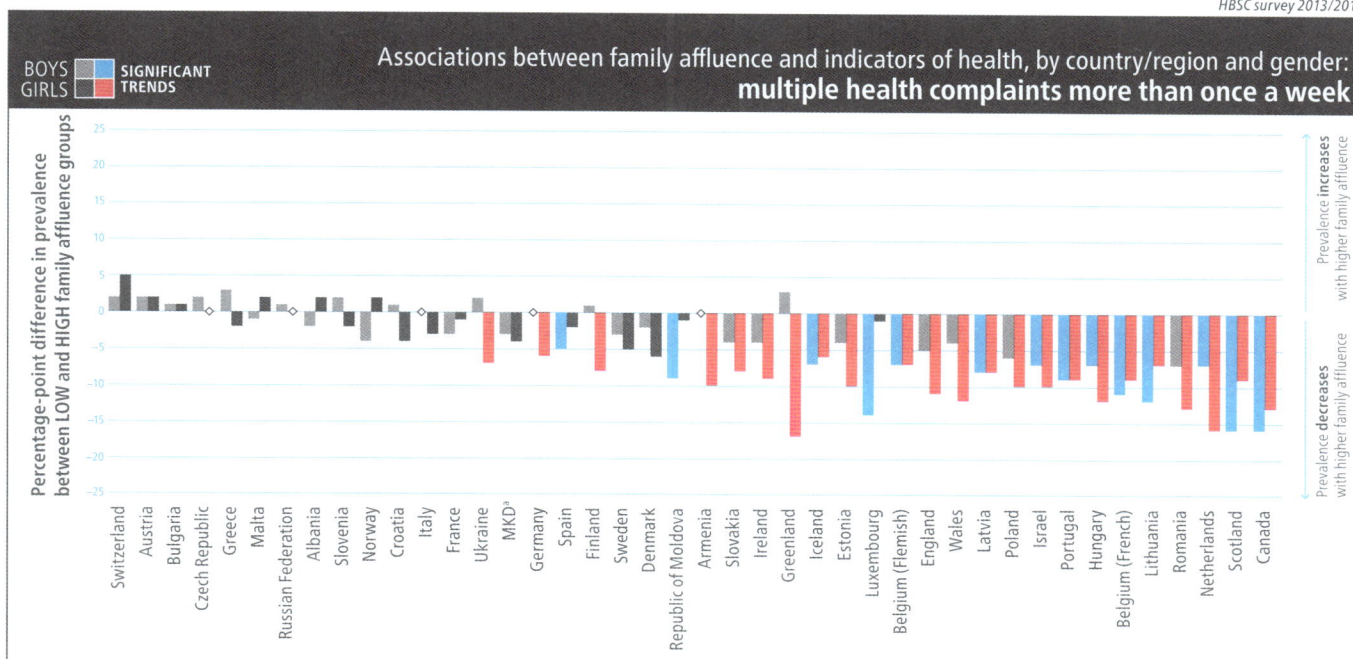

HBSC survey 2013/2014

Associations between family affluence and indicators of health, by country/region and gender:
multiple health complaints more than once a week

BOYS / GIRLS — SIGNIFICANT TRENDS

a The former Yugoslav Republic of Macedonia. *Note:* low- and high-affluence groups represent the lowest 20% and highest 20% in each country. ◇ means less than +/-0.5%.

MEASURE

Young people were asked how often they had experienced the following symptoms in the last six months: headache; stomach ache; backache; feeling low, irritable or bad tempered; feeling nervous; difficulties in getting to sleep; and feeling dizzy. Response options for each symptom ranged from about every day to rarely or never. This presents a nonclinical measure of psychosomatic complaints and a sum-score scale that can be used for cross-national comparison (39).

Supplementary data on headache, stomach ache, feeling low, feeling nervous and sleep difficulties are provided in the Annex.

RESULTS

Findings presented here show the proportions with multiple (two or more) health complaints more than once a week in the past six months.

Age

Prevalence increased with age among girls in all countries and regions and in 14 for boys. The difference between girls aged 11 and 15 was more than 20 percentage points in 16.

Gender

Generally, girls were more likely to report multiple health complaints, with differences in prevalence increasing with age. Six countries showed no significant difference between gender groups at age 11, but gender differences were observed in all at ages 13 and 15.

Family affluence

A significant social gradient in at least one gender was found in 26 countries and regions (14 for boys and 23 for girls), with higher prevalence being associated with low family affluence.

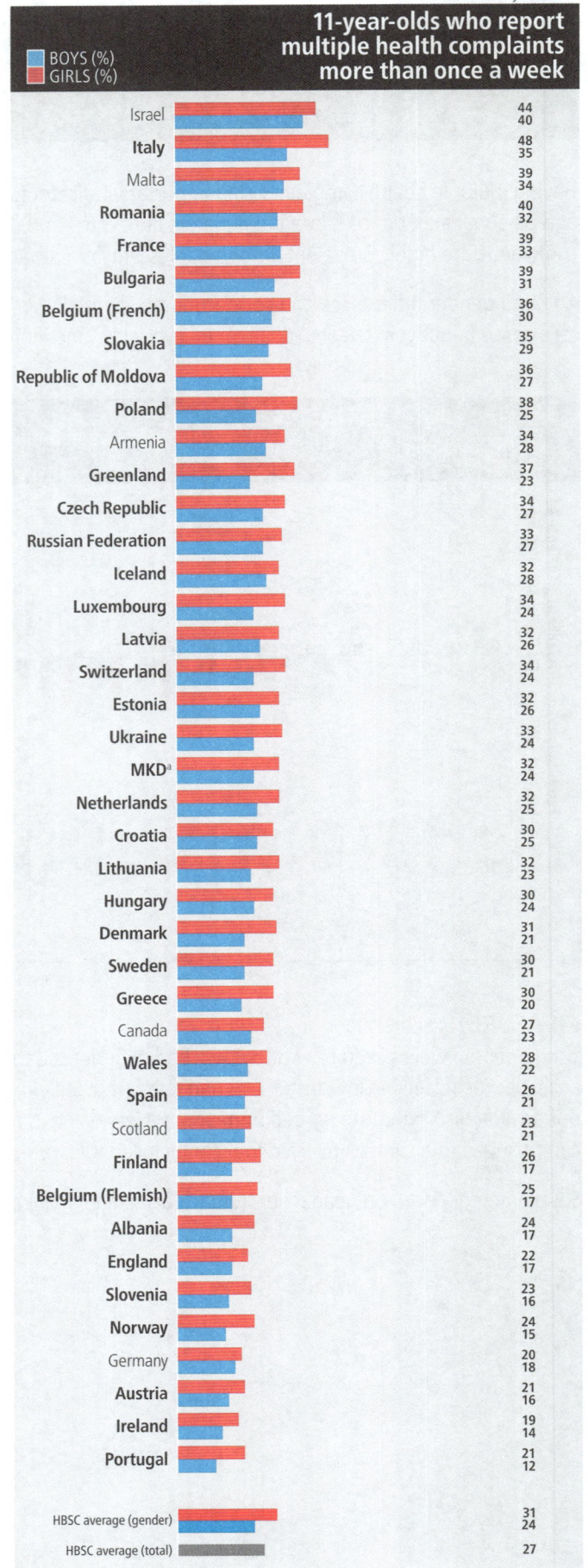

HBSC survey 2013/2014

11-year-olds who report multiple health complaints more than once a week

BOYS (%)
GIRLS (%)

Country	Boys (%)	Girls (%)
Israel	40	44
Italy	35	48
Malta	34	39
Romania	32	40
France	33	39
Bulgaria	31	39
Belgium (French)	30	36
Slovakia	29	35
Republic of Moldova	27	36
Poland	25	38
Armenia	28	34
Greenland	23	37
Czech Republic	27	34
Russian Federation	27	33
Iceland	28	32
Luxembourg	24	34
Latvia	26	32
Switzerland	24	34
Estonia	26	32
Ukraine	24	33
MKD[a]	24	32
Netherlands	25	32
Croatia	25	30
Lithuania	23	32
Hungary	24	30
Denmark	21	31
Sweden	21	30
Greece	20	30
Canada	23	27
Wales	22	28
Spain	21	26
Scotland	21	23
Finland	17	26
Belgium (Flemish)	17	25
Albania	17	24
England	17	22
Slovenia	16	23
Norway	15	24
Germany	18	20
Austria	16	21
Ireland	14	19
Portugal	12	21
HBSC average (gender)	24	31
HBSC average (total)		27

[a] The former Yugoslav Republic of Macedonia.

GROWING UP UNEQUAL: GENDER AND SOCIOECONOMIC
DIFFERENCES IN YOUNG PEOPLE'S HEALTH AND WELL-BEING
PART 2. KEY DATA | CHAPTER 3. HEALTH OUTCOMES
POSITIVE HEALTH: MULTIPLE HEALTH COMPLAINTS

3

13-year-olds who report multiple health complaints more than once a week

HBSC survey 2013/2014

■ BOYS (%)
■ GIRLS (%)

	Girls	Boys
Italy	61	34
Israel	52	40
France	52	34
Bulgaria	50	34
Slovakia	48	32
Malta	48	30
Belgium (French)	48	30
Luxembourg	48	27
MKD[a]	45	30
Greece	48	28
Greenland	48	25
Romania	49	26
Poland	47	28
Sweden	46	27
Armenia	41	29
Czech Republic	43	27
Hungary	44	26
Republic of Moldova	42	28
Iceland	39	29
Latvia	44	23
Croatia	41	26
Lithuania	41	23
Russian Federation	39	23
Netherlands	39	24
Wales	40	23
Spain	40	23
Switzerland	39	23
Scotland	39	23
England	39	22
Estonia	40	22
Belgium (Flemish)	36	25
Ireland	34	22
Finland	37	22
Slovenia	39	19
Canada	38	19
Albania	35	20
Denmark	36	18
Ukraine	32	17
Austria	30	19
Norway	32	16
Germany	31	16
Portugal	31	15
HBSC average (gender)	41	25
HBSC average (total)		33

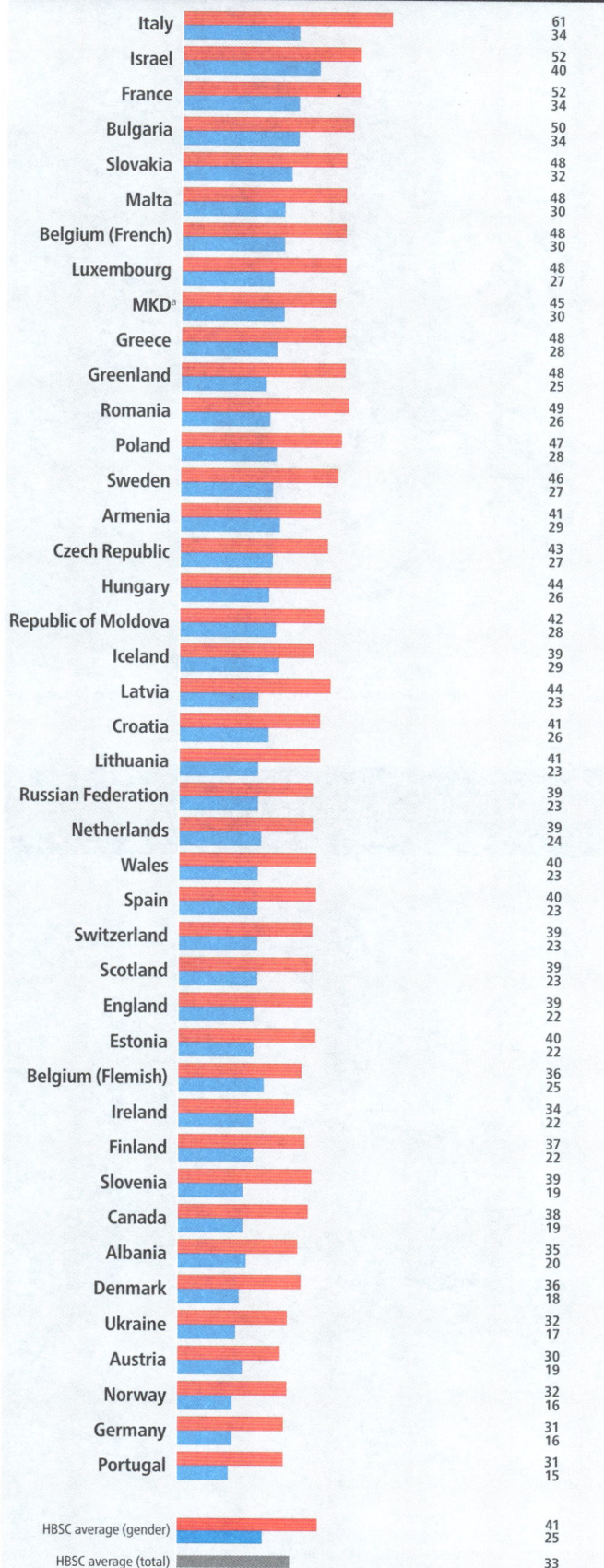

15-year-olds who report multiple health complaints more than once a week

HBSC survey 2013/2014

■ BOYS (%)
■ GIRLS (%)

	Girls	Boys
Malta	65	44
Italy	68	38
Israel	56	43
Bulgaria	60	36
France	60	34
Poland	54	36
Belgium (French)	54	35
Sweden	57	31
Luxembourg	55	32
Ireland	51	29
Latvia	55	29
MKD[a]	53	32
Greece	56	28
Romania	54	26
Scotland	54	29
Albania	52	29
Republic of Moldova	53	29
Armenia	46	33
Hungary	50	29
Slovakia	51	30
Greenland	48	29
England	51	28
Iceland	50	28
Canada	51	27
Czech Republic	48	28
Russian Federation	45	29
Wales	47	27
Lithuania	51	23
Estonia	46	25
Slovenia	48	21
Spain	45	23
Croatia	47	21
Netherlands	46	20
Ukraine	40	22
Switzerland	41	22
Belgium (Flemish)	46	22
Norway	42	19
Finland	39	21
Denmark	39	19
Germany	41	18
Portugal	41	16
Austria	36	18
HBSC average (gender)	50	27
HBSC average (total)		39

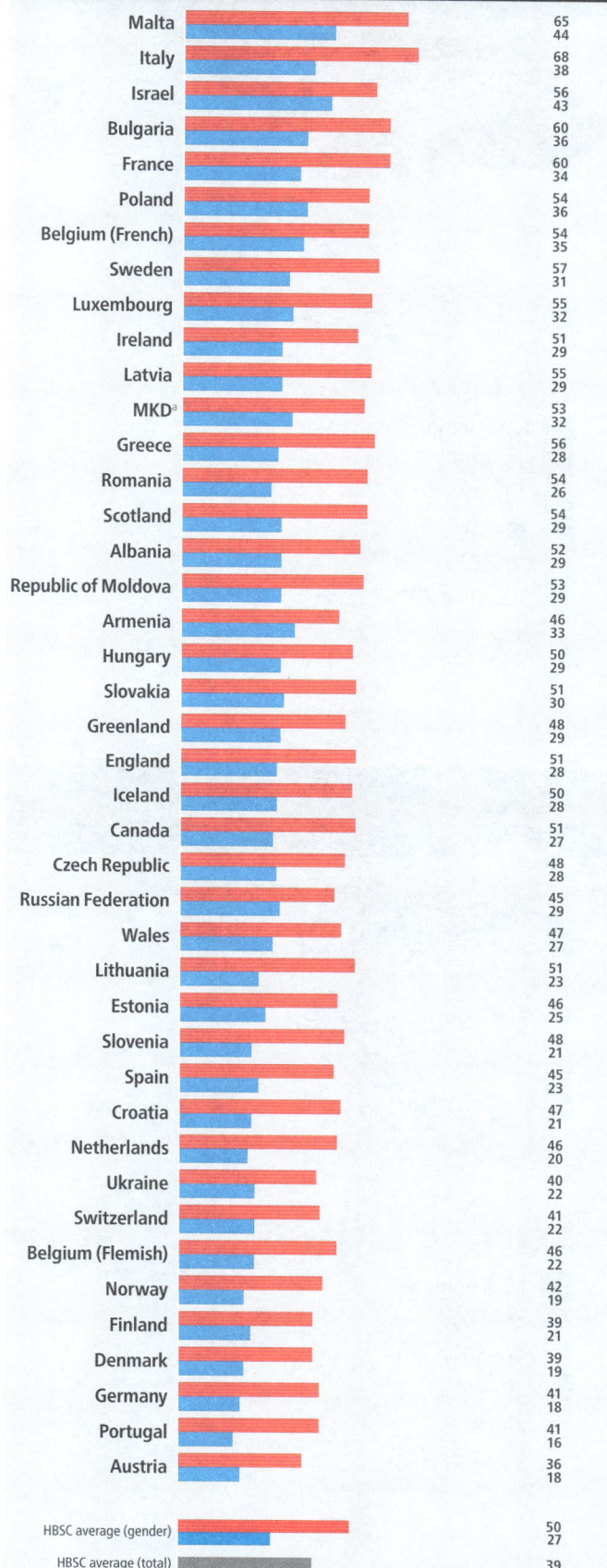

*Note: **indicates** significant gender difference (at p<0.05).*

HBSC survey 2013/2014

15-year-old girls who report multiple health complaints more than once a week

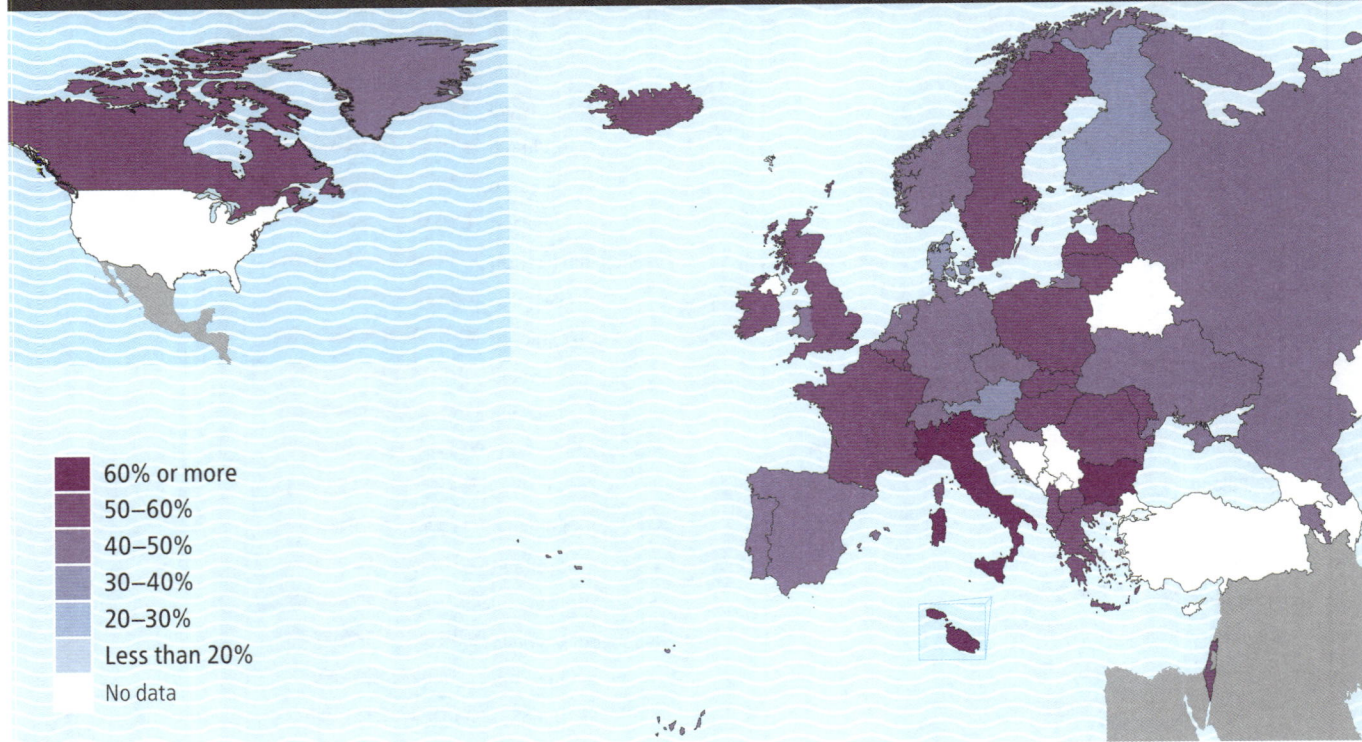

- 60% or more
- 50–60%
- 40–50%
- 30–40%
- 20–30%
- Less than 20%
- No data

Note: HBSC teams provided disaggregated data for Belgium and the United Kingdom; these data appear in the map above.

HBSC survey 2013/2014

15-year-old boys who report multiple health complaints more than once a week

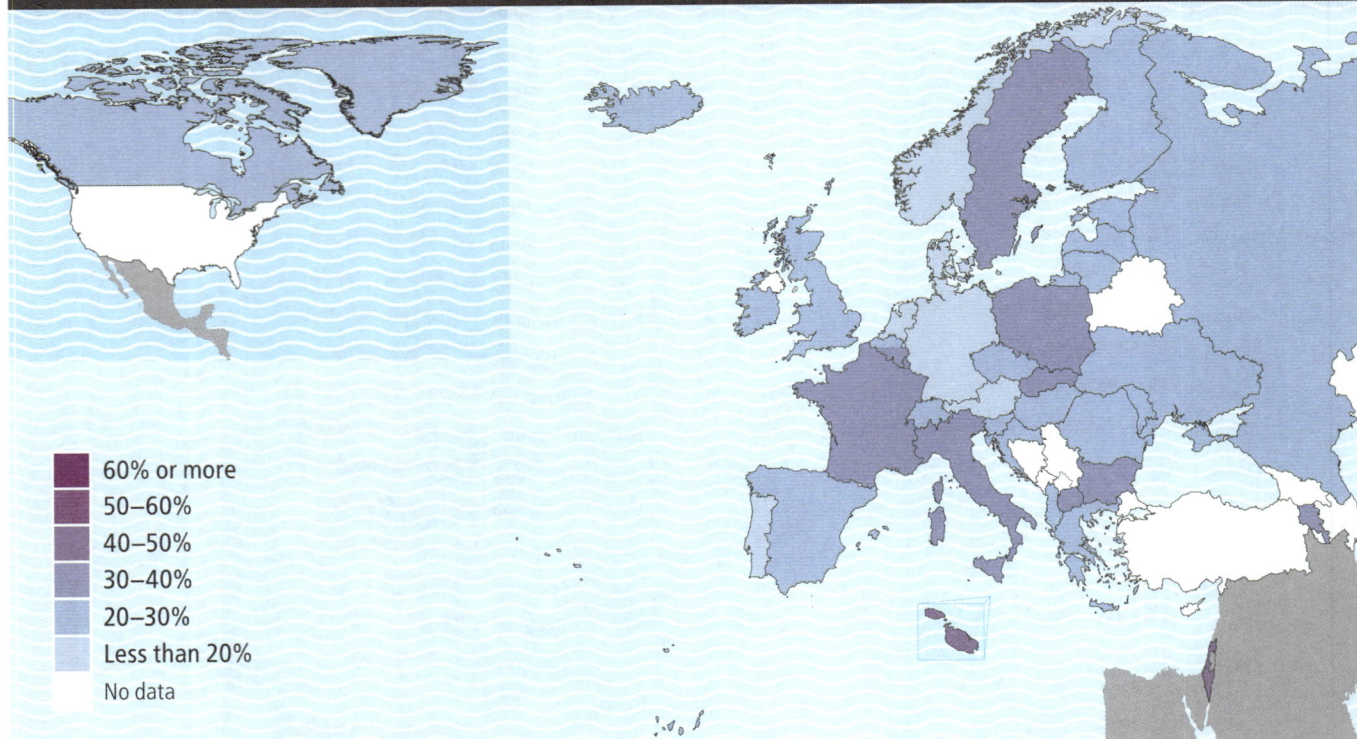

- 60% or more
- 50–60%
- 40–50%
- 30–40%
- 20–30%
- Less than 20%
- No data

Note: HBSC teams provided disaggregated data for Belgium and the United Kingdom; these data appear in the map above.

GROWING UP UNEQUAL: GENDER AND SOCIOECONOMIC
DIFFERENCES IN YOUNG PEOPLE'S HEALTH AND WELL-BEING
PART 2. KEY DATA | CHAPTER 3. HEALTH OUTCOMES
POSITIVE HEALTH

3

POSITIVE HEALTH:
SCIENTIFIC DISCUSSION AND POLICY REFLECTIONS

SCIENTIFIC DISCUSSION

Significant age, gender and social inequalities emerge for all subjective health outcomes (self-rated health, life satisfaction and health complaints) among 11–15-year-old adolescents who attend mainstream education systems.

Adolescents have many common health problems regardless of country or region of residence, but prevalence differs by country/region, age and gender. The prevalence of poor subjective health outcomes increases with age and afflicts girls more than boys, with the gender gap also increasing with age. There is substantial cross-national variation in the prevalence of subjective health outcomes, especially for self-rated health and multiple health complaints.

A consistent significant association emerges between low relative affluence and poor subjective health. Family wealth may have an indirect effect on health, however, and more proximal determinants should be investigated.

The results confirm that the psychosocial dimension of health is very important in the second decade of life, when adolescents undergo many physical, social, psychological and cognitive changes that prepare them for adulthood. Resilience to constant change may differ depending on societal and cultural background.

Poor health outcomes may result in long-term negative effects on everyday functioning and general well-being, leading to social exclusion.

POLICY REFLECTIONS

The burden of deterioration in adolescent subjective health should be recognized in public health policy and practice, taking into account health needs according to age and gender. There is a need to go beyond the provision of services towards the creation of structural changes incorporated in health in all policies (HiAP) or as health impact assessment initiatives (40).

Systematic social inequalities in adolescents (applicable to both genders and for all three subjective health outcomes) are found in eight countries and regions, and no social gradient in only one. Each country and region should review local policies to determine to what extent they address social determinants and how they should be tackled.

Gender differences are found in all measures, with girls reporting lower levels of perceived health and life satisfaction and more frequent health complaints. These increase with age. Efforts need to be made to address this clear gender-difference issue.

Screening and counselling for more sensitive mental health issues should be provided as part of routine preventive care to ensure a balance between physical and mental health (41). In addition to family wealth, other well recognized and interrelated social determinants of health in adolescence (such as access to high-quality education, developing personal skills, social support and safe neighbourhoods) should be addressed to increase understandings of pathways and mechanisms of inequity.

REFERENCES

1. Idler EL, Benyamini Y. Self-rated health and mortality: a review of 27 community studies. J Health Soc Behav. 1997;38(1):21–37.

2. Addressing the socioeconomic determinants of healthy eating habits and physical activity levels among adolescents: report from the 2006 HBSC/WHO Forum. Copenhagen: WHO Regional Office for Europe; 2006 (http://www.euro.who.int/__data/assets/pdf_file/0005/98231/e89375.pdf, accessed 24 August 2015).

3. Breidablik HJ, Meland E, Lydersen S. Self-rated health in adolescence: a multifactorial composite. Scand J Public Health 2008;36(1):12–20.

4. de Matos MG, Barrett P, Dadds M, Shortt A. Anxiety, depression and peer relationships during adolescence: results from the Portuguese national health behaviour in school-aged children survey. Eur J Psychol Educ. 2003;18(1):3–14.

5. Huebner ES, Suldo SM, Smith LC, McKnight CG. Life satisfaction in children and youth: empirical foundations and implications for school psychologists. Psychol Sch. 2004;41(1):81–93.

6. Pavot WG, Diener E. Review of the satisfaction with life scale. Psychol Assess. 1993;5(2):164–72.

7. Edwards LM, Lopez SJ. Perceived family support, acculturation, and life satisfaction in Mexican American youth: a mixed-methods exploration. J Couns Psychol. 2006;53(3):279–87.

8. Gohm CL, Oishi S, Darlington J, Diener E. Culture, parental conflict, parental marital status, and the subjective well-being of young adults. J Marriage Fam. 1998;60(2):319–34.

9. Rask K, Astedt-Kurki P, Paavilainen E, Laippala P. Adolescent subjective well-being and family dynamics. Scand J Caring Sci. 2003;17(2):129–38.

10. Gaspar T. Health-related quality of life in children and adolescents: personal and social factors that promote quality of life. Saarbrücken: Lambert Academic; 2010.

11. Zullig K, Valois R, Huebner ES, Drane JW. Associations among family structure, demographics, and adolescent perceived life satisfaction. J Child Fam Stud. 2005;14(2):195–206.

12. Piko BF. Satisfaction with life, psychosocial health and materialism among Hungarian youth. J Health Psychol. 2006;11(6):827–31.

13. Levin KA, Currie C. Reliability and validity of adapted version of the Cantril ladder for use with adolescent sample. Soc Indic Res. 2014;119(2):1047–63.

14. Hurrelmann K, Lösel F. Basic issues and problem of health in adolescence. In: Hurrelmann K, Lösel F, editors. Health hazards in adolescence. Berlin: Walter de Gruyter; 1990:1–21.

15. Katja R, Paivi AK, Marja-Terttu T, Pekka L. Relationships among adolescent subjective well-being, health behavior, and school satisfaction. J School Health 2002;72(6):243–9.

16. Gobina I, Zaborskis A, Pudule I, Kalnins I, Villerusa A. Bullying and subjective health among adolescents at schools in Latvia and Lithuania. Int J Public Health 2008;53(5):272–6.

17. Torsheim T, Wold B. School-related stress, school support, and somatic complaints: a general population study. J Adolescent Res. 2001;16(3):293–303.

18. Gaspar T, Matos MG, Ribeiro JP, Leal I, Albergaria F. Psychosocial factors related to bullying and victimization in children and adolescents. Health Behav Policy Rev. 2014;1(6):452–9.

19. Due P, Holstein BE, Lynch J, Diderichsen F, Gabhain SN, Scheidt P et al. Bullying and symptoms among school-aged children: international comparative cross sectional study in 28 countries. Eur J Public Health 2005;15(2):128–32.

20. Hjern A, Alfven G, Östberg V. School stressors, psychological complaints and psychosomatic pain. Acta Paediatr. 2008;97(1):112–7.

21. Moreno C, Sánchez-Queija I, Muñoz-Tinoco V, de Matos MG, Dallago L, Bogt TT et al. Cross-national associations between parent and peer communication and psychological complaints. Int J Public Health 2009;54(2):235–42.

22. Eriksson U, Sellstrom E. School demands and subjective health complaints among Swedish schoolchildren: a multilevel study. Scand J Public Health 2010;38(4):344–50.

23. Ottová-Jordan V, Smith OR, Augustine L, Gobina I, Rathmann K, Torsheim T et al. Trends in health complaints from 2002 to 2010 in 34 countries and their association with health behaviours and social context factors at individual and macro-level. Eur J Public Health 2015;25(Suppl. 2):83–9.

24. Berntsson LT, Kohler L. Comparison between 1984 and 1996. Eur J Public Health 2001;11(1):35–42.

25. Santalahti P, Aromma M, Sourander A, Helenius H, Piha J. Have there been changes in children's psychosomatic symptoms? A 10-year comparison from Finland. Pediatrics 2005;115(4):e434–42.

26. Ravens-Sieberer U, Torsheim T, Hetland J, Vollebergh W, Cavallo F, Jericek H et al. Subjective health, symptom load and quality of life of children and adolescents in Europe. Int J Public Health 2009;54(Suppl. 2):151–9.

27. Ottová-Jordan V, Smith OR, Gobina I, Mazur J, Augustine L, Cavallo F et al. Trends in multiple recurrent health complaints in 15-year-olds in 35 countries in Europe, North America and Israel from 1994 to 2010. Eur J Public Health 2015;25(Suppl. 2):24–7.

28. Torsheim T, Ravens-Sieberer U, Hetland J, Välimaa R, Danielson M, Overpeck M. Cross-national variation of gender differences in adolescent subjective health in Europe and North America. Soc Sci Med. 2006;62(4):815–27.

29. Cavallo F, Zambon A, Borraccino A, Raven-Sieberer U, Torsheim T, Lemma P. Girls growing through adolescence have a higher risk of poor health. Qual Life Res. 2006;15(10):1577–85.

30. Holstein BE, Currie C, Boyce W, Damsgaard MT, Gobina I, Kökönyei G et al. Socio-economic inequality in multiple health complaints among adolescents: international comparative study in 37 countries. Int J Public Health 2009;54(Suppl. 2):260–70.

31. Hagquist C. Discrepant trends in mental health complaints among younger and older adolescents in Sweden: an analysis of WHO data 1985–2005. J Adolesc Health 2010;46(3):258–64.

32. Ottova V, Erhart M, Vollebergh W, Kokonyei G, Morgan A, Gobina I et al. The role of individual and macro-level social determinants on young adolescents' psychosomatic complaints. J Early Adolesc. 2012;32(1):126–58.

33. Vingilis E, Wade T, Seeley J. Predictors of adolescent health care utilization. J Adolesc. 2007;30(5):773–800.

34. Shannon RA, Bergren MD, Matthews A. Frequent visitors: somatization in school-age children and implications for school nurses. J Sch Nurs. 2010;26(3):169–82.

35. Gobina I, Välimaa R, Tynjälä J, Villberg J, Villerusa A, Iannotti RJ et al. The medicine use and corresponding subjective health complaints among adolescents, a cross-national survey. Pharmacoepidemiol Drug Saf. 2011;20(4):424–31.

36. Saps M, Seshadri R, Sztainberg M, Schaffer G, Marshall BM, Di Lorenzo C. A prospective school-based study of abdominal pain and other common somatic complaints in children. J Pediatr. 2009;154(3):322–6.

37. Wood JJ, Lynne-Landsman SD, Langer DA, Wood PA, Clark SL, Eddy JM et al. School attendance problems and youth psychopathology: structural cross-lagged regression models in three longitudinal data sets. Child Dev. 2012;83(1):351–66.

38. Erhart M, Ottova V, Gaspar T, Jericek H, Schnohr C, Alikasifoglu M et al. Measuring mental health and well-being of school-children in 15 European countries using the KIDSCREEN–10 Index. Int J Public Health 2009;54(2):160–6.

GROWING UP UNEQUAL: GENDER AND SOCIOECONOMIC
DIFFERENCES IN YOUNG PEOPLE'S HEALTH AND WELL-BEING
PART 2. KEY DATA | CHAPTER 3. HEALTH OUTCOMES
POSITIVE HEALTH

3

39. Ravens-Sieberer U, Erhart M, Torsheim T, Hetland J, Freeman J, Danielson M et al. An international scoring system for self-reported health complaints in adolescents. Eur J Public Health 2008;18(3):294–9.

40. Woolf SH, Purnell JQ, Simon SM, Zimmerman EB, Camberos GJ, Haley A et al. Translating evidence into population health improvement: strategies and barriers. Annu Rev Public Health 2015;36:463–82.

41. Ozer EM, Zahnd EG, Adams SH, Husting SR, Wibbelsman CJ, Norman KP et al. Are adolescents being screened for emotional distress in primary care? J Adolesc Health 2009;44(6):520–7.

GROWING UP UNEQUAL: GENDER AND SOCIOECONOMIC
DIFFERENCES IN YOUNG PEOPLE'S HEALTH AND WELL-BEING
PART 2. KEY DATA | CHAPTER 3. HEALTH OUTCOMES

3

MEDICALLY ATTENDED INJURIES

Injury is a public health concern in adolescence (1) and one of the leading causes of death among young people globally (1,2). Many established individual risk factors and correlates for adolescent injury exist: common examples include substance misuse (3), violence (4), time engaged in sport (5) and SES (6). Trend analysis over the past decade has not shown consistent changes in levels of morbidity despite advances in injury prevention (7).

HBSC survey 2013/2014

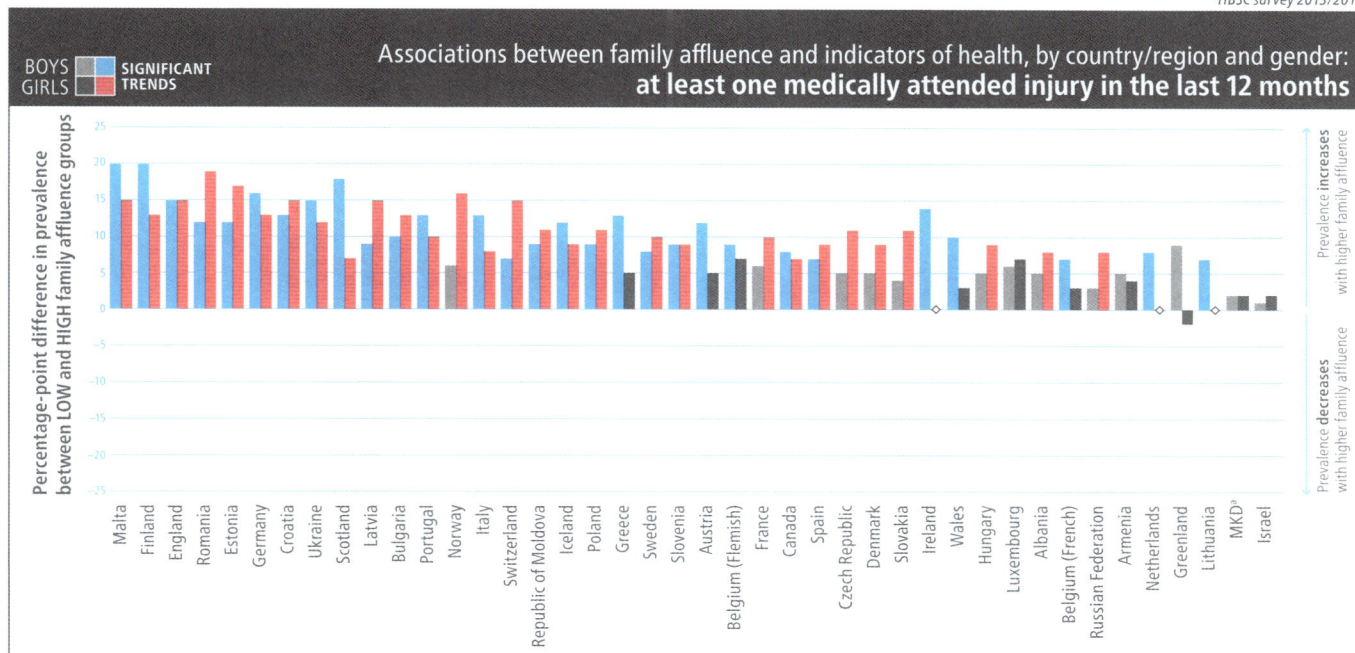

Associations between family affluence and indicators of health, by country/region and gender: **at least one medically attended injury in the last 12 months**

BOYS / GIRLS — SIGNIFICANT TRENDS

ᵃ The former Yugoslav Republic of Macedonia. *Note:* low- and high-affluence groups represent the lowest 20% and highest 20% in each country. ◇ means less than +/-0.5%.

MEASURE

Young people were asked how many times over the last 12 months they had been injured and needed to be treated by a doctor or nurse. Response options ranged from no injury to four times or more.

Supplementary data on prevalence of most serious injury requiring medical treatment, such as placement of a cast, stitches, surgery or hospitalization, are provided in the Annex.

RESULTS

Findings presented here show the proportions who reported having a medically attended injury at least once in the last 12 months.

Age

Overall average prevalence for boys was around 48%, with levels remaining high at ages 11 and 13 and falling slightly by 15. A similar pattern was seen for girls, with an overall average prevalence of 38% and higher levels at 11 and 13, dropping slightly at 15. Prevalence increased with age in a few countries. Cross-national differences in prevalence were large.

Gender

Boys were injured more at all ages in almost all countries and regions.

Family affluence

Differences across affluence status were seen in almost all countries and regions for boys and girls, with injury prevalence associated with high affluence.

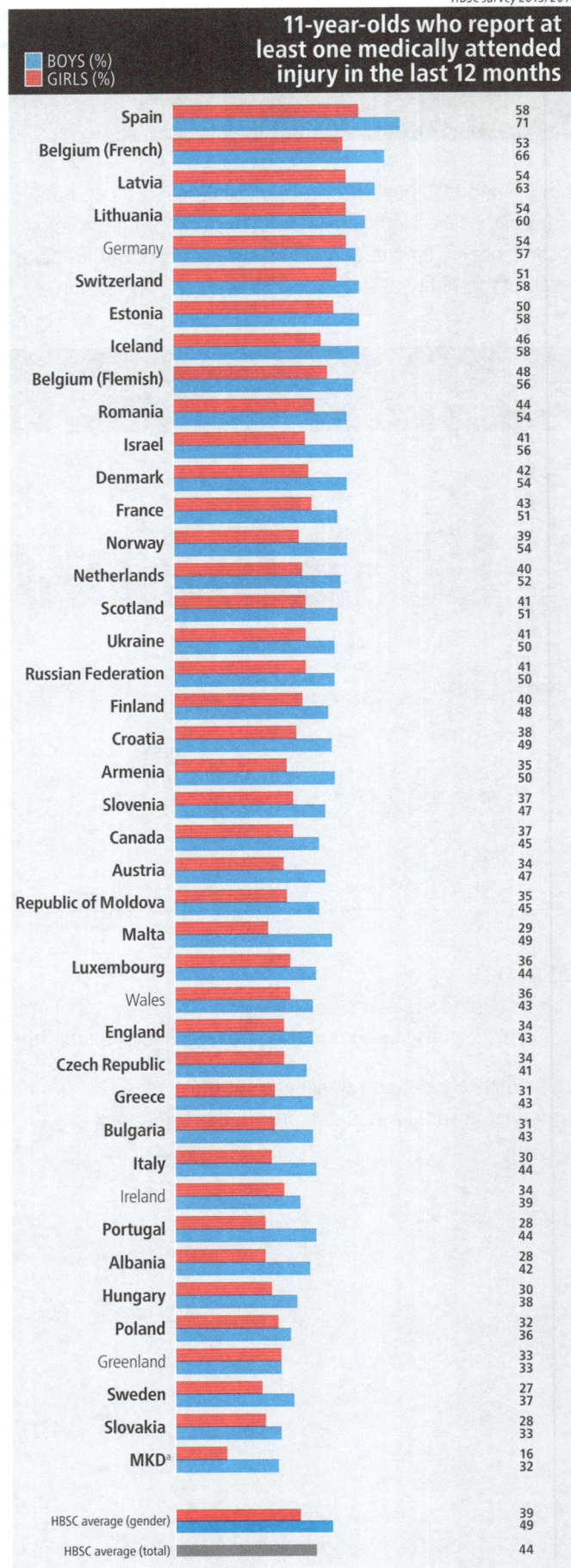

HBSC survey 2013/2014

11-year-olds who report at least one medically attended injury in the last 12 months

BOYS (%)
GIRLS (%)

Country	Girls	Boys
Spain	58	71
Belgium (French)	53	66
Latvia	54	63
Lithuania	54	60
Germany	54	57
Switzerland	51	58
Estonia	50	58
Iceland	46	58
Belgium (Flemish)	48	56
Romania	44	54
Israel	41	56
Denmark	42	54
France	43	51
Norway	39	54
Netherlands	40	52
Scotland	41	51
Ukraine	41	50
Russian Federation	41	50
Finland	40	48
Croatia	38	49
Armenia	35	50
Slovenia	37	47
Canada	37	45
Austria	34	47
Republic of Moldova	35	45
Malta	29	49
Luxembourg	36	44
Wales	36	43
England	34	43
Czech Republic	34	41
Greece	31	43
Bulgaria	31	43
Italy	30	44
Ireland	34	39
Portugal	28	44
Albania	28	42
Hungary	30	38
Poland	32	36
Greenland	33	33
Sweden	27	37
Slovakia	28	33
MKD[a]	16	32
HBSC average (gender)	39	49
HBSC average (total)		44

[a] The former Yugoslav Republic of Macedonia.

GROWING UP UNEQUAL: GENDER AND SOCIOECONOMIC
DIFFERENCES IN YOUNG PEOPLE'S HEALTH AND WELL-BEING
PART 2. KEY DATA | CHAPTER 3. HEALTH OUTCOMES
MEDICALLY ATTENDED INJURIES

3

HBSC survey 2013/2014

13-year-olds who report at least one medically attended injury in the last 12 months

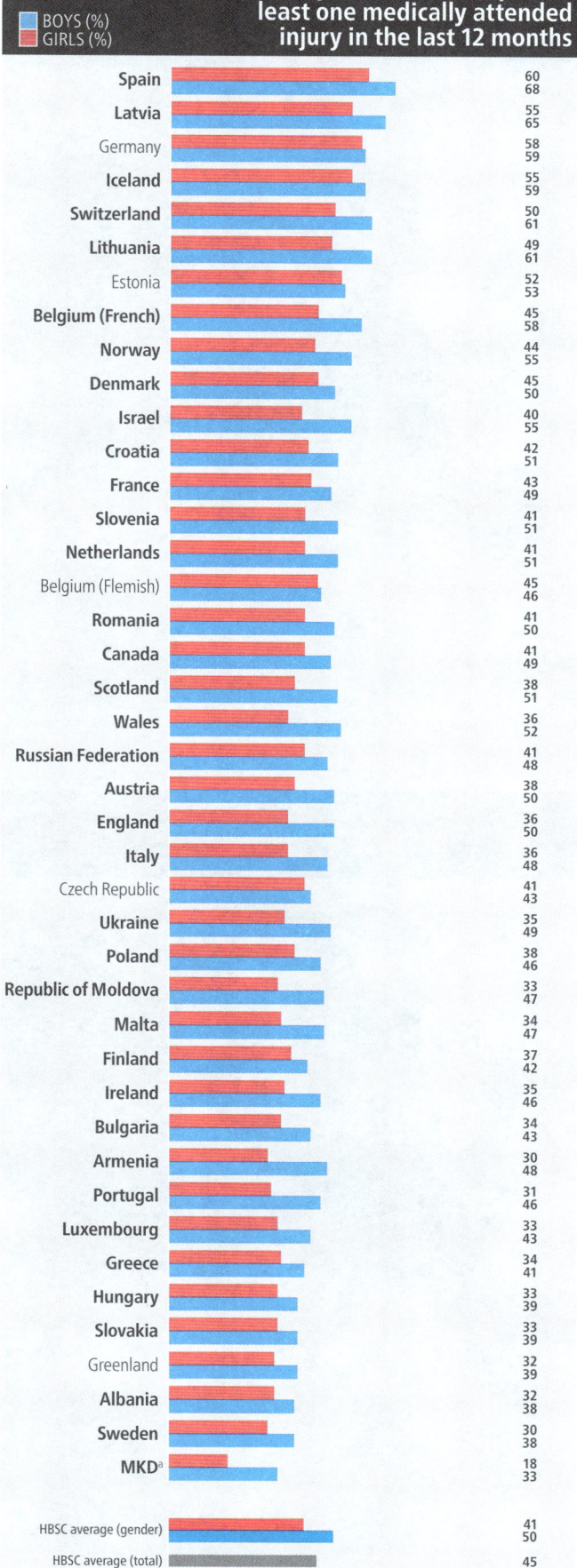

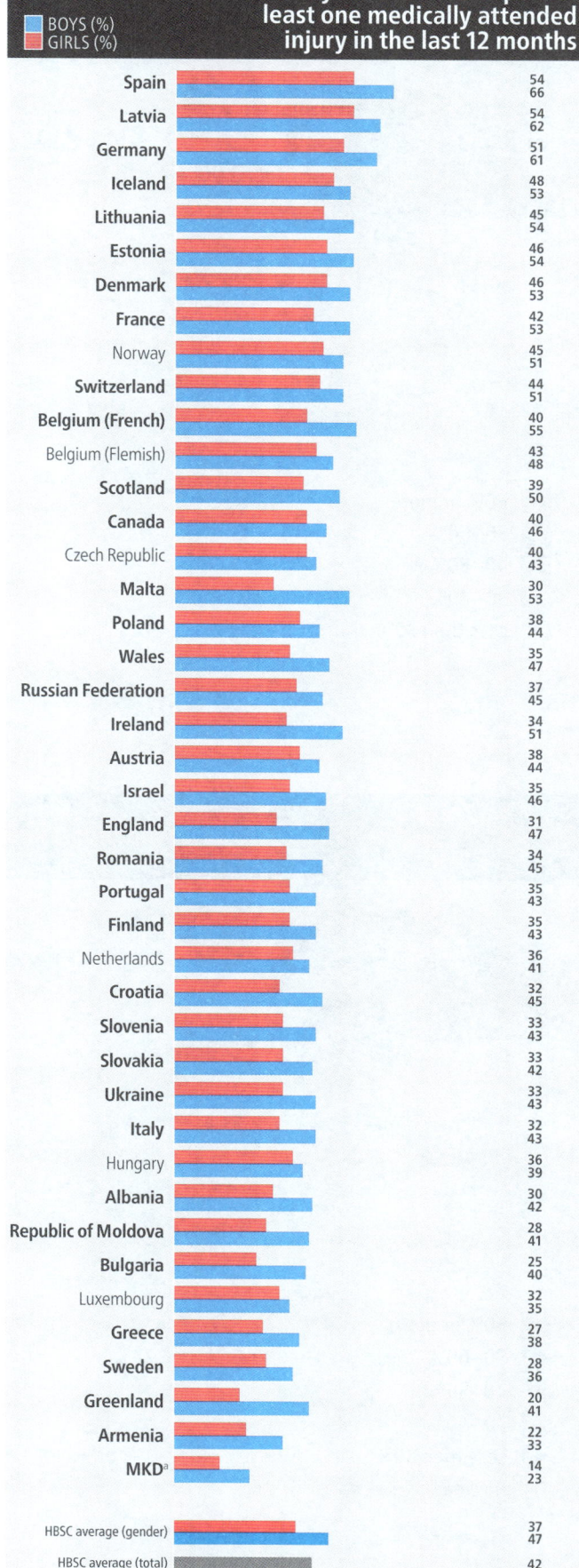

- **BOYS (%)**
- **GIRLS (%)**

Country	Girls	Boys
Spain	60	68
Latvia	55	65
Germany	58	59
Iceland	55	59
Switzerland	50	61
Lithuania	49	61
Estonia	52	53
Belgium (French)	45	58
Norway	44	55
Denmark	45	50
Israel	40	55
Croatia	42	51
France	43	49
Slovenia	41	51
Netherlands	41	51
Belgium (Flemish)	45	46
Romania	41	50
Canada	41	49
Scotland	38	51
Wales	36	52
Russian Federation	41	48
Austria	38	50
England	36	50
Italy	36	48
Czech Republic	41	43
Ukraine	35	49
Poland	38	46
Republic of Moldova	33	47
Malta	34	47
Finland	37	42
Ireland	35	46
Bulgaria	34	43
Armenia	30	48
Portugal	31	46
Luxembourg	33	43
Greece	34	41
Hungary	33	39
Slovakia	33	39
Greenland	32	39
Albania	32	38
Sweden	30	38
MKD[a]	18	33
HBSC average (gender)	41	50
HBSC average (total)		45

HBSC survey 2013/2014

15-year-olds who report at least one medically attended injury in the last 12 months

- **BOYS (%)**
- **GIRLS (%)**

Country	Girls	Boys
Spain	54	66
Latvia	54	62
Germany	51	61
Iceland	48	53
Lithuania	45	54
Estonia	46	54
Denmark	46	53
France	42	53
Norway	45	51
Switzerland	44	51
Belgium (French)	40	55
Belgium (Flemish)	43	48
Scotland	39	50
Canada	40	46
Czech Republic	40	43
Malta	30	53
Poland	38	44
Wales	35	47
Russian Federation	37	45
Ireland	34	51
Austria	38	44
Israel	35	46
England	31	47
Romania	34	45
Portugal	35	43
Finland	35	43
Netherlands	36	41
Croatia	32	45
Slovenia	33	43
Slovakia	33	42
Ukraine	33	43
Italy	32	43
Hungary	36	39
Albania	30	42
Republic of Moldova	28	41
Bulgaria	25	40
Luxembourg	32	35
Greece	27	38
Sweden	28	36
Greenland	20	41
Armenia	22	33
MKD[a]	14	23
HBSC average (gender)	37	47
HBSC average (total)		42

*Note: **indicates** significant gender difference (at p<0.05).*

HBSC survey 2013/2014

15-year-old girls who report at least one medically attended injury in the last 12 months

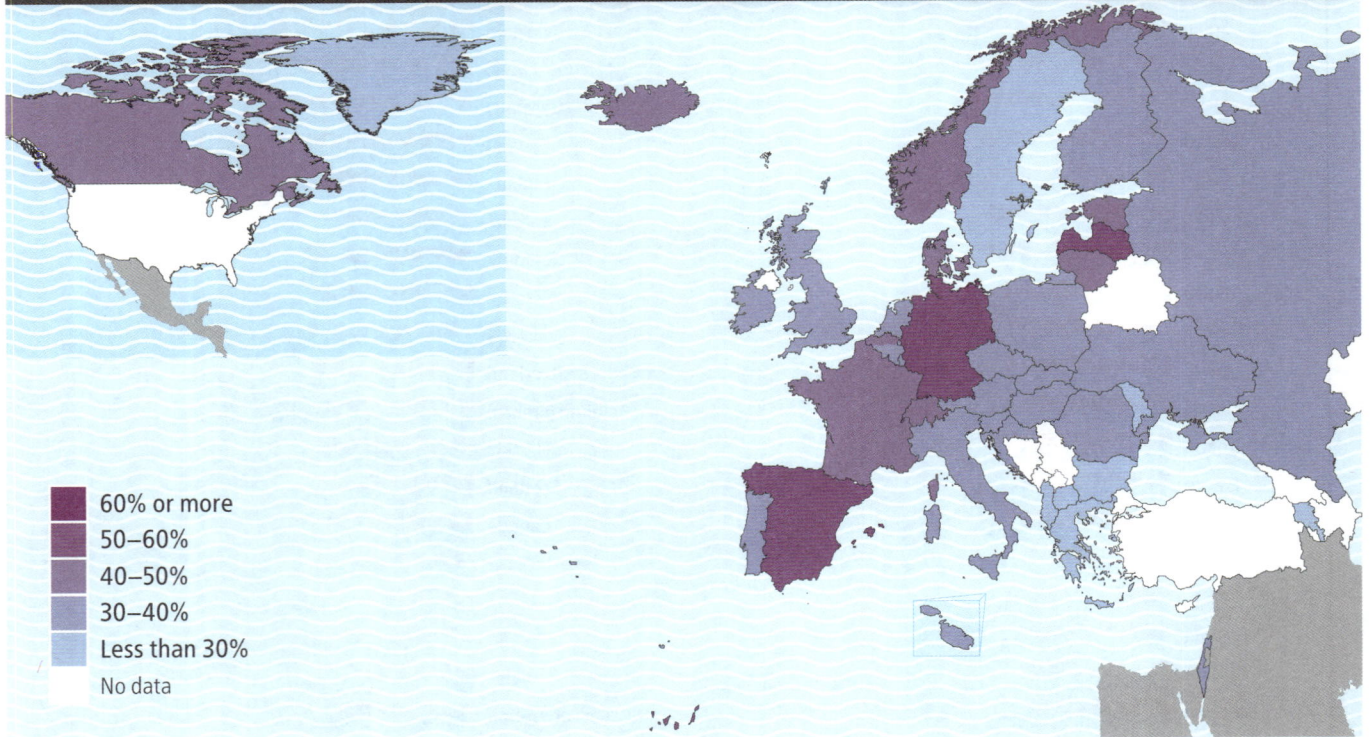

60% or more
50–60%
40–50%
30–40%
Less than 30%
No data

Note: HBSC teams provided disaggregated data for Belgium and the United Kingdom; these data appear in the map above.

HBSC survey 2013/2014

15-year-old boys who report at least one medically attended injury in the last 12 months

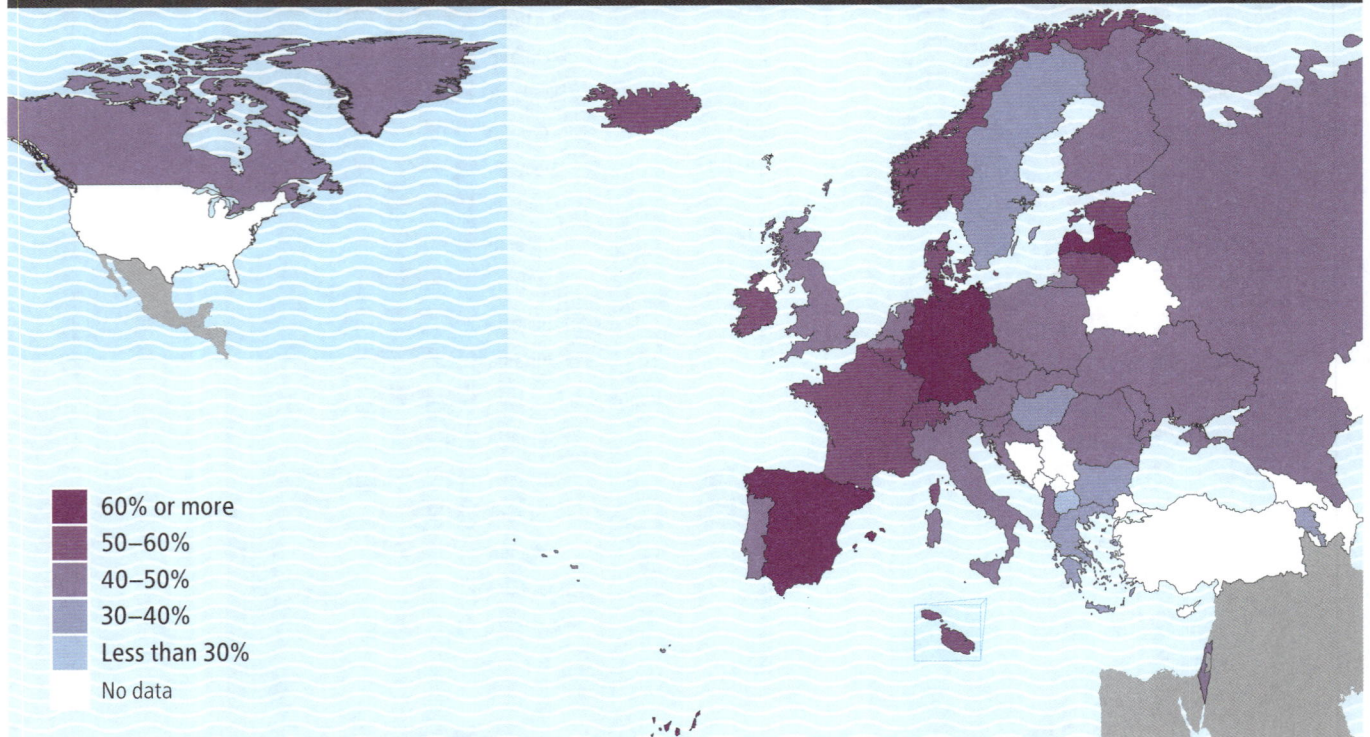

60% or more
50–60%
40–50%
30–40%
Less than 30%
No data

Note: HBSC teams provided disaggregated data for Belgium and the United Kingdom; these data appear in the map above.

GROWING UP UNEQUAL: GENDER AND SOCIOECONOMIC
DIFFERENCES IN YOUNG PEOPLE'S HEALTH AND WELL-BEING
PART 2. KEY DATA | CHAPTER 3. HEALTH OUTCOMES
MEDICALLY ATTENDED INJURIES

3

MEDICALLY ATTENDED INJURIES: SCIENTIFIC DISCUSSION AND POLICY REFLECTIONS

SCIENTIFIC DISCUSSION

Findings from the current survey show that boys sustain more injuries *(8,9)*, levels decrease over the course of adolescence and injuries are more prevalent in those of higher affluence.

Levels have remained relatively constant since the last HBSC survey. Differences related to family affluence and gender may be due to greater involvement of boys and those of higher affluence in sports and better access to medical attention *(3)*.

The known relationship between injuries and involvement in other risk behaviours means the very high prevalence in many countries and regions raises public health concerns. Large cross-national differences in injury levels suggest a need to understand country/regional-level factors that may influence injury prevalence, such as young people's physical activity levels and the availability of safety and prevention programmes.

POLICY REFLECTIONS

Injuries are the leading cause of death among young people aged 5–17 years in the European Region *(10)*. The frequency, severity, potential for death and disability, and costs of these injuries, together with the high success potential of prevention strategies, make injury prevention a key public health goal for improving adolescent health in the future.

Interest in reducing childhood injuries is a shared priority throughout Europe *(11)*. Reports indicate that prevention capacity has improved in several countries and regions *(1)*. Effective prevention strategies for young people include using car seat belts and wearing bicycle and motorcycle helmets, installing residential smoke alarms, reducing misuse of alcohol, strengthening graduated driver licensing laws, promoting policy change, using safety equipment in sports and leisure activities, and protecting adolescents in workplaces *(12)*.

Main macro approaches to preventing injuries among young people include legislation modification, product and environmental adjustments to promote children's safety, supportive home visits from trained professional visitors such as nurses (who can provide family support, suggest improvements in the home environment and offer education and training to parents), promotion of the use of safety devices (including helmets, seat belts and smoke alarms) and education programmes to promote skills development and behaviour change *(13)*. It is important, however, that prevention efforts do not hinder children's participation in physical activity.

REFERENCES

1. Peden M, Oyegbite K, Ozanne-Smith J, Hyder AA, Branche C, Rhaman AKMF et al., editors. World report on child injury prevention. Geneva: World Health Organization; 2008 (http://apps.who.int/iris/bitstream/10665/43851/1/9789241563574_eng.pdf, accessed 24 August 2015).

2. Sethi D, Racioppi F, Baumgarten I, Vida P. Injuries and violence in Europe: why they matter and what can be done. Copenhagen: WHO Regional Office for Europe; 2006 (http://www.euro.who.int/__data/assets/pdf_file/0005/98762/E88037.pdf, accessed 24 August 2015).

3. De Looze ME, Pickett W, Raaijmakers Q, Kuntcshe E, Hublet A, Nic Gabhainn S et al. Early risk behaviors and adolescent injury in 25 European and North American countries: a cross-national consistent relationship. J Early Adolesc. 2012;32(1):104–25.

4. Pickett W, Craig W, Harel Y, Cunningham J, Simpson K, Molcho M et al. Cross-national study of fighting and weapon carrying as determinants of adolescent injury. Paediatrics 2005;116(6):855–63.

5. Molcho M, Harel Y, Pickett W, Schiedt PC, Mazur J, Overpeck MD. The epidemiology of non-fatal injuries among 11, 13 and 15 year old youth in 11 countries: findings from the 1998 WHO–HBSC cross national survey. Inj Control Saf Promot. 2000;13(4):205–11.

6. Pickett W, Molcho M, Simpson K, Janssen I, Kuntsche E, Mazur J et al. Cross-national study of injury and social determinants in adolescents. Inj Prev. 2005;11:213–18.

7. Molcho M, Walsh S, Donnelly P, Gaspar de Matos M, Pickett W. Trends in injury-related mortality and morbidity among adolescents across 30 countries from 2002 to 2010. Eur J Public Health 2015;25(Suppl. 2):33–6.

8. Morrongiello BA, Midgett C, Stanton KL. Gender biases in children's appraisals of injury risk and other children's risk-taking behaviors. J Exp Child Psychol. 2000;77(4):317–36.

9.   Graine MA. Sex differences, effects of sex-stereotype conformity, age and internalisation on risk-taking among pedestrian adolescents. Saf Sci. 2009;47:1277–83.

10. Sethi D, Towner E, Vincenten J, Segui-Gomez M, Racioppi F. European report on child injury prevention. Copenhagen: WHO Regional Office for Europe; 2008 (http://www.who.int/violence_injury_prevention/child/injury/world_report/European_report.pdf, accessed 24 August 2015).

11. MacKay M, Vincenten J. Action planning for child safety: 2010 update on the strategic and coordinated approach to reducing the number one cause of death and disability for children in Europe – injury. Amsterdam: European Child Safety Alliance; 2010 (http://www.childsafetyeurope.org/actionplans/info/action-planning-for-child-safety-update.pdf, accessed 24 August 2015).

12. Sleet DA, Ballesteros MF, Borse NN. A review of unintentional injuries in adolescents. Annu Rev Public Health 2010;31:195–212.

13. Harvey A, Towner E, Peden M, Soori H, Bartolomeos K. Injury prevention and the attainment of child and adolescent health. Bull World Health Organ. 2009;87:390–4.

GROWING UP UNEQUAL: GENDER AND SOCIOECONOMIC
DIFFERENCES IN YOUNG PEOPLE'S HEALTH AND WELL-BEING
PART 2. KEY DATA | CHAPTER 3. HEALTH OUTCOMES

3

BODY WEIGHT:
OVERWEIGHT AND OBESITY

Childhood obesity, a multifactorial disease, is a global epidemic that poses a severe risk to the present and future health of young people *(1)*. Children with a high body mass index (BMI) often become obese adults *(2)*. Childhood obesity is associated with cardiovascular, endocrine, pulmonary, musculoskeletal and gastrointestinal complications and may have psychosocial consequences such as the development of poor self-esteem, depression and eating disorders *(2–8)*.

HBSC survey 2013/2014

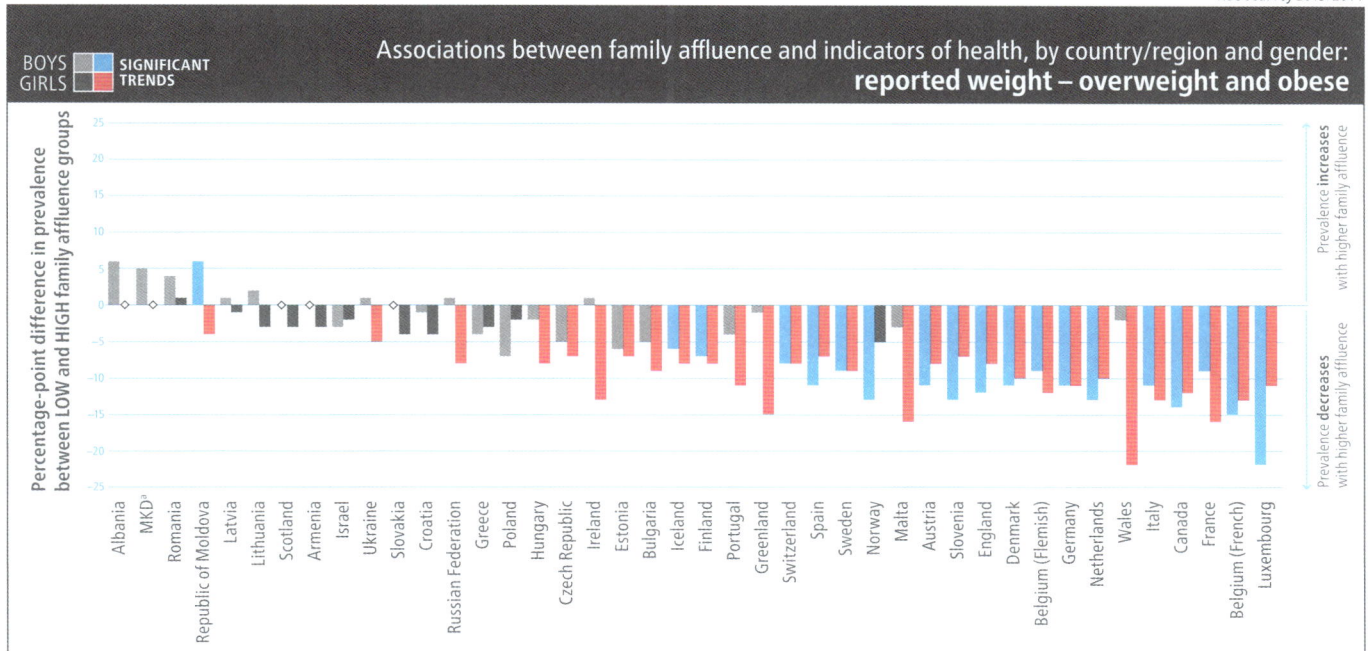

BOYS
GIRLS
SIGNIFICANT TRENDS

Associations between family affluence and indicators of health, by country/region and gender:
reported weight – overweight and obese

Percentage-point difference in prevalence between LOW and HIGH family affluence groups

Prevalence **increases** with higher family affluence

Prevalence **decreases** with higher family affluence

[a] The former Yugoslav Republic of Macedonia. *Note:* low- and high-affluence groups represent the lowest 20% and highest 20% in each country. ◇ means less than +/-0.5%.

MEASURE

Young people were asked how much they weighed without clothes and how tall they were without shoes. These data were (re)coded in centimetres and kilograms respectively to calculate the BMI (weight (kg) divided by height (m[2])).

Supplementary data using the international BMI standards for young people adopted by the International Obesity Task Force (IOTF) (the IOTF BMI cut-off points) *(9)* and rates of missing data per country or region are presented in the Annex.

RESULTS

Findings presented here show the proportion who are overweight or obese based on the WHO child growth curve standards *(10)*.

Age

Generally, overweight and obesity decreased with increasing age.

Gender

Boys tended to have significantly higher prevalence in almost all countries and regions at all ages. The gender difference exceeded 10 percentage points in 11 countries.

Family affluence

Increased prevalence was associated with low family affluence for boys in around half of countries and regions and about two thirds for girls.

HBSC survey 2013/2014

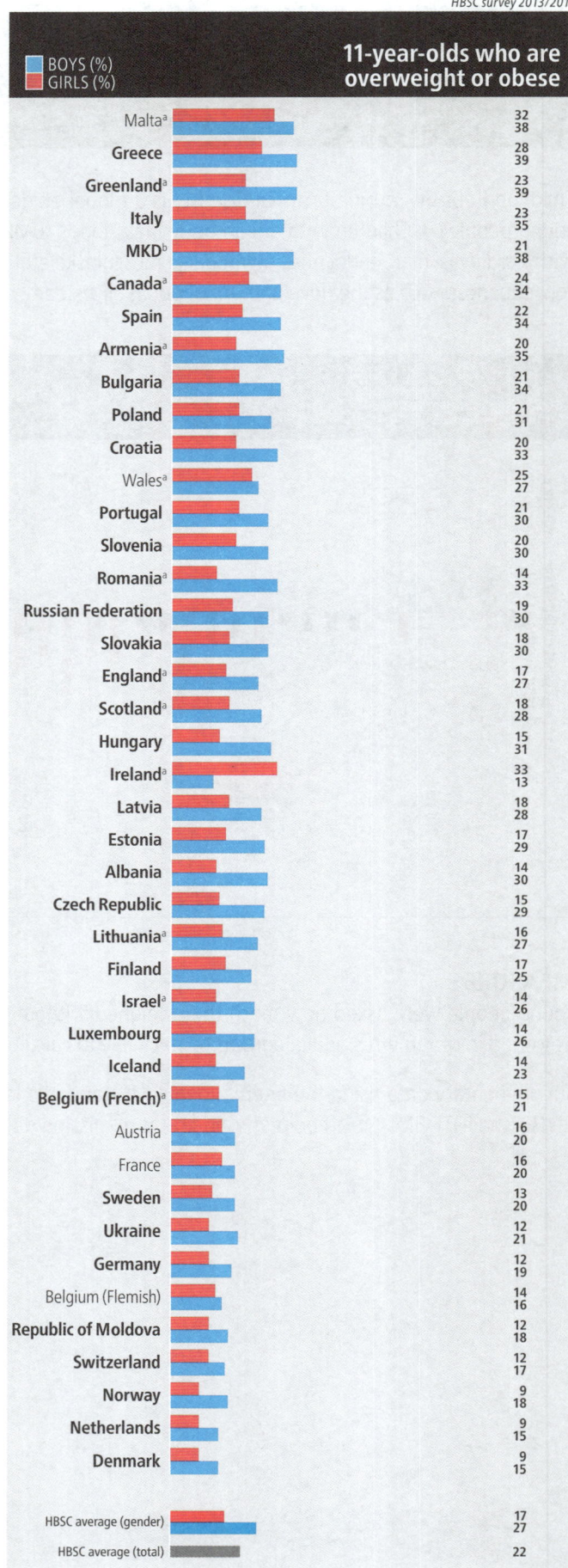

11-year-olds who are overweight or obese

BOYS (%)
GIRLS (%)

Country	Boys	Girls
Malta[a]	32	38
Greece	28	39
Greenland[a]	23	39
Italy	23	35
MKD[b]	21	38
Canada[a]	24	34
Spain	22	34
Armenia[a]	20	35
Bulgaria	21	34
Poland	21	31
Croatia	20	33
Wales[a]	25	27
Portugal	21	30
Slovenia	20	30
Romania[a]	14	33
Russian Federation	19	30
Slovakia	18	30
England[a]	17	27
Scotland[a]	18	28
Hungary	15	31
Ireland[a]	33	13
Latvia	18	28
Estonia	17	29
Albania	14	30
Czech Republic	15	29
Lithuania[a]	16	27
Finland	17	25
Israel[a]	14	26
Luxembourg	14	26
Iceland	14	23
Belgium (French)[a]	15	21
Austria	16	20
France	16	20
Sweden	13	20
Ukraine	12	21
Germany	12	19
Belgium (Flemish)	14	16
Republic of Moldova	12	18
Switzerland	12	17
Norway	9	18
Netherlands	9	15
Denmark	9	15
HBSC average (gender)	17	27
HBSC average (total)	22	

[a] BMI is missing for more than 30% of age-group sample.
[b] The former Yugoslav Republic of Macedonia.

GROWING UP UNEQUAL: GENDER AND SOCIOECONOMIC
DIFFERENCES IN YOUNG PEOPLE'S HEALTH AND WELL-BEING
PART 2. KEY DATA | CHAPTER 3. HEALTH OUTCOMES
BODY WEIGHT: OVERWEIGHT AND OBESITY

3

13-year-olds who are overweight or obese

HBSC survey 2013/2014

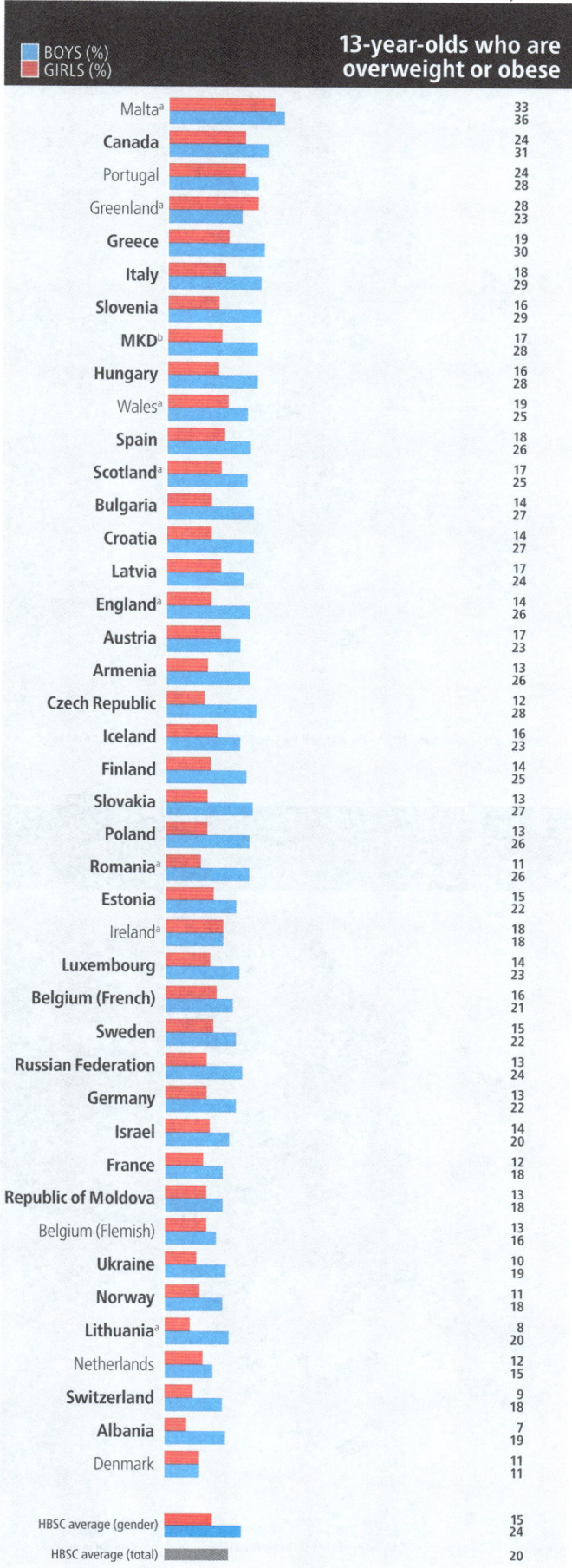

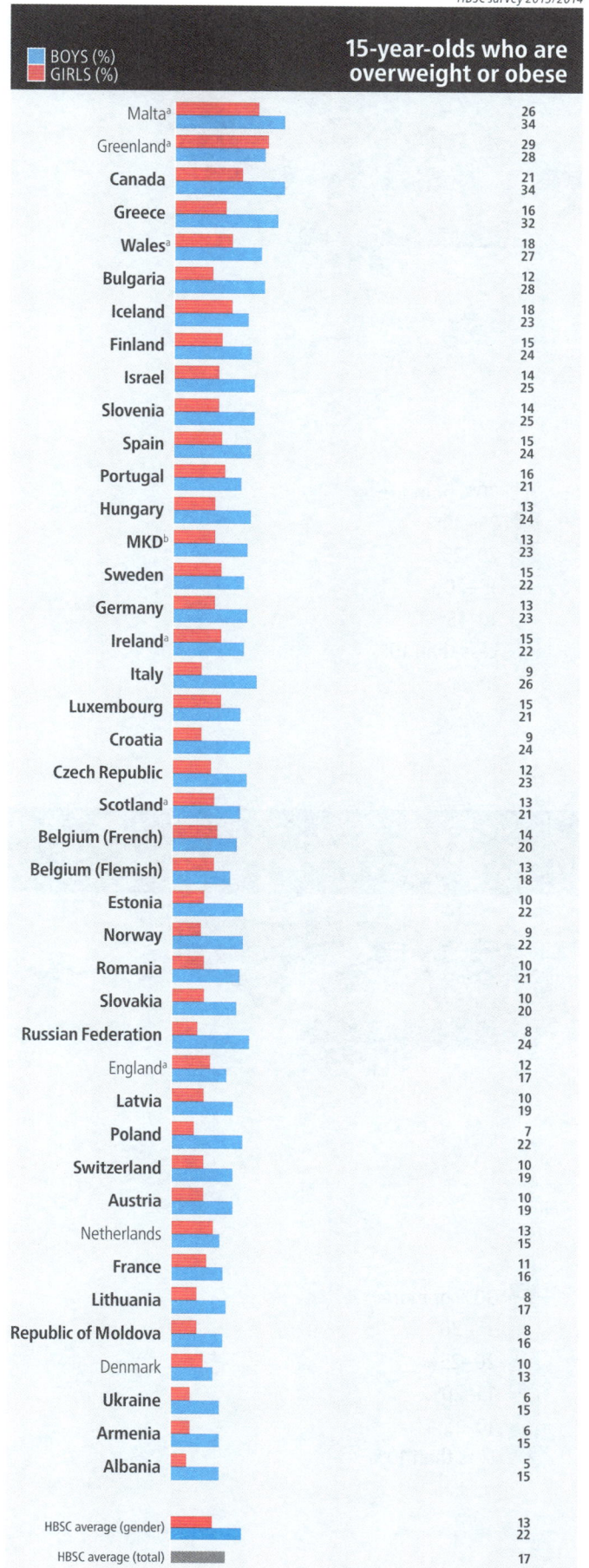

Legend: ■ BOYS (%) ■ GIRLS (%)

Country	Girls (%)	Boys (%)
Malta[a]	33	36
Canada	24	31
Portugal	24	28
Greenland[a]	28	23
Greece	19	30
Italy	18	29
Slovenia	16	29
MKD[b]	17	28
Hungary	16	28
Wales[a]	19	25
Spain	18	26
Scotland[a]	17	25
Bulgaria	14	27
Croatia	14	27
Latvia	17	24
England[a]	14	26
Austria	17	23
Armenia	13	26
Czech Republic	12	28
Iceland	16	23
Finland	14	25
Slovakia	13	27
Poland	13	26
Romania[a]	11	26
Estonia	15	22
Ireland[a]	18	18
Luxembourg	14	23
Belgium (French)	16	21
Sweden	15	22
Russian Federation	13	24
Germany	13	22
Israel	14	20
France	12	18
Republic of Moldova	13	18
Belgium (Flemish)	13	16
Ukraine	10	19
Norway	11	18
Lithuania[b]	8	20
Netherlands	12	15
Switzerland	9	18
Albania	7	19
Denmark	11	11
HBSC average (gender)	15	24
HBSC average (total)		20

15-year-olds who are overweight or obese

HBSC survey 2013/2014

Legend: ■ BOYS (%) ■ GIRLS (%)

Country	Girls (%)	Boys (%)
Malta[a]	26	34
Greenland[a]	29	28
Canada	21	34
Greece	16	32
Wales[a]	18	27
Bulgaria	12	28
Iceland	18	23
Finland	15	24
Israel	14	25
Slovenia	14	25
Spain	15	24
Portugal	16	21
Hungary	13	24
MKD[b]	13	23
Sweden	15	22
Germany	13	23
Ireland[a]	15	22
Italy	9	26
Luxembourg	15	21
Croatia	9	24
Czech Republic	12	23
Scotland[a]	13	21
Belgium (French)	14	20
Belgium (Flemish)	13	18
Estonia	10	22
Norway	9	22
Romania	10	21
Slovakia	10	20
Russian Federation	8	24
England[a]	12	17
Latvia	10	19
Poland	7	22
Switzerland	10	19
Austria	10	19
Netherlands	13	15
France	11	16
Lithuania	8	17
Republic of Moldova	8	16
Denmark	10	13
Ukraine	6	15
Armenia	6	15
Albania	5	15
HBSC average (gender)	13	22
HBSC average (total)		17

Note: **indicates** significant gender difference (at p<0.05).

HBSC survey 2013/2014

15-year-old girls who are overweight or obese

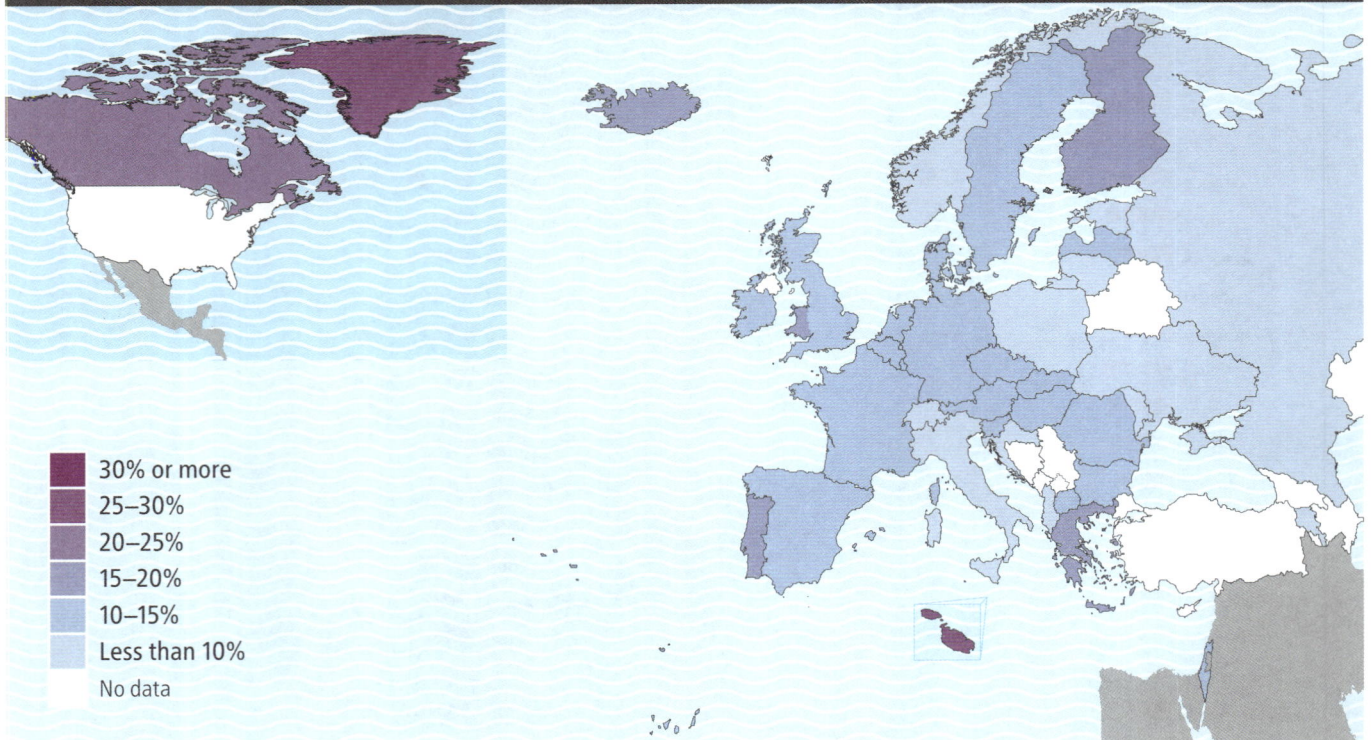

30% or more
25–30%
20–25%
15–20%
10–15%
Less than 10%
No data

Note: HBSC teams provided disaggregated data for Belgium and the United Kingdom; these data appear in the map above.

HBSC survey 2013/2014

15-year-old boys who are overweight or obese

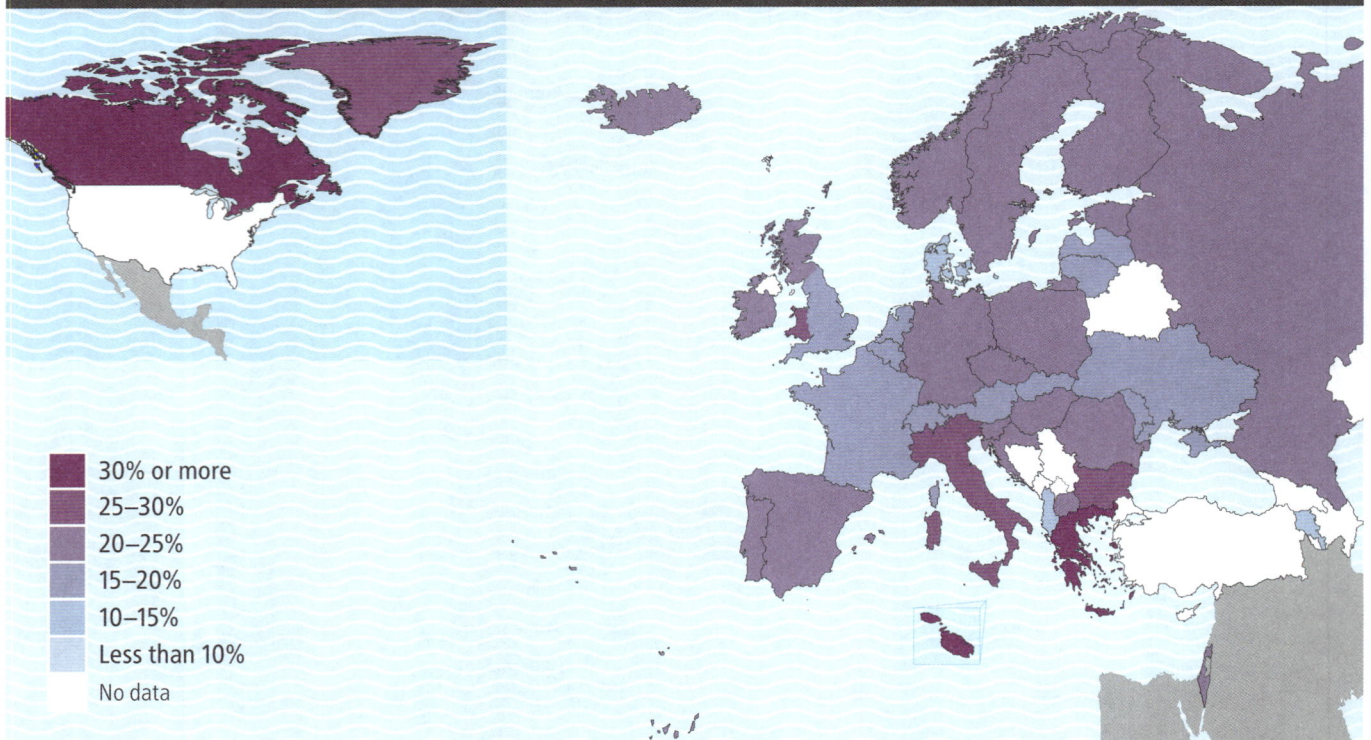

30% or more
25–30%
20–25%
15–20%
10–15%
Less than 10%
No data

Note: HBSC teams provided disaggregated data for Belgium and the United Kingdom; these data appear in the map above.

GROWING UP UNEQUAL: GENDER AND SOCIOECONOMIC
DIFFERENCES IN YOUNG PEOPLE'S HEALTH AND WELL-BEING
PART 2. KEY DATA | CHAPTER 3. HEALTH OUTCOMES

3

BODY WEIGHT: BODY IMAGE

Body image is a psychological construct that is part of self-image. Its importance increases as young people become more body-conscious with the physical changes associated with puberty.

Poor body image among children and adolescents can have severe health-related implications, including reduced levels of physical activity (11), unhealthy eating behaviours (12) and mental health problems such as depression (13).

Prevalence of negative body image increases through early and mid-adolescence and is linked to actual and perceived obesity (14,15). Protective factors include regular physical activity (16), acceptance by peers and family, and good social relationships (17).

HBSC survey 2013/2014

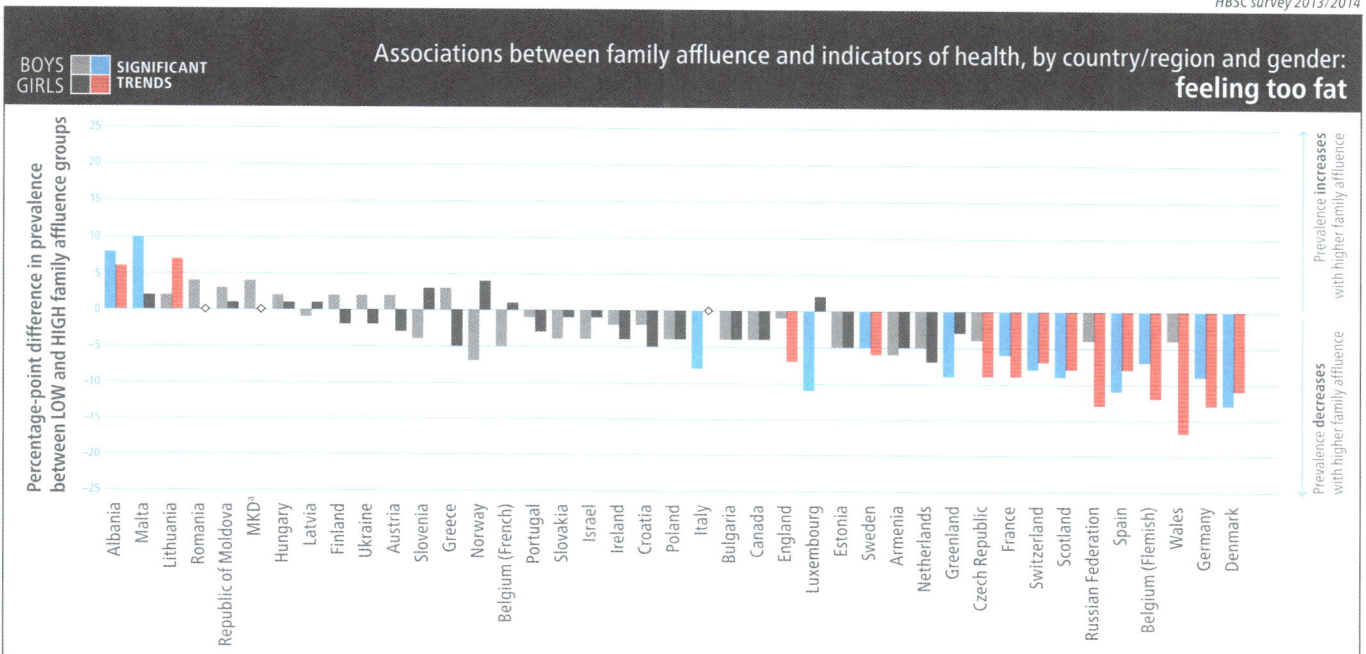

Associations between family affluence and indicators of health, by country/region and gender: **feeling too fat**

ᵃThe former Yugoslav Republic of Macedonia. *Note:* low- and high-affluence groups represent the lowest 20% and highest 20% in each country. ◇ means less than +/-0.5%. No data were received from Iceland.

MEASURE
Young people were asked about how they perceive their body. Response options ranged from much too thin to much too fat.

RESULTS

Findings presented here show the proportions who reported perceiving their body to be too fat, defined as being a bit or much too fat.

Age

Girls aged 15 were significantly more likely than 11-year-olds in almost all countries and regions to report that they were too fat. The difference in prevalence between 11 and 15 was more than 10 percentage points in most and 20 in a few. There was no clear patterning by age for boys, with some showing increased prevalence with age and others the opposite trend.

Gender

Girls aged 15 had significantly higher prevalence in all countries and regions: this was also seen in almost all for 13-year-olds and in most for those aged 11. The size of the gender difference tended to increase with age in most countries and regions.

Family affluence

More than half of the countries and regions showed no significant relationship with family affluence. Where an association was found, the perception of being too fat was more commonly associated with low affluence.

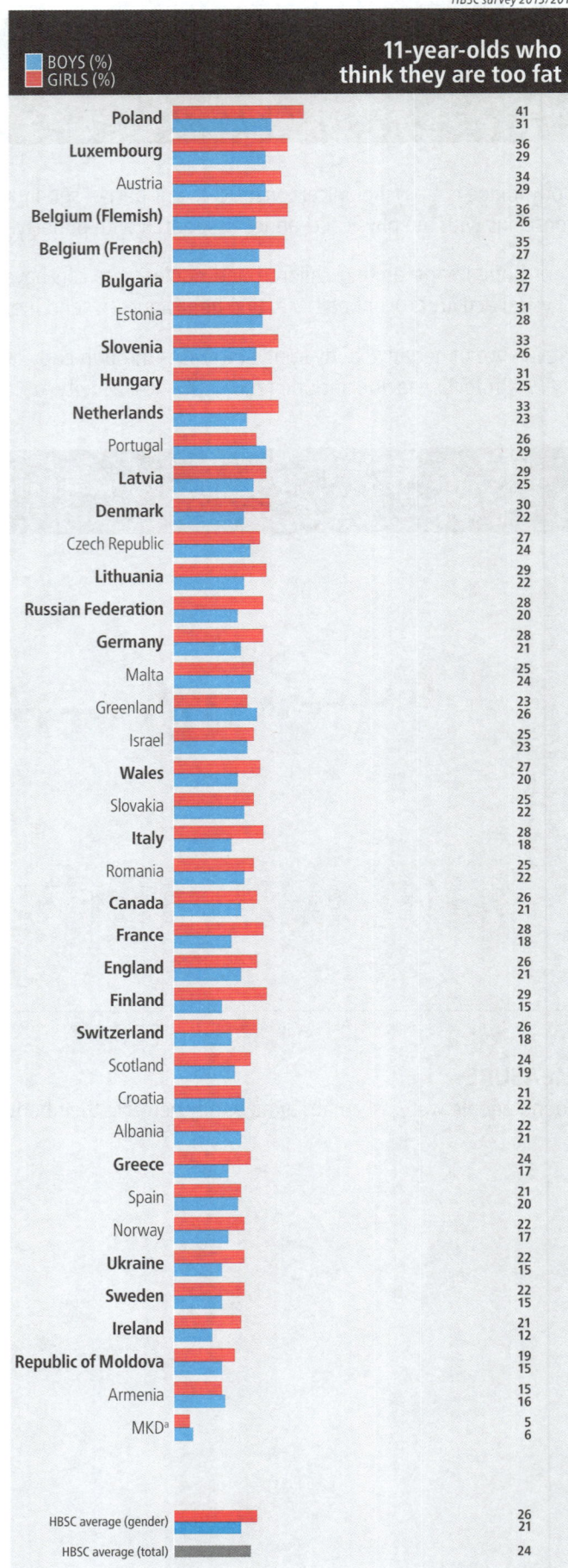

HBSC survey 2013/2014

11-year-olds who think they are too fat

BOYS (%)
GIRLS (%)

Country	Girls	Boys
Poland	41	31
Luxembourg	36	29
Austria	34	29
Belgium (Flemish)	36	26
Belgium (French)	35	27
Bulgaria	32	27
Estonia	31	28
Slovenia	33	26
Hungary	31	25
Netherlands	33	23
Portugal	26	29
Latvia	29	25
Denmark	30	22
Czech Republic	27	24
Lithuania	29	22
Russian Federation	28	20
Germany	28	21
Malta	25	24
Greenland	23	26
Israel	25	23
Wales	27	20
Slovakia	25	22
Italy	28	18
Romania	25	22
Canada	26	21
France	28	18
England	26	21
Finland	29	15
Switzerland	26	18
Scotland	24	19
Croatia	21	22
Albania	22	21
Greece	24	17
Spain	21	20
Norway	22	17
Ukraine	22	15
Sweden	22	15
Ireland	21	12
Republic of Moldova	19	15
Armenia	15	16
MKDᵃ	5	6
HBSC average (gender)	26	21
HBSC average (total)	24	

ᵃ The former Yugoslav Republic of Macedonia.

GROWING UP UNEQUAL: GENDER AND SOCIOECONOMIC
DIFFERENCES IN YOUNG PEOPLE'S HEALTH AND WELL-BEING
PART 2. KEY DATA | CHAPTER 3. HEALTH OUTCOMES
BODY WEIGHT: BODY IMAGE

3

HBSC survey 2013/2014

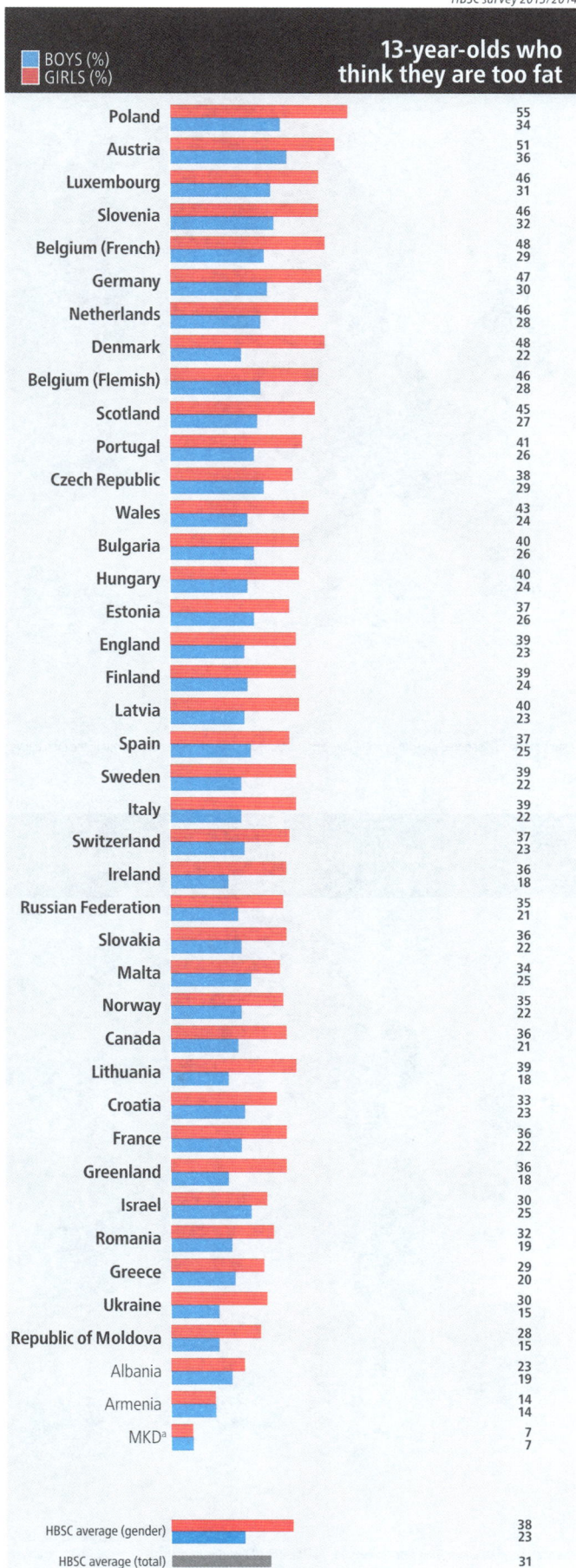

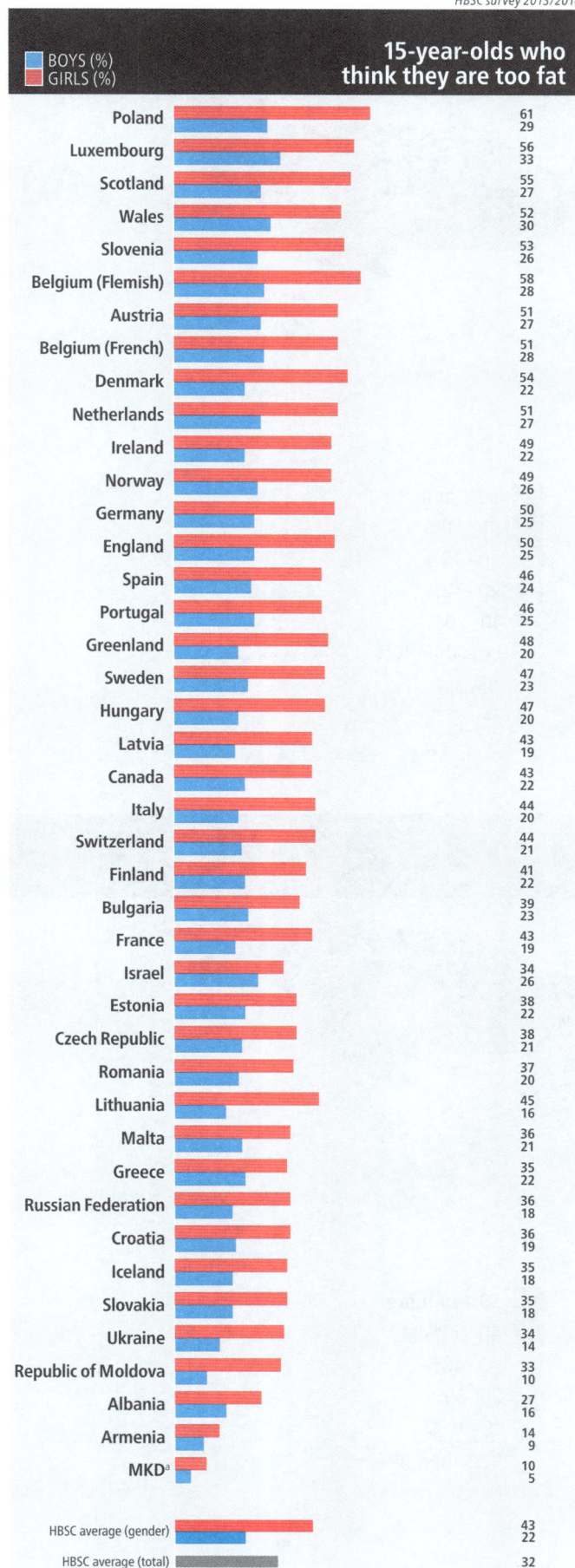

13-year-olds who think they are too fat

■ BOYS (%)
■ GIRLS (%)

Country	Girls	Boys
Poland	55	34
Austria	51	36
Luxembourg	46	31
Slovenia	46	32
Belgium (French)	48	29
Germany	47	30
Netherlands	46	28
Denmark	48	22
Belgium (Flemish)	46	28
Scotland	45	27
Portugal	41	26
Czech Republic	38	29
Wales	43	24
Bulgaria	40	26
Hungary	40	24
Estonia	37	26
England	39	23
Finland	39	24
Latvia	40	23
Spain	37	25
Sweden	39	22
Italy	39	22
Switzerland	37	23
Ireland	36	18
Russian Federation	35	21
Slovakia	36	22
Malta	34	25
Norway	35	22
Canada	36	21
Lithuania	39	18
Croatia	33	23
France	36	22
Greenland	36	18
Israel	30	25
Romania	32	19
Greece	29	20
Ukraine	30	15
Republic of Moldova	28	15
Albania	23	19
Armenia	14	14
MKD[a]	7	7
HBSC average (gender)	38	23
HBSC average (total)	31	

HBSC survey 2013/2014

15-year-olds who think they are too fat

■ BOYS (%)
■ GIRLS (%)

Country	Girls	Boys
Poland	61	29
Luxembourg	56	33
Scotland	55	27
Wales	52	30
Slovenia	53	26
Belgium (Flemish)	58	28
Austria	51	27
Belgium (French)	51	28
Denmark	54	22
Netherlands	51	27
Ireland	49	22
Norway	49	26
Germany	50	25
England	50	25
Spain	46	24
Portugal	46	25
Greenland	48	20
Sweden	47	23
Hungary	47	20
Latvia	43	19
Canada	43	22
Italy	44	20
Switzerland	44	21
Finland	41	22
Bulgaria	39	23
France	43	19
Israel	34	26
Estonia	38	22
Czech Republic	38	21
Romania	37	20
Lithuania	45	16
Malta	36	21
Greece	35	22
Russian Federation	36	18
Croatia	36	19
Iceland	35	18
Slovakia	35	18
Ukraine	34	14
Republic of Moldova	33	10
Albania	27	16
Armenia	14	9
MKD[a]	10	5
HBSC average (gender)	43	22
HBSC average (total)	32	

Note: **indicates** significant gender difference (at p<0.05).
No data were received from Iceland (11- and 13-year-olds).

HBSC survey 2013/2014

15-year-old girls who think they are too fat

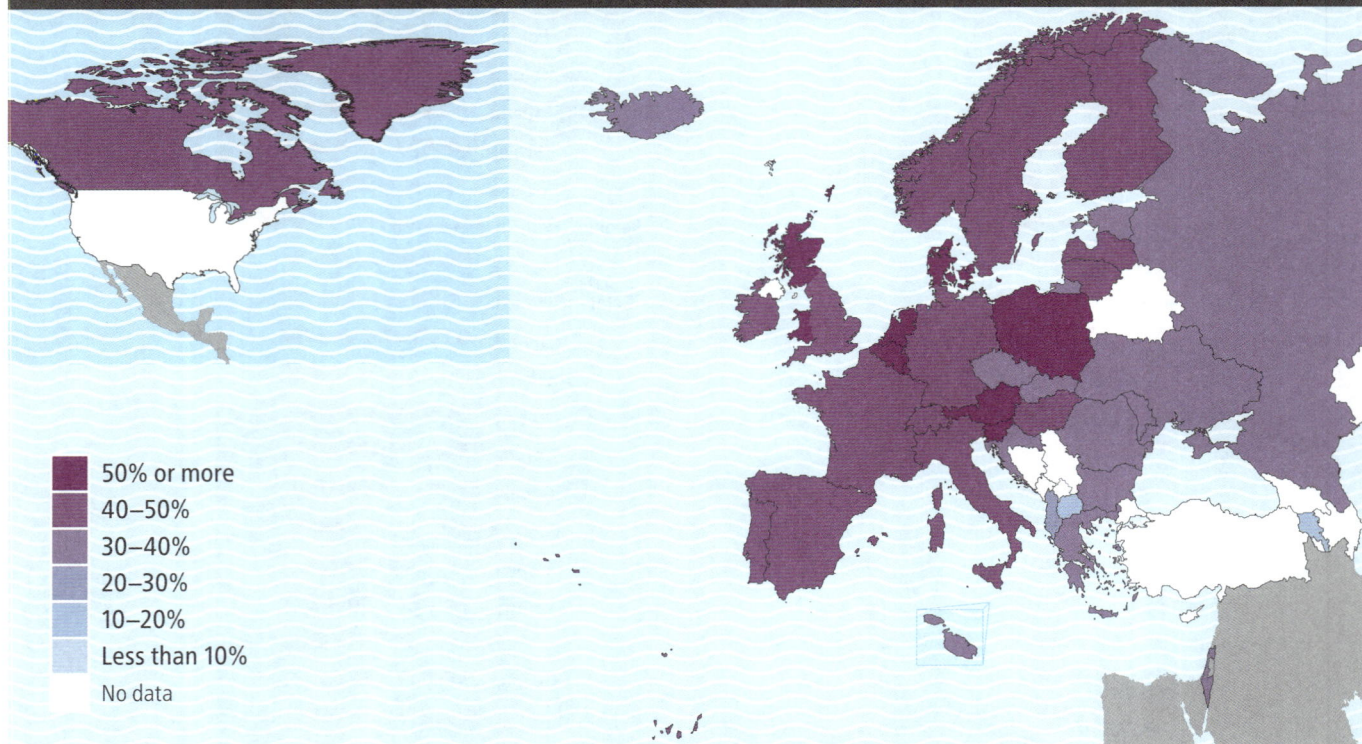

- 50% or more
- 40–50%
- 30–40%
- 20–30%
- 10–20%
- Less than 10%
- No data

Note: HBSC teams provided disaggregated data for Belgium and the United Kingdom; these data appear in the map above.

HBSC survey 2013/2014

15-year-old boys who think they are too fat

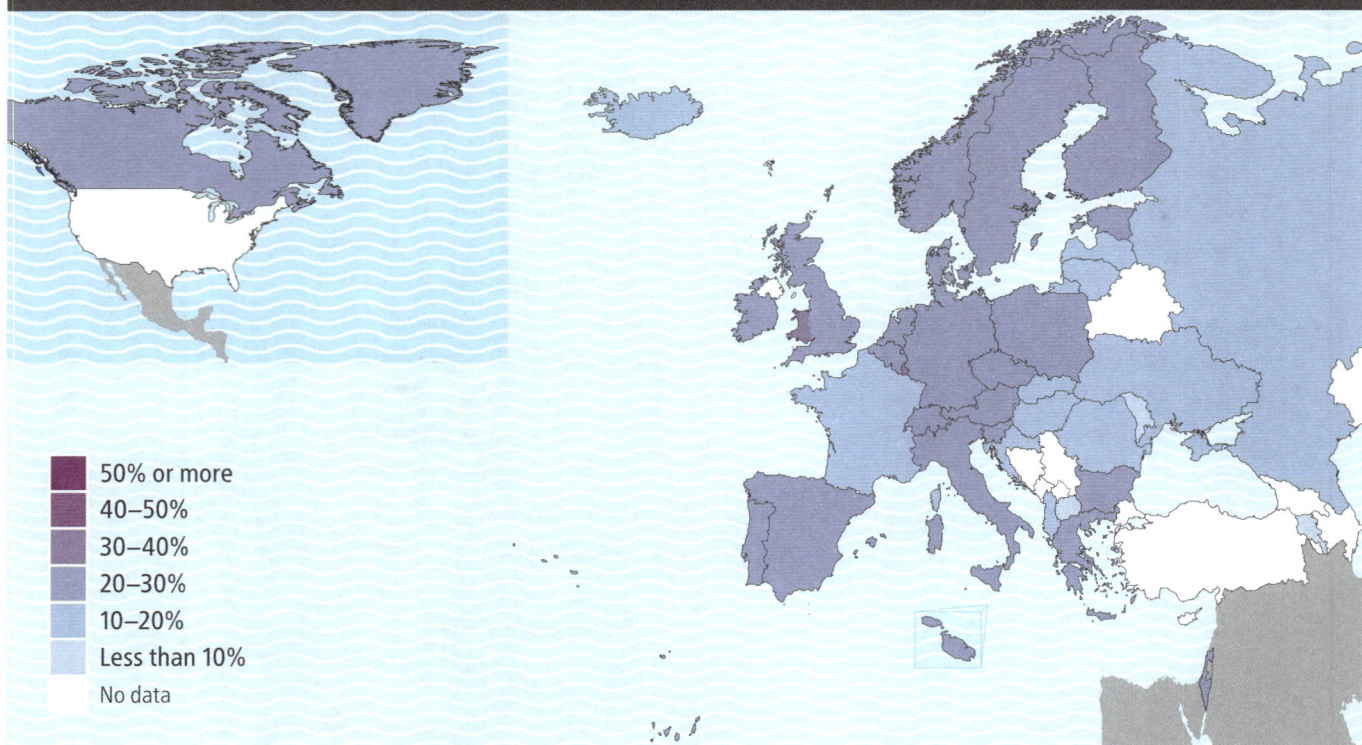

- 50% or more
- 40–50%
- 30–40%
- 20–30%
- 10–20%
- Less than 10%
- No data

Note: HBSC teams provided disaggregated data for Belgium and the United Kingdom; these data appear in the map above.

GROWING UP UNEQUAL: GENDER AND SOCIOECONOMIC
DIFFERENCES IN YOUNG PEOPLE'S HEALTH AND WELL-BEING
PART 2. KEY DATA | CHAPTER 3. HEALTH OUTCOMES

3

BODY WEIGHT:
WEIGHT-REDUCTION BEHAVIOUR

Weight-reduction behaviour is prevalent in adolescence, especially among girls and overweight young people (18). Adolescents often try to lose weight through inappropriate methods that may result in negative health consequences, including nutritional deficiency, growth retardation, delayed sexual maturation, menstrual irregularities and osteoporosis in girls, poor self-esteem and body image, anxiety and disordered eating (19–21).

Excessive dieting is related to substance use (22), depression, and suicide ideation and attempts (23). It may also lead to eating disorders and obesity over time (20,24).

HBSC survey 2013/2014

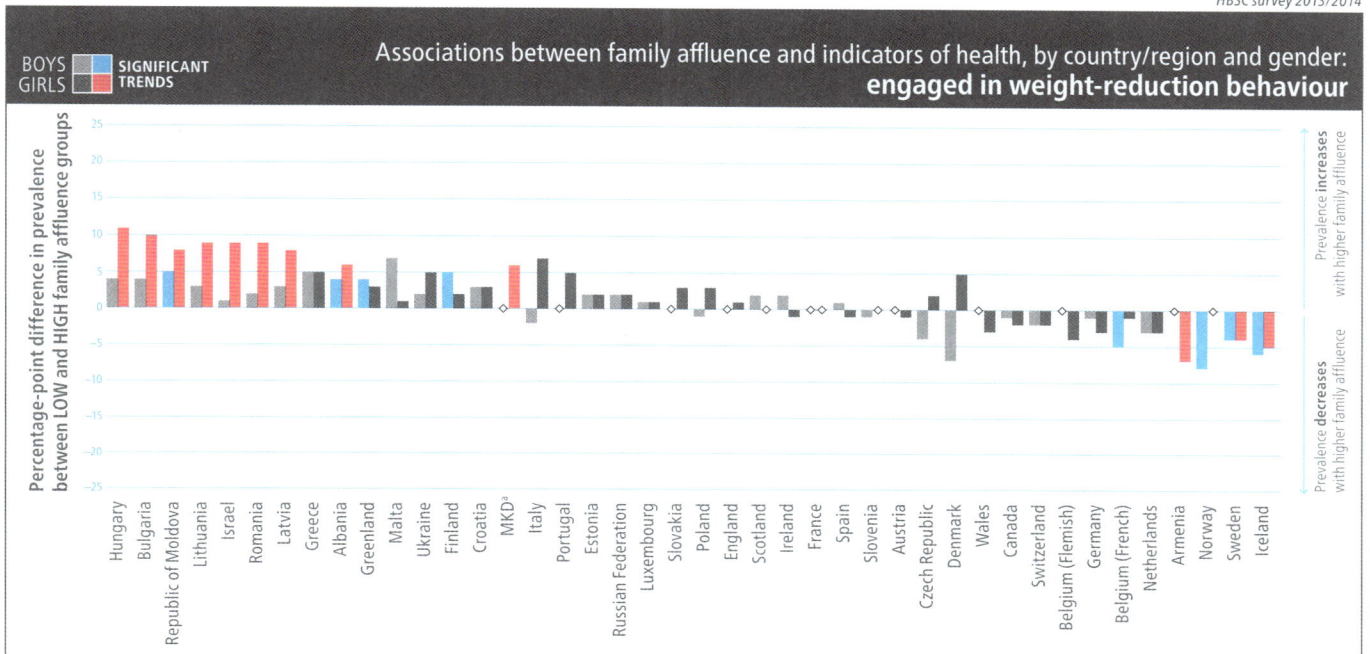

Associations between family affluence and indicators of health, by country/region and gender: **engaged in weight-reduction behaviour**

ª The former Yugoslav Republic of Macedonia. *Note:* low- and high-affluence groups represent the lowest 20% and highest 20% in each country. ◇ means less than +/-0.5%.

MEASURE
Young people were asked whether they are currently on a diet or doing something else to lose weight. Response options were: no, my weight is fine; no, but I should lose some weight; no, I need to put on weight; and yes.

RESULTS

Findings presented here show the proportions engaged in weight-reduction behaviour, meaning they were on a diet or doing something else to lose weight.

Age

Prevalence increased significantly among girls from age 11 to 15 in all but two countries and regions, with differences ranging from 7 to 23 percentage points. Significant trends in boys were evident in a quarter but the direction was opposite to that of girls, with decreases of 3–10 percentage points.

Gender

Girls reported significantly higher prevalence in a quarter of countries and regions for 11-year-olds, in almost all for 13-year-olds and in all for those who were 15. Generally, differences increased between 11 and 13 years and between 13 and 15.

Family affluence

Significant differences were found in about one quarter of countries and regions, but no clear pattern was evident.

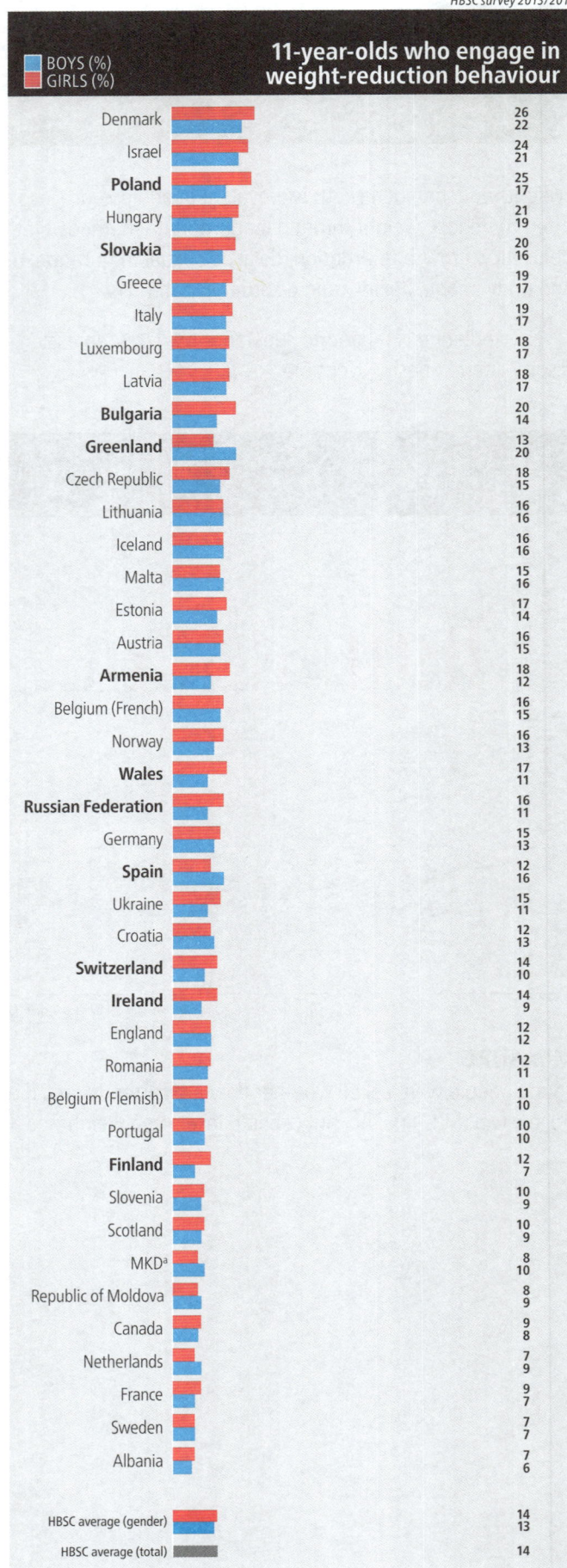

HBSC survey 2013/2014

11-year-olds who engage in weight-reduction behaviour

BOYS (%)
GIRLS (%)

Country	Boys	Girls
Denmark	26	22
Israel	24	21
Poland	25	17
Hungary	21	19
Slovakia	20	16
Greece	19	17
Italy	19	17
Luxembourg	18	17
Latvia	18	17
Bulgaria	20	14
Greenland	13	20
Czech Republic	18	15
Lithuania	16	16
Iceland	16	16
Malta	15	16
Estonia	17	14
Austria	16	15
Armenia	18	12
Belgium (French)	16	15
Norway	16	13
Wales	17	11
Russian Federation	16	11
Germany	15	13
Spain	12	16
Ukraine	15	11
Croatia	12	13
Switzerland	14	10
Ireland	14	9
England	12	12
Romania	12	11
Belgium (Flemish)	11	10
Portugal	10	10
Finland	12	7
Slovenia	10	9
Scotland	10	9
MKD[a]	8	10
Republic of Moldova	8	9
Canada	9	8
Netherlands	7	9
France	9	7
Sweden	7	7
Albania	7	6
HBSC average (gender)	14	13
HBSC average (total)	14	

[a] The former Yugoslav Republic of Macedonia.

GROWING UP UNEQUAL: GENDER AND SOCIOECONOMIC
DIFFERENCES IN YOUNG PEOPLE'S HEALTH AND WELL-BEING
PART 2. KEY DATA | CHAPTER 3. HEALTH OUTCOMES
BODY WEIGHT: WEIGHT-REDUCTION BEHAVIOUR

3

HBSC survey 2013/2014

13-year-olds who engage in weight-reduction behaviour

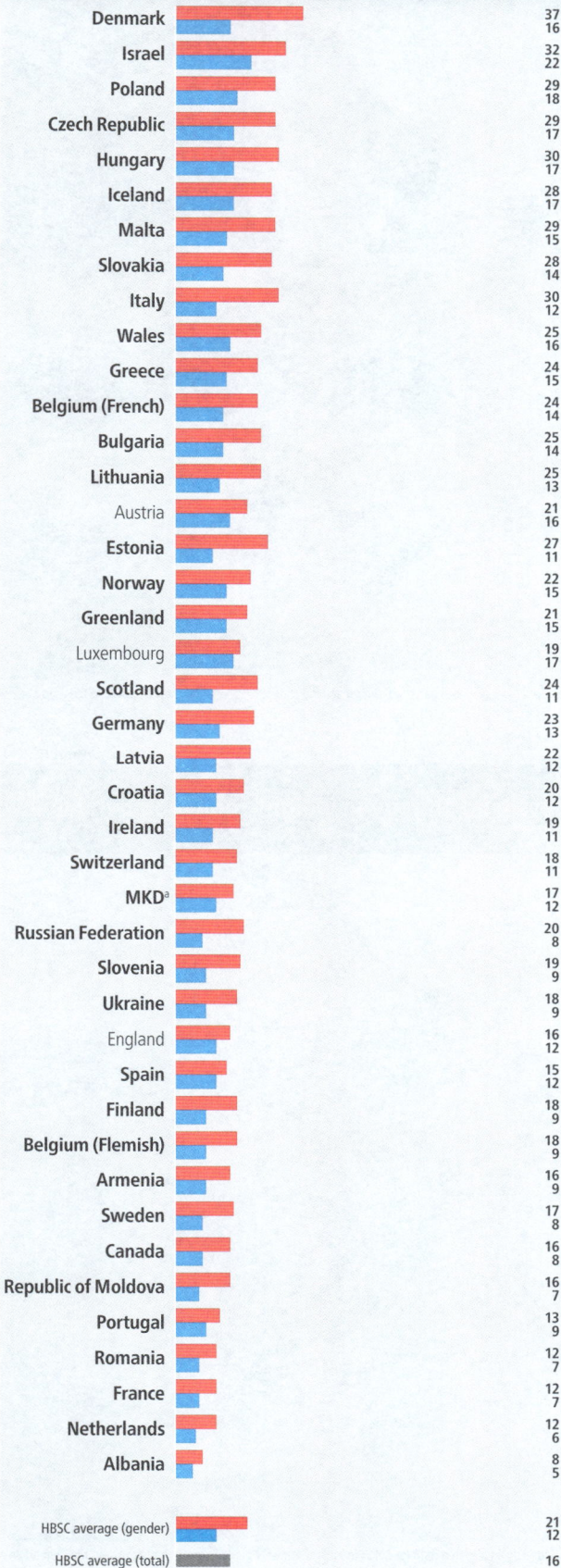

■ BOYS (%)
■ GIRLS (%)

	Girls	Boys
Denmark	37	16
Israel	32	22
Poland	29	18
Czech Republic	29	17
Hungary	30	17
Iceland	28	17
Malta	29	15
Slovakia	28	14
Italy	30	12
Wales	25	16
Greece	24	15
Belgium (French)	24	14
Bulgaria	25	14
Lithuania	25	13
Austria	21	16
Estonia	27	11
Norway	22	15
Greenland	21	15
Luxembourg	19	17
Scotland	24	11
Germany	23	13
Latvia	22	12
Croatia	20	12
Ireland	19	11
Switzerland	18	11
MKD[a]	17	12
Russian Federation	20	8
Slovenia	19	9
Ukraine	18	9
England	16	12
Spain	15	12
Finland	18	9
Belgium (Flemish)	18	9
Armenia	16	9
Sweden	17	8
Canada	16	8
Republic of Moldova	16	7
Portugal	13	9
Romania	12	7
France	12	7
Netherlands	12	6
Albania	8	5
HBSC average (gender)	21	12
HBSC average (total)	16	

HBSC survey 2013/2014

15-year-olds who engage in weight-reduction behaviour

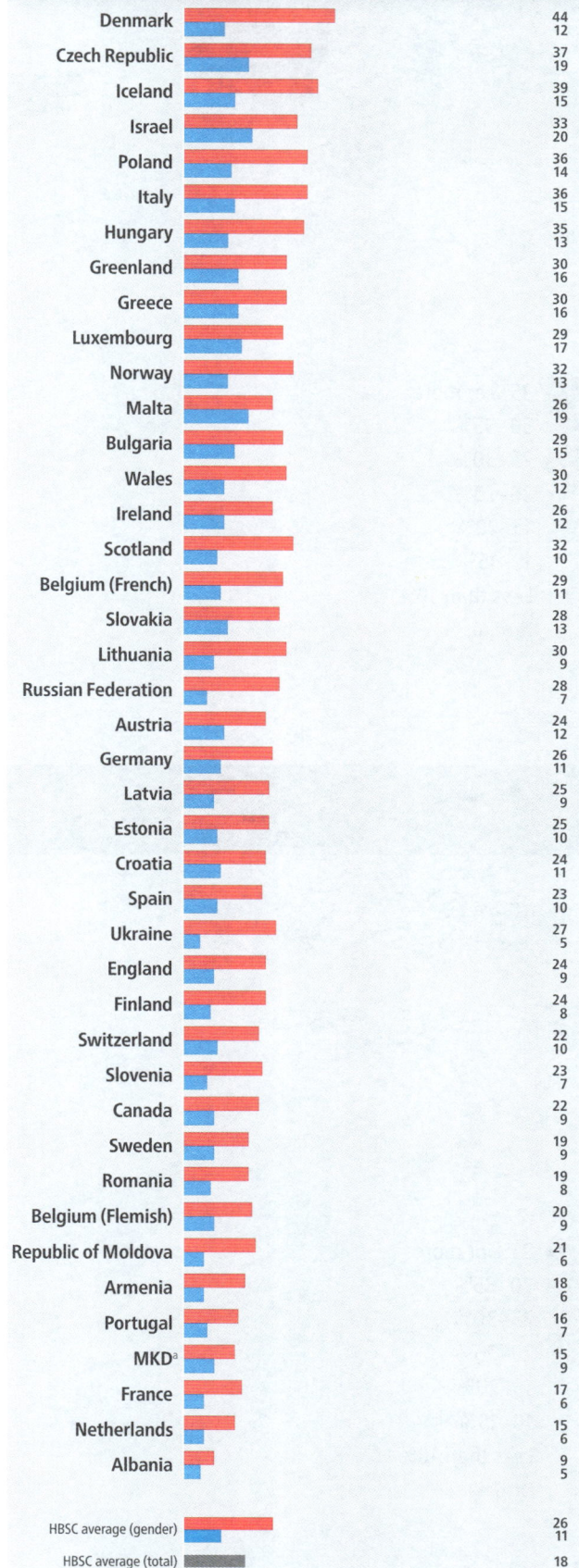

■ BOYS (%)
■ GIRLS (%)

	Girls	Boys
Denmark	44	12
Czech Republic	37	19
Iceland	39	15
Israel	33	20
Poland	36	14
Italy	36	15
Hungary	35	13
Greenland	30	16
Greece	30	16
Luxembourg	29	17
Norway	32	13
Malta	26	19
Bulgaria	29	15
Wales	30	12
Ireland	26	12
Scotland	32	10
Belgium (French)	29	11
Slovakia	28	13
Lithuania	30	9
Russian Federation	28	7
Austria	24	12
Germany	26	11
Latvia	25	9
Estonia	25	10
Croatia	24	11
Spain	23	10
Ukraine	27	5
England	24	9
Finland	24	8
Switzerland	22	10
Slovenia	23	7
Canada	22	9
Sweden	19	9
Romania	19	8
Belgium (Flemish)	20	9
Republic of Moldova	21	6
Armenia	18	6
Portugal	16	7
MKD[a]	15	9
France	17	6
Netherlands	15	6
Albania	9	5
HBSC average (gender)	26	11
HBSC average (total)	18	

Note: **indicates** significant gender difference (at p<0.05).

HBSC survey 2013/2014

15-year-old girls who engage in weight-reduction behaviour

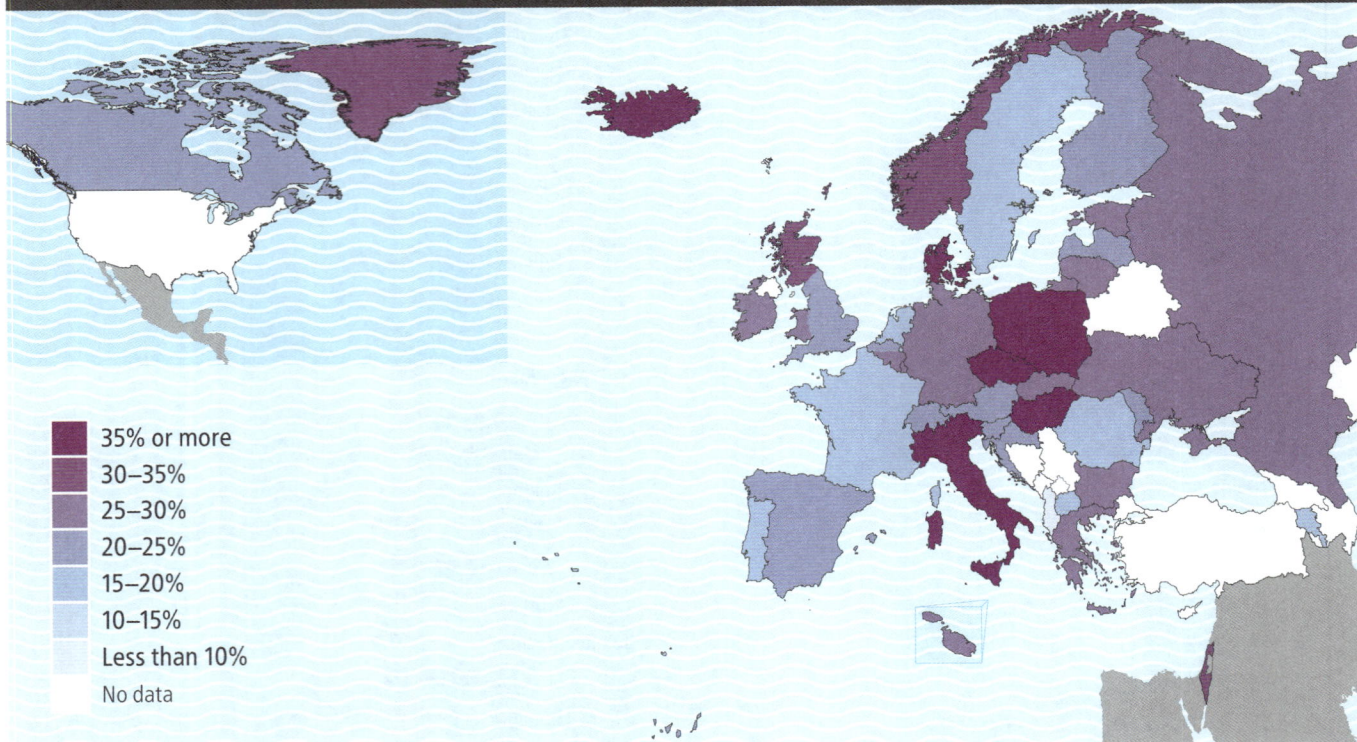

35% or more
30–35%
25–30%
20–25%
15–20%
10–15%
Less than 10%
No data

Note: HBSC teams provided disaggregated data for Belgium and the United Kingdom; these data appear in the map above.

HBSC survey 2013/2014

15-year-old boys who engage in weight-reduction behaviour

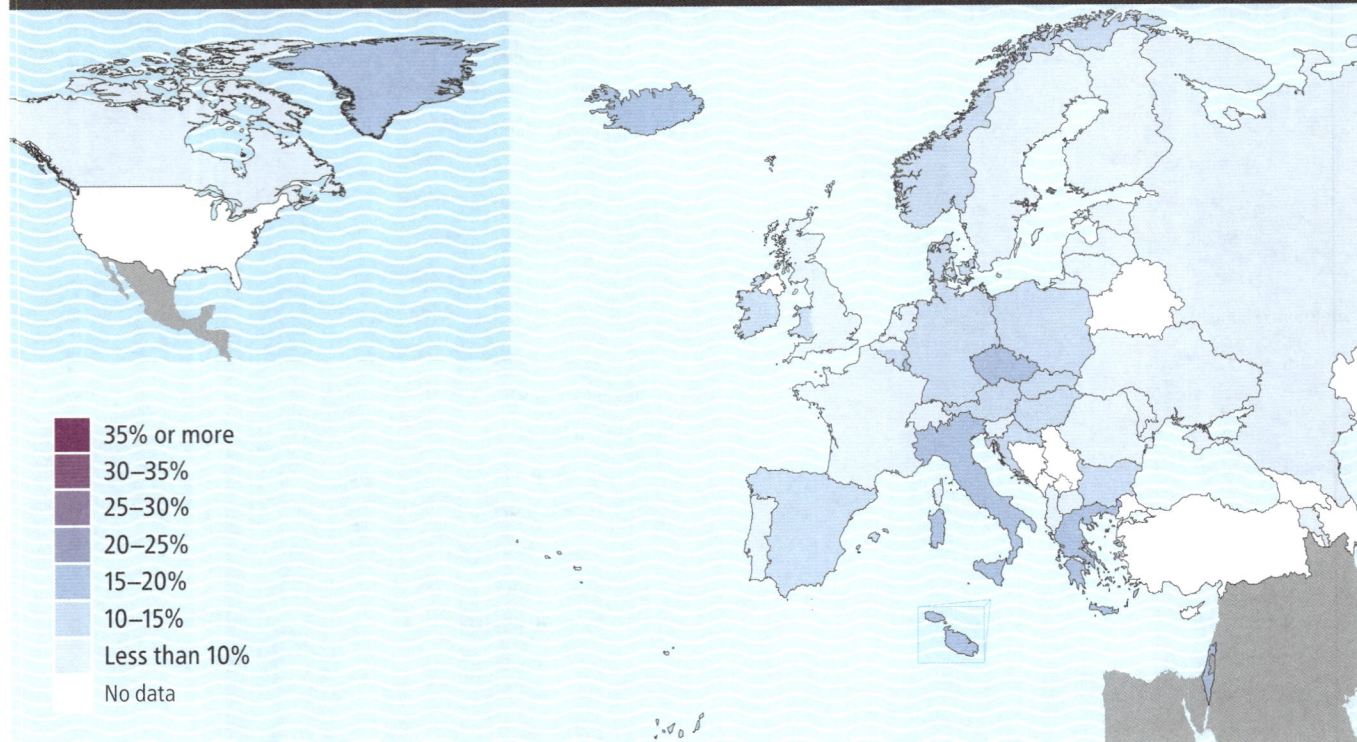

35% or more
30–35%
25–30%
20–25%
15–20%
10–15%
Less than 10%
No data

Note: HBSC teams provided disaggregated data for Belgium and the United Kingdom; these data appear in the map above.

GROWING UP UNEQUAL: GENDER AND SOCIOECONOMIC
DIFFERENCES IN YOUNG PEOPLE'S HEALTH AND WELL-BEING
PART 2. KEY DATA | CHAPTER 3. HEALTH OUTCOMES
BODY WEIGHT

3

BODY WEIGHT:
SCIENTIFIC DISCUSSION AND POLICY REFLECTIONS

SCIENTIFIC DISCUSSION

While overweight and obesity remain stable during adolescence or show a slight decrease with age, perceptions of overweight and dieting behaviour increase markedly in girls during this time. Clear gender differences are apparent, with boys tending to be more overweight in most countries and regions. Higher overweight prevalence is associated with lower affluence in some, but findings must be interpreted with caution due to the self-report nature of height and weight data used to categorize BMI status.

Gender and age patterns in relation to body image and weight-reduction behaviour seem consistent with previous findings: girls are more likely to be discontented with their body weight regardless of country or region. Being female is a stronger predictor for self-perceived fatness and weight-reduction behaviour than BMI or family affluence.

POLICY REFLECTIONS

The prevalence of overweight and obesity is not increasing but remains high in many countries and regions. WHO provides leadership, advocacy and evidence-based recommendations for international action to improve dietary practices and increase physical activity through its global strategy on diet, physical activity and health (25). It also promotes and supports research in priority areas to facilitate programme implementation and evaluation.

A systemic approach is needed to address high overweight and obesity rates and enable young people to have positive thoughts and feelings about their body as a means of improving well-being. Communities, families and individuals need to work together to address this issue. International and national support is needed to protect children and promote health through the provision of healthy and nutritious food, safe neighbourhoods, safe activities and opportunities for physical activity and sports participation. Identification of shared risk and protective factors for overweight and body dissatisfaction can support the development of relevant interventions for a broad spectrum of weight-related problems.

REFERENCES

1. Pulgarón ER. Childhood obesity: a review of increased risk for physical and psychological comorbidities. Clin Ther. 2013;35(1):18–32.

2. Mamun AA, O'Callaghan MJ, Cramb SM, Najman JM, Williams GM, Bor W. Childhood behavioral problems predict young adults' BMI and obesity: evidence from a birth cohort study. Obesity (Silver Spring) 2009;17(4):761–6.

3. Freedman DS, Mei Z, Srinivasan SR, Berenson GS, Dietz WH. Cardiovascular risk factors and excess adiposity among overweight children and adolescents: the Bogalusa Heart Study. J Pediatr. 2007;150(1):12–17.e2.

4. Koebnick C, Getahun D, Smith N, Porter AH, Der-Sarkissian JK, Jacobsen SJ. Extreme childhood obesity is associated with increased risk for gastroesophageal reflux disease in a large population-based study. Int J Pediatr Obes. 2011;6(2–2):e257–63.

5. Norris AL, Steinberger J, Steffen LM, Metzig AM, Schwarzenberg SJ, Kelly AS. Circulating oxidized LDL and inflammation in extreme pediatric obesity. Obesity (Silver Spring) 2011;19(7):1415–9.

6. Van Emmerik NM, Renders CM, van de Veer M, van Buuren S, van der Baan-Slootweg OH, Kist-van Holthe JE et al. High cardiovascular risk in severely obese young children and adolescents. Arch Dis Child. 2012; 97(9):818–21.

7. Udomittipong K, Chierakul N, Ruttanaumpawan P, Chotinaiwattarakul W, Susiva C, Mahoran K et al. Severe obesity is a risk factor for severe obstructive sleep apnea in obese children. J Med Assoc Thai. 2011;94(11):1346–51.

8. Scholtens S, Wijga AH, Seidell JC, Brunekreef B, de Jongste JC, Gehring U et al. Overweight and changes in weight status during childhood in relation to asthma symptoms at 8 years of age. J Allergy Clin Immunol. 2009;123(6):1312–8.

9. Cole TJ, Lobstein T. Extended international (IOTF) body mass index cut-offs for thinness, overweight and obesity. Pediatr Obes. 2012;7(4):284–94. doi:10.1111/j.2047-6310.2012.00064.x.

10. The WHO child growth standards [website]. Geneva: World Health Organization; 2015 (http://www.who.int/childgrowth/standards/en/, accessed 24 August 2015).

11. Grogan S. Body image and health: contemporary perspectives. J Health Psychol. 2006;11:523–30.

12. Tremblay L, Lariviere M. The influences of puberty onset, body mass index, and pressure to be thin on disordered eating behaviors in children and adolescents. Eat Behav. 2009;10(2):75–83.

13. Xie B, Unger J, Gallaher B, Anderson Johnson C, Wu Q, Chu C-P. Overweight, body image, and depression in Asian and Hispanic adolescents. Am J Health Behav. 2010;34:476–88.

14. Fenton C, Brooks F, Spencer NH, Morgan A. Sustaining a positive body image in adolescence: an assets-based analysis. Health Soc Care Community 2010;18:189–98.

15. Bucchianieri MM, Arikian AJ, Hannan PJ, Eisenberg ME, Neumark-Sztainer D. Body dissatisfaction from adolescence to young adulthood: findings from a 10-year longitudinal study. Body Image 2013;10(1):1–7.

16. Monteiro Gaspar M, Amarala TF, Oliveiraa BMPM, Borgesa N. Protective effect of physical activity on dissatisfaction with body image in children – a cross-sectional study. Psychol Sport Exerc. 2011;12(5):563–69.

17. Barker ET, Galambos NL. Body dissatisfaction of adolescent girls and boys: risk and resource factors. J Early Adolesc. 2003;23:141–65.

18. Ojala K, Vereecken C, Välimaa R, Currie C, Villberg J, Tynjälä J et al. Attempts to lose weight among overweight and non-overweight adolescents: a cross-national survey. Int J Behav Nutr & Phys Act. 2007;4:50.

19. Canadian Pediatric Society. Dieting in adolescence. Paediatr Child Health 2004;9(7):487–91.

20. Neumark-Sztainer D, Wall M, Guo J, Story M, Haines J, Eisenberg M. Obesity, disordered eating, and eating disorders in a longitudinal study of adolescents: how do dieters fare 5 years later? J Am Diet Assoc. 2006;106:559–68.

21. Espinoza P, Penelo E, Raich RM. Disordered eating behaviors and body image in a longitudinal pilot study of adolescent girls: what happens 2 years later? Body Image 2010;7(1):70–3.

22. Carroll SL, Lee RE, Kaur H, Harris KJ, Strother ML, Huang TT-K. Smoking, weight loss intention and obesity-promoting behaviors in college students. J Am Coll Nutr. 2006;25(4):348–53.

23. Crow S, Eisenberg ME, Story M, Neumark-Sztainer D. Suicidal behaviour in adolescents: relationship to weight status, weight control behaviours and body dissatisfaction. Int J Eat Disord. 2008;41(1):82–7.

24. Neumark-Sztainer D, Wall M, Haines J, Story M, Eisenberg ME. Why does dieting predict weight gain in adolescents? Findings from Project EAT-II: a 5-year longitudinal study. J Am Diet Assoc. 2007;107(3):448–55.

25. Global strategy on diet, physical activity and health [website]. Geneva: World Health Organization; 2015 (http://www.who.int/dietphysicalactivity/en/, accessed 24 August 2015).

GROWING UP UNEQUAL: GENDER AND SOCIOECONOMIC
DIFFERENCES IN YOUNG PEOPLE'S HEALTH AND WELL-BEING
PART 2. KEY DATA | CHAPTER 4. HEALTH BEHAVIOURS

4

HEALTH BEHAVIOURS

EATING BEHAVIOUR
ORAL HEALTH
ENERGY EXPENDITURE

"Doing at least one sport a day is easy enough – if you have a dog you could even take it out for a walk as it is exercising!"

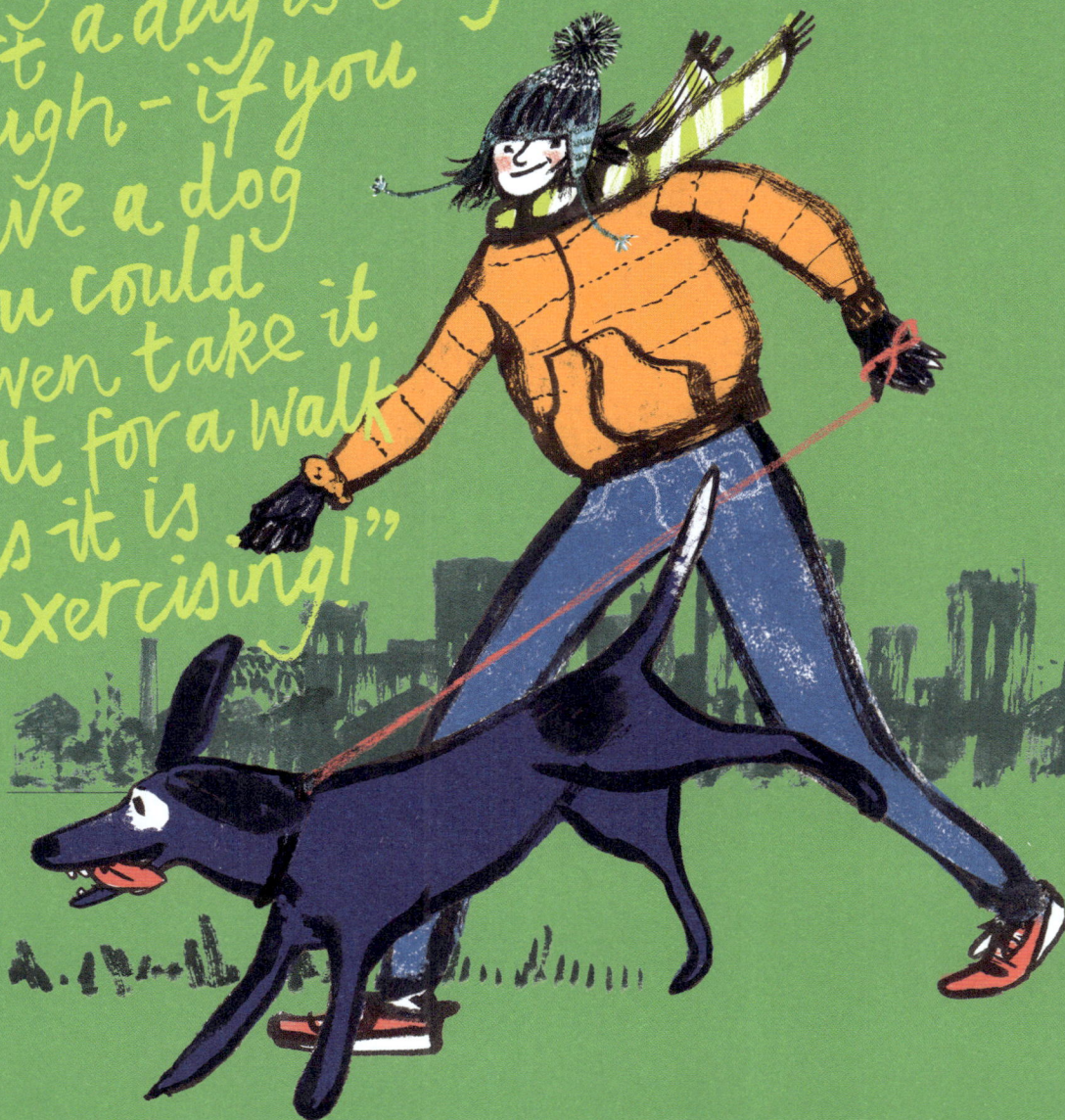

QUOTES FROM YOUNG PEOPLE ON HEALTH BEHAVIOURS

"I see frequently young people that do not have breakfast and causes vary. Some of them are not hungry in the morning. For others, and this scares me, it is because they are on a diet because they feel overweight. It is not the right way to lose weight. And furthermore, why do we have to be slaves to a thin body image?"

"I think eating breakfast in the morning is really important, as in the day, you will get hungry, and have headaches and your brain won't be able to work properly. In the mornings of school, it is even more important to eat breakfast for these reasons."

"I have the telly switched on because I don't want to feel lonely."

GROWING UP UNEQUAL: GENDER AND SOCIOECONOMIC
DIFFERENCES IN YOUNG PEOPLE'S HEALTH AND WELL-BEING
PART 2. KEY DATA | CHAPTER 4. HEALTH BEHAVIOURS

4

EATING BEHAVIOUR: BREAKFAST CONSUMPTION

Cross-sectional and longitudinal studies show that breakfast consumption is inversely related to BMI and overweight in children and adolescents (1–5). Eating breakfast is thought to reduce snacking and consumption of energy-rich foods of poor nutrient density. Regular and healthy breakfast habits in childhood can track into adulthood (6–9). It is assumed that skipping breakfast can affect school performance, but this area requires further in-depth research (10).

HBSC survey 2013/2014

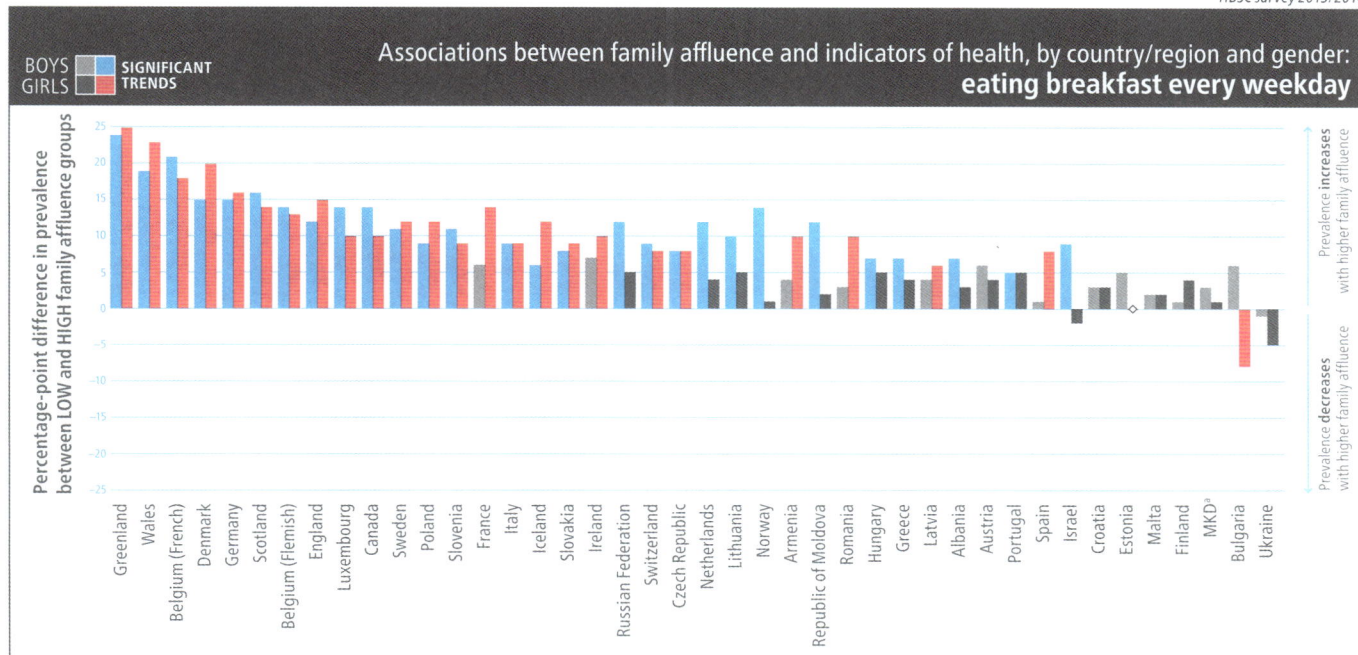

Associations between family affluence and indicators of health, by country/region and gender: **eating breakfast every weekday**

BOYS / GIRLS — SIGNIFICANT TRENDS

Percentage-point difference in prevalence between LOW and HIGH family affluence groups

Prevalence **increases** with higher family affluence / Prevalence **decreases** with higher family affluence

Countries (left to right): Greenland, Wales, Belgium (French), Denmark, Germany, Scotland, Belgium (Flemish), England, Luxembourg, Canada, Sweden, Poland, Slovenia, France, Italy, Iceland, Slovakia, Ireland, Russian Federation, Switzerland, Czech Republic, Netherlands, Lithuania, Norway, Armenia, Republic of Moldova, Romania, Hungary, Greece, Latvia, Albania, Austria, Portugal, Spain, Israel, Croatia, Estonia, Malta, Finland, MKD[a], Bulgaria, Ukraine

[a] The former Yugoslav Republic of Macedonia. *Note*: low- and high-affluence groups represent the lowest 20% and highest 20% in each country. ◇ means less than +/-0.5%.

MEASURE

Young people were asked how often they eat breakfast, defined as more than a glass of milk or fruit juice, on school days and at weekends.

RESULTS

Findings presented here show the proportions reporting eating breakfast every weekday.

Age

In general, older children were less likely to eat breakfast daily. The highest rate across each age group for boys and girls of 80% or more was found in the Netherlands and Portugal and the lowest of under 50% overall in Slovenia, although not among 11-year-olds.

Gender

Girls in most countries and regions were less likely to eat breakfast daily, and gender differences tended to increase with age. The largest differences were found in England (13- and 15-year-olds), France (15-year-olds), Greenland (13-year-olds) and Wales (13- and 15-year-olds).

Family affluence

Young people from higher-affluence families (especially boys) had higher consumption rates in most countries and regions.

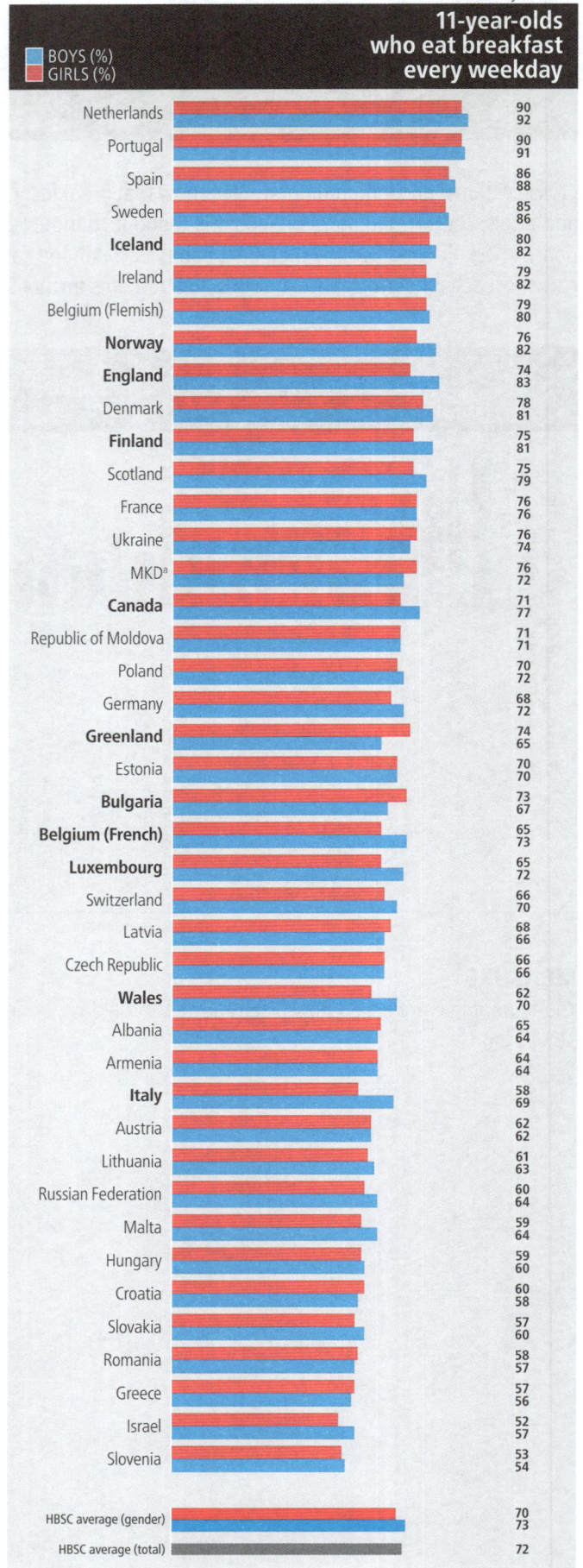

HBSC survey 2013/2014

11-year-olds who eat breakfast every weekday

BOYS (%)
GIRLS (%)

Country	Girls	Boys
Netherlands	90	92
Portugal	90	91
Spain	86	88
Sweden	85	86
Iceland	80	82
Ireland	79	82
Belgium (Flemish)	79	80
Norway	76	82
England	74	83
Denmark	78	81
Finland	75	81
Scotland	75	79
France	76	76
Ukraine	76	74
MKD[a]	76	72
Canada	71	77
Republic of Moldova	71	71
Poland	70	72
Germany	68	72
Greenland	74	65
Estonia	70	70
Bulgaria	73	67
Belgium (French)	65	73
Luxembourg	65	72
Switzerland	66	70
Latvia	68	66
Czech Republic	66	66
Wales	62	70
Albania	65	64
Armenia	64	64
Italy	58	69
Austria	62	62
Lithuania	61	63
Russian Federation	60	64
Malta	59	64
Hungary	59	60
Croatia	60	58
Slovakia	57	60
Romania	58	57
Greece	57	56
Israel	52	57
Slovenia	53	54
HBSC average (gender)	70	73
HBSC average (total)		72

[a] The former Yugoslav Republic of Macedonia.

GROWING UP UNEQUAL: GENDER AND SOCIOECONOMIC
DIFFERENCES IN YOUNG PEOPLE'S HEALTH AND WELL-BEING
PART 2. KEY DATA | CHAPTER 4. HEALTH BEHAVIOURS
EATING BEHAVIOUR: BREAKFAST CONSUMPTION

4

13-year-olds who eat breakfast every weekday

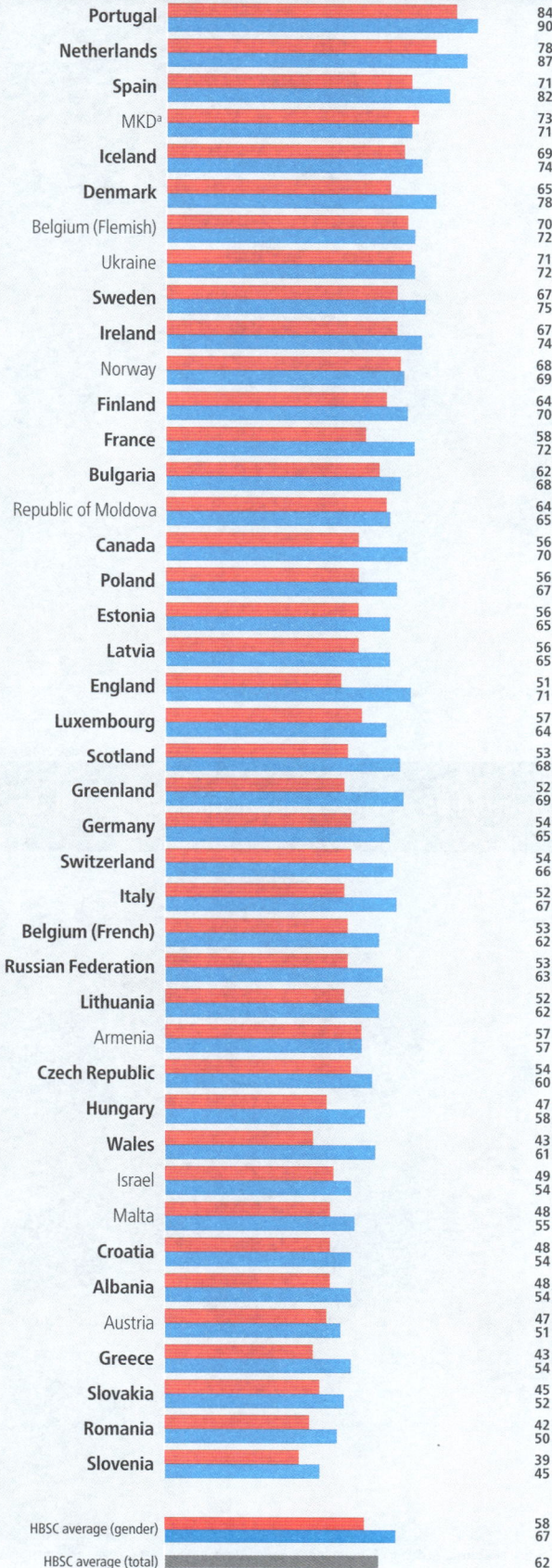

HBSC survey 2013/2014

- **BOYS (%)**
- **GIRLS (%)**

Country	Girls	Boys
Portugal	84	90
Netherlands	78	87
Spain	71	82
MKDª	73	71
Iceland	69	74
Denmark	65	78
Belgium (Flemish)	70	72
Ukraine	71	72
Sweden	67	75
Ireland	67	74
Norway	68	69
Finland	64	70
France	58	72
Bulgaria	62	68
Republic of Moldova	64	65
Canada	56	70
Poland	56	67
Estonia	56	65
Latvia	56	65
England	51	71
Luxembourg	57	64
Scotland	53	68
Greenland	52	69
Germany	54	65
Switzerland	54	66
Italy	52	67
Belgium (French)	53	62
Russian Federation	53	63
Lithuania	52	62
Armenia	57	57
Czech Republic	54	60
Hungary	47	58
Wales	43	61
Israel	49	54
Malta	48	55
Croatia	48	54
Albania	48	54
Austria	47	51
Greece	43	54
Slovakia	45	52
Romania	42	50
Slovenia	39	45
HBSC average (gender)	58	67
HBSC average (total)		62

15-year-olds who eat breakfast every weekday

HBSC survey 2013/2014

- **BOYS (%)**
- **GIRLS (%)**

Country	Girls	Boys
Portugal	73	86
Netherlands	71	81
Denmark	66	74
Iceland	63	75
Spain	63	75
Ukraine	64	71
Ireland	62	73
MKDª	65	63
Belgium (Flemish)	55	70
Finland	62	64
Norway	57	67
Estonia	58	66
Sweden	58	65
Bulgaria	56	66
Republic of Moldova	57	63
Latvia	55	64
Poland	56	62
Russian Federation	51	65
England	48	64
Germany	52	59
France	46	64
Italy	50	61
Belgium (French)	50	59
Switzerland	52	56
Lithuania	50	58
Canada	48	59
Greenland	56	50
Wales	44	59
Malta	50	53
Greece	47	54
Scotland	43	57
Armenia	46	55
Luxembourg	45	54
Israel	45	52
Czech Republic	44	53
Croatia	44	52
Austria	42	52
Hungary	35	50
Slovakia	38	46
Albania	34	48
Slovenia	38	42
Romania	36	40
HBSC average (gender)	52	62
HBSC average (total)		57

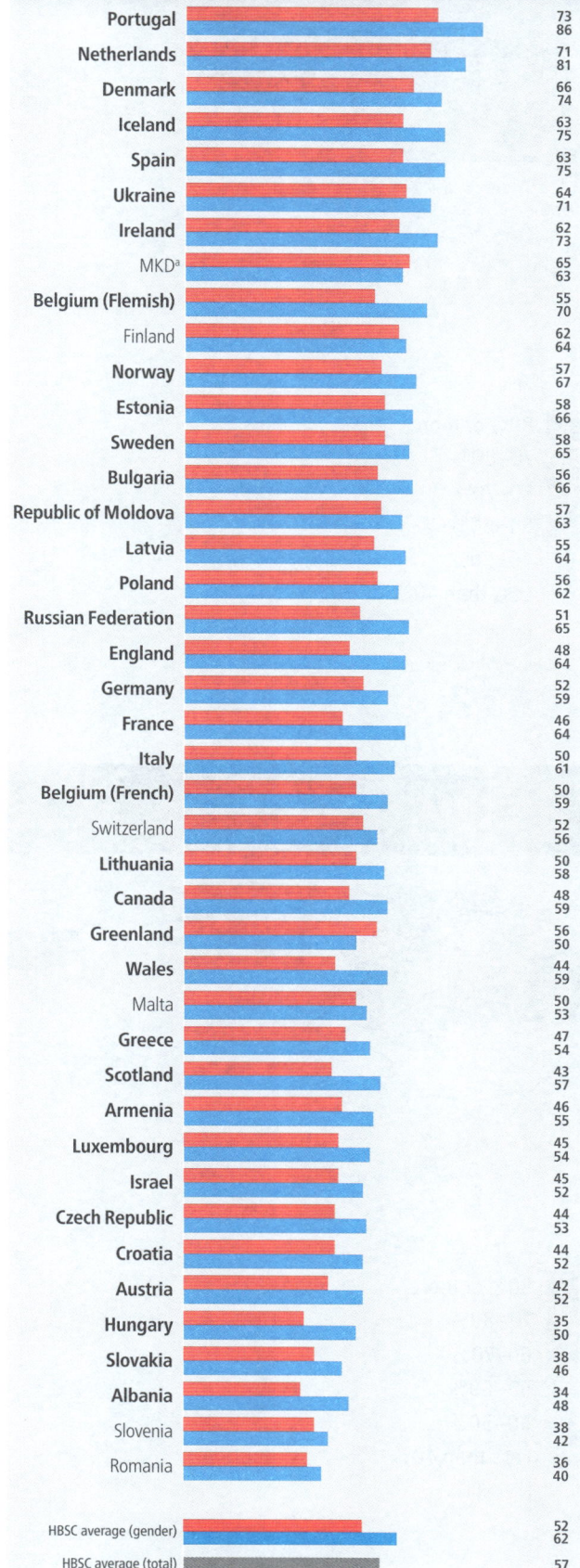

Note: **indicates** significant gender difference (at p<0.05).

HBSC survey 2013/2014

15-year-old girls who eat breakfast every weekday

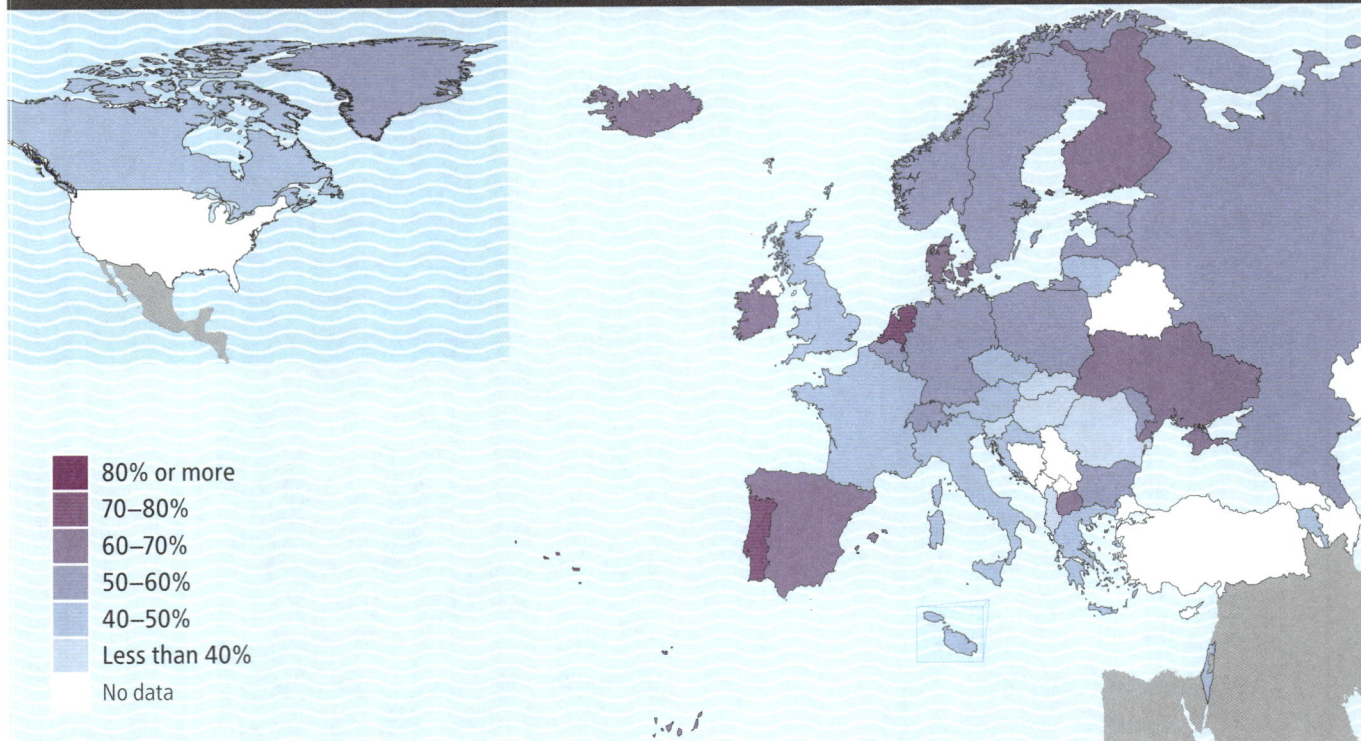

80% or more
70–80%
60–70%
50–60%
40–50%
Less than 40%
No data

Note: HBSC teams provided disaggregated data for Belgium and the United Kingdom; these data appear in the map above.

HBSC survey 2013/2014

15-year-old boys who eat breakfast every weekday

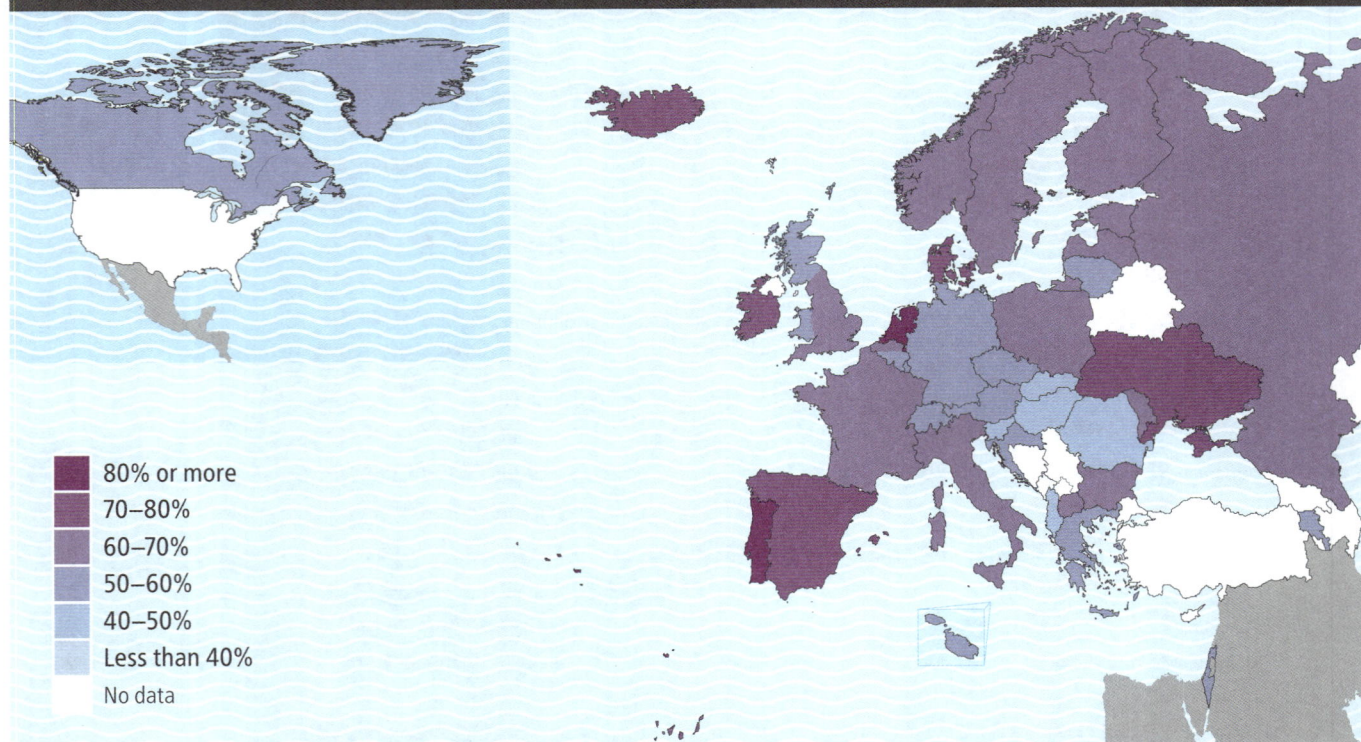

80% or more
70–80%
60–70%
50–60%
40–50%
Less than 40%
No data

Note: HBSC teams provided disaggregated data for Belgium and the United Kingdom; these data appear in the map above.

GROWING UP UNEQUAL: GENDER AND SOCIOECONOMIC
DIFFERENCES IN YOUNG PEOPLE'S HEALTH AND WELL-BEING
PART 2. KEY DATA | CHAPTER 4. HEALTH BEHAVIOURS

4

EATING BEHAVIOUR: FRUIT CONSUMPTION

Fruit consumption is linked to positive health in the short and long term, with a well established decreased risk of chronic diseases evident *(11–13)*. Recommendations on consumption vary across countries and regions, with eating five or more portions of fruit and vegetables daily tending to be advised *(14)*. Increasing adolescents' fruit intakes requires policy and environmental responses and targeted interventions at school and home. Dietary habits in adolescence track into adulthood *(15)*.

HBSC survey 2013/2014

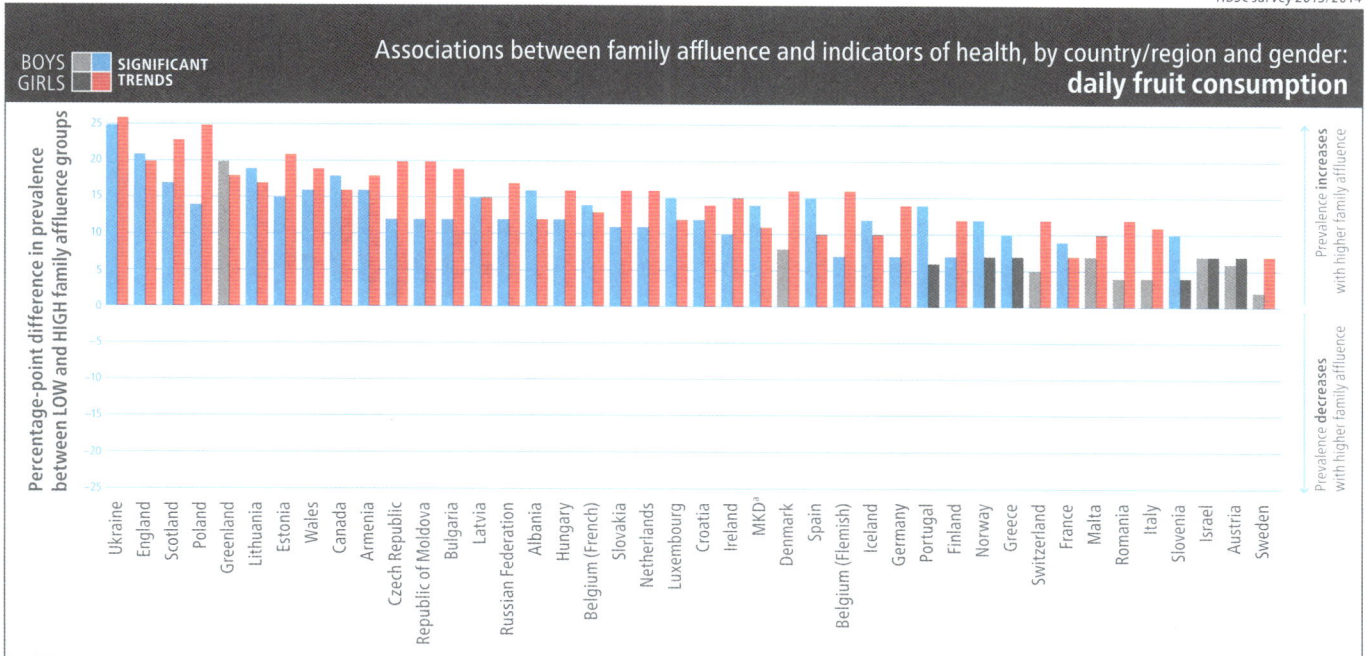

Associations between family affluence and indicators of health, by country/region and gender: **daily fruit consumption**

ª The former Yugoslav Republic of Macedonia. *Note:* low- and high-affluence groups represent the lowest 20% and highest 20% in each country.

MEASURE

Young people were asked how often they eat fruit. Response options ranged from never to every day, more than once.

Supplementary data on daily vegetable consumption are provided in the Annex.

RESULTS

Findings presented here show the proportions who reported eating fruit at least once a day.

Age

Daily fruit consumption decreased with age among boys in 38 countries and regions, with differences between 11- and 15-year-olds of 3–24 percentage points (Iceland and Austria, respectively). It also decreased with age for girls aged 11–15 in 32, with percentage-point differences ranging from 0.5 in Denmark to 20 in Hungary.

Gender

Overall, girls reported eating fruit more frequently. Gender differences were significant in two thirds of countries and regions in each age group. Frequency of intake was lowest in Greenland and highest among 15-year-old girls in Armenia.

Family affluence

Fruit consumption was higher among children from high-affluence families in almost all countries and regions. It was lower among boys (significant in 33) and girls (significant in 36) from low-affluence families relative to those of high affluence.

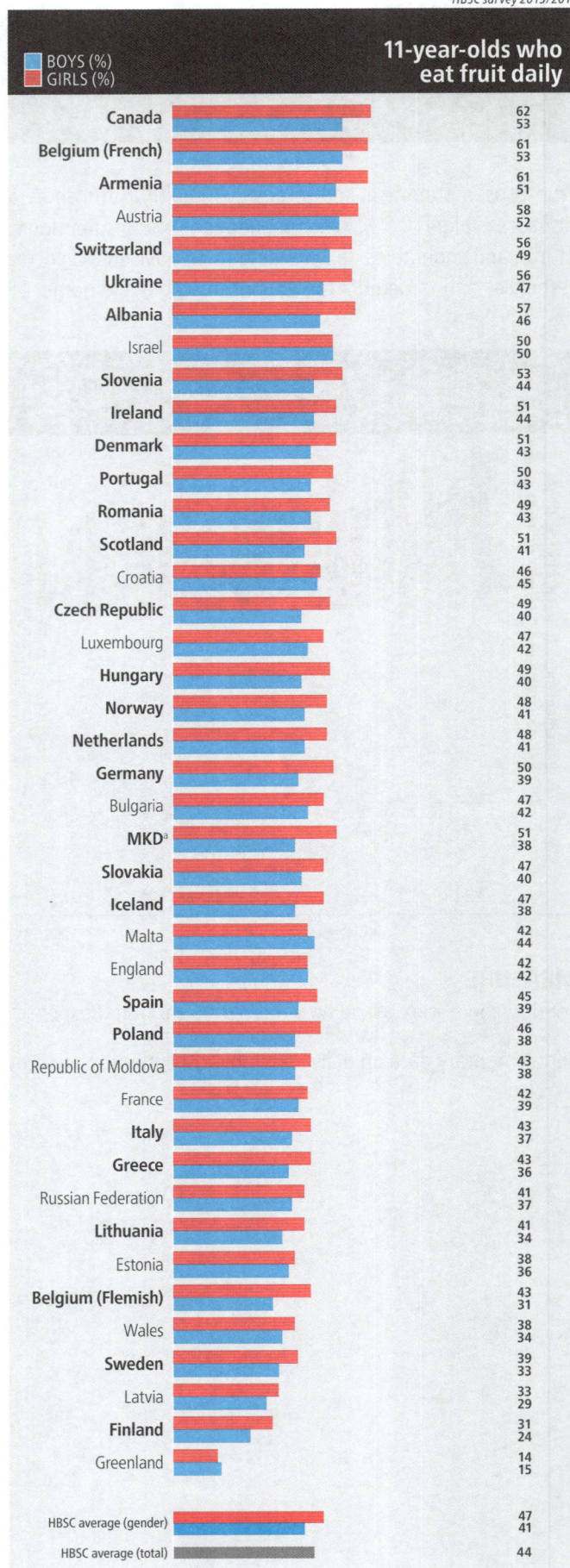

HBSC survey 2013/2014

11-year-olds who eat fruit daily

BOYS (%)
GIRLS (%)

Country	Boys (%)	Girls (%)
Canada	53	62
Belgium (French)	53	61
Armenia	51	61
Austria	52	58
Switzerland	49	56
Ukraine	47	56
Albania	46	57
Israel	50	50
Slovenia	44	53
Ireland	44	51
Denmark	43	51
Portugal	43	50
Romania	43	49
Scotland	41	51
Croatia	45	46
Czech Republic	40	49
Luxembourg	42	47
Hungary	40	49
Norway	41	48
Netherlands	41	48
Germany	39	50
Bulgaria	42	47
MKD[a]	38	51
Slovakia	40	47
Iceland	38	47
Malta	44	42
England	42	42
Spain	39	45
Poland	38	46
Republic of Moldova	38	43
France	39	42
Italy	37	43
Greece	36	43
Russian Federation	37	41
Lithuania	34	41
Estonia	36	38
Belgium (Flemish)	31	43
Wales	34	38
Sweden	33	39
Latvia	29	33
Finland	24	31
Greenland	15	14
HBSC average (gender)	41	47
HBSC average (total)		44

[a] The former Yugoslav Republic of Macedonia.

GROWING UP UNEQUAL: GENDER AND SOCIOECONOMIC
DIFFERENCES IN YOUNG PEOPLE'S HEALTH AND WELL-BEING
PART 2. KEY DATA | CHAPTER 4. HEALTH BEHAVIOURS
EATING BEHAVIOUR: FRUIT CONSUMPTION

4

13-year-olds who eat fruit daily

HBSC survey 2013/2014

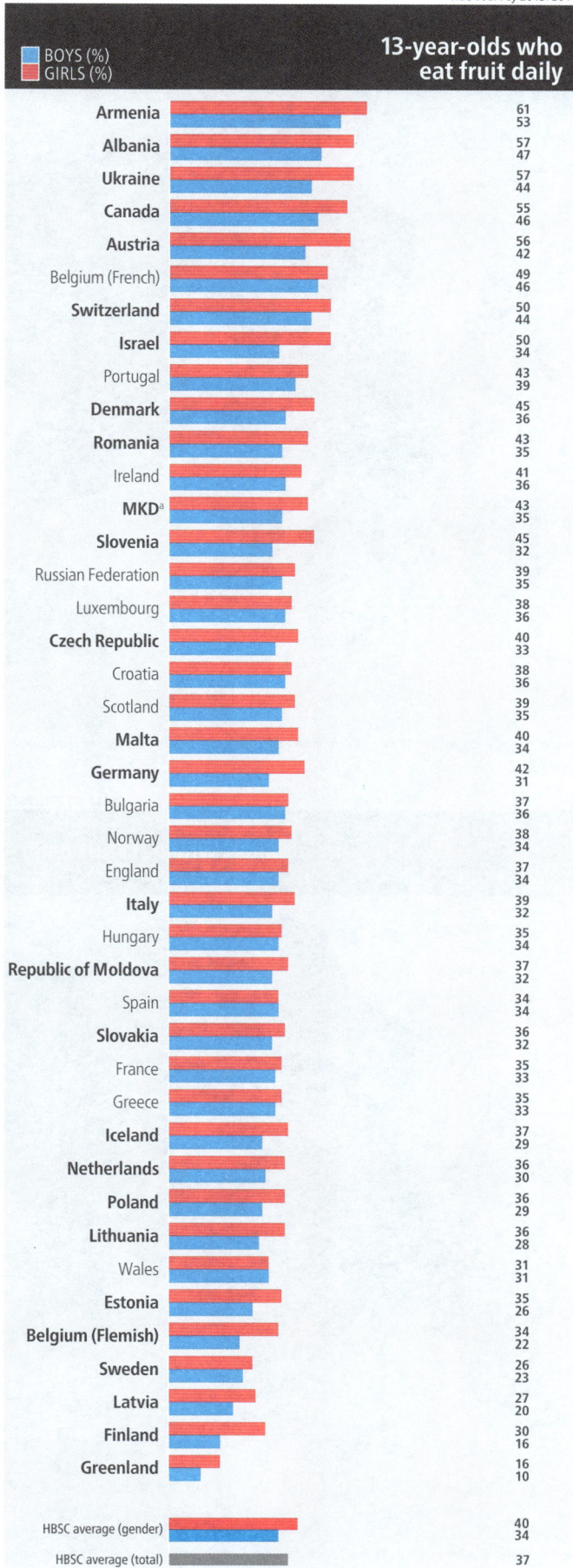

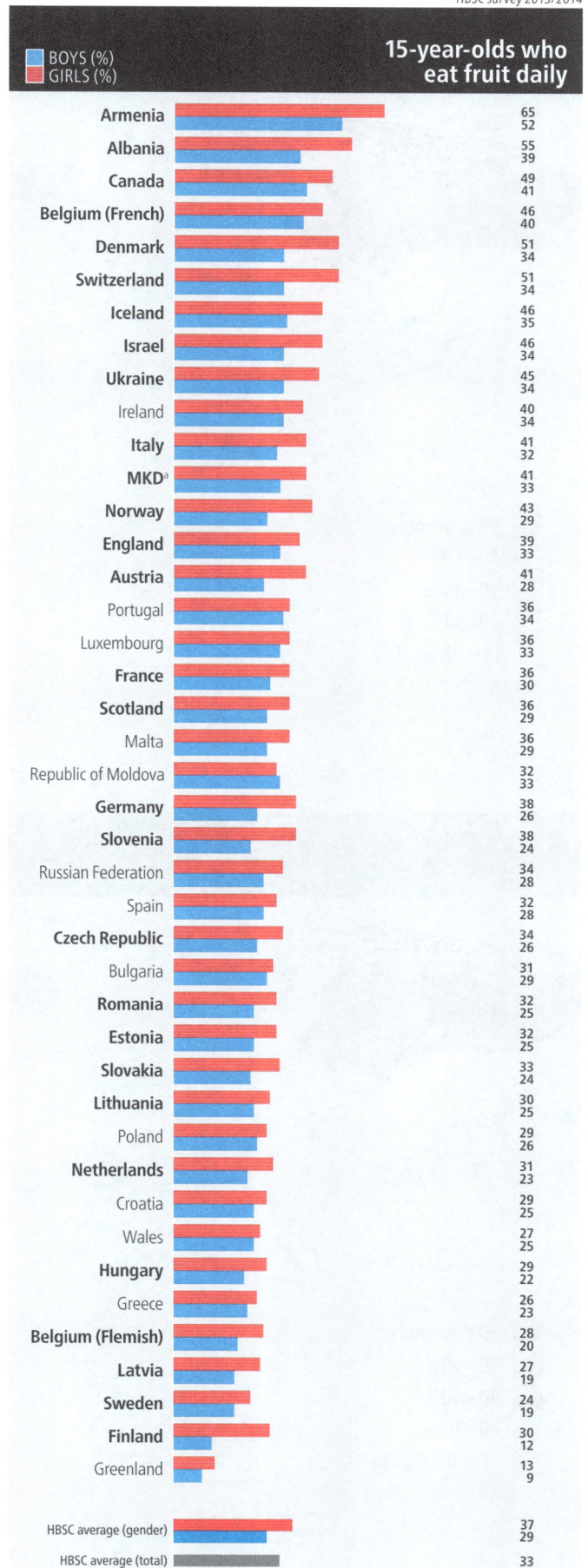

- BOYS (%)
- GIRLS (%)

Country	Girls	Boys
Armenia	61	53
Albania	57	47
Ukraine	57	44
Canada	55	46
Austria	56	42
Belgium (French)	49	46
Switzerland	50	44
Israel	50	34
Portugal	43	39
Denmark	45	36
Romania	43	35
Ireland	41	36
MKDª	43	35
Slovenia	45	32
Russian Federation	39	35
Luxembourg	38	36
Czech Republic	40	33
Croatia	38	36
Scotland	39	35
Malta	40	34
Germany	42	31
Bulgaria	37	36
Norway	38	34
England	37	34
Italy	39	32
Hungary	35	34
Republic of Moldova	37	32
Spain	34	34
Slovakia	36	32
France	35	33
Greece	35	33
Iceland	37	29
Netherlands	36	30
Poland	36	29
Lithuania	36	28
Wales	31	31
Estonia	35	26
Belgium (Flemish)	34	22
Sweden	26	23
Latvia	27	20
Finland	30	16
Greenland	16	10
HBSC average (gender)	40	34
HBSC average (total)	37	

15-year-olds who eat fruit daily

HBSC survey 2013/2014

- BOYS (%)
- GIRLS (%)

Country	Girls	Boys
Armenia	65	52
Albania	55	39
Canada	49	41
Belgium (French)	46	40
Denmark	51	34
Switzerland	51	34
Iceland	46	35
Israel	46	34
Ukraine	45	34
Ireland	40	34
Italy	41	32
MKDª	41	33
Norway	43	29
England	39	33
Austria	41	28
Portugal	36	34
Luxembourg	36	33
France	36	30
Scotland	36	29
Malta	36	29
Republic of Moldova	32	33
Germany	38	26
Slovenia	38	24
Russian Federation	34	28
Spain	32	28
Czech Republic	34	26
Bulgaria	31	29
Romania	32	25
Estonia	32	25
Slovakia	33	24
Lithuania	30	25
Poland	29	26
Netherlands	31	23
Croatia	29	25
Wales	27	25
Hungary	29	22
Greece	26	23
Belgium (Flemish)	28	20
Latvia	27	19
Sweden	24	19
Finland	30	12
Greenland	13	9
HBSC average (gender)	37	29
HBSC average (total)	33	

*Note: **indicates** significant gender difference (at p<0.05).*

HBSC survey 2013/2014

15-year-old girls who eat fruit daily

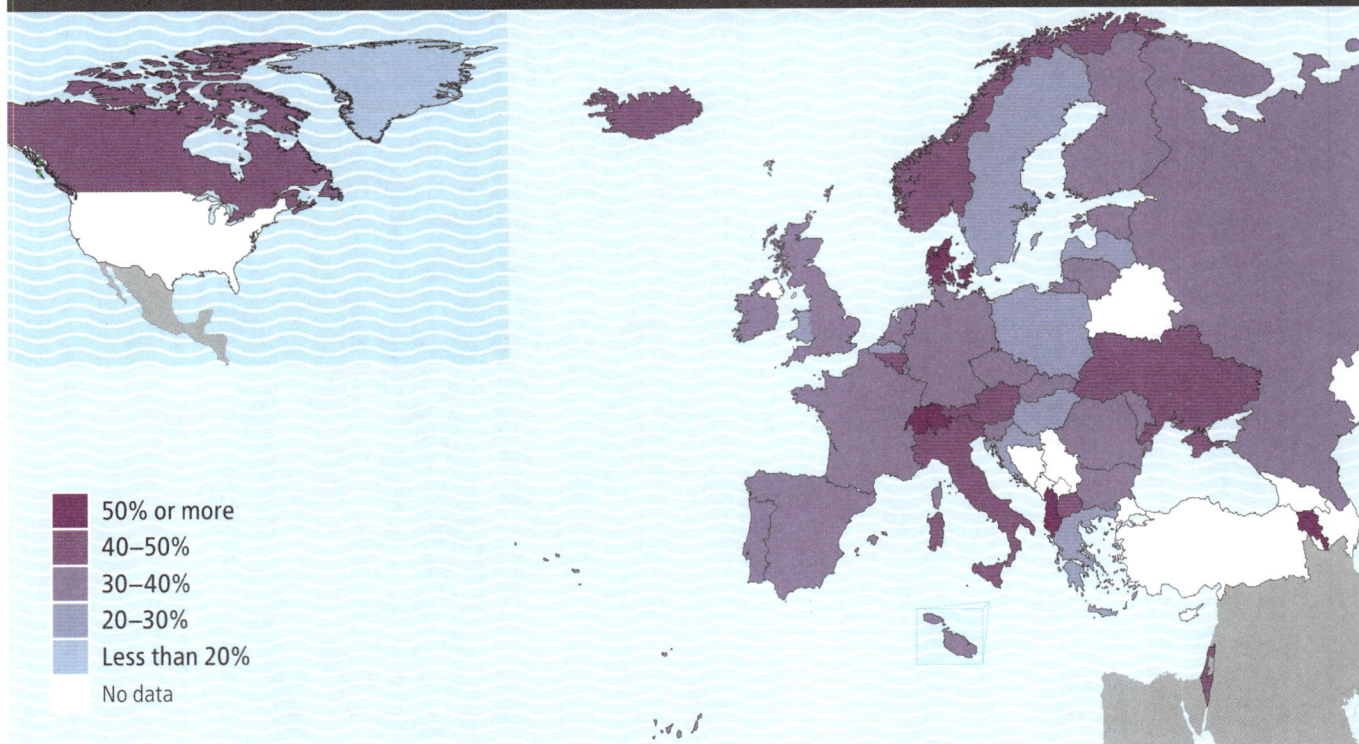

50% or more
40–50%
30–40%
20–30%
Less than 20%
No data

Note: HBSC teams provided disaggregated data for Belgium and the United Kingdom; these data appear in the map above.

HBSC survey 2013/2014

15-year-old boys who eat fruit daily

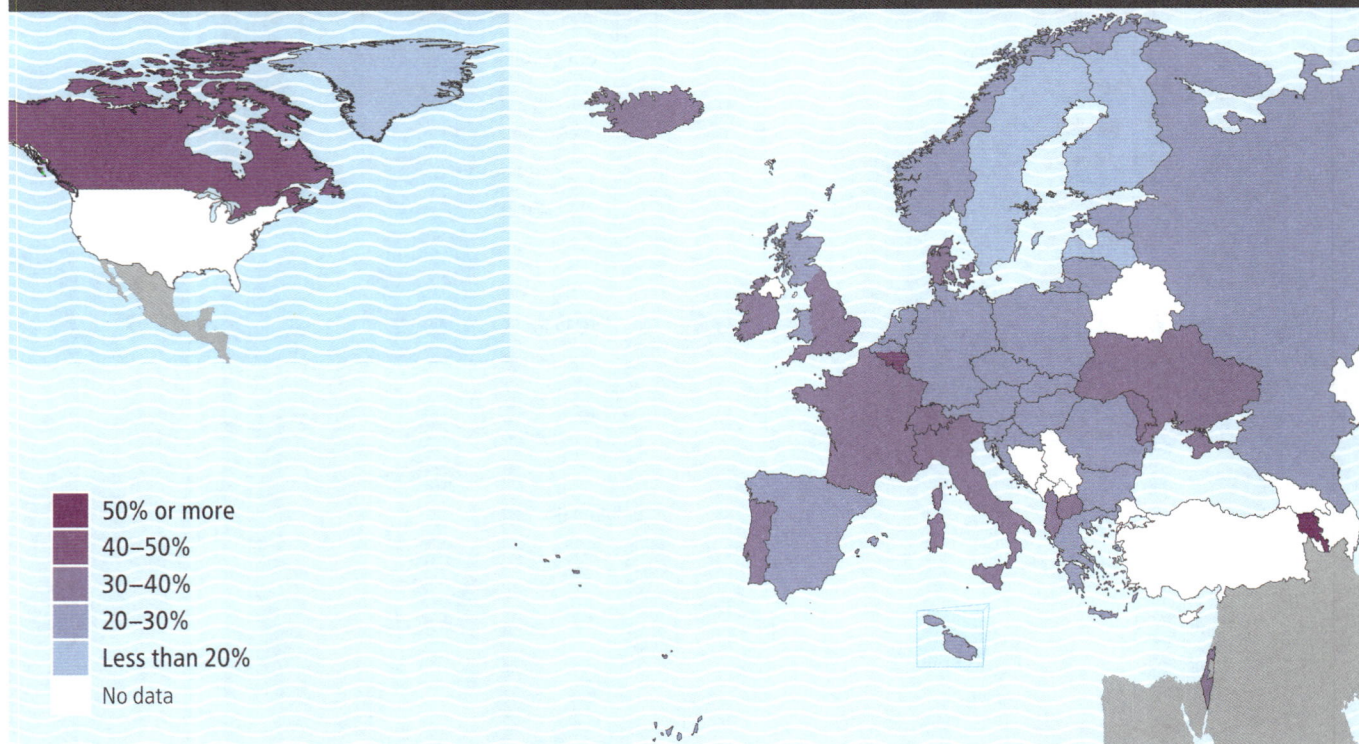

50% or more
40–50%
30–40%
20–30%
Less than 20%
No data

Note: HBSC teams provided disaggregated data for Belgium and the United Kingdom; these data appear in the map above.

GROWING UP UNEQUAL: GENDER AND SOCIOECONOMIC
DIFFERENCES IN YOUNG PEOPLE'S HEALTH AND WELL-BEING
PART 2. KEY DATA | CHAPTER 4. HEALTH BEHAVIOURS

4

EATING BEHAVIOUR:
SOFT-DRINK CONSUMPTION

Intake of soft drinks among adolescents is a matter of concern *(16,17)* and is higher than in other age groups *(17,18)*. It is associated with a greater risk of weight gain *(19)*, obesity *(20–22)* and chronic diseases *(23,24)* and directly affects dental health by providing excessive amounts of sugars *(25)*.

Consumption is correlated with taste preferences *(26)*, high availability of products *(27)* and parents and peers' attitudes *(28–30)*. Soft drinks provide high energy intake in liquid form that contributes to increasing the simple-carbohydrate content of the diet and reducing other nutrients *(31,32)*.

HBSC survey 2013/2014

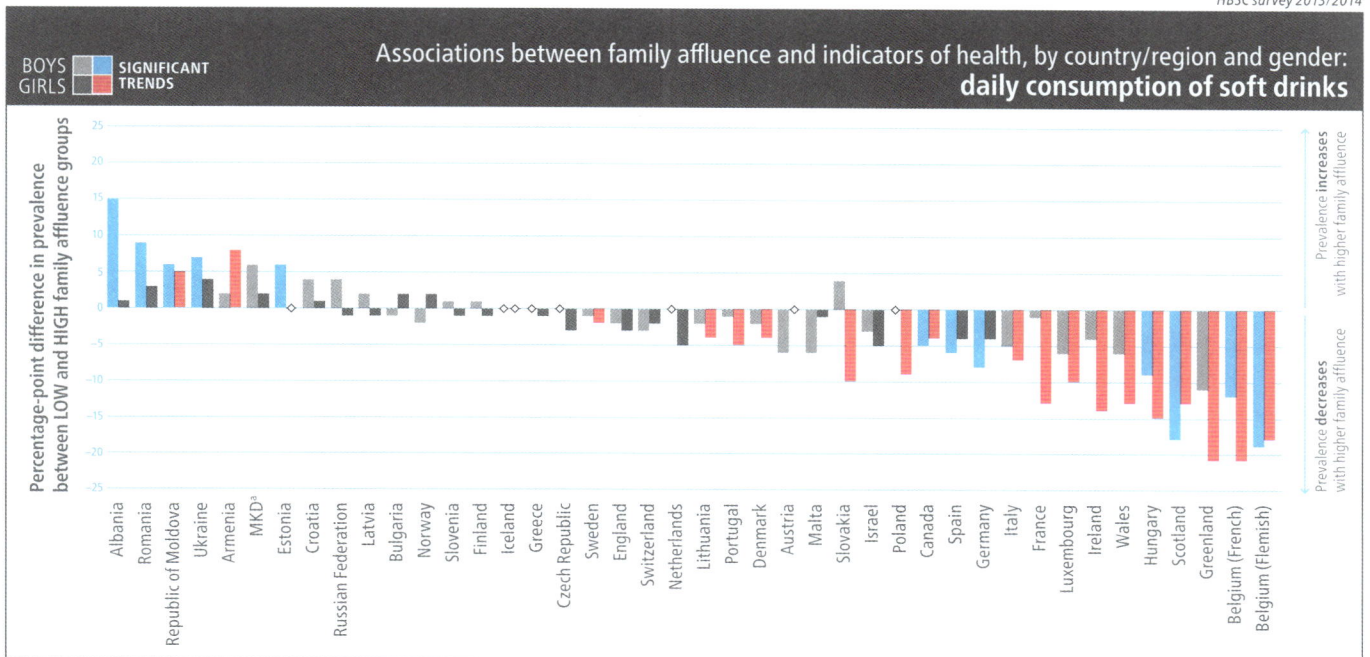

BOYS
GIRLS
SIGNIFICANT TRENDS

Associations between family affluence and indicators of health, by country/region and gender:
daily consumption of soft drinks

[a] The former Yugoslav Republic of Macedonia. *Note:* low- and high-affluence groups represent the lowest 20% and highest 20% in each country. ◇ means less than +/-0.5%.

MEASURE

Participants were asked how often they drink sugared soft drinks, with response categories ranging from never to every day, more than once.

Supplementary data on daily sweets consumption are provided in the Annex.

RESULTS

Findings presented here show the proportions reporting that they consumed soft drinks at least once a day.

Age

Daily consumption increased with age for boys in 23 countries and regions, with differences between 11- and 15-year-olds of 4–23 percentage points (Iceland and the Netherlands, respectively). For girls, it increased with age in 16: percentage-point differences between 11- and 15-year-olds ranged from 1 (Wales) to 22 (Greenland).

Gender

Boys generally reported greater daily consumption across all age groups, except for 11-year-olds in Ireland and 13-year-olds in Israel (girls were more likely to report it). Gender differences in each age group were significant in more than half of countries and regions, with average differences increasing with age.

Family affluence

The relationship between family affluence and soft-drink consumption was not consistent across countries and regions. It was significantly associated for boys in 12: seven had a negative relationship (low affluence, high consumption) and five a positive (high affluence, high consumption). For girls, there was a significant association in 19, with consumption being higher among low-affluence groups in most.

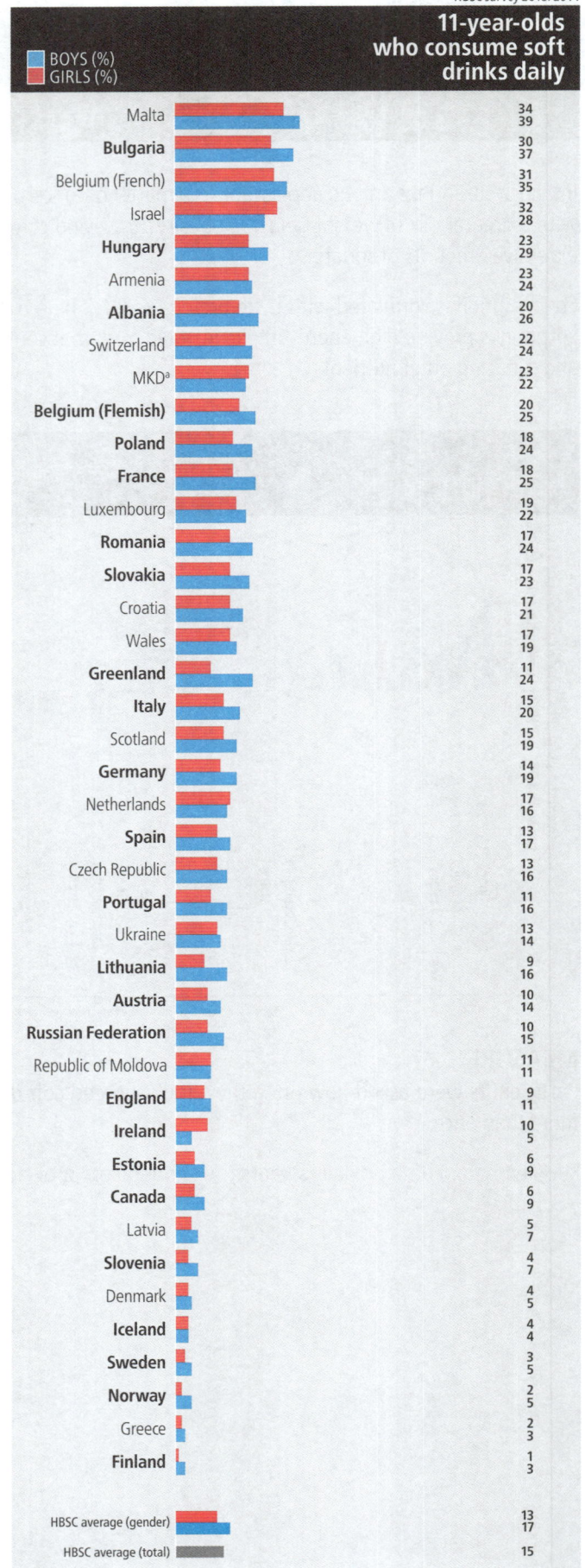

HBSC survey 2013/2014

11-year-olds who consume soft drinks daily

BOYS (%)
GIRLS (%)

Country	Boys	Girls
Malta	34	39
Bulgaria	30	37
Belgium (French)	31	35
Israel	32	28
Hungary	23	29
Armenia	23	24
Albania	20	26
Switzerland	22	24
MKD[a]	23	22
Belgium (Flemish)	20	25
Poland	18	24
France	18	25
Luxembourg	19	22
Romania	17	24
Slovakia	17	23
Croatia	17	21
Wales	17	19
Greenland	11	24
Italy	15	20
Scotland	15	19
Germany	14	19
Netherlands	17	16
Spain	13	17
Czech Republic	13	16
Portugal	11	16
Ukraine	13	14
Lithuania	9	16
Austria	10	14
Russian Federation	10	15
Republic of Moldova	11	11
England	9	11
Ireland	10	5
Estonia	6	9
Canada	6	9
Latvia	5	7
Slovenia	4	7
Denmark	4	5
Iceland	4	4
Sweden	3	5
Norway	2	5
Greece	2	3
Finland	1	3
HBSC average (gender)	13	17
HBSC average (total)		15

[a] The former Yugoslav Republic of Macedonia.

GROWING UP UNEQUAL: GENDER AND SOCIOECONOMIC
DIFFERENCES IN YOUNG PEOPLE'S HEALTH AND WELL-BEING
PART 2. KEY DATA | CHAPTER 4. HEALTH BEHAVIOURS
EATING BEHAVIOUR: SOFT-DRINK CONSUMPTION

4

13-year-olds who consume soft drinks daily

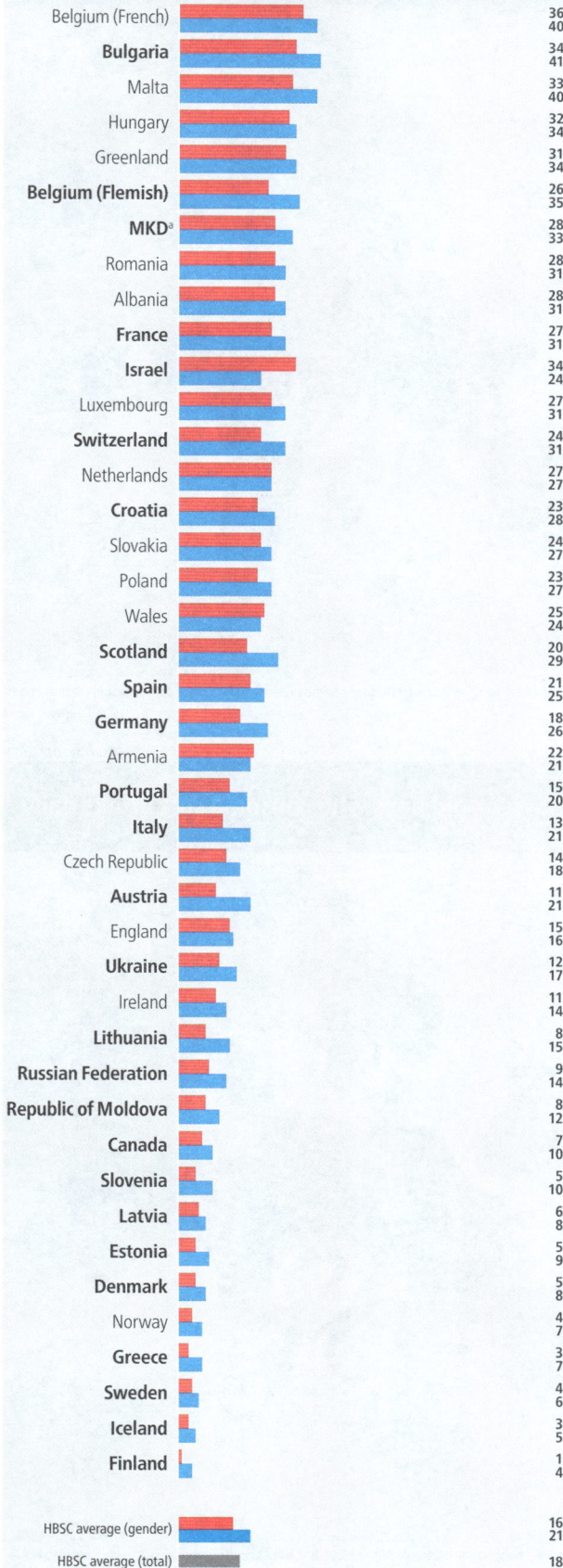

HBSC survey 2013/2014

■ BOYS (%)
■ GIRLS (%)

Country	Girls	Boys
Belgium (French)	36	40
Bulgaria	34	41
Malta	33	40
Hungary	32	34
Greenland	31	34
Belgium (Flemish)	26	35
MKD[a]	28	33
Romania	28	31
Albania	28	31
France	27	31
Israel	34	24
Luxembourg	27	31
Switzerland	24	31
Netherlands	27	27
Croatia	23	28
Slovakia	24	27
Poland	23	27
Wales	25	24
Scotland	20	29
Spain	21	25
Germany	18	26
Armenia	22	21
Portugal	15	20
Italy	13	21
Czech Republic	14	18
Austria	11	21
England	15	16
Ukraine	12	17
Ireland	11	14
Lithuania	8	15
Russian Federation	9	14
Republic of Moldova	8	12
Canada	7	10
Slovenia	5	10
Latvia	6	8
Estonia	5	9
Denmark	5	8
Norway	4	7
Greece	3	7
Sweden	4	6
Iceland	3	5
Finland	1	4
HBSC average (gender)	16	21
HBSC average (total)		18

15-year-olds who consume soft drinks daily

HBSC survey 2013/2014

■ BOYS (%)
■ GIRLS (%)

Country	Girls	Boys
Malta	39	37
Belgium (French)	34	41
MKD[a]	35	40
Greenland	33	42
Netherlands	29	39
Belgium (Flemish)	28	37
Luxembourg	27	40
Bulgaria	30	34
Israel	31	33
Hungary	32	30
France	28	35
Albania	26	35
Switzerland	23	36
Scotland	24	32
Slovakia	25	29
Romania	24	30
Croatia	24	26
Poland	20	27
Armenia	21	25
Germany	16	26
Wales	18	23
Spain	18	23
Portugal	18	22
Austria	15	24
England	13	18
Czech Republic	14	17
Ukraine	12	17
Italy	12	16
Ireland	13	14
Republic of Moldova	10	12
Canada	7	14
Lithuania	7	13
Norway	5	13
Russian Federation	7	10
Slovenia	6	8
Denmark	5	8
Greece	4	9
Latvia	5	8
Sweden	5	7
Iceland	3	8
Estonia	3	7
Finland	1	5
HBSC average (gender)	16	22
HBSC average (total)		19

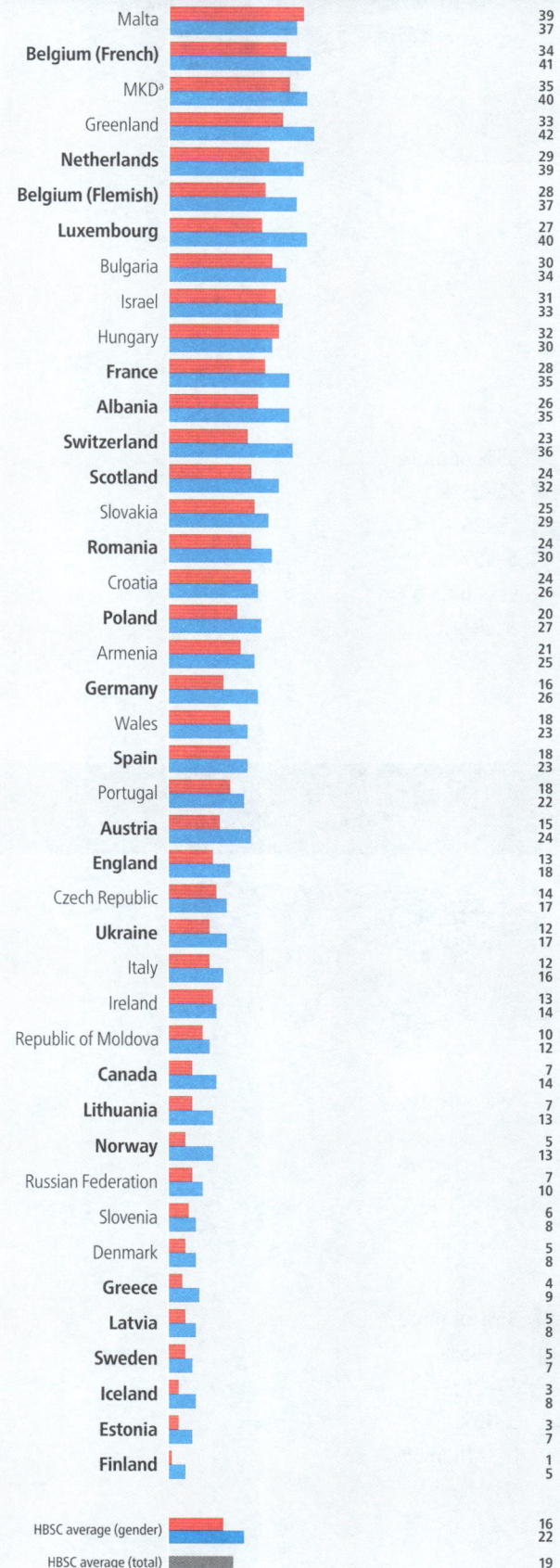

Note: **indicates** significant gender difference (at p<0.05).

HBSC survey 2013/2014

15-year-old girls who consume soft drinks daily

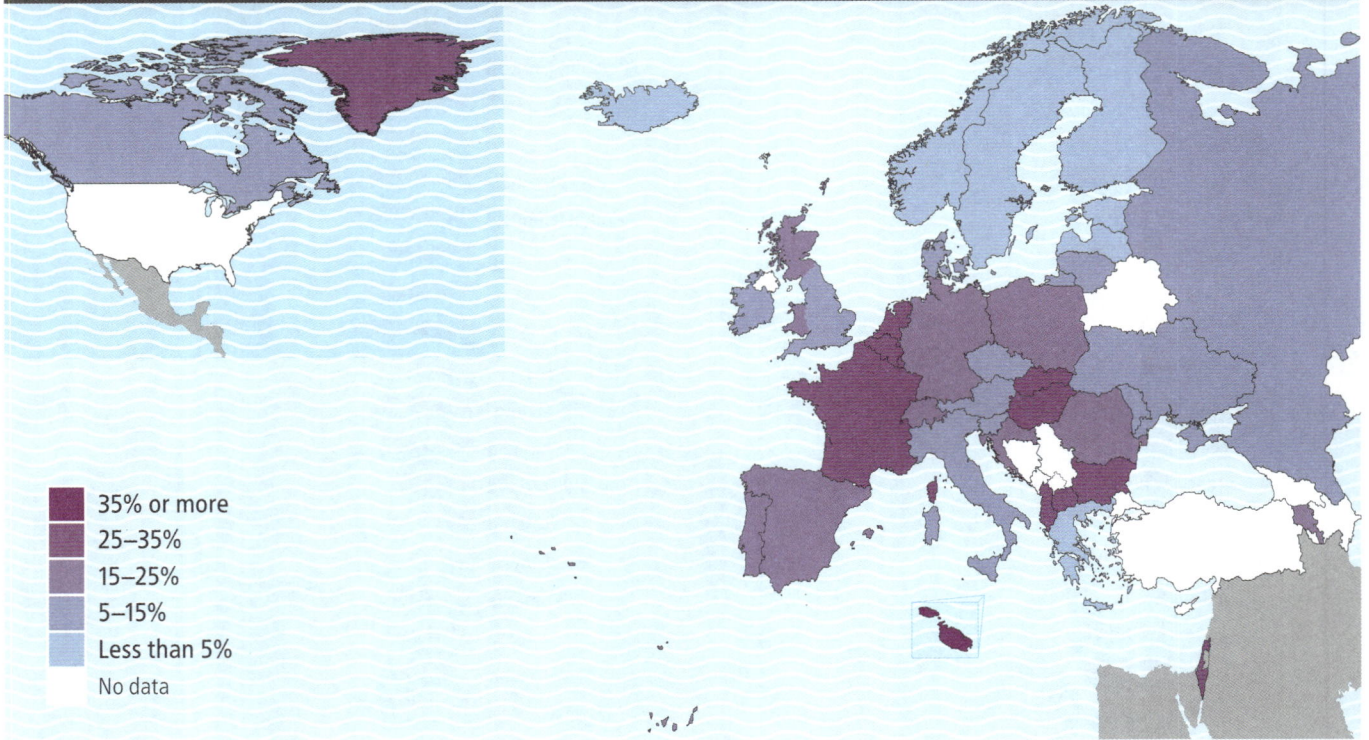

- 35% or more
- 25–35%
- 15–25%
- 5–15%
- Less than 5%
- No data

Note: HBSC teams provided disaggregated data for Belgium and the United Kingdom; these data appear in the map above.

HBSC survey 2013/2014

15-year-old boys who consume soft drinks daily

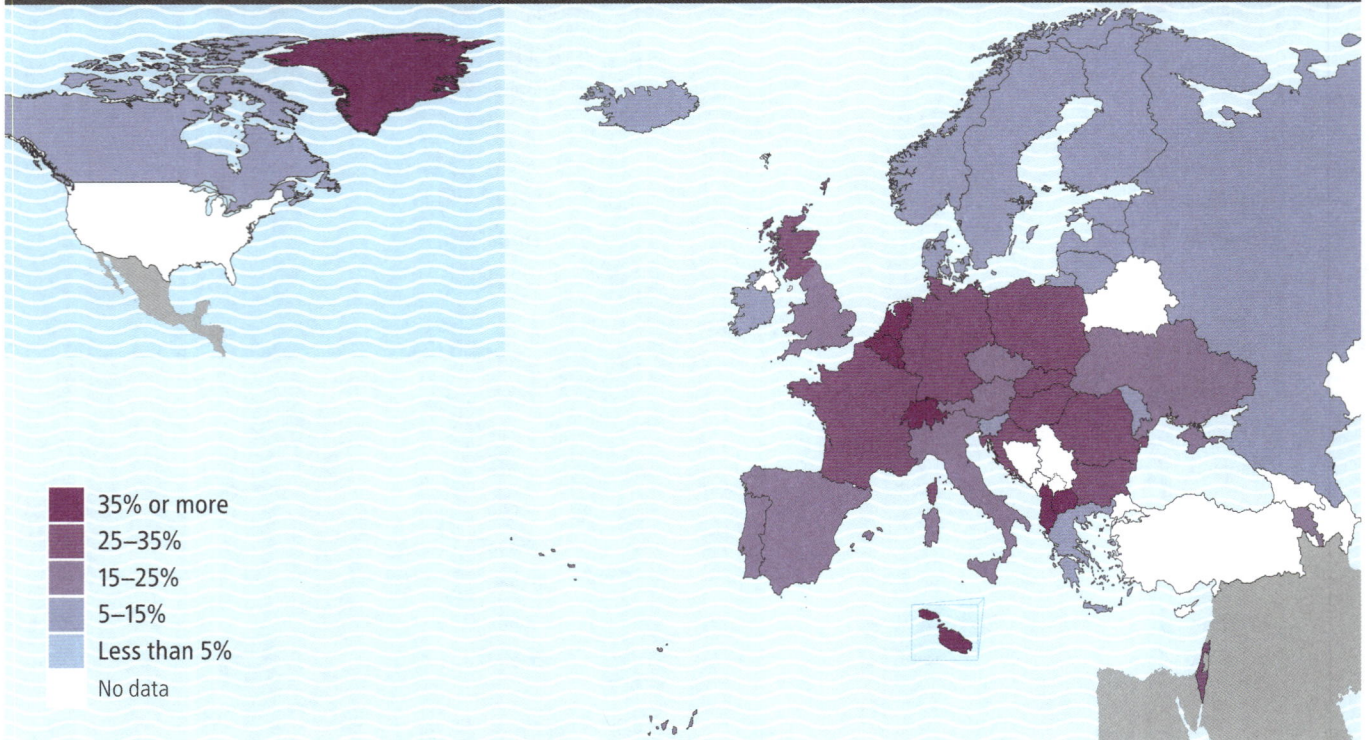

- 35% or more
- 25–35%
- 15–25%
- 5–15%
- Less than 5%
- No data

Note: HBSC teams provided disaggregated data for Belgium and the United Kingdom; these data appear in the map above.

GROWING UP UNEQUAL: GENDER AND SOCIOECONOMIC
DIFFERENCES IN YOUNG PEOPLE'S HEALTH AND WELL-BEING
PART 2. KEY DATA | CHAPTER 4. HEALTH BEHAVIOURS

4

EATING BEHAVIOUR:
EVENING MEALS WITH FAMILY

Studies indicate that a regular family meal is associated with healthier diets for children and adolescents (33–38). Some have also found a positive dietary effect of family meals over time (39–41).

Family meals may offer an opportunity for parents to provide healthy choices and present an example of healthy eating (42,43), or have a family conversation about food (34). In addition, they may contribute to the development of regular eating patterns, support young people's positive psychosocial development (33) and help parents to notice whether or not their child is taking an adequate diet (44).

HBSC survey 2013/2014

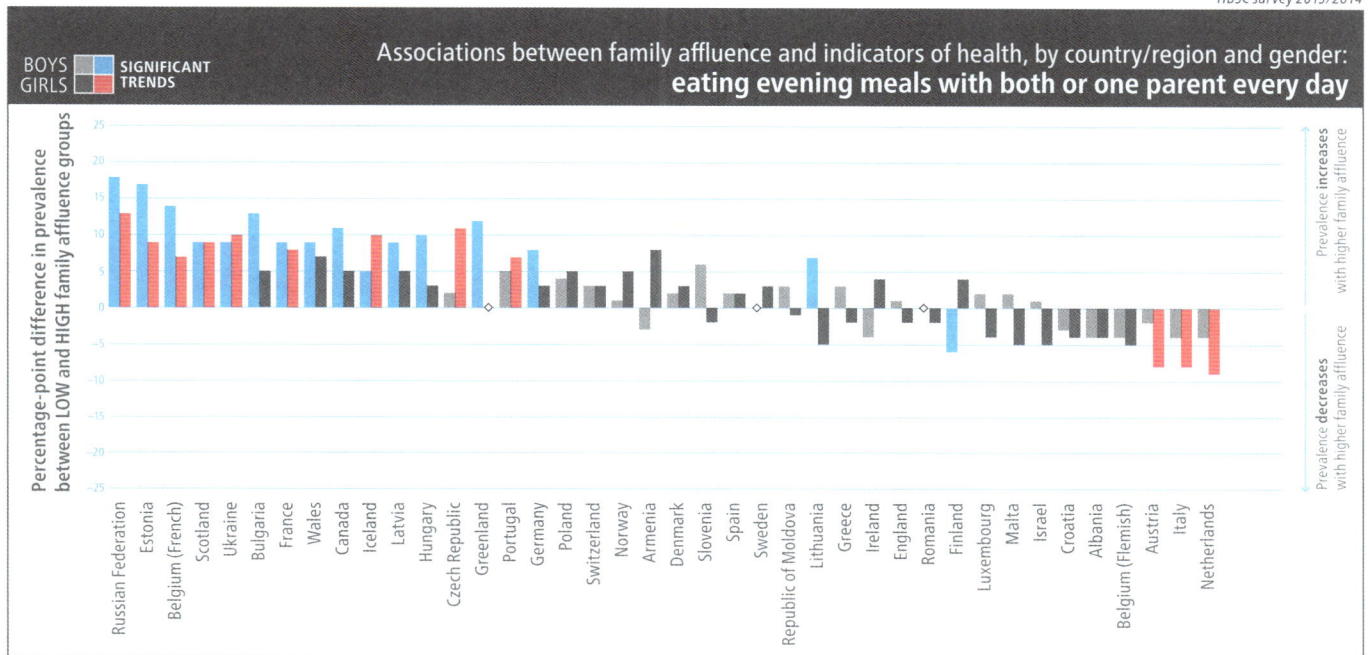

Associations between family affluence and indicators of health, by country/region and gender: **eating evening meals with both or one parent every day**

Note: low- and high-affluence groups represent the lowest 20% and highest 20% in each country. ◇ means less than +/-0.5%.
No data were received from Slovakia and the former Yugoslav Republic of Macedonia.

MEASURE
Young people were asked how often they eat an evening meal with both or one parent.

Supplementary data on eating breakfast with mother or father every day are provided in the Annex.

RESULTS

Findings presented here show the proportions reporting eating evening meals with both or one parent every day.

Age

Prevalence ranged from 88% of 11-year-old girls in Portugal to 13% of 15-year-old girls in Finland and Poland. A significant decrease with age was seen among boys in 35 countries and regions, with the largest difference between 11- and 15-year-olds being 29 percentage points (Austria). It decreased significantly with age for girls in 39, the largest being 32 percentage points (Austria, Hungary and Sweden).

Gender

No significant difference was seen in most countries and regions. Among 11-year-olds, more girls reported family meals in nine countries and regions and more boys in two. By age 15, the respective numbers were five for boys and two for girls.

Family affluence

Daily evening meals with parents tended to be more common among young people from high-affluence families. A higher prevalence was seen among high-affluence boys in 15, with the opposite relationship in only one. For girls, the respective figures were nine and three.

HBSC survey 2013/2014

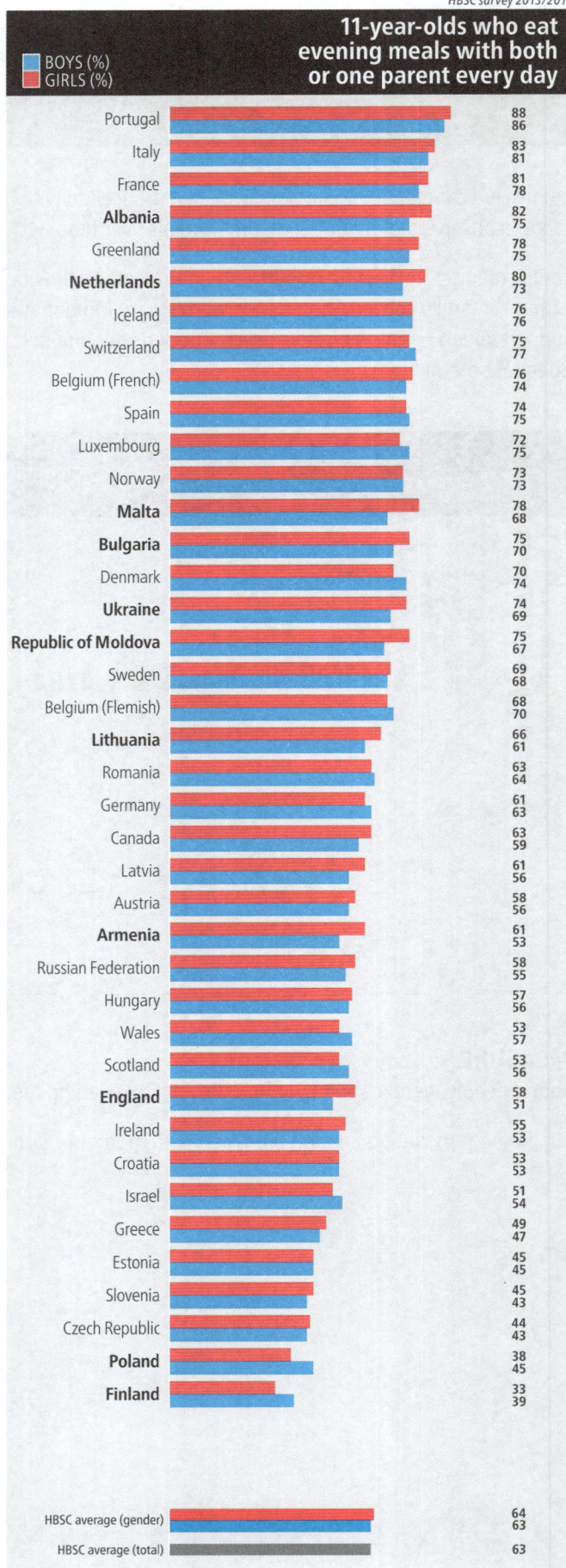

11-year-olds who eat evening meals with both or one parent every day

BOYS (%)
GIRLS (%)

Country	Girls	Boys
Portugal	88	86
Italy	83	81
France	81	78
Albania	82	75
Greenland	78	75
Netherlands	80	73
Iceland	76	76
Switzerland	75	77
Belgium (French)	76	74
Spain	74	75
Luxembourg	72	75
Norway	73	73
Malta	78	68
Bulgaria	75	70
Denmark	70	74
Ukraine	74	69
Republic of Moldova	75	67
Sweden	69	68
Belgium (Flemish)	68	70
Lithuania	66	61
Romania	63	64
Germany	61	63
Canada	63	59
Latvia	61	56
Austria	58	56
Armenia	61	53
Russian Federation	58	55
Hungary	57	56
Wales	53	57
Scotland	53	56
England	58	51
Ireland	55	53
Croatia	53	53
Israel	51	54
Greece	49	47
Estonia	45	45
Slovenia	45	43
Czech Republic	44	43
Poland	38	45
Finland	33	39
HBSC average (gender)	64	63
HBSC average (total)		63

ª The former Yugoslav Republic of Macedonia.

GROWING UP UNEQUAL: GENDER AND SOCIOECONOMIC
DIFFERENCES IN YOUNG PEOPLE'S HEALTH AND WELL-BEING
PART 2. KEY DATA | CHAPTER 4. HEALTH BEHAVIOURS
EATING BEHAVIOUR: EVENING MEALS WITH FAMILY

4

13-year-olds who eat evening meals with both or one parent every day

HBSC survey 2013/2014

- BOYS (%)
- GIRLS (%)

Country	Girls	Boys
Portugal	86	81
Italy	81	84
Albania	84	77
France	81	78
Belgium (French)	77	74
Netherlands	75	74
Spain	73	73
Greenland	71	72
Luxembourg	68	72
Belgium (Flemish)	68	70
Switzerland	70	67
Republic of Moldova	67	66
Denmark	64	68
Iceland	64	67
Malta	66	65
Norway	63	68
Ukraine	68	61
Bulgaria	65	63
Romania	56	57
Armenia	59	51
Canada	54	55
Germany	52	55
Sweden	50	57
Lithuania	51	53
Russian Federation	51	51
Wales	48	52
England	49	50
Scotland	48	50
Ireland	50	48
Latvia	47	45
Austria	45	45
Hungary	40	45
Croatia	42	42
Israel	45	34
Greece	40	40
Estonia	29	39
Slovenia	31	31
Poland	30	32
Czech Republic	29	32
Finland	21	23
HBSC average (gender)	56	57
HBSC average (total)		56

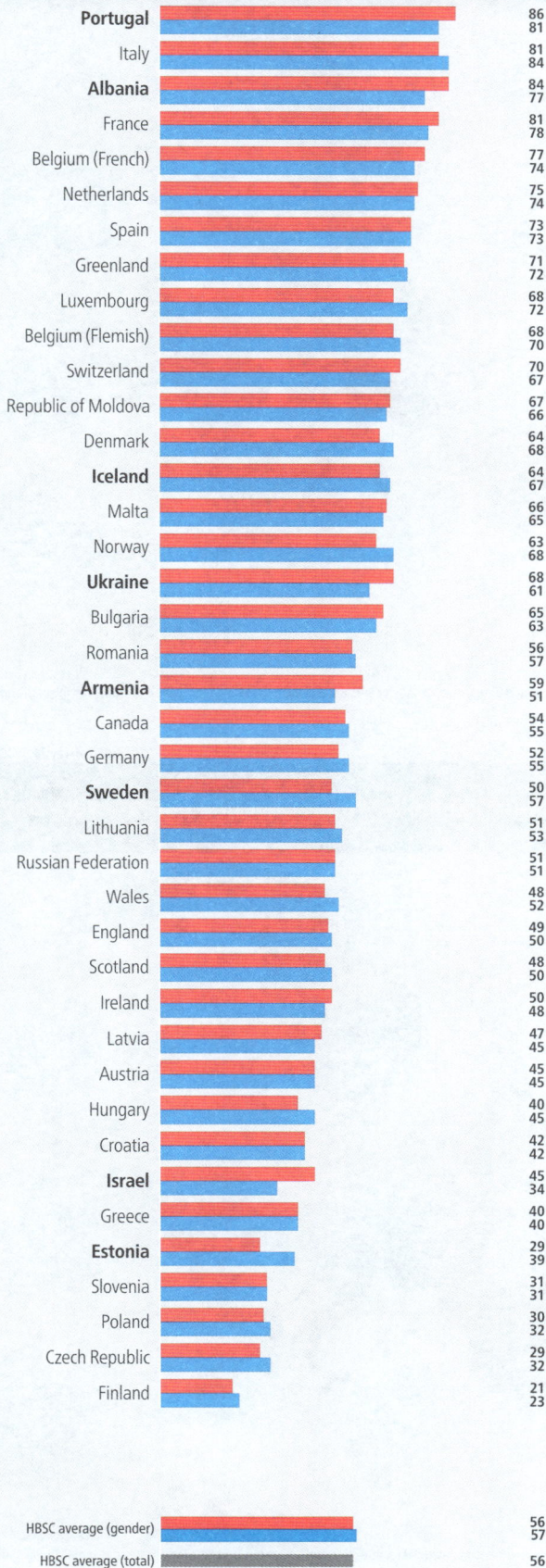

15-year-olds who eat evening meals with both or one parent every day

HBSC survey 2013/2014

- BOYS (%)
- GIRLS (%)

Country	Girls	Boys
Portugal	80	79
Albania	76	73
Italy	73	70
Belgium (French)	72	70
France	68	68
Netherlands	65	68
Greenland	58	68
Luxembourg	60	60
Spain	59	59
Republic of Moldova	59	60
Switzerland	57	61
Belgium (Flemish)	57	58
Armenia	61	52
Iceland	52	59
Ukraine	54	51
Norway	52	51
Malta	52	51
MKD[a]	53	48
Denmark	47	53
Bulgaria	50	45
England	43	44
Canada	41	45
Ireland	41	44
Scotland	42	41
Lithuania	38	43
Wales	38	43
Russian Federation	39	40
Germany	39	40
Sweden	37	41
Romania	39	39
Croatia	32	35
Latvia	32	33
Israel	31	29
Greece	27	33
Austria	26	27
Hungary	25	27
Estonia	21	23
Slovenia	17	20
Czech Republic	17	19
Poland	13	20
Slovakia	14	16
Finland	13	16
HBSC average (gender)	44	46
HBSC average (total)		45

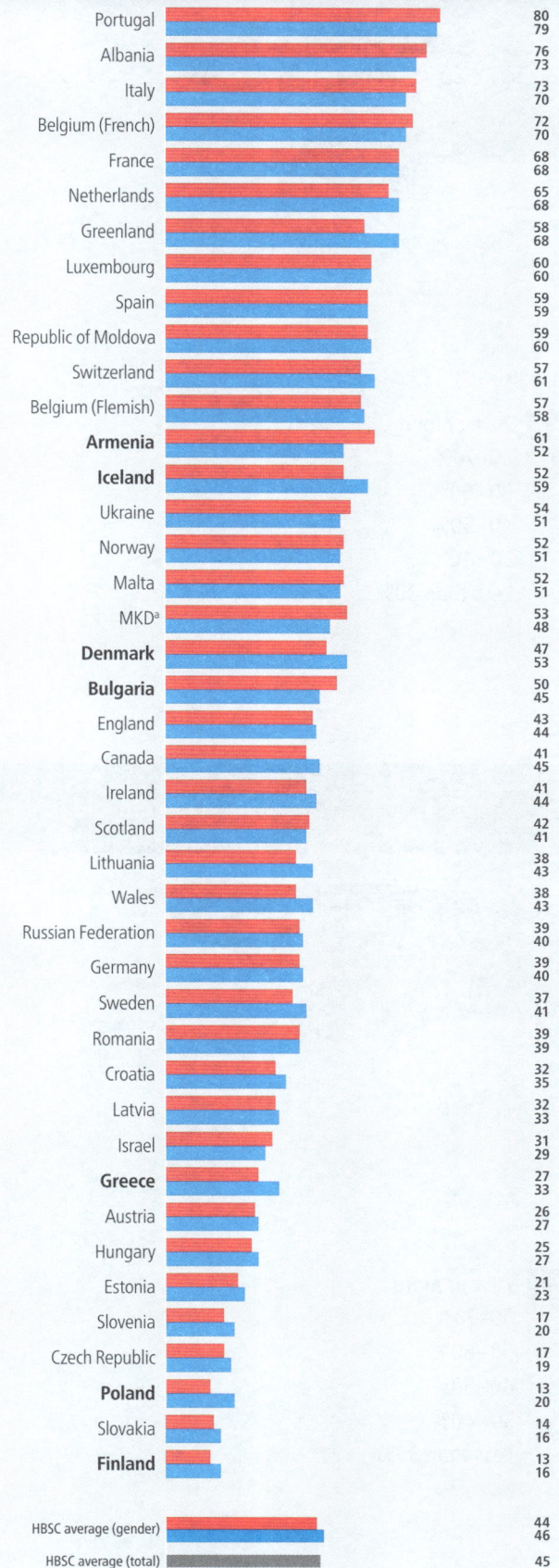

Note: **indicates** significant gender difference (at p<0.05). No data were received from Slovakia (11- and 13-year-olds) and the former Yugoslav Republic of Macedonia (11- and 13-year-olds).

HBSC survey 2013/2014

15-year-old girls who eat evening meals with both or one parent every day

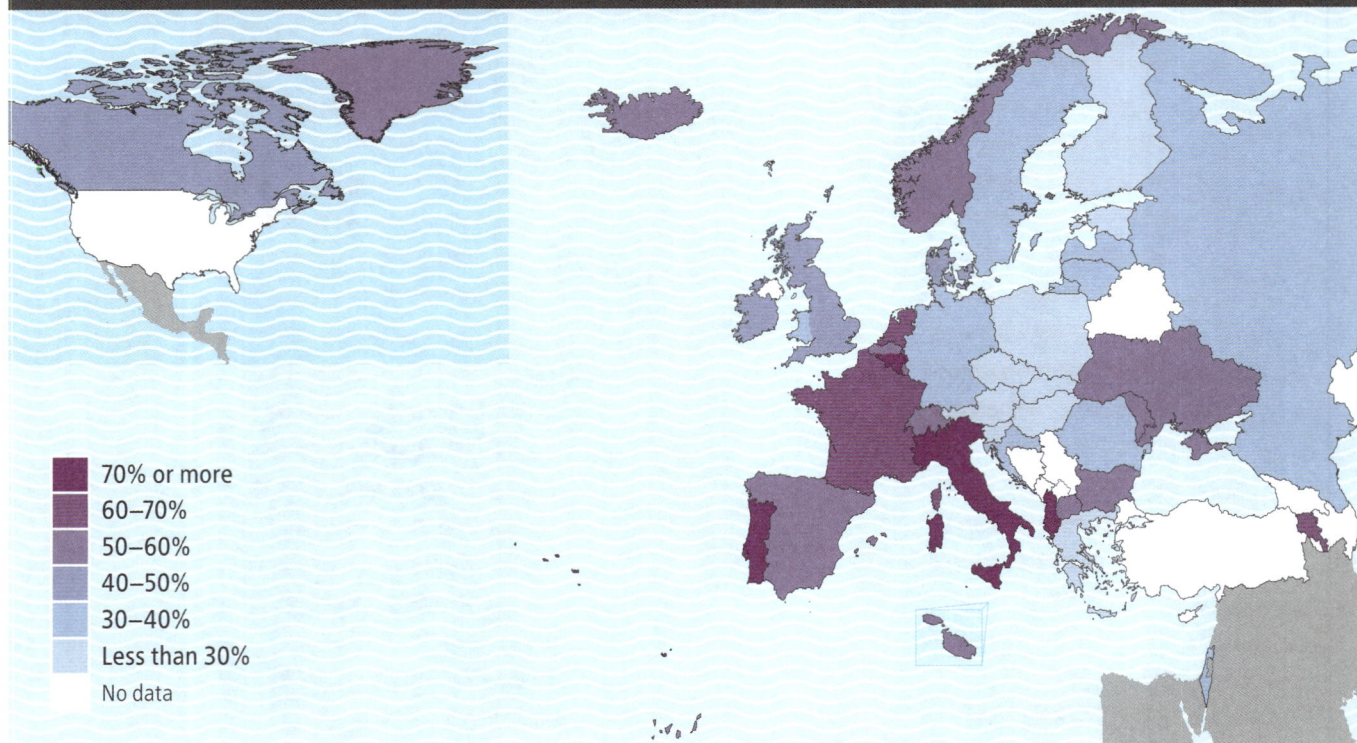

70% or more
60–70%
50–60%
40–50%
30–40%
Less than 30%
No data

Note: HBSC teams provided disaggregated data for Belgium and the United Kingdom; these data appear in the map above.

HBSC survey 2013/2014

15-year-old boys who eat evening meals with both or one parent every day

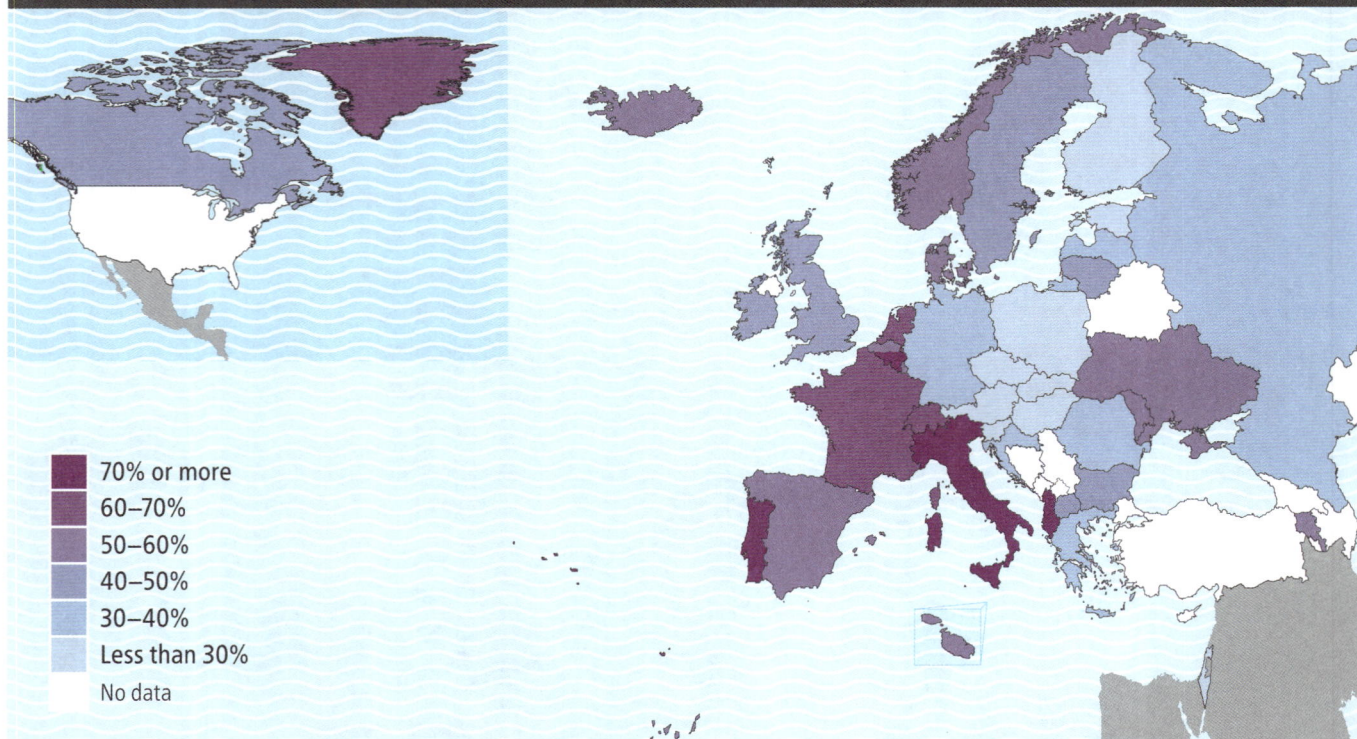

70% or more
60–70%
50–60%
40–50%
30–40%
Less than 30%
No data

Note: HBSC teams provided disaggregated data for Belgium and the United Kingdom; these data appear in the map above.

GROWING UP UNEQUAL: GENDER AND SOCIOECONOMIC
DIFFERENCES IN YOUNG PEOPLE'S HEALTH AND WELL-BEING
PART 2. KEY DATA | CHAPTER 4. HEALTH BEHAVIOURS
EATING BEHAVIOUR

4

EATING BEHAVIOUR:
SCIENTIFIC DISCUSSION AND POLICY REFLECTIONS

SCIENTIFIC DISCUSSION

Skipping breakfast continues to be common among young people *(45)*. Daily breakfast consumption is less frequent among girls, in families with lower affluence and in older children, which is consistent with the literature *(1,45,46)*. Greater autonomy among older children and reduced family environmental influence may contribute to these findings *(47,48)*.

Fruit intake is higher among girls, those from high-affluence families and younger children; again, this is consistent with previous findings *(49)*. Greater independence of food choice among older children may play a role *(50)*. Gender difference might be attributable to girls choosing healthier diets *(51)* and family affluence differences may reflect food environments within and across countries and regions.

Boys generally report greater soft-drink consumption, with intakes increasing significantly with age in just over half of countries and regions against just over a third for girls. Similar to other food and dietary items of interest, greater independence in food choice among older children may play a role *(50)*. Determinants of soft-drink consumption include gender, dieting, accessibility and modelling, which may explain some of the findings *(52)*. The relationship with family affluence is largely inverse for girls but mixed for boys. Food choice is influenced by a number of social and economic factors and luxury items (including soft drinks) may only be affordable in some countries and regions for families with greater material wealth *(53)*. Patterning by family affluence in the Baltic states and eastern European region is consistent with previous HBSC reports *(54)*.

The decrease by age in having a daily evening meal with parents is clear. Gender differences are present in only a few countries and regions. High family affluence is positively associated with evening meals in one third for boys and a quarter for girls, which is consistent with findings on family meals *(37)*. Family meal frequency and context is diverse across countries and regions.

POLICY REFLECTIONS

Food choice is determined by multiple factors, so approaches to improving dietary habits among adolescents must be diverse. Support from policy and practice at environmental, community, family and local levels is necessary, with multisectoral action being important. The socioeconomic gradient found in most indicators must also be addressed, ensuring that schoolchildren from all walks of life benefit from interventions.

Policy actions have included food labelling, food-based dietary guidelines, school programmes (vending machines and fruit schemes), salt reduction/reformulation, restriction on marketing of food with high fat, sugar and salt content to children, and taxes on sugar-sweetened beverages. School fruit schemes, food-based guidelines and labelling have been implemented more successfully than other policy actions, some of which have been only partially implemented or not at all *(55)*.

REFERENCES

1. Affenito SG. Breakfast: a missed opportunity. J Am Diet Assoc. 2007;107:565–69.

2. Haug E, Rasmussen M, Samdal O, Iannotti R, Kelly C, Borraccino A et al. Overweight in school-aged children and its relation with demographic and lifestyle factors: results from the WHO-collaborative Health Behaviour in School-aged Children (HBSC) Study. Int J Public Health 2009;54(2):167–79.

3. Keski-Rahkonen A, Kaprio J, Rissanen A, Virkkunen M, Rose RJ. Breakfast skipping and health-compromising behaviors in adolescents and adults. Eur J Clin Nutr. 2003;57:842–53.

4. Rampersaud GC, Pereira MA, Girard BL, Adams J, Metzl JD. Review – breakfast habits, nutritional status, body weight, and academic performance in children and adolescents. J Am Diet Assoc. 2005;105:743–60.

5. Deshmukh-Taskar PR, Nicklas TA, O'Neil CE, Keast DR, Radcliffe JD, Cho S. The relationship of breakfast skipping and type of breakfast consumption with nutrient intake and weight status in children and adolescents: the National Health and Nutrition Examination Survey 1999–2006. J Am Diet Assoc. 2010;110(6):869–78.

6. Leidy HJ, Ortinau LC, Douglas SM, Hoertel HA. Beneficial effects of a higher-protein breakfast on the appetitive, hormonal, and neural signals controlling energy intake regulation in overweight/obese, "breakfast-skipping", late-adolescent girls. Am J Clin Nutr. 2013;97(4):677–88.

7. Pearson N, Biddle SJ, Gorely T. Family correlates of breakfast consumption among children and adolescents. A systematic review. Appetite 2009;52(1):1–7.

8. Merten MJ, Williams AL, Shriver LH. Breakfast consumption in adolescence and young adulthood: parental presence, community context, and obesity. J Am Diet Assoc. 2009;109(8):1384–91.

9. Pedersen TP, Holstein BE, Flachs EM, Rasmussen M. Meal frequencies in early adolescence predict meal frequencies in late adolescence and early adulthood. BMC Public Health 2013;13(1):445.

10. Hoyland AI, Dye L, Lawton CL. A systematic review of the effect of breakfast on the cognitive performance of children and adolescents. Nutr Res Rev. 2009;22(2):220–43. doi: 10.1017/S0954422409990175.

11. Vainio H, Weiderpass E. Fruit and vegetables in cancer prevention. Nutr Cancer 2006;54:111–42.

12. He FJ, Nowson CA, Lucas M, MacGregor GA. Increased consumption of fruit and vegetables is related to a reduced risk of coronary heart disease: meta-analysis of cohort studies. J Hum Hypertens. 2007;21:717–28.

13. He FJ, Nowson CA, MacGregor GA. Fruit and vegetable consumption and stroke: meta-analysis of cohort studies. Lancet 2006;367:320–6.

14. Yngve A, Wolf A, Poortvliet E, Elmadfa I, Brug J, Ehrenblad B et al. Fruit and vegetable intake in a sample of 11-year-old children in 9 European countries: the Pro Children Cross-sectional Survey. Ann Nutr Metab. 2005;49:236–45.

15. Lien N, Lytle LA, Klepp KI. Stability in consumption of fruit, vegetables, and sugary foods in a cohort from age 14 to age 21. Prevent Med. 2001;33:217–26.

16. Han E, Powell LM. Consumption patterns of sugar-sweetened beverages in the United States. J Acad Nutr Diet 2013;113:43–53.

17. Duffey KJ, Huybrechts I, Mouratidou T, Libuda L, Kersting M, De Vriendt T et al. Beverage consumption among European adolescents in the HELENA study. Eur J Clin Nutr. 2012; 66(2):244–52. doi:10.1038/ejcn.2011.166.

18. Ozen AE, Bibiloni MD, Pons A, Tur JA. Fluid intake from beverages across age groups: a systematic review. J Hum Nutr Diet. 2014;28(5):417–42. doi:10.1111/jhn.12250.

19. Malik VS, Pan A, Willett WC, Hu FB. Sugar-sweetened beverages and weight gain in children and adults: a systematic review and meta-analysis. Am J Clin Nutr. 2013;98(4):1084–102. doi:10.3945/ajcn.113.058362.

20. Trumbo PR, Rivers CR. Systematic review of the evidence for an association between sugar-sweetened beverage consumption and risk of obesity. Nutr Rev. 2014;72(9):566–74. doi:10.1111/nure.12128.

21. Sahoo K, Sahoo B, Choudhury AK, Sofi NY, Kumar R, Bhadoria A. Childhood obesity: causes and consequences. J Family Med Prim Care 2015;4(2):187–92. doi:10.4103/2249-4863.154628.

22. Bigornia SJ, LaValley MP, Noel SE, Moore LL, Ness AR, Newby PK. Sugar-sweetened beverage consumption and central and total adiposity in older children: a prospective study accounting for dietary reporting errors. Public Health Nutr. 2015;18:1155–63. doi:10.1017/S1368980014001700.

23. Basu S, McKee M, Galea G, Stuckler D. Relationship of soft drink consumption to global overweight, obesity, and diabetes: a cross-national analysis of 75 countries. Am J Public Health 2013;103(11):2071–77. doi:10.2105/AJPH.2012.300974.

24. Greenwood DC, Threapleton DE, Evans CEL, Cleghorn CL, Nykjaer C, Woodhead C et al. Association between sugar-sweetened and artificially sweetened soft drinks and type 2 diabetes: systematic review and dose–response meta-analysis of prospective studies. Br J Nutr. 2014;112:725–34. doi:10.1017/S0007114514001329.

25. Hasselkvist A, Johansson A, Johansson AK. Association between soft drink consumption, oral health and some lifestyle factors in Swedish adolescents. Acta Odontol Scand. 2014;72(8):1039–46. doi:10.3109/00016357.2014.946964.

26. Low YQ, Lacy K, Keast R. The role of sweet taste in satiation and satiety. Nutrients 2014;6(9):3431–50. doi:10.3390/nu6093431.

27. Grimm GC, Harnack L, Story M. Factors associated with soft drink consumption in school-aged children. J Am Diet Assoc. 2004;104:1244–9.

28. Pettigrew S, Jongenelis M, Chapman K, Miller C. Factors influencing the frequency of children's consumption of soft drinks. Appetite 2015;91:393–8. doi:10.1016/j.appet.2015.04.080.

29. Bere E, Glomnes ES, te Velde SJ, Klepp K-I. Determinants of adolescents' soft drink consumption. Public Health Nutr. 2007;11(1):49–56. doi:10.1017/S1368980007000122.

30. Stok FM, de Vet E, de Wit JB, Luszczynska A, Safron M, de Ridder DT. The proof is in the eating: subjective peer norms are associated with adolescents' eating behavior. Public Health Nutr. 2015;18(6):1044–51. doi:10.1017/S1368980014001268.

31. Reedy J, Krebs-Smith SM. Dietary sources of energy, solid fats, and added sugars among children and adolescents in the United States. J Am Diet Assoc. 2010;110(10):1477–84. doi:10.1016/j.jada.2010.07.010.

32. Vartanian LR, Schwartz MB, Brownell KD. Effects of soft drink consumption on nutrition and health: a systematic review and meta-analysis. Am J Public Health 2007;97(4):667–75.

33. Neumark-Sztainer D, Hannan PJ, Story M, Croll J, Perry CL. Family meal patterns: associations with sociodemographic characteristics and improved dietary intake among adolescents. J Am Diet Assoc. 2003;103(3):317–22.

34. Gillman MW, Rifas-Shiman SL, Frazier AL, Rockett HR, Camargo CA Jr, Field AE et al. Family dinner and diet quality among older children and adolescents. Arch Fam Med. 2000;9(3):235–40.

35. Haapalahti M, Mykkanen H, Tikkanen S, Kokkonen J. Meal patterns and food use in 10- to 11-year-old Finnish children. Public Health Nutr. 2003;6(4):365–70.

36. Videon TM, Manning CK. Influences on adolescent eating patterns: the importance of family meals. J Adolesc Health 2003;32(5):365–73.

37. Neumark-Sztainer D, Larson NI, Fulkerson JA, Eisenberg ME, Story M. Family meals and adolescents: what have we learned from Project EAT (Eating Among Teens)? Public Health Nutr. 2010;13(7):1113–21.

38. Utter J, Denny S, Robinson E, Fleming T, Ameratunga S, Grant S. Family meals among New Zealand young people: relationships with eating behaviors and body mass index. J Nutr Educ Behav. 2013;45(1):3–11.

GROWING UP UNEQUAL: GENDER AND SOCIOECONOMIC
DIFFERENCES IN YOUNG PEOPLE'S HEALTH AND WELL-BEING
PART 2. KEY DATA | CHAPTER 4. HEALTH BEHAVIOURS
EATING BEHAVIOUR

4

39. Larson NI, Neumark-Sztainer D, Hannan PJ, Story M. Family meals during adolescence are associated with higher diet quality and healthful meal patterns during young adulthood. J Am Diet Assoc. 2007;107(9):1502–10.

40. Larson NI, Neumark-Sztainer DR, Story MT, Wall MM, Harnack LJ, Eisenberg ME. Fast food intake: longitudinal trends during the transition to young adulthood and correlates of intake. J Adolesc Health 2008;43(1):79–86.

41. Burgess-Champoux TL, Larson N, Neumark-Sztainer D, Hannan PJ, Story M. Are family meal patterns associated with overall diet quality during the transition from early to middle adolescence? J Nutr Educ Behav. 2009;41(2):79–86.

42. Kelsey KS, Campbell MK, Vanata DF. Parent and adolescent girls' preferences for parental involvement in adolescent health promotion programs. J Am Diet Assoc. 1998;98(8):906–7.

43. Neumark-Sztainer D, Story M, Perry C, Casey MA. Factors influencing food choices of adolescents: findings from focus-group discussions with adolescents. J Am Diet Assoc. 1999; 99(8):929–37.

44. Neumark-Sztainer D, Wall M, Story M, Fulkerson JA. Are family meal patterns associated with disordered eating behaviors among adolescents? J Adolesc Health 2004;35(5):350–9.

45. Vereecken C, Dupuy M, Rasmussen M, Kelly C, Nansel T.R, Al Sabbah H et al. Breakfast consumption and its socio-demographic and lifestyle correlates in schoolchildren in 41 countries participating in the HBSC study. Int J Public Health 2009;54(Suppl. 2):180–90. doi: 10.1007/s00038-009-5409-5.

46. Deshmukh-Taskar PR, Nicklas TA, O'Neil CE, Keast DR, Radcliffe JD, Cho S. The relationship of breakfast skipping and type of breakfast consumption with nutrient intake and weight status in children and adolescents: the National Health and Nutrition Examination Survey 1999–2006. J Am Diet Assoc 2010;110(6):869–78. doi:10.1016/j.jada.2010.03.023.

47. Pearson N, Biddle SJ, Gorely T. Family correlates of breakfast consumption among children and adolescents. A systematic review. Appetite 2009;52(1):1–7.

48. Pearson N, MacFarlane A, Crawford D, Biddle SJ. Family circumstance and adolescent dietary behaviours. Appetite 2009;52(3):668–74.

49. Vereecken C, Pedersen TP, Ojala K, Krolner R, Dzielska A, Ahluwalia N et al. Fruit and vegetable consumption trends among adolescents from 2002 to 2010 in 33 countries. Eur J Public Health 2015;25(Suppl. 2):16–9. doi:10.1093/eurpub/ckv012.

50. Fitzgerald A, Heary C, Nixon E, Kelly C. Factors influencing the food choices of Irish children and adolescents: a qualitative investigation. Health Promot Int. 2010;25(3):289–98. doi:10.1093/heapro/daq021.

51. Wardle J, Robb KA, Johnson F, Griffith J, Brunner E, Power C et al. Socioeconomic variation in attitudes to eating and weight in female adolescents. Health Psychol. 2004;23(3):275–82.

52. Bere E, Glomnes ES, te Velde SJ, Klepp KI. Determinants of adolescents' soft drink consumption. Public Health Nutr. 2008;11(1):49–56.

53. Vereecken CA, Inchley J, Subramanian SV, Hublet A, Maes L. The relative influence of individual and contextual socio-economic status on consumption of fruit and soft drinks among adolescents in Europe. Eur J Public Health 2005;15(3):224–32.

54. Currie C, Zanotti C, Morgan A, Currie D, de Looze M, Roberts C et al., editors. Social determinants of health and well-being among young people. Health Behaviour in School-aged Children (HBSC) study: international report from the 2009/2010 survey. Copenhagen: WHO Regional Office for Europe; 2012 (Health Policy for Children and Adolescents, No. 6; http://www.euro.who.int/en/what-we-publish/abstracts/socialdeterminants-of-health-and-well-being-among-young-people.-health-behaviour-in-schoolaged-children-hbsc-study, accessed 24 August 2015).

55. Marketing of foods high in fat, salt and sugar to children: update 2012–2013. Copenhagen: WHO Regional Office for Europe; 2013 (http://www.euro.who.int/__data/assets/pdf_file/0019/191125/e96859.pdf, accessed 24 August 2015).

GROWING UP UNEQUAL: GENDER AND SOCIOECONOMIC
DIFFERENCES IN YOUNG PEOPLE'S HEALTH AND WELL-BEING
PART 2. KEY DATA | CHAPTER 4. HEALTH BEHAVIOURS

4

ORAL HEALTH

Oral diseases have a strong association with cardiovascular and respiratory disease, diabetes and cancer, and poor oral hygiene with cardiovascular disease, hypertension, diabetes and metabolic syndrome (1,2).

Twice-a-day toothbrushing is the main self-care method to remove plaque and prevent the most prevalent noncommunicable diseases, periodontal disease and dental caries (3). Toothbrushing frequency has increased among schoolchildren in many countries and regions but still lags far behind the recommended twice a day in most, especially among boys (4).

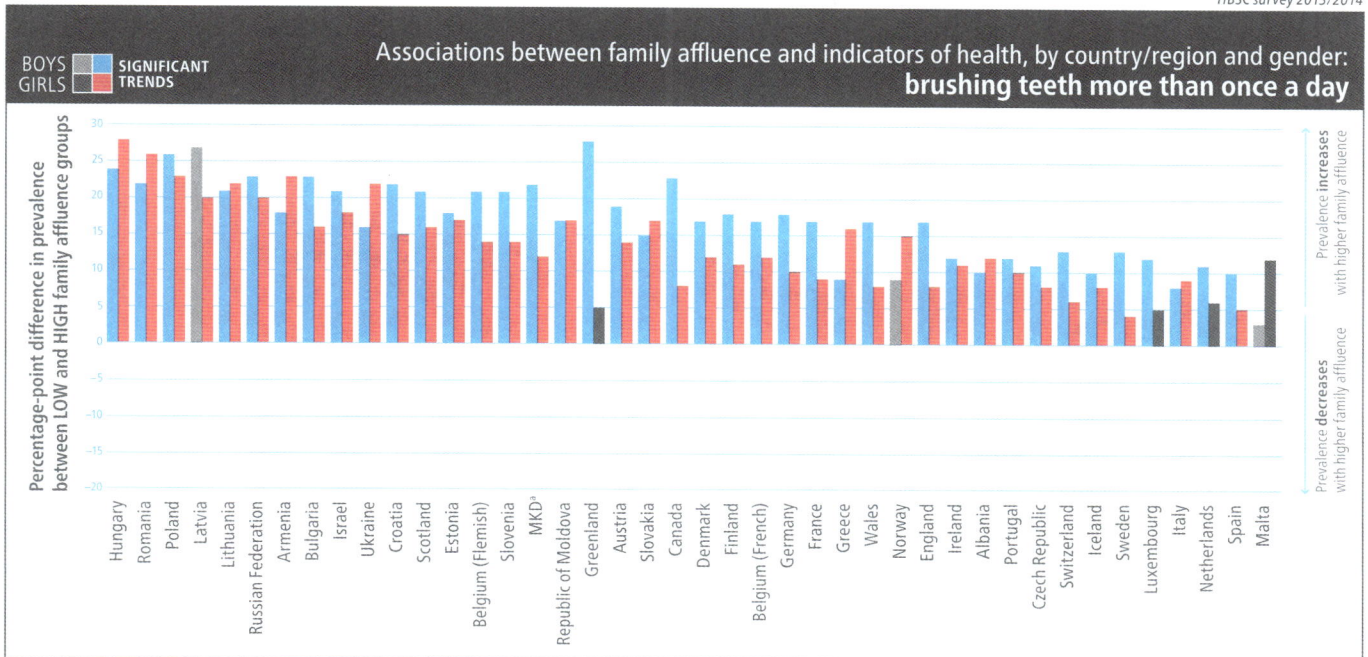

HBSC survey 2013/2014

Associations between family affluence and indicators of health, by country/region and gender:
brushing teeth more than once a day

ª The former Yugoslav Republic of Macedonia. *Note:* low- and high-affluence groups represent the lowest 20% and highest 20% in each country.

MEASURE

Young people were asked how often they brush their teeth. Response options ranged from never to more than once a day.

RESULTS

Findings presented here show the proportions who reported brushing their teeth more than once a day.

Age

Prevalence was higher among 15-year-old girls than 11-year-olds in around half of countries and regions. Toothbrushing tended to decrease with age for boys, with about half of countries and regions showing a significant decrease between 11 and 15 years.

Percentage-point differences between 11- and 15-year-olds varied from +6 to −16 for boys and +20 to −4 for girls.

Gender

Girls brushed their teeth more than once a day more often than boys in most countries and regions. This gender difference was evident across all age groups and increased with increasing age. A difference of more than 15 percentage points was found in one country among 11-year-olds, 16 among those who were 13, and 33 for 15-year-olds.

Family affluence

Prevalence of toothbrushing was associated with higher affluence in almost all countries and regions, with the exception of three for boys and four for girls.

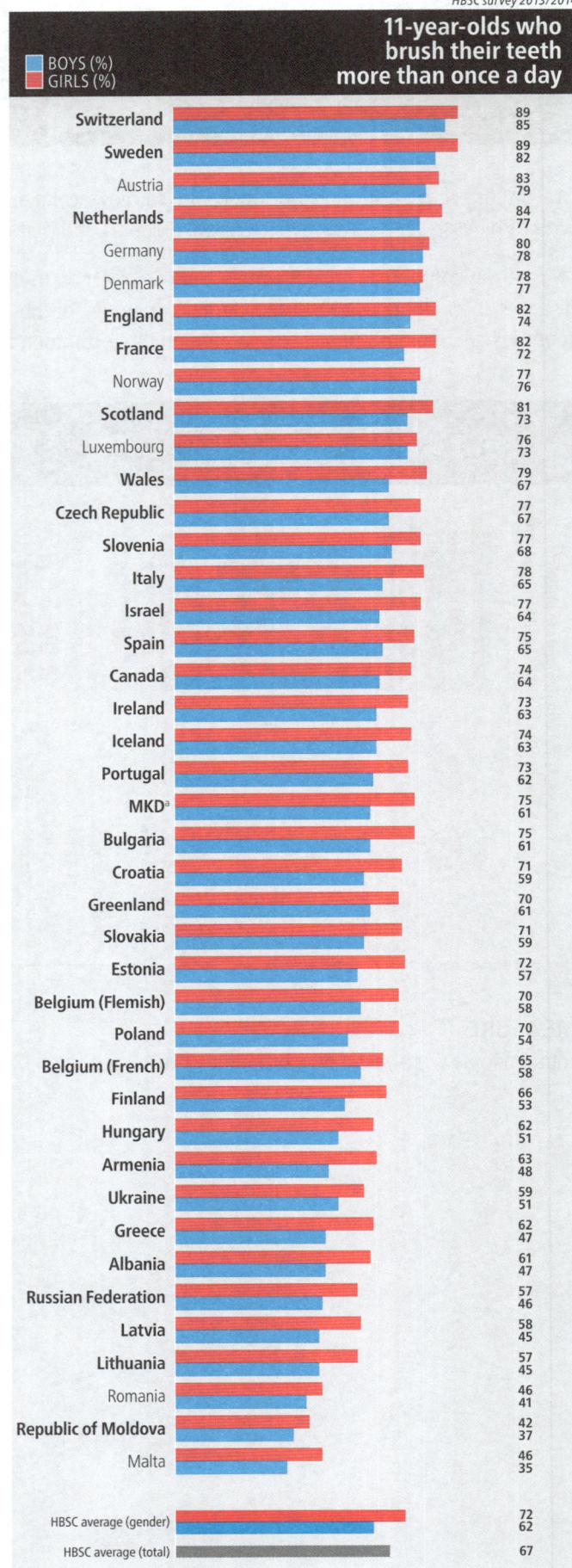

HBSC survey 2013/2014

11-year-olds who brush their teeth more than once a day

BOYS (%)
GIRLS (%)

Country	Girls	Boys
Switzerland	89	85
Sweden	89	82
Austria	83	79
Netherlands	84	77
Germany	80	78
Denmark	78	77
England	82	74
France	82	72
Norway	77	76
Scotland	81	73
Luxembourg	76	73
Wales	79	67
Czech Republic	77	67
Slovenia	77	68
Italy	78	65
Israel	77	64
Spain	75	65
Canada	74	64
Ireland	73	63
Iceland	74	63
Portugal	73	62
MKD[a]	75	61
Bulgaria	75	61
Croatia	71	59
Greenland	70	61
Slovakia	71	59
Estonia	72	57
Belgium (Flemish)	70	58
Poland	70	54
Belgium (French)	65	58
Finland	66	53
Hungary	62	51
Armenia	63	48
Ukraine	59	51
Greece	62	47
Albania	61	47
Russian Federation	57	46
Latvia	58	45
Lithuania	57	45
Romania	46	41
Republic of Moldova	42	37
Malta	46	35
HBSC average (gender)	72	62
HBSC average (total)		67

[a] The former Yugoslav Republic of Macedonia.

GROWING UP UNEQUAL: GENDER AND SOCIOECONOMIC
DIFFERENCES IN YOUNG PEOPLE'S HEALTH AND WELL-BEING
PART 2. KEY DATA | CHAPTER 4. HEALTH BEHAVIOURS
ORAL HEALTH

4

13-year-olds who brush their teeth more than once a day

HBSC survey 2013/2014

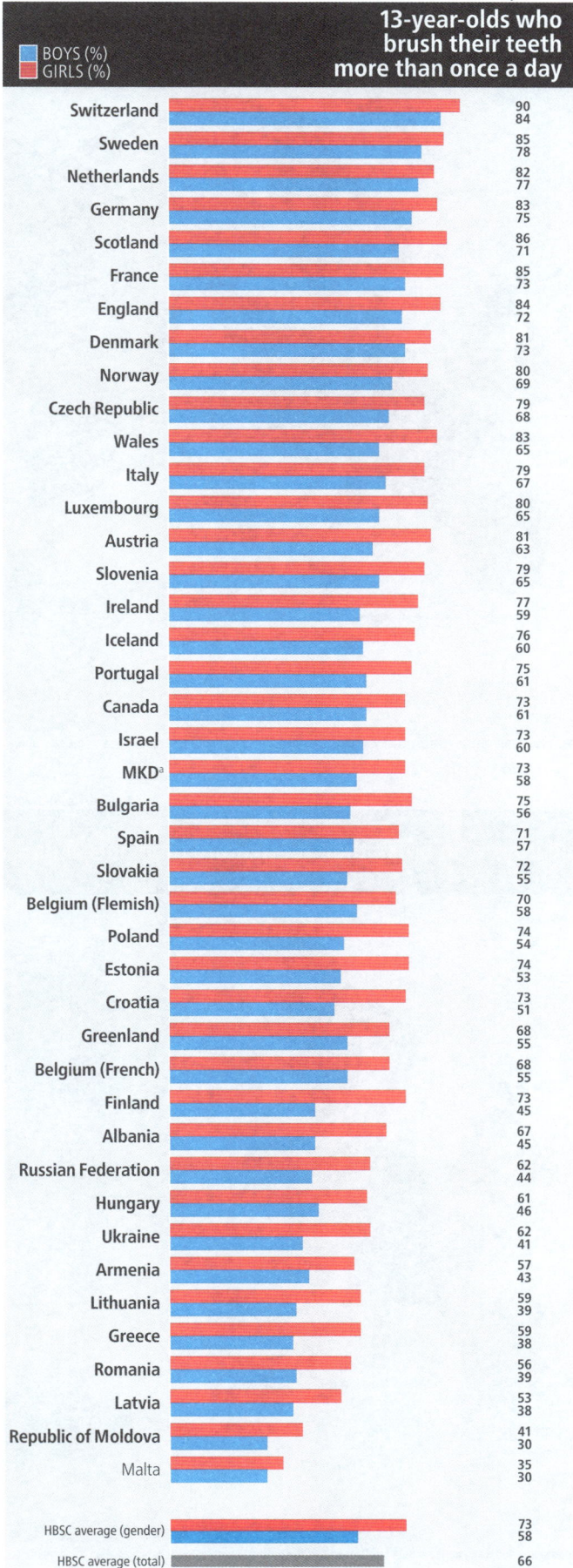

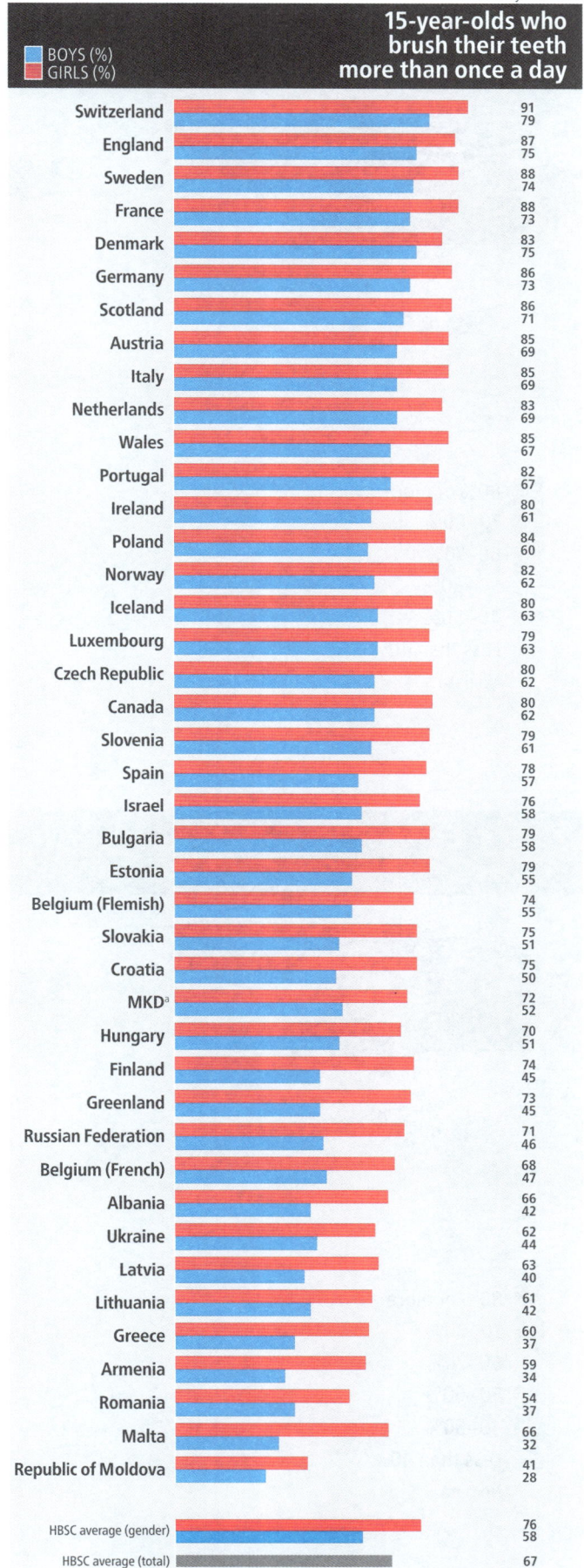

BOYS (%)
GIRLS (%)

Country	Girls	Boys
Switzerland	90	84
Sweden	85	78
Netherlands	82	77
Germany	83	75
Scotland	86	71
France	85	73
England	84	72
Denmark	81	73
Norway	80	69
Czech Republic	79	68
Wales	83	65
Italy	79	67
Luxembourg	80	65
Austria	81	63
Slovenia	79	65
Ireland	77	59
Iceland	76	60
Portugal	75	61
Canada	73	61
Israel	73	60
MKD[a]	73	58
Bulgaria	75	56
Spain	71	57
Slovakia	72	55
Belgium (Flemish)	70	58
Poland	74	54
Estonia	74	53
Croatia	73	51
Greenland	68	55
Belgium (French)	68	55
Finland	73	45
Albania	67	45
Russian Federation	62	44
Hungary	61	46
Ukraine	62	41
Armenia	57	43
Lithuania	59	39
Greece	59	38
Romania	56	39
Latvia	53	38
Republic of Moldova	41	30
Malta	35	30
HBSC average (gender)	73	58
HBSC average (total)	66	

15-year-olds who brush their teeth more than once a day

HBSC survey 2013/2014

BOYS (%)
GIRLS (%)

Country	Girls	Boys
Switzerland	91	79
England	87	75
Sweden	88	74
France	88	73
Denmark	83	75
Germany	86	73
Scotland	86	71
Austria	85	69
Italy	85	69
Netherlands	83	69
Wales	85	67
Portugal	82	67
Ireland	80	61
Poland	84	60
Norway	82	62
Iceland	80	63
Luxembourg	79	63
Czech Republic	80	62
Canada	80	62
Slovenia	79	61
Spain	78	57
Israel	76	58
Bulgaria	79	58
Estonia	79	55
Belgium (Flemish)	74	55
Slovakia	75	51
Croatia	75	50
MKD[a]	72	52
Hungary	70	51
Finland	74	45
Greenland	73	45
Russian Federation	71	46
Belgium (French)	68	47
Albania	66	42
Ukraine	62	44
Latvia	63	40
Lithuania	61	42
Greece	60	37
Armenia	59	34
Romania	54	37
Malta	66	32
Republic of Moldova	41	28
HBSC average (gender)	76	58
HBSC average (total)	67	

Note: **indicates** significant gender difference (at p<0.05).

HBSC survey 2013/2014

15-year-old girls who brush their teeth more than once a day

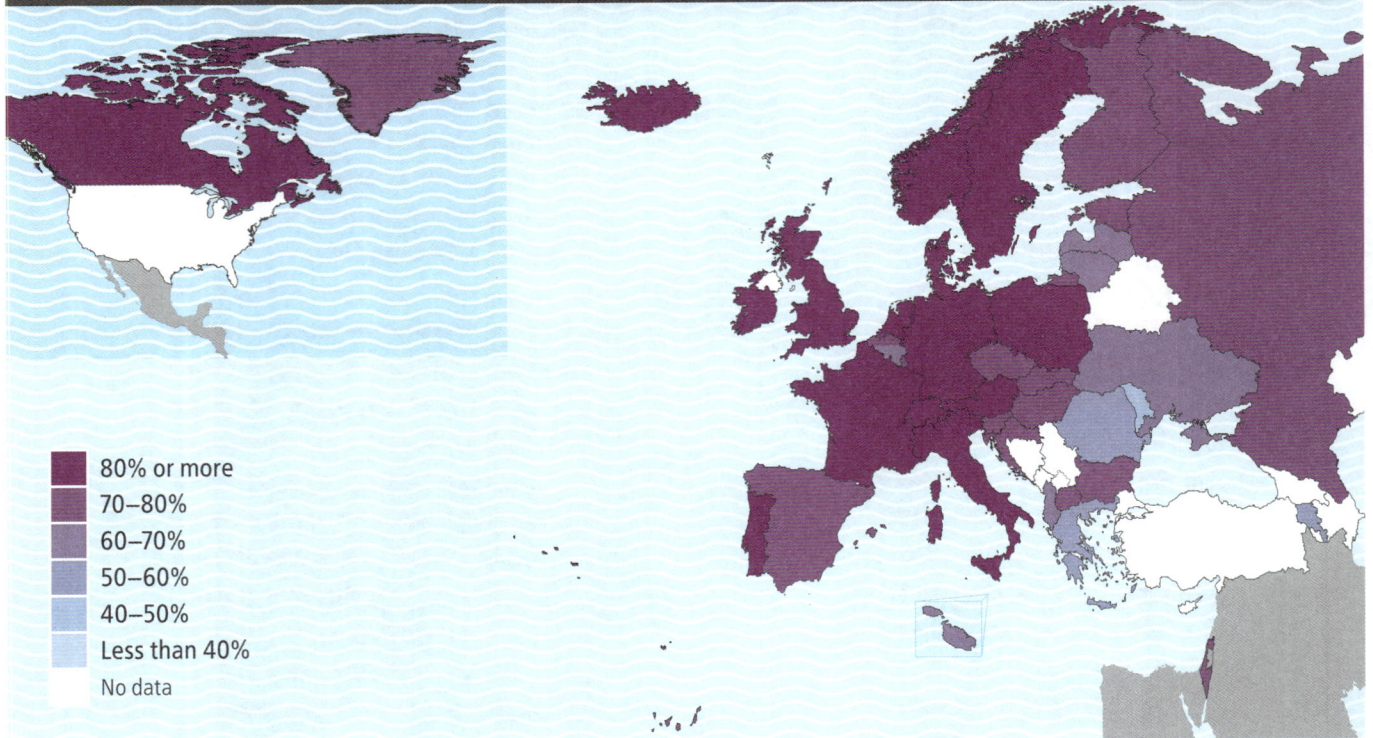

- 80% or more
- 70–80%
- 60–70%
- 50–60%
- 40–50%
- Less than 40%
- No data

Note: HBSC teams provided disaggregated data for Belgium and the United Kingdom; these data appear in the map above.

HBSC survey 2013/2014

15-year-old boys who brush their teeth more than once a day

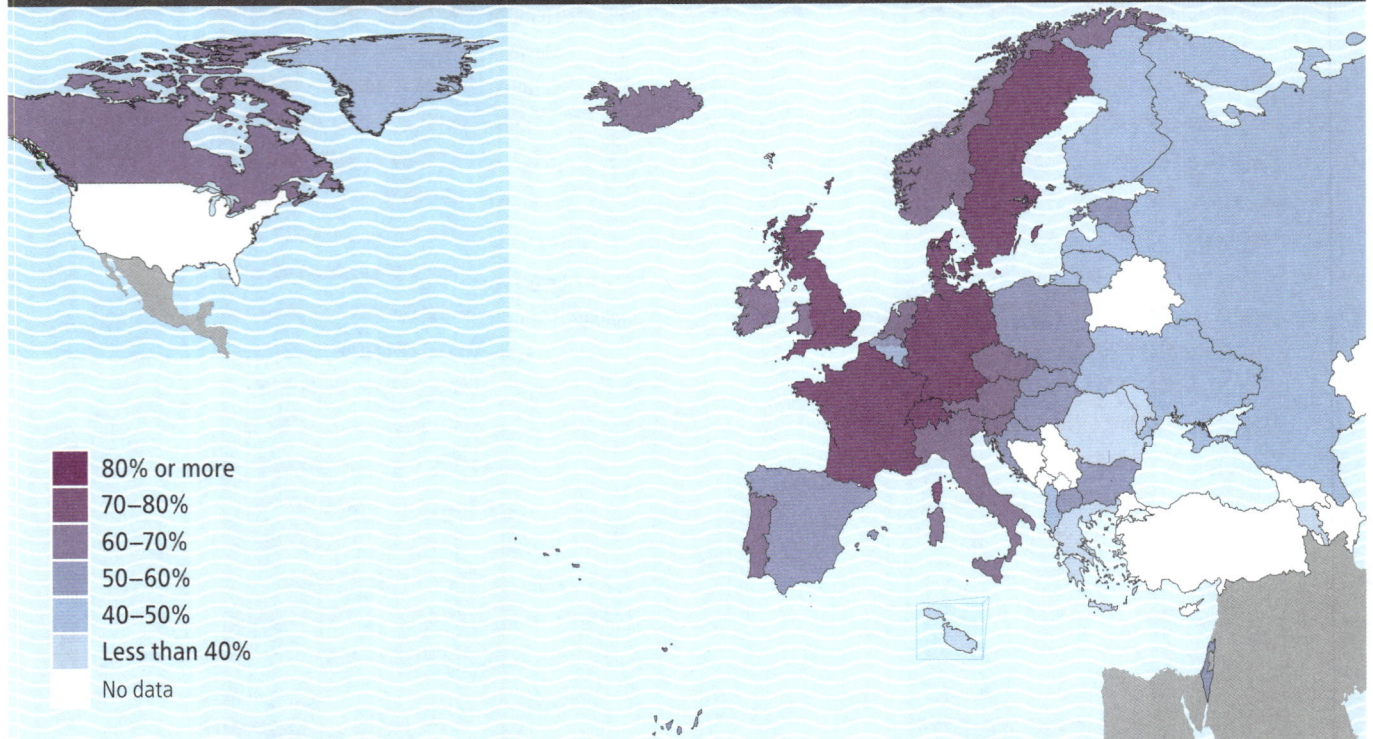

- 80% or more
- 70–80%
- 60–70%
- 50–60%
- 40–50%
- Less than 40%
- No data

Note: HBSC teams provided disaggregated data for Belgium and the United Kingdom; these data appear in the map above.

GROWING UP UNEQUAL: GENDER AND SOCIOECONOMIC
DIFFERENCES IN YOUNG PEOPLE'S HEALTH AND WELL-BEING
PART 2. KEY DATA | CHAPTER 4. HEALTH BEHAVIOURS
ORAL HEALTH

4

ORAL HEALTH:
SCIENTIFIC DISCUSSION AND POLICY REFLECTIONS

SCIENTIFIC DISCUSSION

Results confirm earlier findings suggesting that girls brush their teeth more frequently across all age groups and in all countries and regions (4). Recent data show a positive trend, with improvements in toothbrushing frequency in many countries (4).

Older girls have better brushing habits, a finding that is reversed among boys (which again is similar to earlier findings (4)). Family affluence is strongly linked with toothbrushing frequency: brushing more than once a day is associated with higher affluence, reflecting findings from earlier work (5).

Toothbrushing frequency is lowest in eastern and southern European countries.

POLICY REFLECTIONS

Toothbrushing habits are established quite early in life (6,7), so the family plays an important role in determining behaviour (8). Once formed, habits are difficult to change (6,7). Interventions focusing on parents and young children are therefore required.

Recognizing that younger boys brush less regularly, many countries and regions have targeted this group for oral health promotion. It is encouraging that the toothbrushing habits of 11-year-olds have improved (4), which may in time lead to an increase in brushing in older adolescents and adults, but 15-year-old boys currently brush less often than 11-year-olds.

Boys have consistently shown lower toothbrushing frequency. Public health policies and campaigns should therefore address the specific health needs of boys and girls and disseminate gender-specific and gender-sensitive health messages (9).

Evidence suggests that poor toothbrushing habits are often accompanied by other health-detrimental behaviours such as regular smoking (10), unhealthy eating habits and low levels of physical activity (11), which are common risk factors for several noncommunicable diseases (12). Consequently, oral health promotion should be integrated within general health promotion (13).

HBSC findings highlight socioeconomic and sociodemographic inequalities in oral health behaviour (4,5). Socioeconomic inequalities also exist in the experience of oral diseases between and within countries and regions (13,14). Public health plans and actions for reducing social inequalities in oral health have been established in many (13), but greater political will is needed to ensure sufficient resources for implementation.

Oral diseases are highly prevalent worldwide and poor oral health is a severe public health problem (13). Investing more in health promotion and prevention of oral diseases will reduce prevalence and contribute to the overall health of children and young people (15).

REFERENCES

1. de Oliveira C, Watt R, Hamer M. Toothbrushing, inflammation, and risk of cardiovascular disease: results from Scottish Health Survey. Br Med J. 2010;340:c2451. doi:10.1136/bmj.c2451.

2. Kobayashi Y, Niu K, Guan L, Momma H, Guo H, Cui Y et al. Oral health behavior and metabolic syndrome and its components in adults. J Dent Res. 2012;91(5):479–84.

3. Löe H. Oral hygiene in the prevention of caries and periodontal disease. Int Dent J. 2000;50(3):129–39.

4. Honkala S, Vereecken C, Niclasen B, Honkala E. Trends in toothbrushing in 20 countries or regions between 1994 and 2010. Eur J Public Health 2015;25(Suppl. 2):20–3.

5. Maes L, Vereecken C, Vanobbergen J, Honkala S. Tooth brushing and social characteristics of families in 32 countries. Int Dent J. 2006;56(3):159–67.

6. Kuusela S, Honkala E, Rimpelä A. Toothbrushing frequency between the ages of 12 and 18 years – longitudinal prospective studies of Finnish adolescents. Community Dent Health 1996;13(1):34–9.

7. Åstrøm AN. Stability of oral health-related behaviour in a Norwegian cohort between the ages of 15 and 23 years. Community Dent Oral Epidemiol. 2004;32(5):354–62.

8. Levin KA, Currie C. Adolescent toothbrushing and the home environment: sociodemographic factors, family relationships and mealtime routines and disorganisation. Community Dent Oral Epidemiol. 2010;38(1):10–8.

9.   European strategy for child and adolescent health and development. Gender tool. Copenhagen: WHO Regional Office for Europe; 2007 (http://www. euro.who.int/__data/assets/pdf_file/0020/76511/EuroStrat_Gender_tool.pdf, accessed 24 August 2015).

10. Honkala S, Honkala E, Newton T, Rimpelä A. Toothbrushing and smoking among adolescents – aggregation of health damaging behaviors. J Clin Periodontol. 2011;38(5):442–8.

11. Sanders AE, Spencer AJ, Stewart JF. Clustering of risk behaviours for oral and general health. Community Dent Health 2005;22(3):133–40.

12. Sheiham A, Watt R. The common risk factor approach: a rational basis for promoting oral health. Community Dent Oral Epidemiol. 2000;28(6):399–406.

13. Petersen PE, Kwan S. Equity, social determinants and public health programmes – the case of oral health. Community Dent Oral Epidemiol. 2011;39(6):481–7

14. Schwendicke F, Dörfer CE, Schlattmann P, Page LF, Thomson WM, Paris S. Socioeconomic inequality and caries: a systematic review and meta-analysis. J Dent Res. 2015;94(1):10–8.

15. Investing in children: the European child and adolescent health strategy 2015–2020. Copenhagen: WHO Regional Office for Europe; 2014 (http://www.pnsd.msssi.gob.es/novedades/pdf/Investing_in_children_European_strategy.pdf, accessed 24 August 2015).

GROWING UP UNEQUAL: GENDER AND SOCIOECONOMIC
DIFFERENCES IN YOUNG PEOPLE'S HEALTH AND WELL-BEING
PART 2. KEY DATA | CHAPTER 4. HEALTH BEHAVIOURS

4

PHYSICAL ACTIVITY AND SEDENTARY BEHAVIOUR: MODERATE-TO-VIGOROUS PHYSICAL ACTIVITY

The benefits of moderate-to-vigorous physical activity (MVPA) to adolescents' physical, mental and social health and their academic achievements are well documented *(1,2)*. Globally, levels of MVPA were stable over the last decade, but only a minority of young people meet the current worldwide recommendation of 60 minutes per day *(3,4)*. The establishment of healthy patterns of physical activity during childhood and adolescence is important as physical activity tracks moderately during adolescence and from adolescence to adulthood *(5)*, but levels are declining among young people *(4)*.

HBSC survey 2013/2014

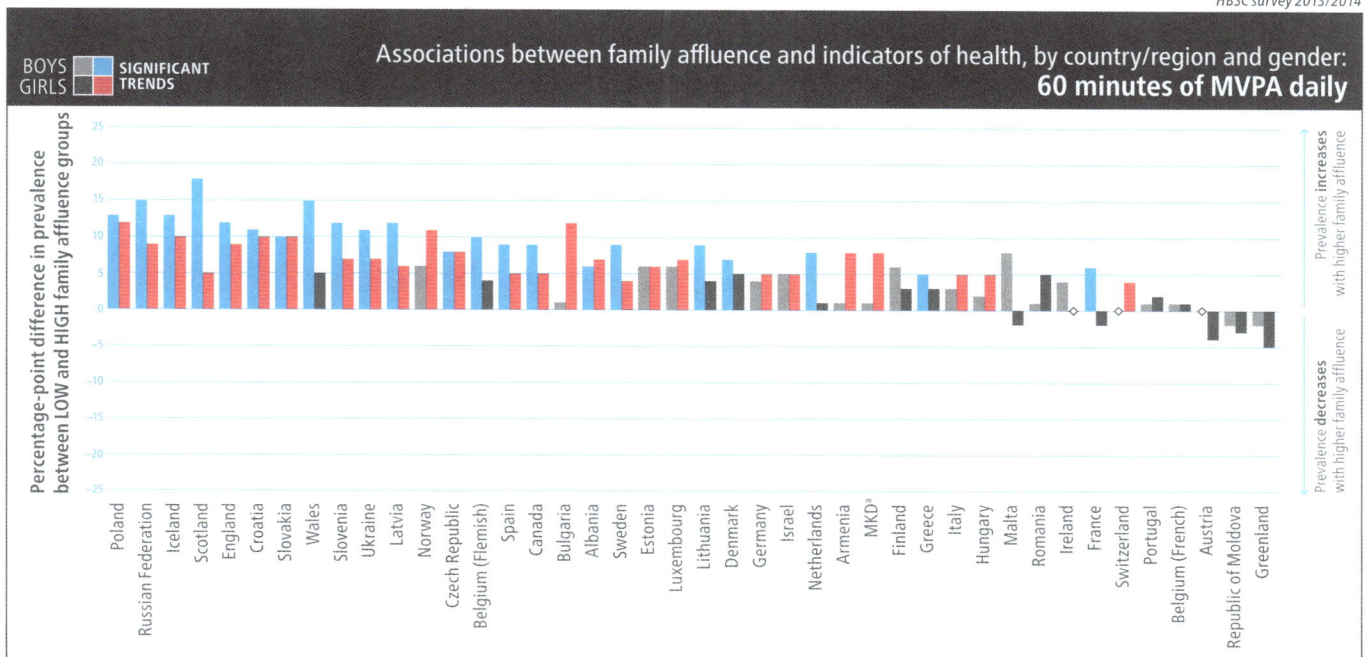

Associations between family affluence and indicators of health, by country/region and gender:
60 minutes of MVPA daily

ᵃ The former Yugoslav Republic of Macedonia. *Note:* low- and high-affluence groups represent the lowest 20% and highest 20% in each country. ◇ means less than +/-0.5%.

MEASURE

Young people were asked to report the number of days over the past week during which they were physically active for a total of at least 60 minutes. The question was introduced by text defining MVPA as any activity that increases the heart rate and makes the person get out of breath some of the time, with examples provided.

Supplementary data on participating in vigorous physical activity for two or more hours a week are provided in the Annex.

RESULTS

Findings presented here show the proportions reporting daily MVPA of at least one hour.

Age

Daily MVPA decreased with age among boys and girls. A significant decrease between ages 11 and 15 was observed among boys in 33 countries and regions, with a difference of up to 25 percentage points. A decrease was seen in 35 for girls, with a difference of up to 22 percentage points. The average difference was 9 percentage points for boys and 10 for girls.

Gender

Boys reported at least 60 minutes of MVPA per day more often. Gender differences were significant across all age groups and in nearly all countries and regions, with the largest being found among 13-year-olds in Ireland, Luxembourg, Portugal and Spain.

Family affluence

High-affluence boys and girls were more likely to achieve 60 minutes of MVPA daily in more than half of countries and regions. The difference between high- and low-affluence groups was 10 percentage points or less in most.

HBSC survey 2013/2014

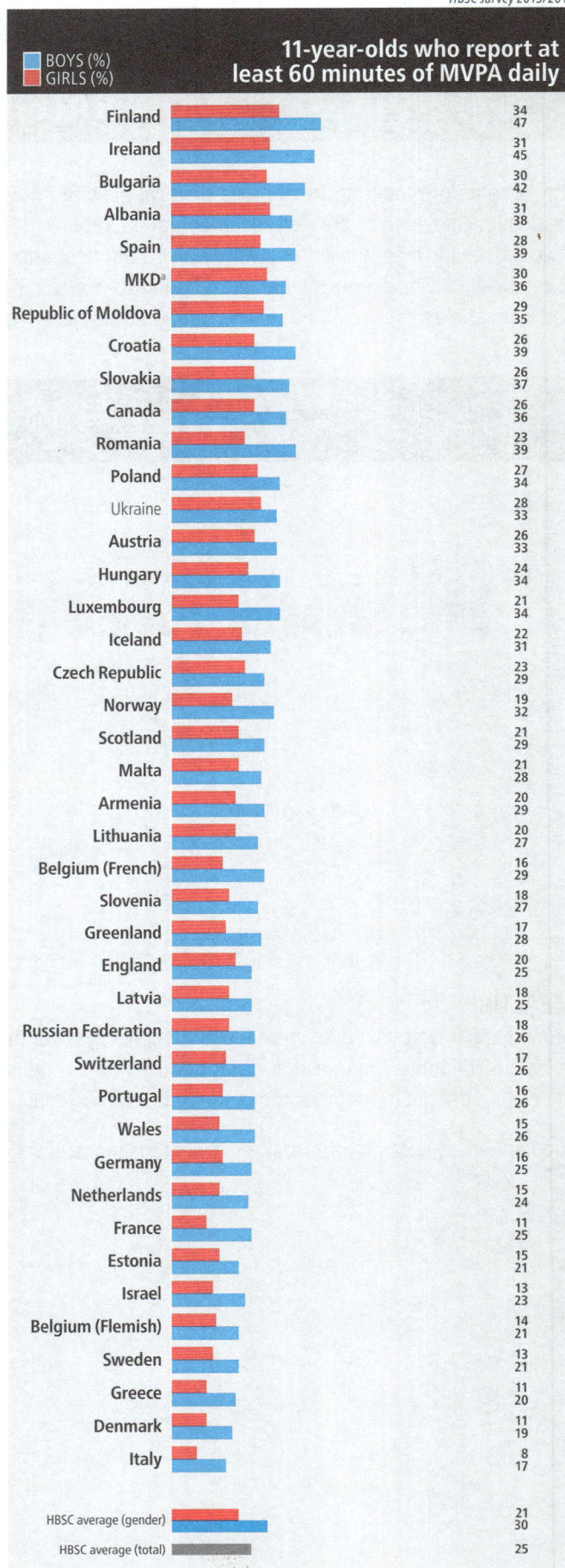

11-year-olds who report at least 60 minutes of MVPA daily

BOYS (%) / GIRLS (%)

Country	BOYS (%)	GIRLS (%)
Finland	47	34
Ireland	45	31
Bulgaria	42	30
Albania	38	31
Spain	39	28
MKD[a]	36	30
Republic of Moldova	35	29
Croatia	39	26
Slovakia	37	26
Canada	36	26
Romania	39	23
Poland	34	27
Ukraine	33	28
Austria	33	26
Hungary	34	24
Luxembourg	34	21
Iceland	31	22
Czech Republic	29	23
Norway	32	19
Scotland	29	21
Malta	28	21
Armenia	29	20
Lithuania	27	20
Belgium (French)	29	16
Slovenia	27	18
Greenland	28	17
England	25	20
Latvia	25	18
Russian Federation	26	18
Switzerland	26	17
Portugal	26	16
Wales	26	15
Germany	25	16
Netherlands	24	15
France	25	11
Estonia	21	15
Israel	23	13
Belgium (Flemish)	21	14
Sweden	21	13
Greece	20	11
Denmark	19	11
Italy	17	8
HBSC average (gender)	30	21
HBSC average (total)	25	

[a] The former Yugoslav Republic of Macedonia.

GROWING UP UNEQUAL: GENDER AND SOCIOECONOMIC
DIFFERENCES IN YOUNG PEOPLE'S HEALTH AND WELL-BEING
PART 2. KEY DATA | CHAPTER 4. HEALTH BEHAVIOURS
PHYSICAL ACTIVITY AND SEDENTARY BEHAVIOUR: MODERATE-TO-VIGOROUS PHYSICAL ACTIVITY

4

13-year-olds who report at least 60 minutes of MVPA daily

HBSC survey 2013/2014

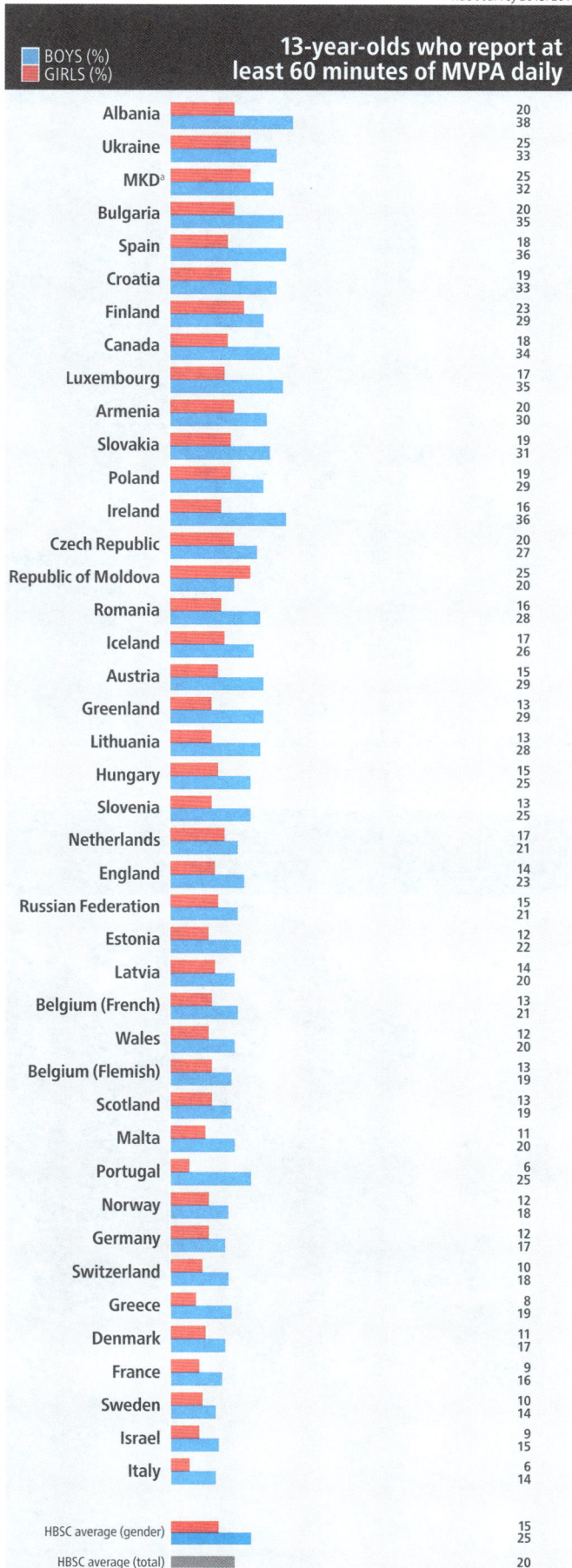

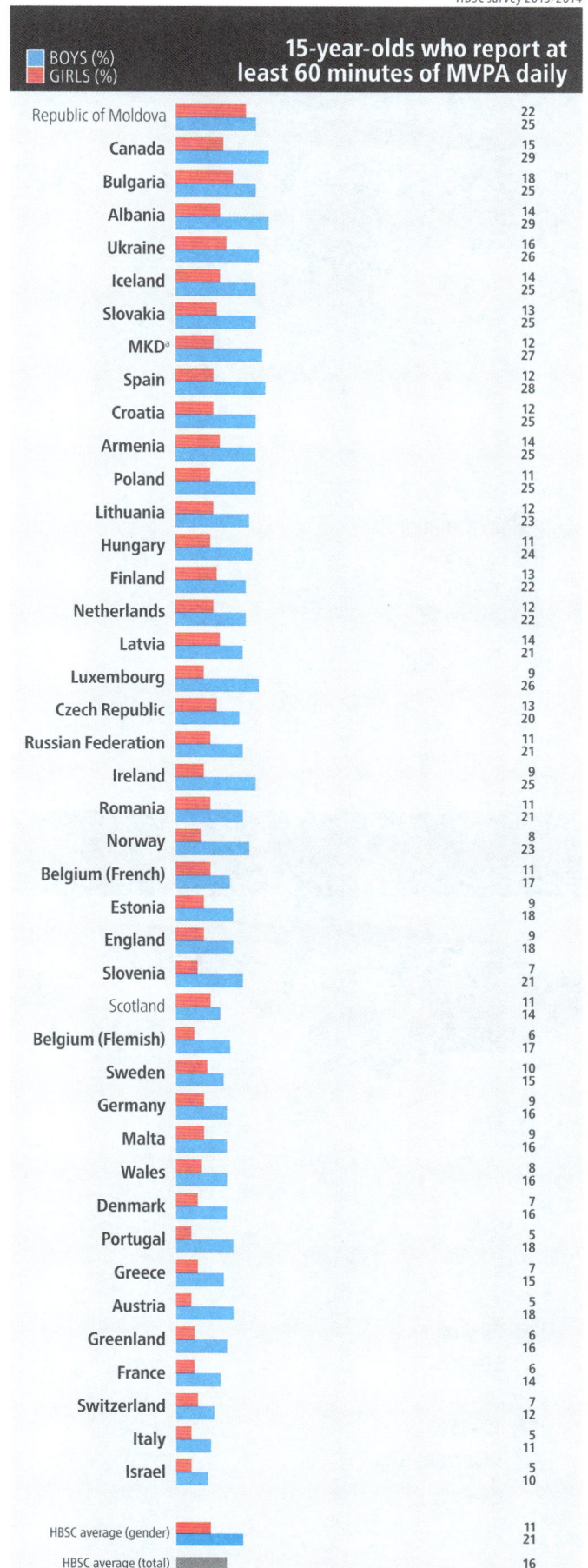

Country	Boys (%)	Girls (%)
Albania	38	20
Ukraine	33	25
MKD[a]	32	25
Bulgaria	35	20
Spain	36	18
Croatia	33	19
Finland	29	23
Canada	34	18
Luxembourg	35	17
Armenia	30	20
Slovakia	31	19
Poland	29	19
Ireland	36	16
Czech Republic	27	20
Republic of Moldova	20	25
Romania	28	16
Iceland	26	17
Austria	29	15
Greenland	29	13
Lithuania	28	13
Hungary	25	15
Slovenia	25	13
Netherlands	21	17
England	23	14
Russian Federation	21	15
Estonia	22	12
Latvia	20	14
Belgium (French)	21	13
Wales	20	12
Belgium (Flemish)	19	13
Scotland	19	13
Malta	20	11
Portugal	25	6
Norway	18	12
Germany	17	12
Switzerland	18	10
Greece	19	8
Denmark	17	11
France	16	9
Sweden	14	10
Israel	15	9
Italy	14	6
HBSC average (gender)	25	15
HBSC average (total)	20	

15-year-olds who report at least 60 minutes of MVPA daily

HBSC survey 2013/2014

Country	Boys (%)	Girls (%)
Republic of Moldova	25	22
Canada	29	15
Bulgaria	25	18
Albania	29	14
Ukraine	26	16
Iceland	25	14
Slovakia	25	13
MKD[a]	27	12
Spain	28	12
Croatia	25	12
Armenia	25	14
Poland	25	11
Lithuania	23	12
Hungary	24	11
Finland	22	13
Netherlands	22	12
Latvia	21	14
Luxembourg	26	9
Czech Republic	20	13
Russian Federation	21	11
Ireland	25	9
Romania	21	11
Norway	23	8
Belgium (French)	17	11
Estonia	18	9
England	18	9
Slovenia	21	7
Scotland	14	11
Belgium (Flemish)	17	6
Sweden	15	10
Germany	16	9
Malta	16	9
Wales	16	8
Denmark	16	7
Portugal	18	5
Greece	15	7
Austria	18	5
Greenland	16	6
France	14	6
Switzerland	12	7
Italy	11	5
Israel	10	5
HBSC average (gender)	21	11
HBSC average (total)	16	

Note: **indicates** significant gender difference (at p<0.05).

HBSC survey 2013/2014

15-year-old girls who report at least 60 minutes of MVPA daily

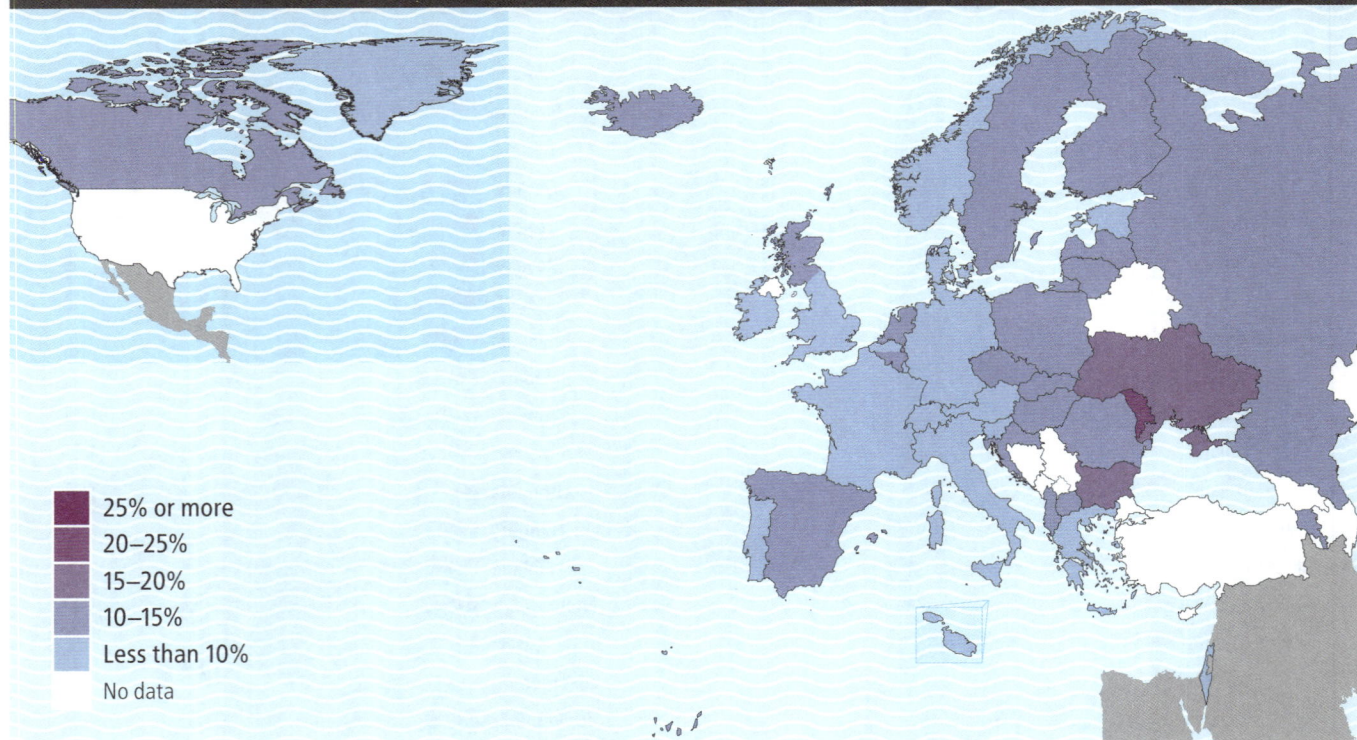

- 25% or more
- 20–25%
- 15–20%
- 10–15%
- Less than 10%
- No data

Note: HBSC teams provided disaggregated data for Belgium and the United Kingdom; these data appear in the map above.

HBSC survey 2013/2014

15-year-old boys who report at least 60 minutes of MVPA daily

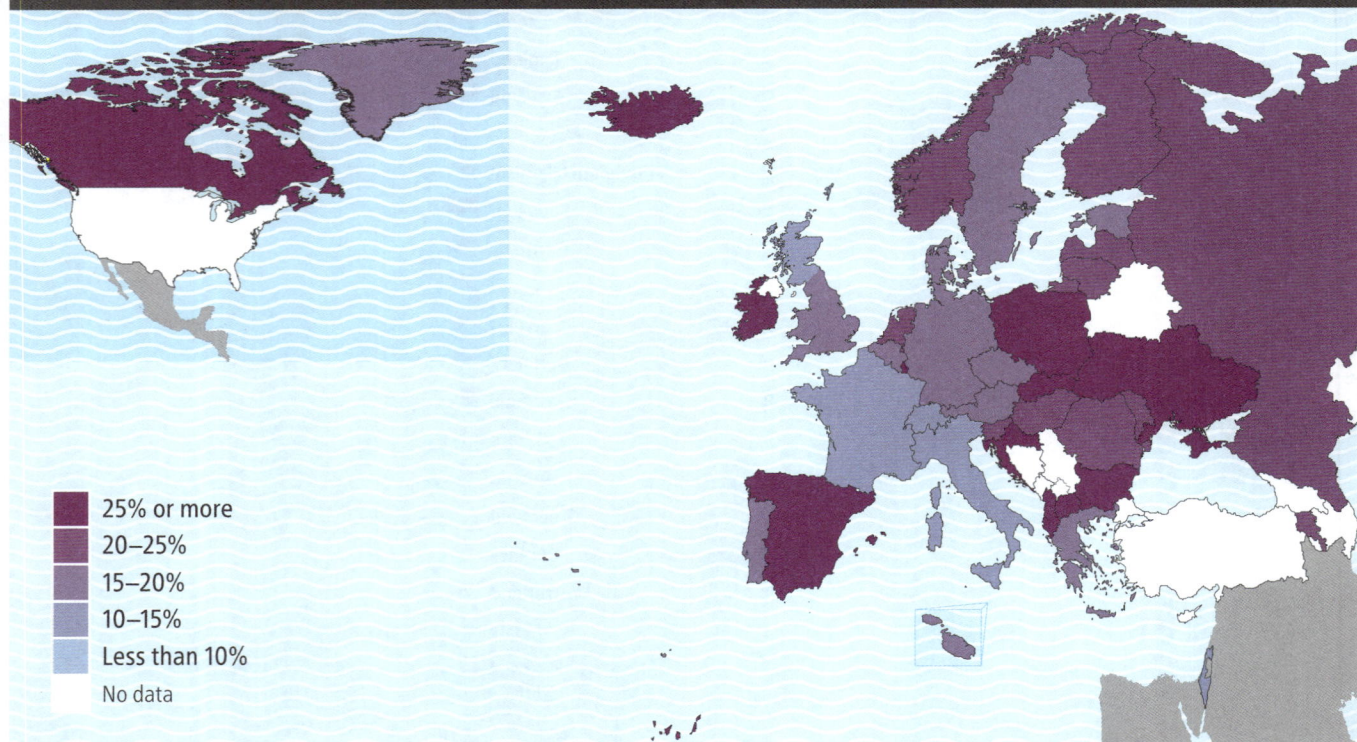

- 25% or more
- 20–25%
- 15–20%
- 10–15%
- Less than 10%
- No data

Note: HBSC teams provided disaggregated data for Belgium and the United Kingdom; these data appear in the map above.

GROWING UP UNEQUAL: GENDER AND SOCIOECONOMIC
DIFFERENCES IN YOUNG PEOPLE'S HEALTH AND WELL-BEING
PART 2. KEY DATA | CHAPTER 4. HEALTH BEHAVIOURS

4

PHYSICAL ACTIVITY AND SEDENTARY BEHAVIOUR: WATCHING TELEVISION

Engaging in screen-time behaviours such as watching television is an important sedentary behaviour, although it is acknowledged that non-screen-time behaviours (like passive travel, reading, sitting and chatting with friends and sitting in class) also contribute to total sedentary time (6,7).

Watching television is often associated with a range of adverse psychosocial (depression and poor academic performance) and physical (lower physical fitness and more musculoskeletal pain) health outcomes independent of MVPA in children, adolescents and adults (8,9). Adolescents tend to spend a lot of time watching television, a behaviour that tracks moderately from childhood to adulthood (10). Current guidelines recommend that young people should limit their recreational screen time to no more than two hours per day (11,12).

HBSC survey 2013/2014

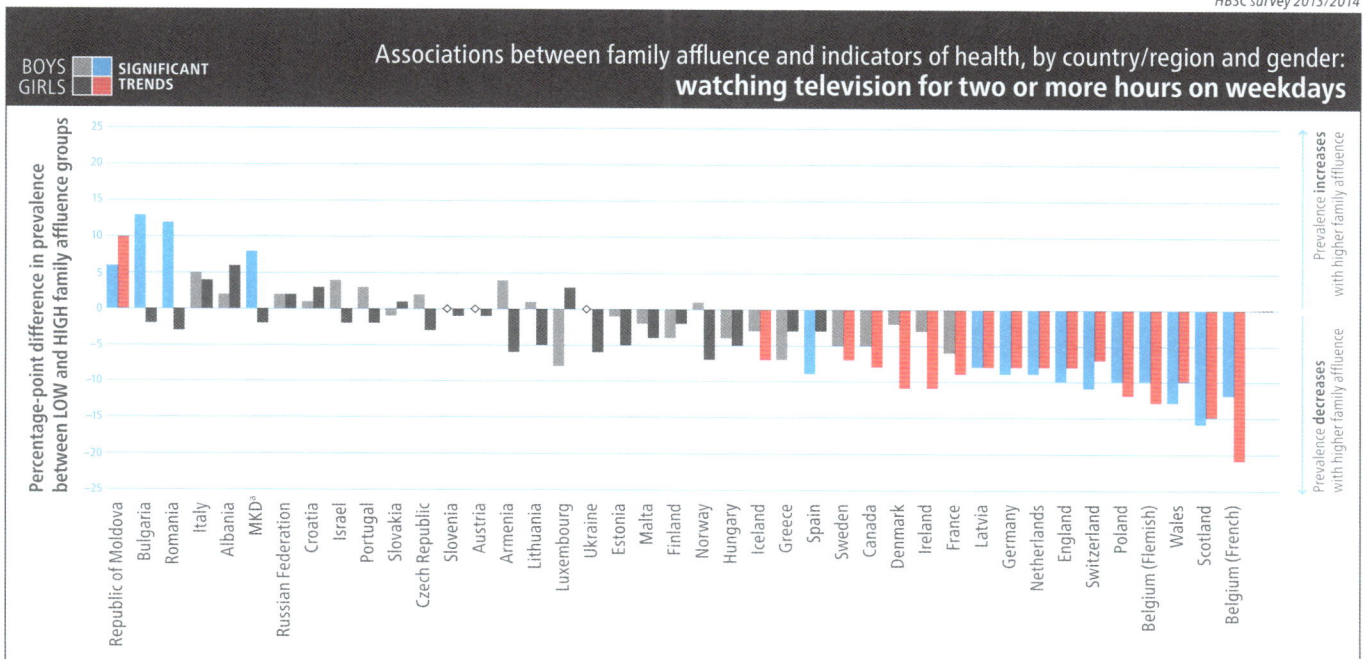

Associations between family affluence and indicators of health, by country/region and gender: watching television for two or more hours on weekdays

BOYS
GIRLS
SIGNIFICANT TRENDS

ᵃ The former Yugoslav Republic of Macedonia. *Note*: low- and high-affluence groups represent the lowest 20% and highest 20% in each country. ◇ means less than +/-0.5%. No data were received from Greenland.

MEASURE

Young people were asked how many hours a day in their free time they usually spend watching television, videos (including YouTube or similar services), DVDs and other screen entertainments on weekdays.

Supplementary data on time spent playing computer games and using a computer for email, internet or homework on weekdays are provided in the Annex.

RESULTS

Findings presented here show the proportions reporting watching television for two or more hours on weekdays.

Age

Daily television-viewing of two hours or more increased with age in both genders across almost all countries and regions, with an age difference (11–15 years) of up to 29 percentage points in girls and up to 26 in boys. The average difference was 13 for boys and 16 for girls.

Gender

At age 11, boys were more likely to watch television in over half of countries and regions. Gender differences were usually less than 10 percentage points across all age groups and tended to decrease with age. At age 13, television-viewing was higher among girls in two countries (Bulgaria and Israel).

Family affluence

Boys and girls from low-affluence families tended to have higher prevalence. The difference was less than 10 percentage points in most countries and regions and was significant in about two fifths.

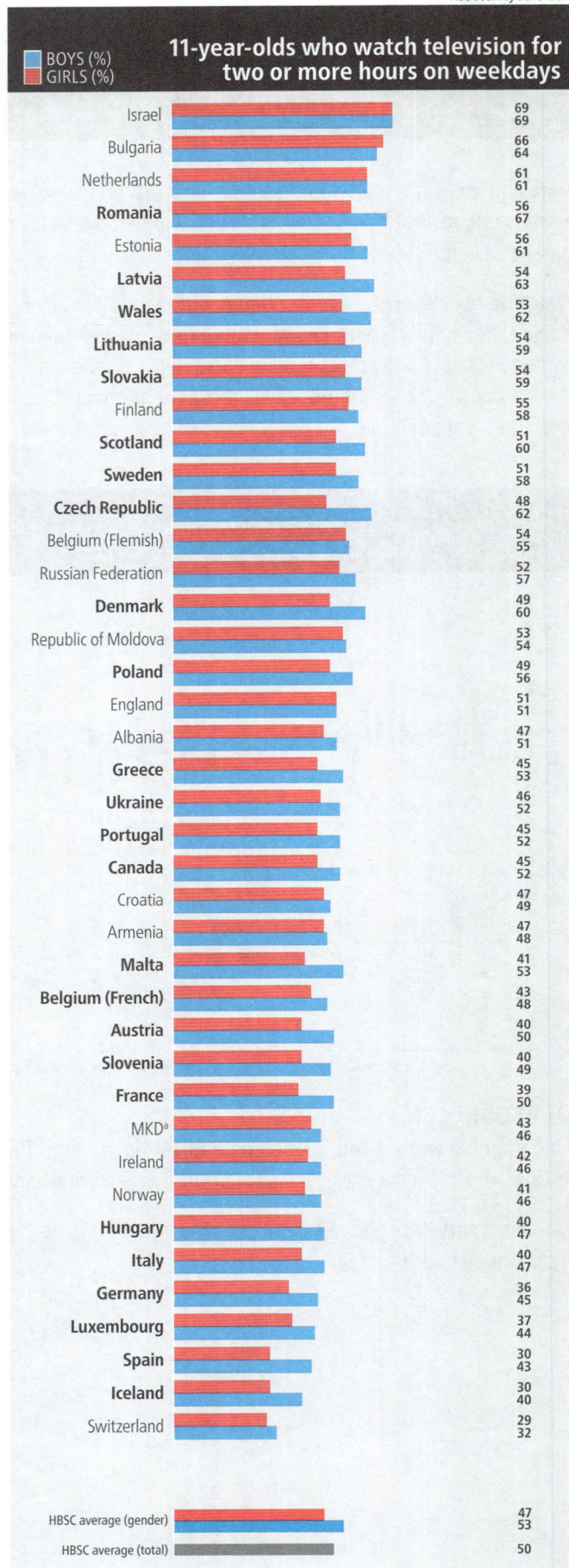

HBSC survey 2013/2014

11-year-olds who watch television for two or more hours on weekdays

BOYS (%)
GIRLS (%)

Country	Girls	Boys
Israel	69	69
Bulgaria	66	64
Netherlands	61	61
Romania	56	67
Estonia	56	61
Latvia	54	63
Wales	53	62
Lithuania	54	59
Slovakia	54	59
Finland	55	58
Scotland	51	60
Sweden	51	58
Czech Republic	48	62
Belgium (Flemish)	54	55
Russian Federation	52	57
Denmark	49	60
Republic of Moldova	53	54
Poland	49	56
England	51	51
Albania	47	51
Greece	45	53
Ukraine	46	52
Portugal	45	52
Canada	45	52
Croatia	47	49
Armenia	47	48
Malta	41	53
Belgium (French)	43	48
Austria	40	50
Slovenia	40	49
France	39	50
MKD[a]	43	46
Ireland	42	46
Norway	41	46
Hungary	40	47
Italy	40	47
Germany	36	45
Luxembourg	37	44
Spain	30	43
Iceland	30	40
Switzerland	29	32
HBSC average (gender)	47	53
HBSC average (total)		50

[a] The former Yugoslav Republic of Macedonia.

GROWING UP UNEQUAL: GENDER AND SOCIOECONOMIC
DIFFERENCES IN YOUNG PEOPLE'S HEALTH AND WELL-BEING
PART 2. KEY DATA | CHAPTER 4. HEALTH BEHAVIOURS
PHYSICAL ACTIVITY AND SEDENTARY BEHAVIOUR: WATCHING TELEVISION

4

13-year-olds who watch television for two or more hours on weekdays

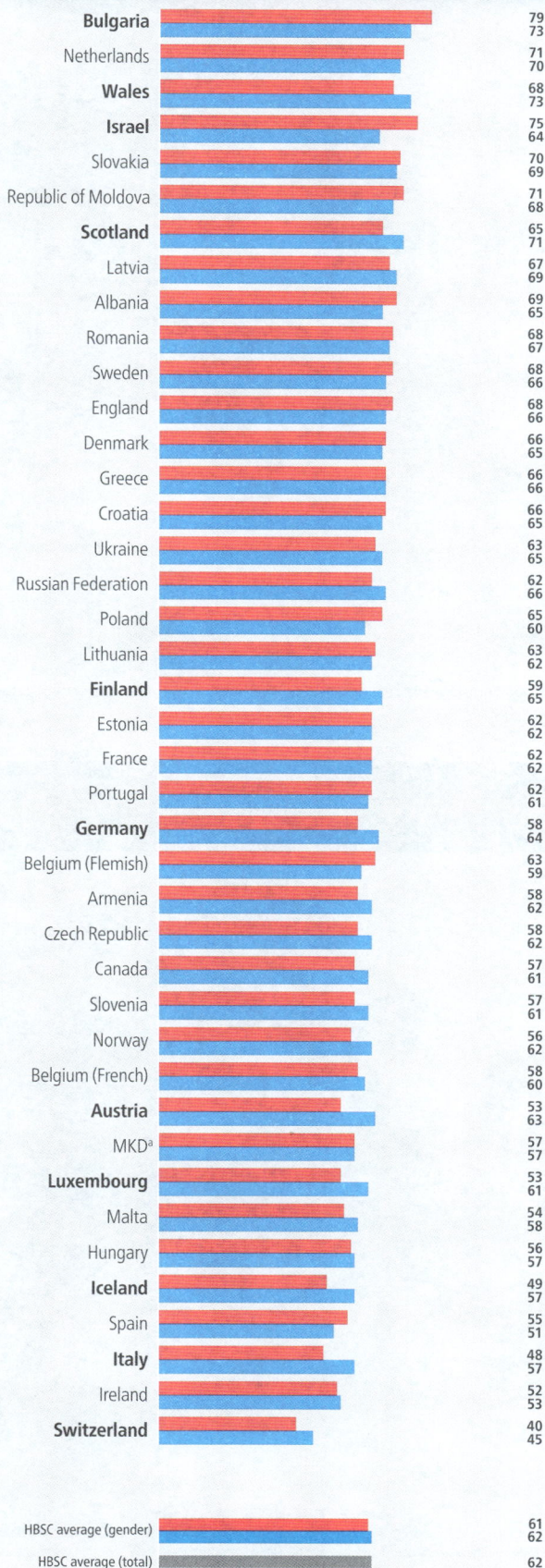

HBSC survey 2013/2014

Legend: BOYS (%) — blue; GIRLS (%) — red

Country	Boys (%)	Girls (%)
Bulgaria	73	79
Netherlands	70	71
Wales	73	68
Israel	64	75
Slovakia	69	70
Republic of Moldova	68	71
Scotland	71	65
Latvia	69	67
Albania	65	69
Romania	67	68
Sweden	66	68
England	66	68
Denmark	65	66
Greece	66	66
Croatia	65	66
Ukraine	65	63
Russian Federation	66	62
Poland	60	65
Lithuania	62	63
Finland	65	59
Estonia	62	62
France	62	62
Portugal	61	62
Germany	64	58
Belgium (Flemish)	59	63
Armenia	62	58
Czech Republic	62	58
Canada	61	57
Slovenia	61	57
Norway	62	56
Belgium (French)	60	58
Austria	63	53
MKD[a]	57	57
Luxembourg	61	53
Malta	58	54
Hungary	57	56
Iceland	57	49
Spain	51	55
Italy	57	48
Ireland	53	52
Switzerland	45	40
HBSC average (gender)	62	61
HBSC average (total)	62	

15-year-olds who watch television for two or more hours on weekdays

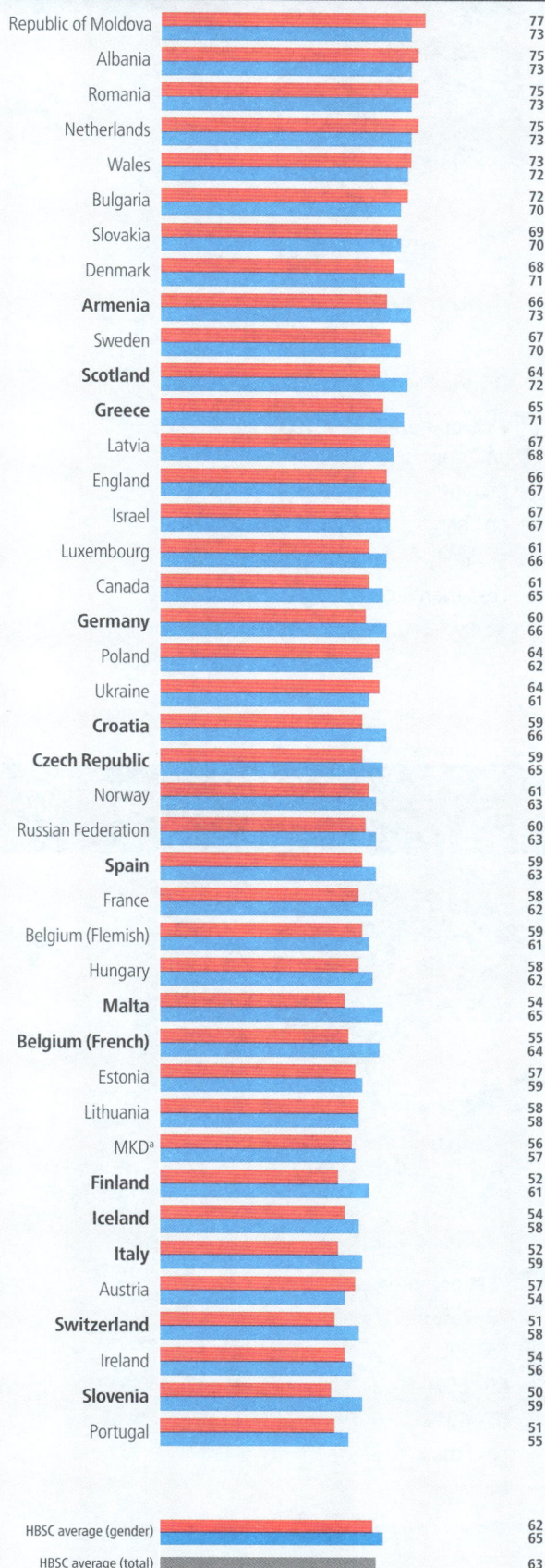

HBSC survey 2013/2014

Legend: BOYS (%) — blue; GIRLS (%) — red

Country	Boys (%)	Girls (%)
Republic of Moldova	73	77
Albania	73	75
Romania	73	75
Netherlands	73	75
Wales	72	73
Bulgaria	70	72
Slovakia	70	69
Denmark	71	68
Armenia	73	66
Sweden	70	67
Scotland	72	64
Greece	71	65
Latvia	68	67
England	67	66
Israel	67	67
Luxembourg	66	61
Canada	65	61
Germany	66	60
Poland	62	64
Ukraine	61	64
Croatia	66	59
Czech Republic	65	59
Norway	63	61
Russian Federation	63	60
Spain	63	59
France	62	58
Belgium (Flemish)	61	59
Hungary	62	58
Malta	65	54
Belgium (French)	64	55
Estonia	59	57
Lithuania	58	58
MKD[a]	57	56
Finland	61	52
Iceland	58	54
Italy	59	52
Austria	54	57
Switzerland	58	51
Ireland	56	54
Slovenia	59	50
Portugal	55	51
HBSC average (gender)	65	62
HBSC average (total)	63	

Note: **indicates** significant gender difference (at p<0.05). No data were received from Greenland.

HBSC survey 2013/2014

15-year-old girls who watch television for two or more hours on weekdays

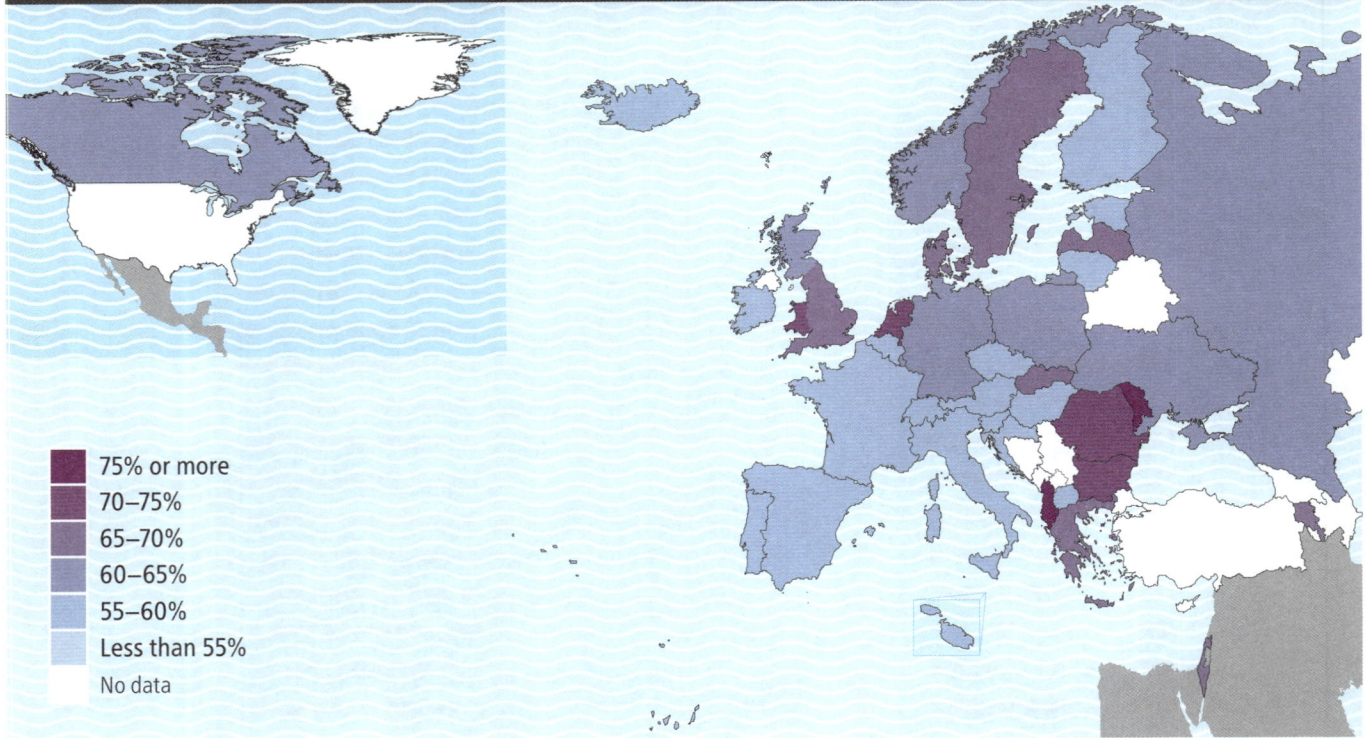

- 75% or more
- 70–75%
- 65–70%
- 60–65%
- 55–60%
- Less than 55%
- No data

Note: HBSC teams provided disaggregated data for Belgium and the United Kingdom; these data appear in the map above.

HBSC survey 2013/2014

15-year-old boys who watch television for two or more hours on weekdays

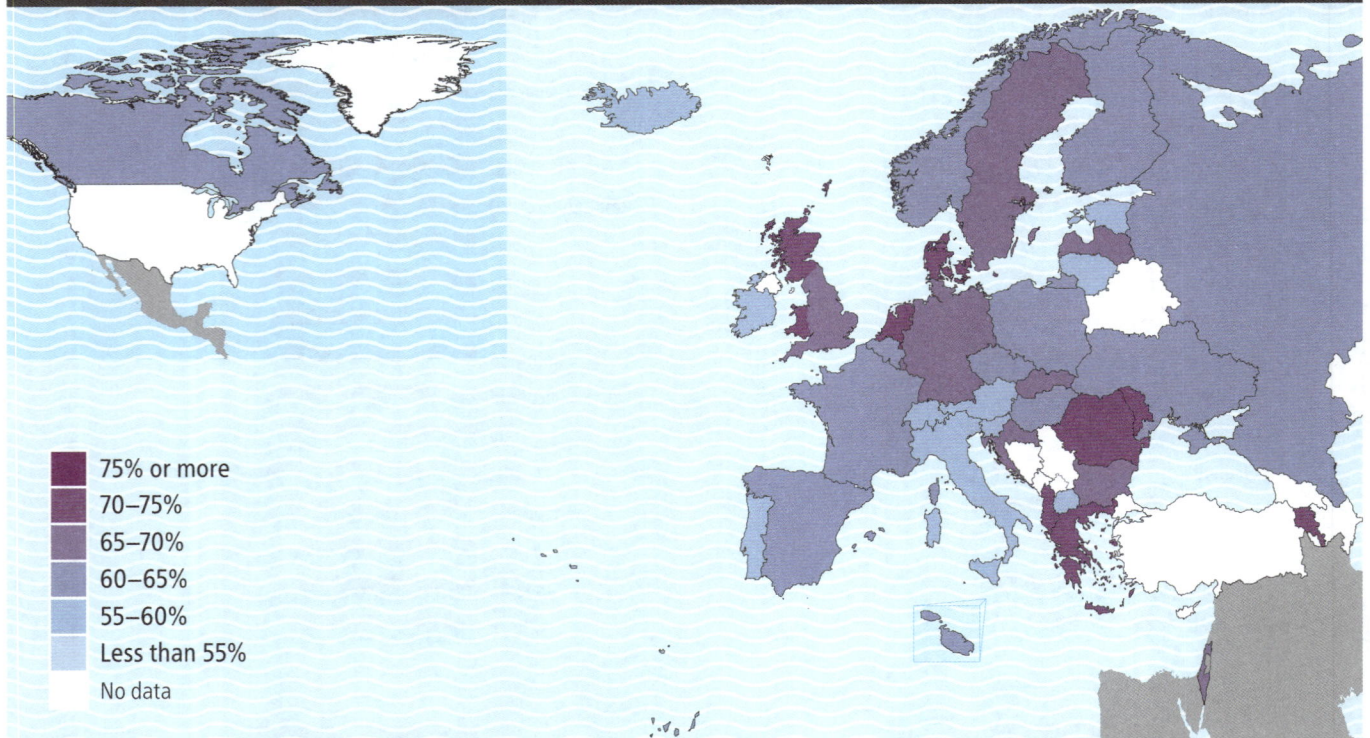

- 75% or more
- 70–75%
- 65–70%
- 60–65%
- 55–60%
- Less than 55%
- No data

Note: HBSC teams provided disaggregated data for Belgium and the United Kingdom; these data appear in the map above.

GROWING UP UNEQUAL: GENDER AND SOCIOECONOMIC
DIFFERENCES IN YOUNG PEOPLE'S HEALTH AND WELL-BEING
PART 2. KEY DATA | CHAPTER 4. HEALTH BEHAVIOURS
PHYSICAL ACTIVITY AND SEDENTARY BEHAVIOUR

4

PHYSICAL ACTIVITY AND SEDENTARY BEHAVIOUR: SCIENTIFIC DISCUSSION AND POLICY REFLECTIONS

SCIENTIFIC DISCUSSION

MVPA levels are generally low and decline through adolescence, with screen-time activities such as watching television and using social media playing an increasingly prominent role in adolescents' lives. Interventions that reflect age-specific needs and preferences should aim to promote MVPA levels and reduce screen-time behaviours.

Girls are less physically active in most countries and regions. The gender gap has not changed very much over time, suggesting that girls should be targeted with gender-sensitive approaches and interventions (4).

Studies show that television-viewing has declined in the last decade, but the reduction is more than compensated by time spent with other screen devices (such as smartphones, tablet PCs and computers). Gender patterns for use of these devices differ, with girls tending to use computers for social purposes and boys for gaming. Consequently, interventions should reflect the complexity of screen-time behaviours (12).

More research is needed to increase understanding of how physical activity patterns and sedentary behaviours are interrelated (13), and to learn more about the relationship between different screen-time and sedentary behaviours and their negative and positive health effects in adolescents (14).

POLICY REFLECTIONS

International strategies and interventions focusing on increasing physical activity and reducing screen-time behaviours in adolescents should take into account age, gender and socioeconomic differences and be focused on different levels of influence (intrapersonal, interpersonal, community and policy). Guidelines for adolescents should be complemented by similar support for stakeholders such as local and municipal representatives, head teachers, teachers and parents, and should reflect local environments and languages. Most important, they should advocate for a more active lifestyle.

The WHO European physical activity strategy (15) and other strategies should be supported by policy action at national, regional and local levels to tackle insufficient levels of MVPA. Action should be intersectoral, comprehensive, targeted at different environments (including schools, health care settings, transport systems and recreational facilities) and be linked to key stakeholders' budgets (national, provincial and/or local).

REFERENCES

1. Janssen I, Leblanc AG. Systematic review of the health benefits of physical activity and fitness in school-aged children and youth. Int J Behav Nutr Phys Act. 2010;7:40.

2. Singh A, Uijtdewilligen L, Twisk JW, van Mechelen W, Chinapaw MJ. Physical activity and performance at school: a systematic review of the literature including methodological quality assessment. Arch Pediatr Adolesc Med. 2012;166(1):49–55.

3. Hallal PC, Andersen LB, Bull FC, Guthold R, Haskell W, Ekelund U. Global physical activity levels: surveillance progress, pitfalls, and prospects. Lancet 2012;380(9838):247–57.

4. Kalman M, Inchley J, Sigmundova D, Iannotti RJ, Tynjala J, Hamrik Z et al. Secular trends in moderate-to-vigorous physical activity in 32 countries from 2002 to 2010: a cross-national perspective. Eur J Public Health 2015;25:S37–S40.

5. Telama R. Tracking of physical activity from childhood to adulthood: a review. Obes Facts 2009;2(3):187–95.

6. Klitsie T, Corder K, Visscher TLS, Atkin AJ, Jones AP, van Sluijs et al. Children's sedentary behaviour: descriptive epidemiology and associations with objectively-measured sedentary time. BMC Public Health 2013;13:1092.

7. Olds TS, Maher CA, Ridley K, Kittel DM. Descriptive epidemiology of screen and non-screen sedentary time in adolescents: a cross sectional study. Int J Behav Nutr Phys Act. 2010;7:92.

8. de Rezende LF, Rodrigues Lopes M, Rey-López JP, Matsudo VK, Luiz-Odo C. Sedentary behavior and health outcomes: an overview of systematic reviews. PLoS ONE 2014; 9(8):e105620.

9. Costigan SA, Barnett L, Plotnikoff RC, Lubans DR. The health indicators associated with screen-based sedentary behavior among adolescent girls: a systematic review. J Adolesc Health 2013;52(4):382–92.

10. Biddle SJ, Pearson N, Ross GM, Braithwaite R. Tracking of sedentary behaviours of young people: a systematic review. Prev Med. 2010;51(5):345–51.

11. Tremblay MS, Leblanc AG, Janssen I, Kho ME, Hicks A, Murumets K et al. Canadian sedentary behaviour guidelines for children and youth. Appl Physiol Nutr Metab. 2011;36(1):59–64.

12. American Academy of Pediatrics. Policy statement. Children, adolescents, and the media. Pediatrics 2013;132(5):958–61.

13. Bucksch J, Inchley J, Hamrik Z, Finne E, Kolip P. Trends in television time, non-gaming PC use and moderate-to-vigorous physical activity among German adolescents 2002–2010. BMC Public Health 2014;14:351.

14. Leech RM, McNaughton SA, Timperio A. The clustering of diet, physical activity and sedentary behavior in children and adolescents: a review. Int J Behav Nutr Phys Act. 2014;11:4.

15. Physical activity strategy for the WHO European Region 2016–2025. Copenhagen: WHO Regional Office for Europe; 2015 (EUR/RC65/9; http://www.euro.who.int/__data/assets/pdf_file/0010/282961/65wd09e_PhysicalActivityStrategy_150474.pdf, accessed 24 August 2015).

GROWING UP UNEQUAL: GENDER AND SOCIOECONOMIC
DIFFERENCES IN YOUNG PEOPLE'S HEALTH AND WELL-BEING
PART 2. KEY DATA | CHAPTER 5. RISK BEHAVIOURS

5

RISK BEHAVIOURS

TOBACCO USE
ALCOHOL USE
CANNABIS USE
SEXUAL BEHAVIOUR
FIGHTING
BULLYING

"I think cyberbullying is a problem because it means anyone can bully anyone."

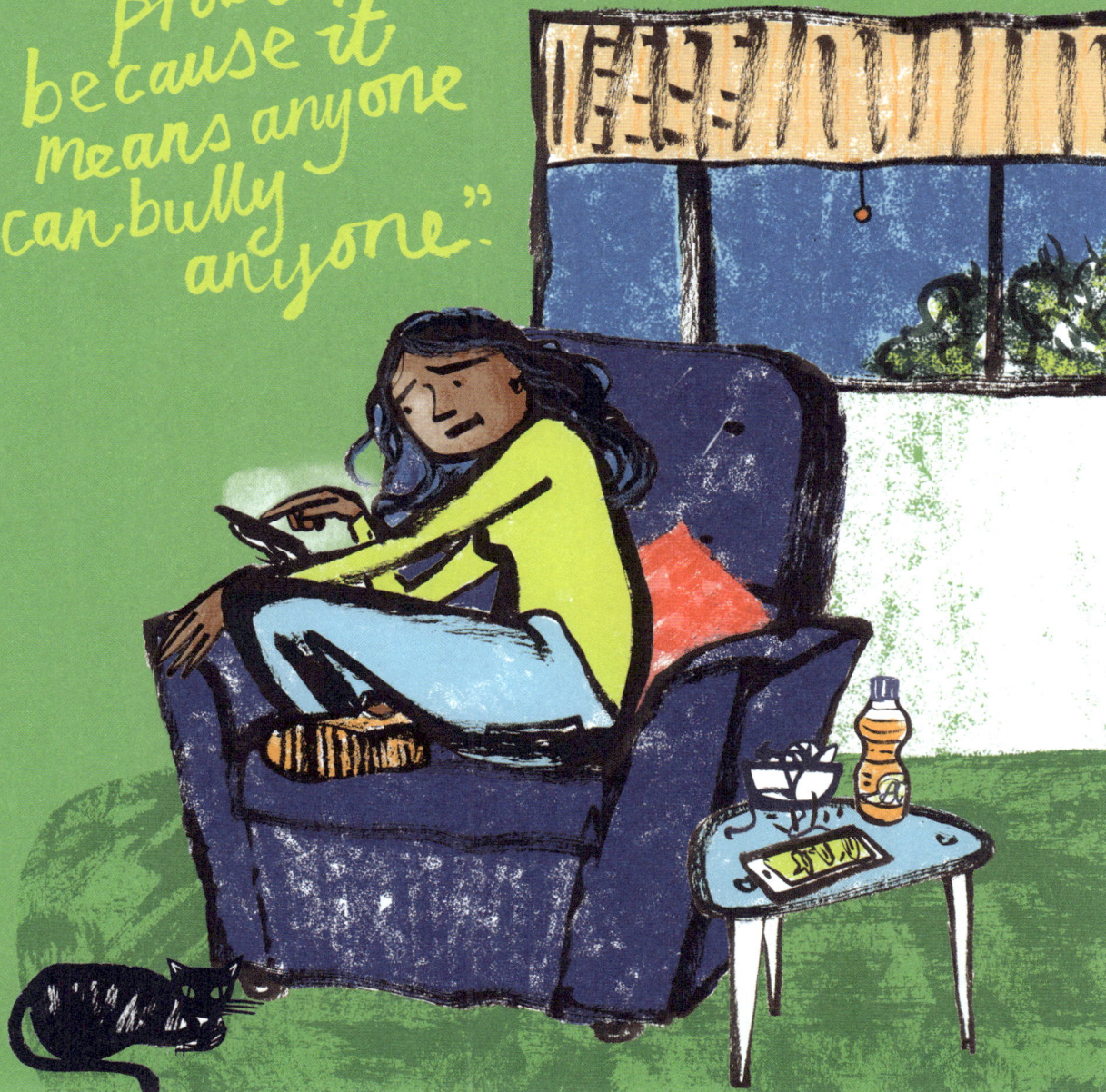

QUOTES FROM YOUNG PEOPLE ON RISK BEHAVIOURS

"Bullying is hard to deal with."

"If you are being cyberbullied and you don't know who by, then it is awful because it could be anybody around you. That is a big problem and so I think people should be trying to come up with ways to stop people from cyberbullying each other."

"There are too many taboos about this issue [sexuality] and that should not happen. Young people have to feel comfortable talking about sexuality to be able to control their future and assure a safer future."

GROWING UP UNEQUAL: GENDER AND SOCIOECONOMIC
DIFFERENCES IN YOUNG PEOPLE'S HEALTH AND WELL-BEING
PART 2. KEY DATA | CHAPTER 5. RISK BEHAVIOURS

5

TOBACCO USE

Tobacco use is the most common preventable cause of premature loss of health worldwide, accounting for almost 6 million deaths annually (including more than 600 000 due to environmental tobacco smoke) *(1)*. Tobacco use, particularly cigarette smoking, is the largest cause of health inequalities based on socioeconomic differences *(2)*: in adolescence, smoking initiation seems to be higher among those from disadvantaged backgrounds *(3)*.

Adolescence is a crucial age for initiation and development of tobacco use, so exact epidemiological data are necessary to support evidence-based preventive interventions *(4)*.

Active cigarette smoking by adolescents has immediate adverse health consequences, including addiction, reduced lung function and impaired lung growth, and asthma *(4)*.

MEASURES

Tobacco initiation
Young people were asked at what age they first smoked a cigarette, defined as more than a puff.

Weekly smoking
Young people were asked how often they smoke tobacco. Response options ranged from never to every day.

Supplementary data on daily smoking and having ever smoked are provided in the Annex.

HBSC survey 2013/2014

BOYS **GIRLS** | **SIGNIFICANT TRENDS**

Associations between family affluence and indicators of health, by country/region and gender:
first cigarette smoked at age 13 or younger

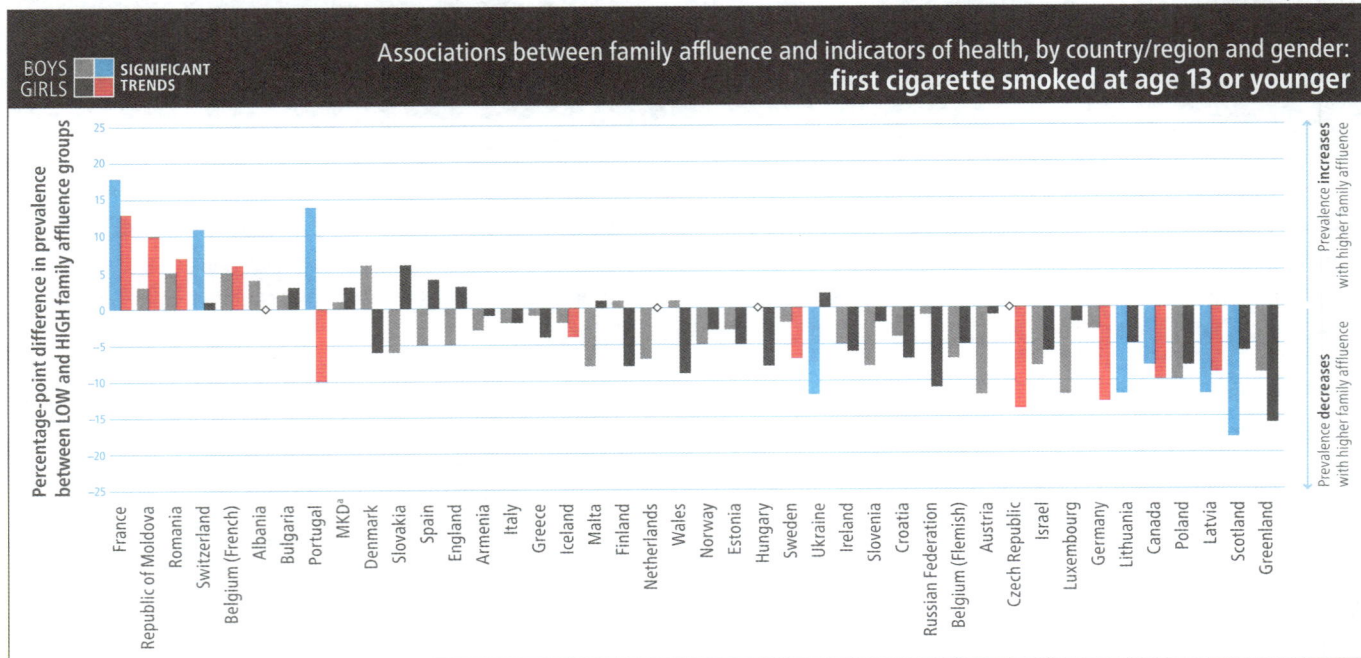

^a The former Yugoslav Republic of Macedonia. *Note:* low- and high-affluence groups represent the lowest 20% and highest 20% in each country. ◇ means less than +/-0.5%.

HBSC survey 2013/2014

BOYS **GIRLS** | **SIGNIFICANT TRENDS**

Associations between family affluence and indicators of health, by country/region and gender:
weekly smoking

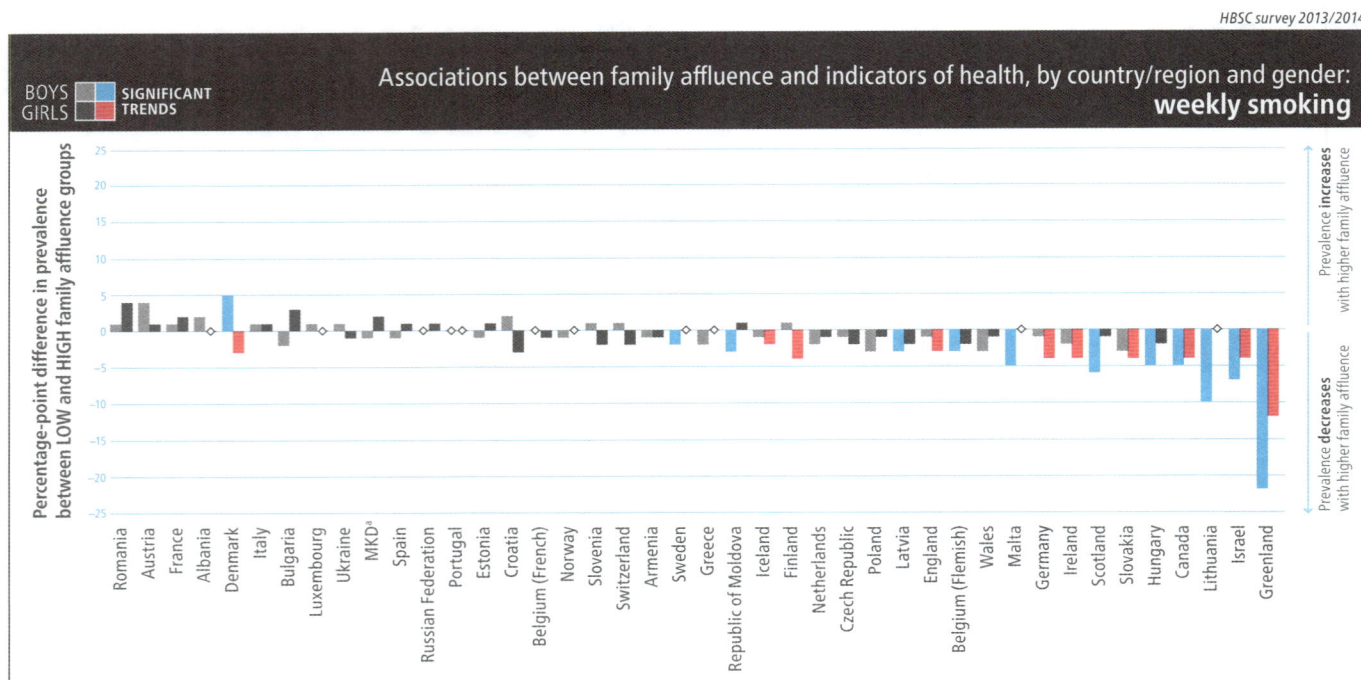

^a The former Yugoslav Republic of Macedonia. *Note:* low- and high-affluence groups represent the lowest 20% and highest 20% in each country. ◇ means less than +/-0.5%.

GROWING UP UNEQUAL: GENDER AND SOCIOECONOMIC
DIFFERENCES IN YOUNG PEOPLE'S HEALTH AND WELL-BEING
PART 2. KEY DATA | CHAPTER 5. RISK BEHAVIOURS
TOBACCO USE

5

RESULTS

Tobacco initiation

Findings presented here show the proportions who reported first smoking a cigarette at age 13 or younger.

Age

Only data for 15-year-olds are reported.

Gender

No gender difference in early onset was observed in more than half of countries and regions. It was more prevalent in boys in the 18 countries in which a significant gender difference was observed.

Family affluence

Family affluence was not significantly related to early onset in most countries and regions, but a significant association was observed for boys in eight: it was more prevalent in low-affluence groups in five and high-affluence in three. For girls, a significant association was found in 11, with higher prevalence among high-affluence girls in four and low-affluence in seven.

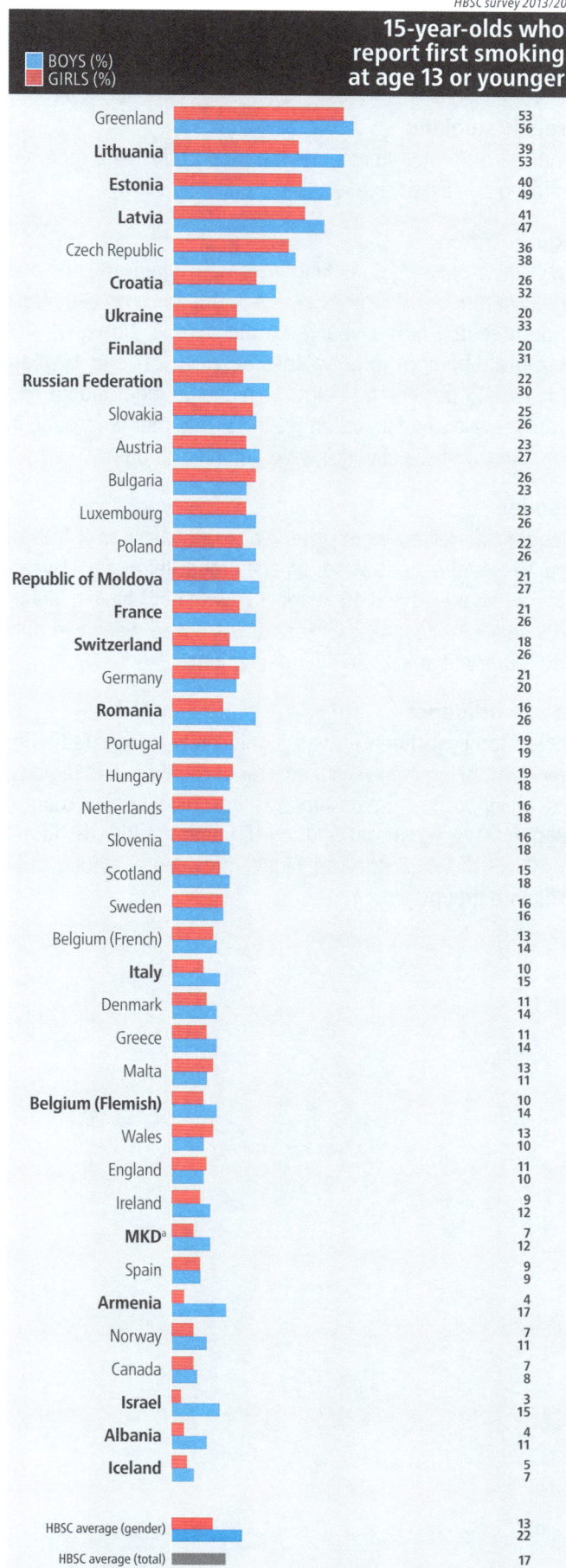

HBSC survey 2013/2014

15-year-olds who report first smoking at age 13 or younger

BOYS (%)
GIRLS (%)

	Girls	Boys
Greenland	53	56
Lithuania	39	53
Estonia	40	49
Latvia	41	47
Czech Republic	36	38
Croatia	26	32
Ukraine	20	33
Finland	20	31
Russian Federation	22	30
Slovakia	25	26
Austria	23	27
Bulgaria	26	23
Luxembourg	23	26
Poland	22	26
Republic of Moldova	21	27
France	21	26
Switzerland	18	26
Germany	21	20
Romania	16	26
Portugal	19	19
Hungary	19	18
Netherlands	16	18
Slovenia	16	18
Scotland	15	18
Sweden	16	16
Belgium (French)	13	14
Italy	10	15
Denmark	11	14
Greece	11	14
Malta	13	11
Belgium (Flemish)	10	14
Wales	13	10
England	11	10
Ireland	9	12
MKD[a]	7	12
Spain	9	9
Armenia	4	17
Norway	7	11
Canada	7	8
Israel	3	15
Albania	4	11
Iceland	5	7
HBSC average (gender)	13	22
HBSC average (total)	17	

[a] The former Yugoslav Republic of Macedonia. *Note:* **indicates** significant gender difference (at p<0.05). This question was asked only of a subset of 15-year-olds in Belgium (French).

RESULTS

Weekly smoking

Findings presented here show the proportions who reported smoking at least once a week.

Age

Prevalence of weekly smoking increased significantly by age in all countries and regions except in one for boys (Armenia) and three for girls (Albania, Armenia and Norway). The absolute difference in prevalence between 11- and 15-year-olds was 15 percentage points or higher in eight (about one fifth). Prevalence of less than 5% in 15-year-olds was found in five countries (two of which were among girls only).

Gender

Gender differences were observed in a quarter to a fifth of countries and regions across all age groups (eight for 11-year-olds, 11 at age 13 and 10 at age 15), with boys having higher prevalence in most cases. More girls smoked weekly in only one country at age 13 and in three when 15.

Family affluence

Lower family affluence was significantly associated with weekly smoking in boys in a quarter of countries and regions, but an opposite relationship was observed in one country (Denmark). A significant relationship among girls was found in 10, all of which showed higher prevalence among low-affluence groups.

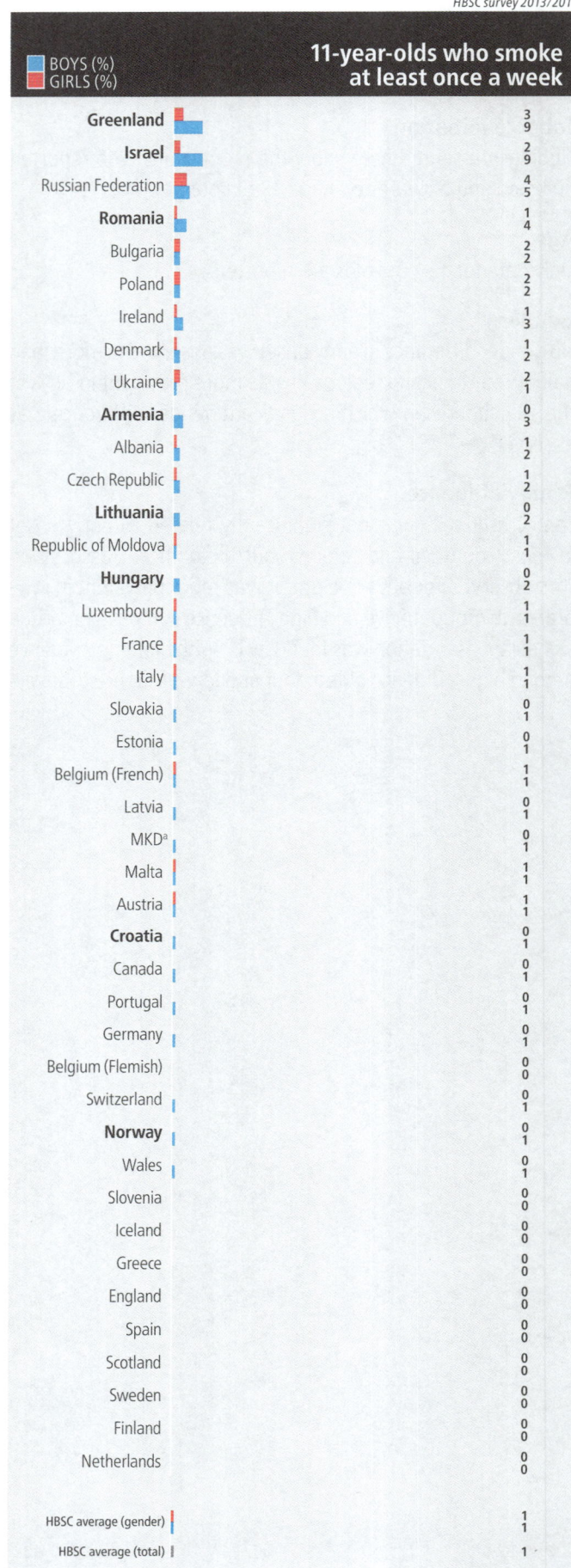

HBSC survey 2013/2014

11-year-olds who smoke at least once a week

BOYS (%)
GIRLS (%)

	Boys	Girls
Greenland	3	9
Israel	2	9
Russian Federation	4	5
Romania	1	4
Bulgaria	2	2
Poland	2	2
Ireland	1	3
Denmark	1	2
Ukraine	2	1
Armenia	0	3
Albania	1	2
Czech Republic	1	2
Lithuania	0	2
Republic of Moldova	1	1
Hungary	0	2
Luxembourg	1	1
France	1	1
Italy	1	1
Slovakia	0	1
Estonia	0	1
Belgium (French)	1	1
Latvia	0	1
MKD[a]	0	1
Malta	1	1
Austria	1	1
Croatia	0	1
Canada	0	1
Portugal	0	1
Germany	0	1
Belgium (Flemish)	0	0
Switzerland	0	1
Norway	0	1
Wales	0	1
Slovenia	0	0
Iceland	0	0
Greece	0	0
England	0	0
Spain	0	0
Scotland	0	0
Sweden	0	0
Finland	0	0
Netherlands	0	0
HBSC average (gender)	1	1
HBSC average (total)	1	

[a] The former Yugoslav Republic of Macedonia.

GROWING UP UNEQUAL: GENDER AND SOCIOECONOMIC
DIFFERENCES IN YOUNG PEOPLE'S HEALTH AND WELL-BEING
PART 2. KEY DATA | CHAPTER 5. RISK BEHAVIOURS
TOBACCO USE

5

13-year-olds who smoke at least once a week

HBSC survey 2013/2014

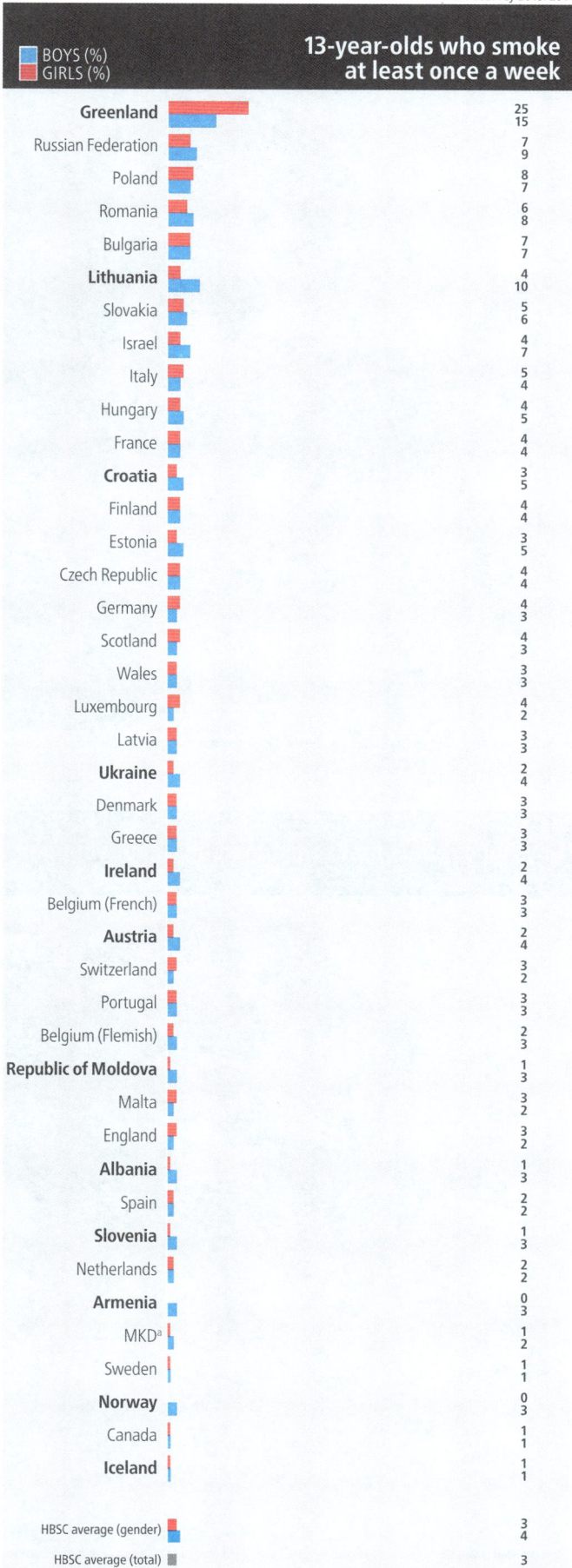

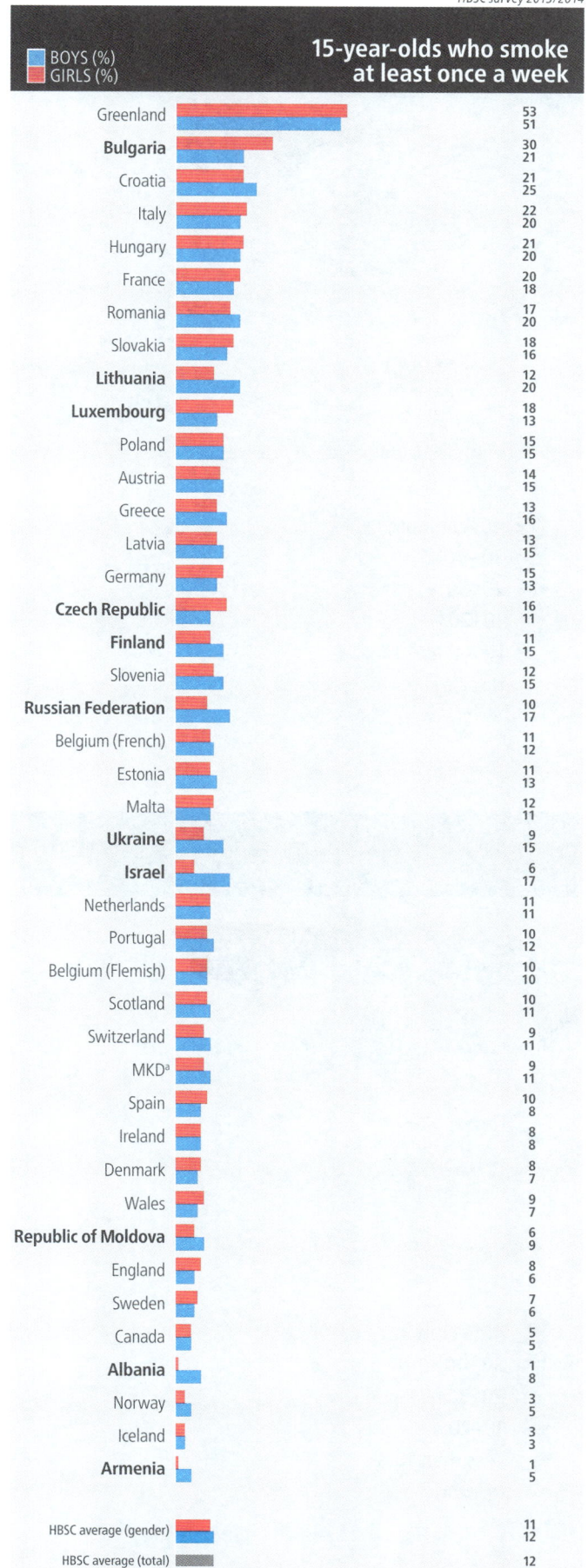

■ BOYS (%)
■ GIRLS (%)

Country	Girls (%)	Boys (%)
Greenland	25	15
Russian Federation	7	9
Poland	8	7
Romania	6	8
Bulgaria	7	7
Lithuania	4	10
Slovakia	5	6
Israel	4	7
Italy	5	4
Hungary	4	5
France	4	4
Croatia	3	5
Finland	4	4
Estonia	3	5
Czech Republic	4	4
Germany	4	3
Scotland	4	3
Wales	3	3
Luxembourg	4	2
Latvia	3	3
Ukraine	2	4
Denmark	3	
Greece	3	3
Ireland	2	4
Belgium (French)	3	3
Austria	2	4
Switzerland	3	2
Portugal	3	3
Belgium (Flemish)	2	3
Republic of Moldova	1	3
Malta	3	2
England	3	2
Albania	1	3
Spain	2	2
Slovenia	1	3
Netherlands	2	
Armenia	0	3
MKD[a]	1	2
Sweden	1	1
Norway	0	3
Canada	1	1
Iceland	1	1
HBSC average (gender)	3	4
HBSC average (total)	3	

15-year-olds who smoke at least once a week

HBSC survey 2013/2014

■ BOYS (%)
■ GIRLS (%)

Country	Girls (%)	Boys (%)
Greenland	53	51
Bulgaria	30	21
Croatia	21	25
Italy	22	20
Hungary	21	20
France	20	18
Romania	17	20
Slovakia	18	16
Lithuania	12	20
Luxembourg	18	13
Poland	15	15
Austria	14	15
Greece	13	16
Latvia	13	15
Germany	15	13
Czech Republic	16	11
Finland	11	15
Slovenia	12	15
Russian Federation	10	17
Belgium (French)	11	12
Estonia	11	13
Malta	12	11
Ukraine	9	15
Israel	6	17
Netherlands	11	11
Portugal	10	12
Belgium (Flemish)	10	10
Scotland	10	11
Switzerland	9	11
MKD[a]	9	11
Spain	10	8
Ireland	8	8
Denmark	8	7
Wales	9	7
Republic of Moldova	6	9
England	8	6
Sweden	7	6
Canada	5	5
Albania	1	8
Norway	3	5
Iceland	3	3
Armenia	1	5
HBSC average (gender)	11	12
HBSC average (total)	12	

*Note: **indicates** significant gender difference (at p<0.05). 0 means less than +/-0.5%.*

HBSC survey 2013/2014

15-year-old girls who report first smoking at age 13 or younger

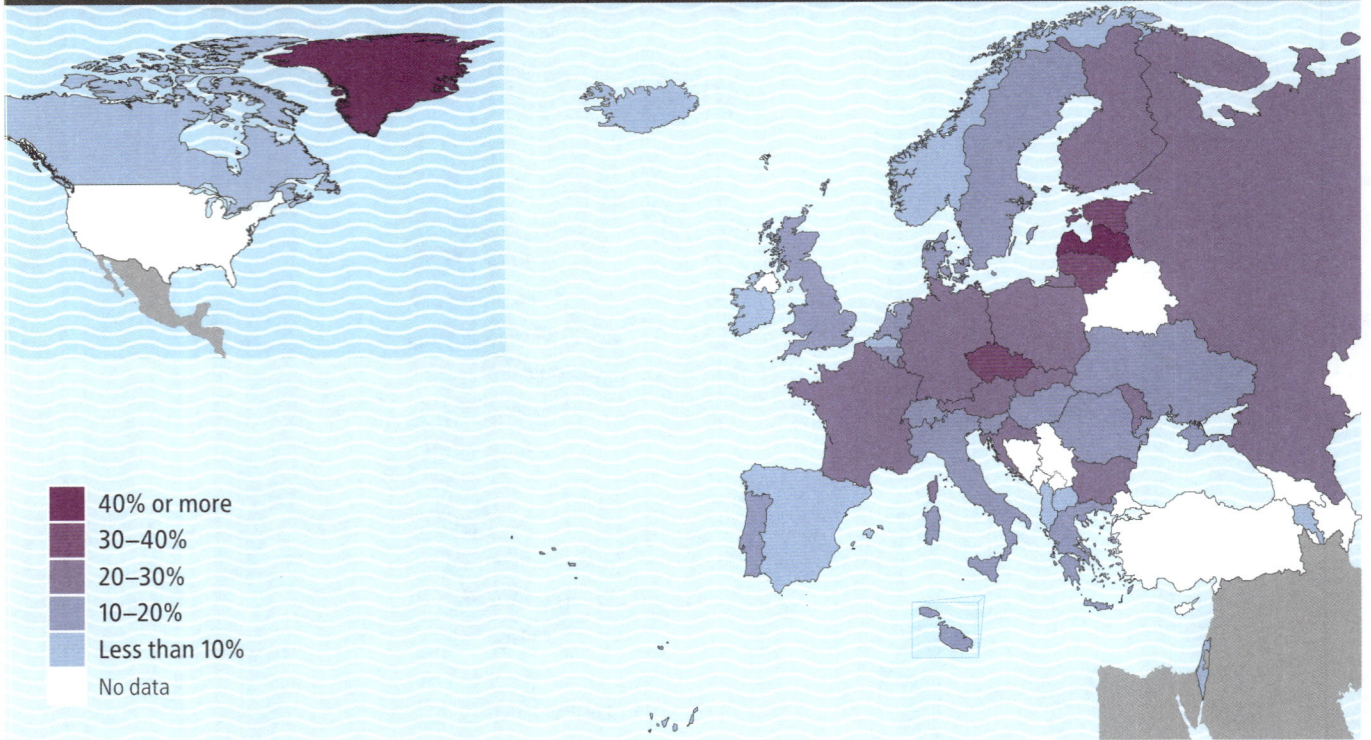

40% or more
30–40%
20–30%
10–20%
Less than 10%
No data

Note: HBSC teams provided disaggregated data for Belgium and the United Kingdom; these data appear in the map above.

HBSC survey 2013/2014

15-year-old boys who report first smoking at age 13 or younger

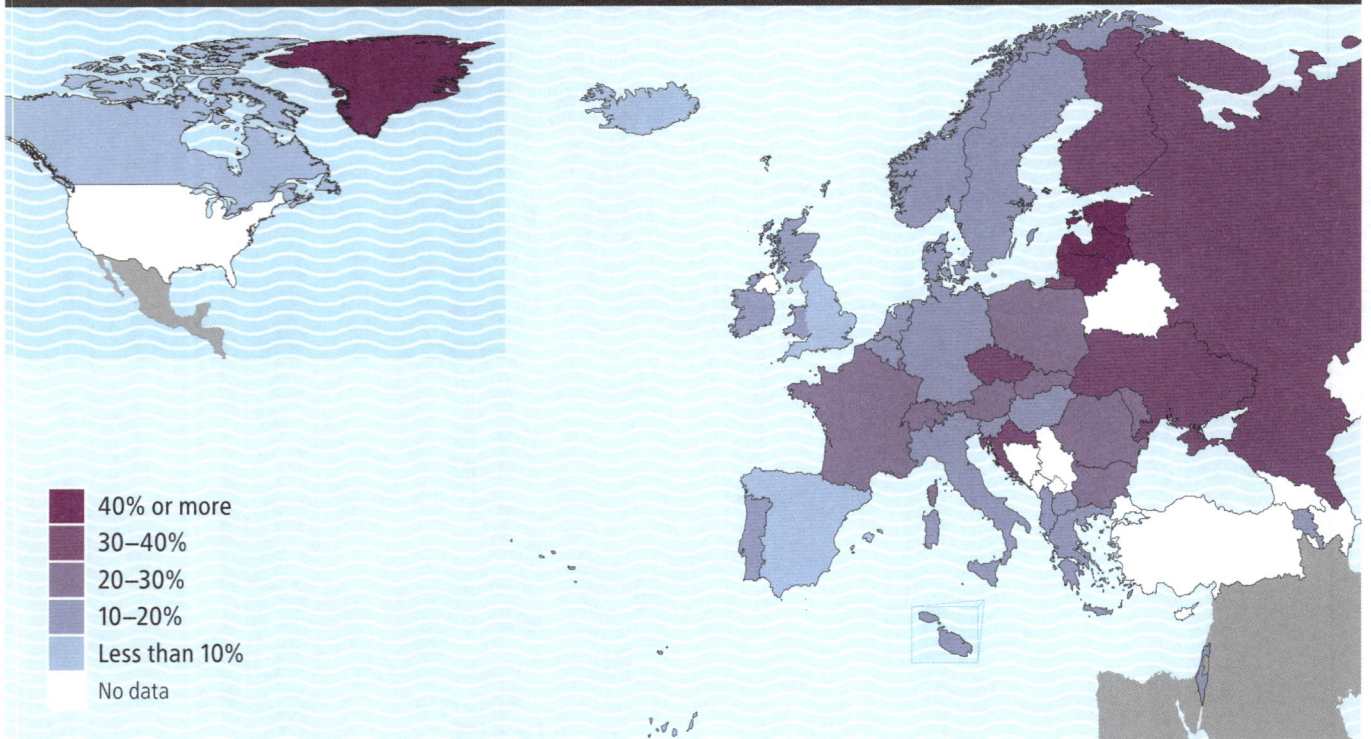

40% or more
30–40%
20–30%
10–20%
Less than 10%
No data

Note: HBSC teams provided disaggregated data for Belgium and the United Kingdom; these data appear in the map above.

GROWING UP UNEQUAL: GENDER AND SOCIOECONOMIC
DIFFERENCES IN YOUNG PEOPLE'S HEALTH AND WELL-BEING
PART 2. KEY DATA | CHAPTER 5. RISK BEHAVIOURS
TOBACCO USE

5

HBSC survey 2013/2014

15-year-old girls who smoke at least once a week

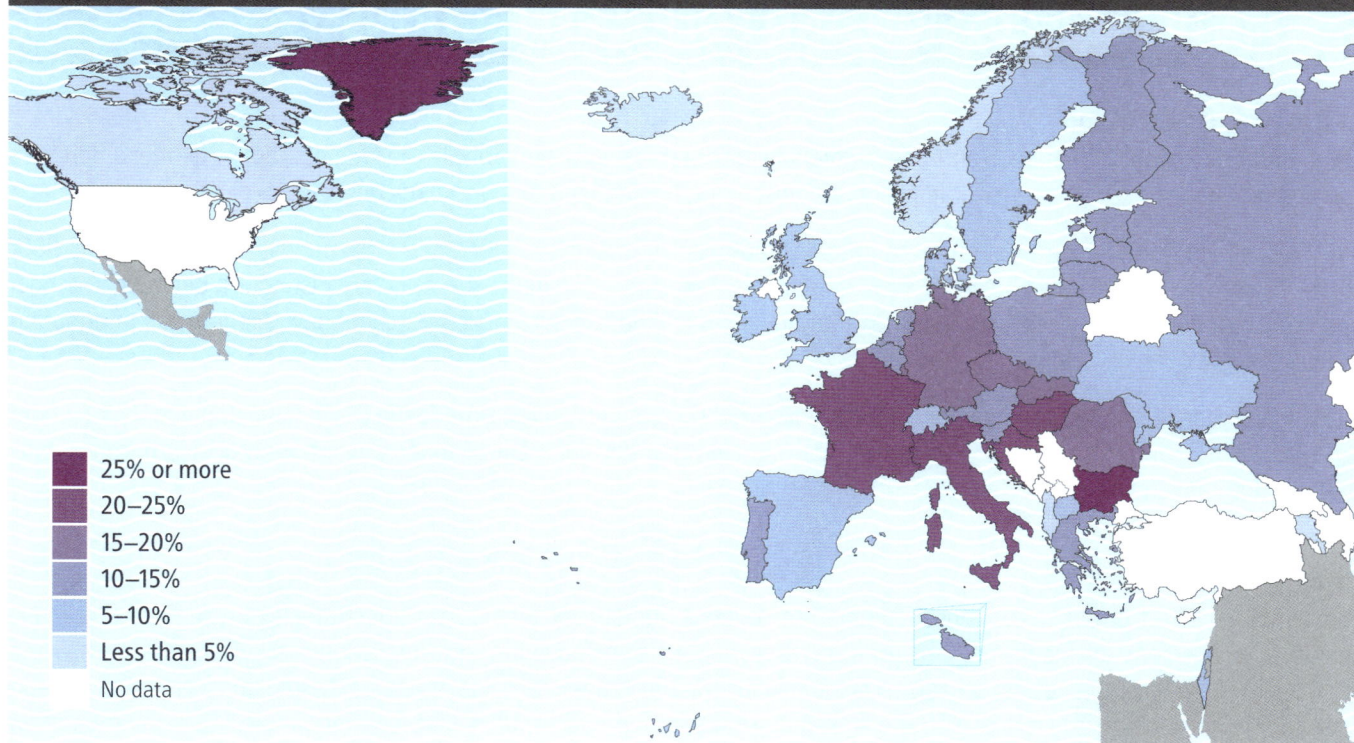

- 25% or more
- 20–25%
- 15–20%
- 10–15%
- 5–10%
- Less than 5%
- No data

Note: HBSC teams provided disaggregated data for Belgium and the United Kingdom; these data appear in the map above.

HBSC survey 2013/2014

15-year-old boys who smoke at least once a week

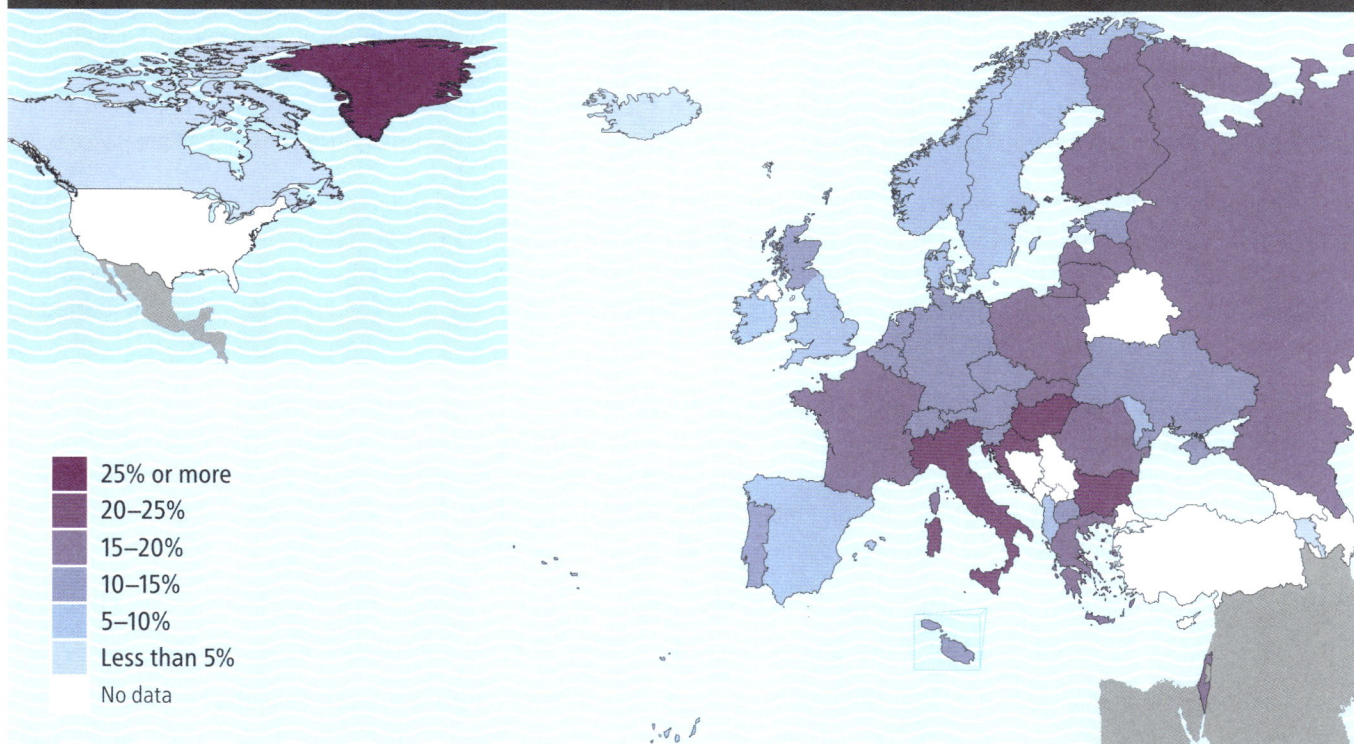

- 25% or more
- 20–25%
- 15–20%
- 10–15%
- 5–10%
- Less than 5%
- No data

Note: HBSC teams provided disaggregated data for Belgium and the United Kingdom; these data appear in the map above.

TOBACCO USE:
SCIENTIFIC DISCUSSION AND POLICY REFLECTIONS

SCIENTIFIC DISCUSSION

Large variations in tobacco initiation and weekly smoking are observed between countries and regions, but no gender differences can be seen in most. Where gender differences are present, more boys tend to report early onset and weekly smoking.

Smoking remains high in some countries and regions, but weekly smoking has declined in comparison to the previous HBSC survey in almost all (5). It should be noted, however, that the measures used in the survey do not distinguish between in-school and out-of-school smoking: research indicates that adolescents who use substances at school have higher risks of adopting other health-risk behaviours (6).

The link between SES and smoking among adolescents is not uniform, unlike the situation in the general population, for whom SES plays a more important role (2,7). It seems that initiation and development of tobacco use during adolescence are only partially determined by SES.

POLICY REFLECTIONS

The combined effect of public awareness-raising interventions and stricter tobacco-control strategies implemented in many countries and regions (including tax and price increases, public smoking bans, and restrictions on advertising and selling sites) seem to be having an effect on adolescent smoking. The data show, however, that weekly smoking increases with age, especially in boys, who also start earlier. The challenge is to scale-up interventions that focus on preventing experimentation among young people and experimenters becoming weekly smokers as well as to develop policies to restrict their access to tobacco products through commercial sources (8). The WHO Framework Convention on Tobacco Control (9) addresses the issue of tobacco sales to and by minors.

Interventions should be comprehensive (integrated), flexible and have sufficient reach (all young people), frequency (throughout the school curriculum, for example) and duration (sustainable over time). The challenge is to promote the creation of as many tobacco-free youth environments as possible by, for instance, introducing policies on tobacco-free schools. Given that adolescents spend much of their time in school settings in which they are exposed to all kinds of risk factors associated with smoking, it is important that policies are introduced to create tobacco-free social environments in schools. The same applies to family environments, with some countries having introduced measures such as banning smoking in cars in which children are passengers.

Effective interventions are those that are clearly communicated, provide unequivocal rules and penalties for those violating them, and are applicable to all involved in young people's social environments – they do not, for instance, promote designated smoking areas for adults and teachers. Lack of integrated policies may lead to negative consequences: creation of tobacco-free school environments, for instance, may be successful in curbing smoking at school but will have little effect if not supported by similar policies in other environments.

Policies should aim to reach at-risk groups with attention-grabbing messages presented in the most efficient and effective way. HBSC and other studies show that young people increasingly use electronic social media to interact and access information, so innovative interventions that make use of new communication technologies should be designed to disseminate tobacco countermarketing (the use of commercial marketing tactics to produce attitudinal and behavioural changes). Measurement and evaluation of interventions that make use of new communication technologies are critical to building an evidence base.

There is some evidence from research in the United States involving young people and adults that interventions have differential effects by SES. Mass-media anti-tobacco campaigns, for instance, have higher impacts among people of low SES.

The equalizing of traditional gender differences in tobacco use through increased prevalence of smoking among girls in some countries and regions, particularly in central and eastern Europe and Greenland, raises cause for concern. Specific issues relating to women's smoking should be reflected in preventive measures, including smoking's effects on appearance and fertility and the risk of thromboembolic complications when practised concurrently with taking hormonal contraceptives (10,11).

GROWING UP UNEQUAL: GENDER AND SOCIOECONOMIC
DIFFERENCES IN YOUNG PEOPLE'S HEALTH AND WELL-BEING
PART 2. KEY DATA | CHAPTER 5. RISK BEHAVIOURS
TOBACCO USE

5

REFERENCES

1. WHO report on the global tobacco epidemic, 2011. Warning about the dangers of tobacco. Geneva: World Health Organization; 2011 (http://www.who.int/tobacco/global_report/2011/en/, accessed 24 August 2015).

2. Kunst A, Giskes K, Mackenbach J. Socioeconomic inequalities in smoking in the European Union. Applying an equity lens to tobacco control policies. Rotterdam: Department of Public Health, Erasmus Medical Center; 2004 (http://old.ensp.org/files/ensp_socioeconomic_inequalities_in_smoking_in_eu.pdf, accessed 24 August 2015).

3. Hiscock R, Bauld L, Amos A, Fidler JA, Munafo M. Socioeconomic status and smoking: a review. Ann NY Acad Sci. 2012;1248:107–23.

4. Preventing tobacco use among youth and young adults: a report of the Surgeon General. Rockville (MD): US Department of Health and Human Services; 2012 (http://www.surgeongeneral.gov/library/reports/preventing-youth-tobacco-use/full-report.pdf, accessed 24 August 2015).

5. Currie C, Zanotti C, Morgan A, Currie D, de Looze M, Roberts C et al., editors. Social determinants of health and well-being among young people. Health Behaviour in School-aged Children (HBSC) study: international report from the 2009/2010 survey. Copenhagen: WHO Regional Office for Europe; 2012 (Health Policy for Children and Adolescents, No. 6; http://www.euro.who.int/en/what-we-publish/abstracts/socialdeterminants-of-health-and-well-being-among-young-people.-health-behaviour-in-schoolaged-children-hbsc-study, accessed 24 August 2015).

6. Dudovitz RN, McCoy K, Chung PJ. At-school substance use as a marker for serious health risks. Acad Pediatr. 2015;15:41–6.

7. Lidegaard Ø. Hormonal contraception, thrombosis and age. Expert Opin Drug Saf. 2014;13(10):1353–60. doi:10.1517/14740338.2014.950654.

8. Gendall P, Hoek J, Marsh L, Edwards R, Healey B. Youth tobacco access: trends and policy implications. BMJ Open 2014;4:e004631. doi:10.1136/bmjopen-2013-004631.

9. WHO Framework Convention on Tobacco Control [website]. Geneva: World Health Organization; 2015 (http://www.who.int/fctc/en, accessed 24 August 2015).

10. The health consequences of smoking – 50 years of progress. A report of the Surgeon General. Rockville (MD): US Department of Health and Human Services; 2014 (http://ash.org/wp-content/uploads/2014/01/full-report.pdf, accessed 24 August 2015).

11. Mackenbach JP. Health inequalities: Europe in profile. London: Department of Health; 2006 (http://ec.europa.eu/health/ph_determinants/socio_economics/documents/ev_060302_rd06_en.pdf, accessed 24 August 2015).

GROWING UP UNEQUAL: GENDER AND SOCIOECONOMIC
DIFFERENCES IN YOUNG PEOPLE'S HEALTH AND WELL-BEING
PART 2. KEY DATA | CHAPTER 5. RISK BEHAVIOURS

5

ALCOHOL USE

Adolescence is a period of discovery and experimentation during which many young people start to explore what they perceive as adult behaviours, such as drinking alcohol. This may be interpreted as a natural, perhaps even healthy, curiosity about transitioning to adult life in which alcohol is used, but not misused. A combination of factors that include not understanding the limits for safe alcohol consumption and requiring less alcohol to experience drunkenness means that for some adolescents, experimentation can turn into excessive rates of use, with the physical, mental and social risks this brings.

Alcohol is one of the most widely available and most commonly used drugs for adolescents *(1,2)*. Young people may use alcohol to fulfil social and personal needs, intensify contacts with peers and initiate new relationships *(3)*. Adolescent alcohol use nevertheless constitutes a major public health concern in many European and North American countries and regions. Risky drinking, including early and frequent drinking and drunkenness, is associated with adverse psychological, social and physical health consequences, including academic failure, violence, accidents, injury, use of other substances and unprotected sexual intercourse *(4)*. It has also been suggested that drinking alcohol during adolescence may negatively affect brain development and functioning, although research on this topic is still in a preliminary phase *(5)*.

MEASURES

Weekly drinking
Young people were asked how often they drink any alcoholic beverage and were given a list of drinks: beer, wine, spirits, alcopops or any other drink that contains alcohol. Response options ranged from never to every day.

Drunkenness initiation
Young people were asked at what age they first got drunk.

Drunkenness
Young people were asked whether they had ever had so much alcohol that they were really drunk. Response options ranged from never to more than 10 times.

Supplementary data on first alcohol use at age 13 or younger and drinking beer, alcopops, wine or spirits at least once a week are provided in the Annex.

HBSC survey 2013/2014

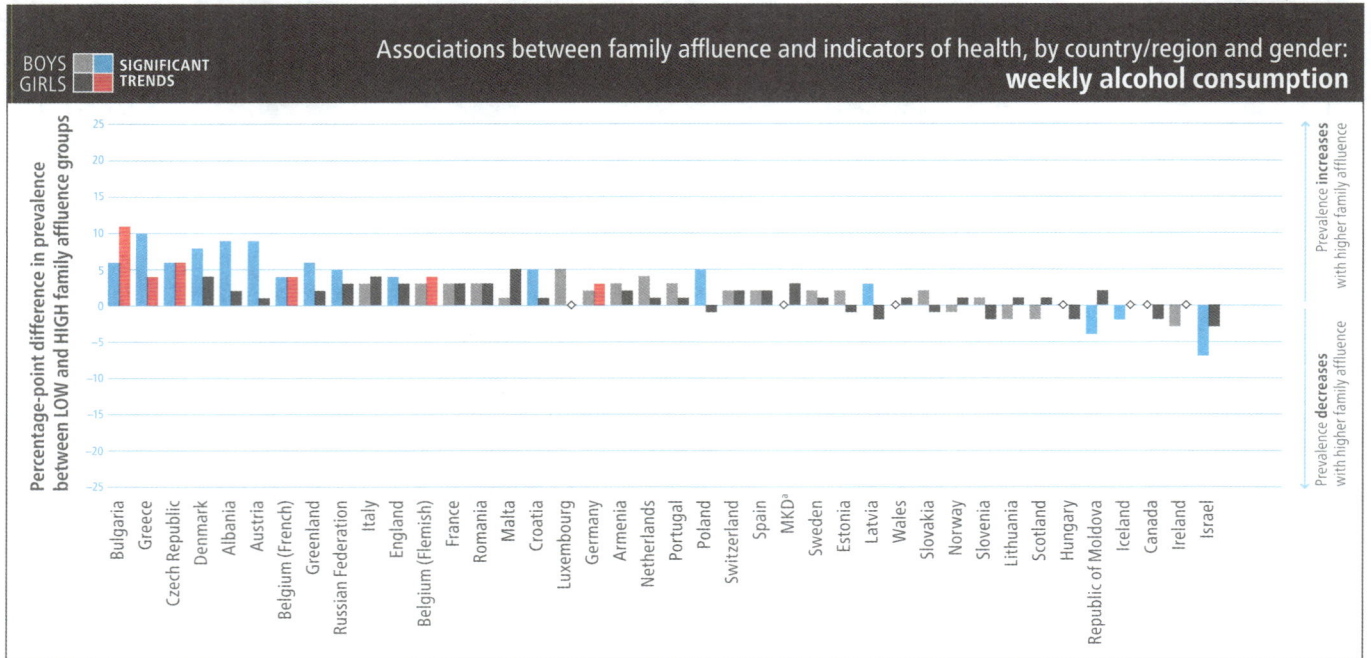

BOYS
GIRLS

SIGNIFICANT
TRENDS

Associations between family affluence and indicators of health, by country/region and gender:
weekly alcohol consumption

Percentage-point difference in prevalence between LOW and HIGH family affluence groups

Prevalence **increases** with higher family affluence

Prevalence **decreases** with higher family affluence

[Countries along x-axis: Bulgaria, Greece, Czech Republic, Denmark, Albania, Austria, Belgium (French), Greenland, Russian Federation, Italy, England, Belgium (Flemish), France, Romania, Malta, Croatia, Luxembourg, Germany, Armenia, Netherlands, Portugal, Poland, Switzerland, Spain, MKD[a], Sweden, Estonia, Latvia, Wales, Slovakia, Norway, Slovenia, Lithuania, Scotland, Hungary, Republic of Moldova, Iceland, Canada, Ireland, Israel]

[a] The former Yugoslav Republic of Macedonia. *Note:* low- and high-affluence groups represent the lowest 20% and highest 20% in each country. ◇ means less than +/-0.5%.
No data were received from Finland and Ukraine.

HBSC survey 2013/2014

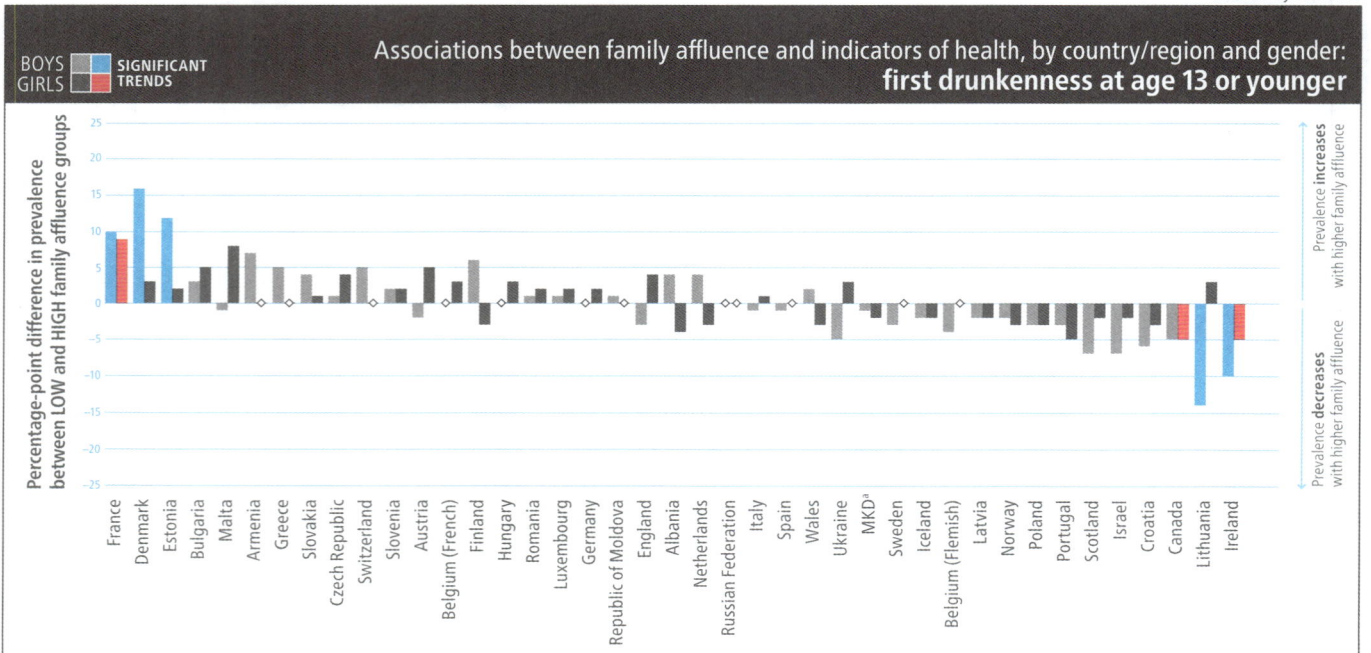

BOYS
GIRLS

SIGNIFICANT
TRENDS

Associations between family affluence and indicators of health, by country/region and gender:
first drunkenness at age 13 or younger

Percentage-point difference in prevalence between LOW and HIGH family affluence groups

Prevalence **increases** with higher family affluence

Prevalence **decreases** with higher family affluence

[Countries along x-axis: France, Denmark, Estonia, Bulgaria, Malta, Armenia, Greece, Slovakia, Czech Republic, Switzerland, Slovenia, Austria, Belgium (French), Finland, Hungary, Romania, Luxembourg, Germany, Republic of Moldova, England, Albania, Netherlands, Russian Federation, Italy, Spain, Wales, Ukraine, MKD[a], Sweden, Iceland, Belgium (Flemish), Latvia, Norway, Poland, Portugal, Scotland, Israel, Croatia, Canada, Lithuania, Ireland]

[a] The former Yugoslav Republic of Macedonia. *Note:* low- and high-affluence groups represent the lowest 20% and highest 20% in each country. ◇ means less than +/-0.5%.
No data were received from Greenland.

GROWING UP UNEQUAL: GENDER AND SOCIOECONOMIC
DIFFERENCES IN YOUNG PEOPLE'S HEALTH AND WELL-BEING
PART 2. KEY DATA | CHAPTER 5. RISK BEHAVIOURS
ALCOHOL USE

5

HBSC survey 2013/2014

Associations between family affluence and indicators of health, by country/region and gender: having been drunk on two or more occasions

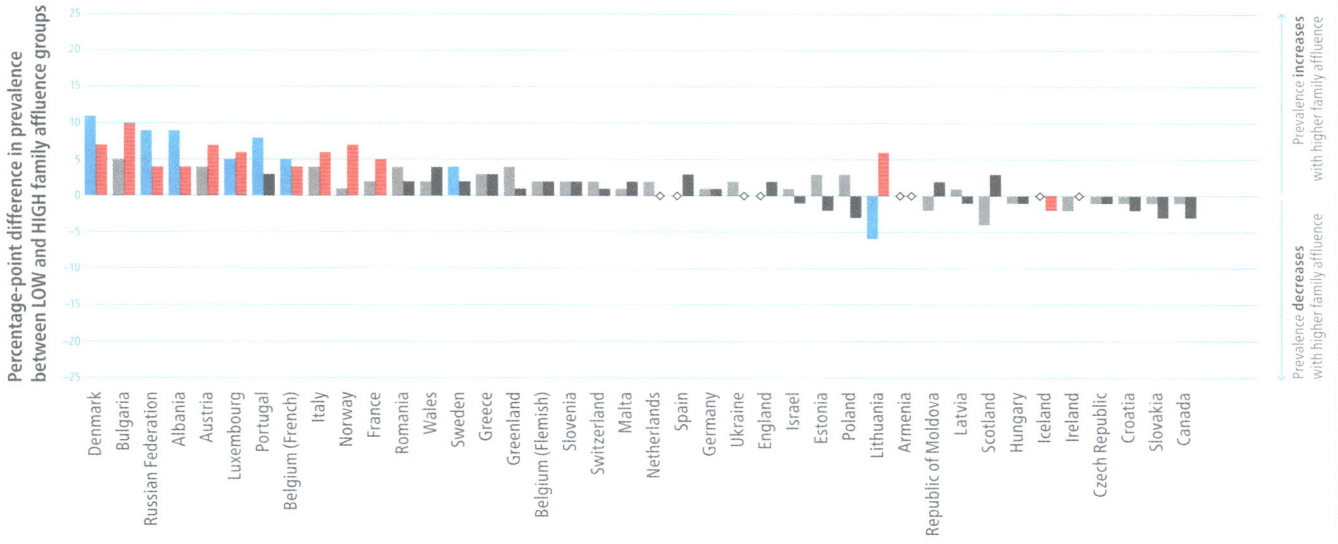

Note: low- and high-affluence groups represent the lowest 20% and highest 20% in each country. ◇ means less than +/-0.5%.
No data were received from Finland and the former Yugoslav Republic of Macedonia.

RESULTS

Weekly drinking

Findings presented here show the proportions who reported drinking any alcoholic beverage at least every week.

Age Prevalence increased significantly between ages 11 and 15 in almost all countries and regions for boys and girls. Increases were particularly large between ages 13 and 15.

Gender Overall, weekly drinking was more common among boys. The gender difference increased with age: at age 15, the difference was greater than 10 percentage points in 12 countries and regions.

Family affluence Family affluence was associated with weekly drinking in 16 countries and regions for boys and six for girls. It was higher among high-affluence groups in most, but three countries and regions showed the opposite relationship among boys.

Drunkenness initiation

Findings presented here show the proportions who reported first getting drunk at age 13 or younger.

Age Data are presented for 15-year-olds only.

Gender Boys were more likely to report first drunkenness at or before age 13 in less than half of countries and regions. Gender differences of 10 percentage points or more were found in three (Croatia, Lithuania and Romania).

Family affluence No significant association was found with family affluence in most countries and regions. In those that showed an association, no clear overall pattern emerged.

Drunkenness

Findings presented here show the proportions who reported having been drunk on two or more occasions.

Age Prevalence increased significantly and substantially between ages 11 and 15 for boys and girls in all countries and regions, with the exception of girls in Armenia.

Gender A significant gender difference was found in less than half of countries and regions, with boys more likely to report it. Girls reported it more often in Greenland (11-year-olds), Scotland (13-year-olds) and England (15-year-olds).

Family affluence An association was found in eight countries and regions for boys and 12 for girls. Drunkenness was more prevalent among high-affluence groups in most, but the opposite relationship was evident in Lithuania for boys and Iceland for girls.

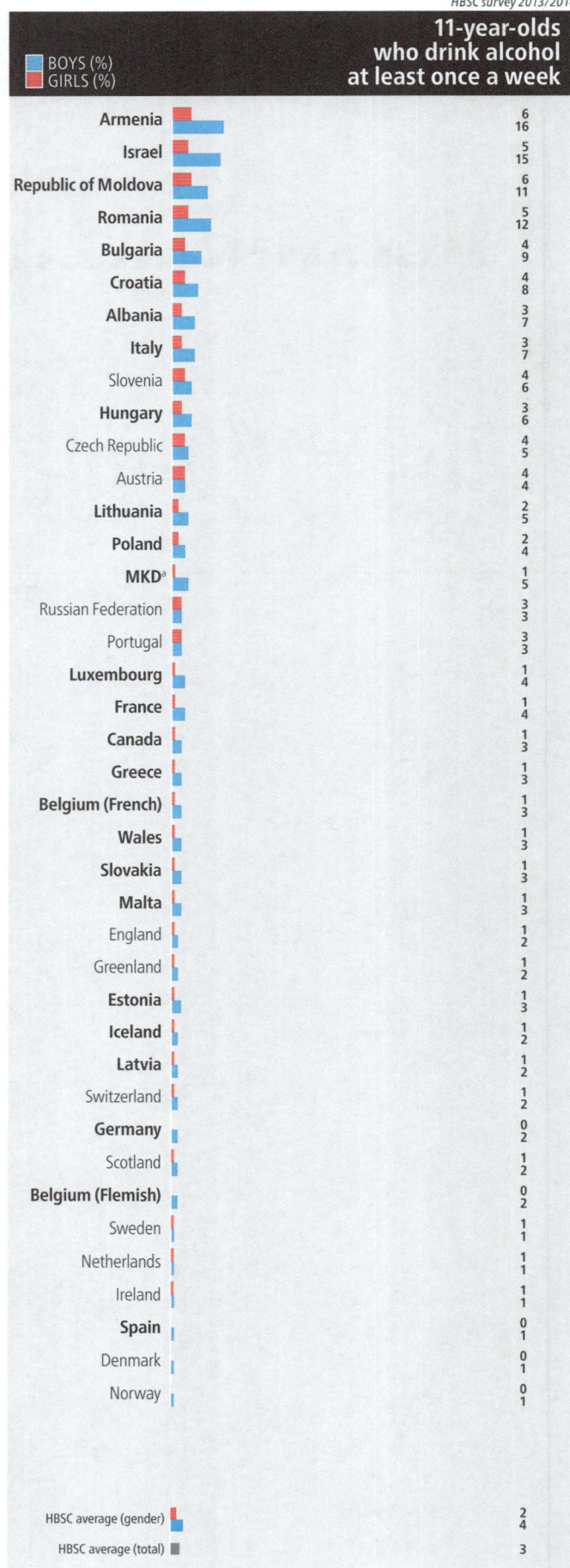

HBSC survey 2013/2014

11-year-olds who drink alcohol at least once a week

■ BOYS (%)
■ GIRLS (%)

Country/region	Boys	Girls
Armenia	6	16
Israel	5	15
Republic of Moldova	6	11
Romania	5	12
Bulgaria	4	9
Croatia	4	8
Albania	3	7
Italy	3	7
Slovenia	4	6
Hungary	3	6
Czech Republic	4	5
Austria	4	4
Lithuania	2	5
Poland	2	4
MKD[a]	1	5
Russian Federation	3	3
Portugal	3	3
Luxembourg	1	4
France	1	4
Canada	1	3
Greece	1	3
Belgium (French)	1	3
Wales	1	3
Slovakia	1	3
Malta	1	3
England	1	2
Greenland	1	2
Estonia	1	3
Iceland	1	2
Latvia	1	2
Switzerland	1	2
Germany	0	2
Scotland	1	2
Belgium (Flemish)	0	2
Sweden	1	1
Netherlands	1	1
Ireland	1	1
Spain	0	1
Denmark	0	1
Norway	0	1
HBSC average (gender)	2	4
HBSC average (total)	3	

[a] The former Yugoslav Republic of Macedonia.

GROWING UP UNEQUAL: GENDER AND SOCIOECONOMIC
DIFFERENCES IN YOUNG PEOPLE'S HEALTH AND WELL-BEING
PART 2. KEY DATA | CHAPTER 5. RISK BEHAVIOURS
ALCOHOL USE

5

13-year-olds who drink alcohol at least once a week

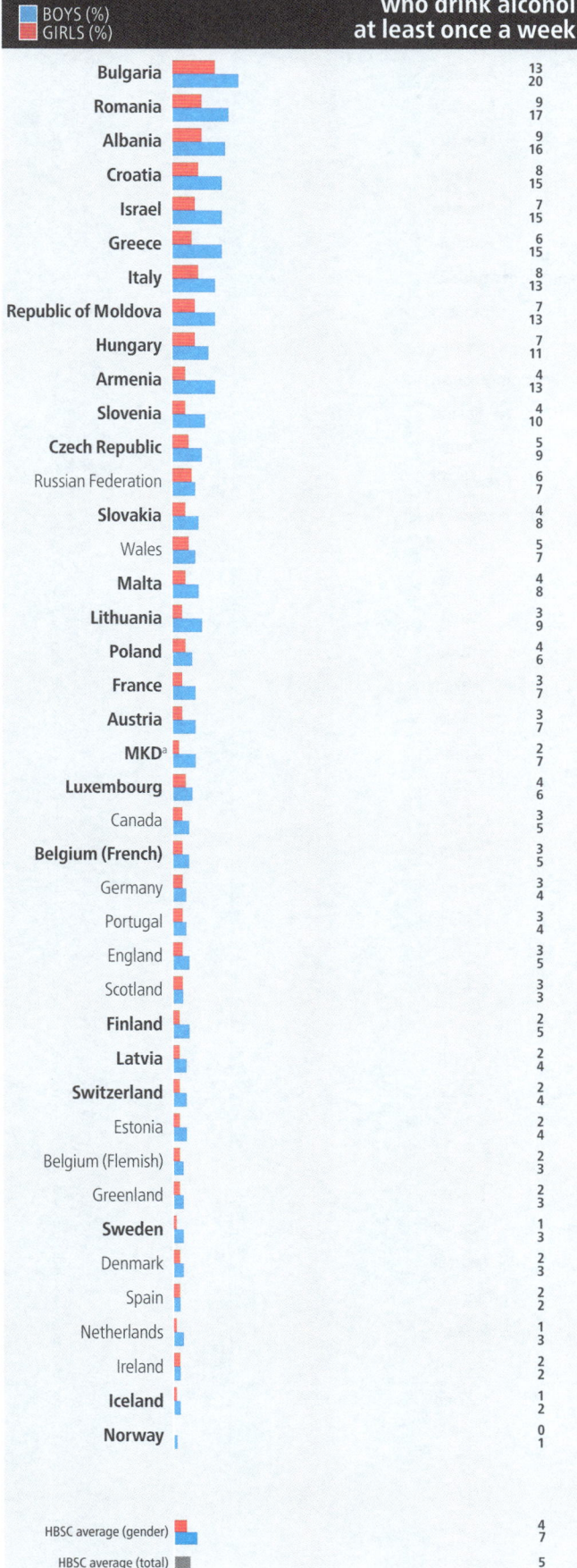

HBSC survey 2013/2014

- BOYS (%)
- GIRLS (%)

Country	Boys	Girls
Bulgaria	13	20
Romania	9	17
Albania	9	16
Croatia	8	15
Israel	7	15
Greece	6	15
Italy	8	13
Republic of Moldova	7	13
Hungary	7	11
Armenia	4	13
Slovenia	4	10
Czech Republic	5	9
Russian Federation	6	7
Slovakia	4	8
Wales	5	7
Malta	4	8
Lithuania	3	9
Poland	4	6
France	3	7
Austria	3	7
MKD[a]	2	7
Luxembourg	4	6
Canada	3	5
Belgium (French)	3	5
Germany	3	4
Portugal	3	4
England	3	5
Scotland	3	3
Finland	2	5
Latvia	2	4
Switzerland	2	4
Estonia	2	4
Belgium (Flemish)	2	3
Greenland	2	3
Sweden	1	3
Denmark	2	3
Spain	2	2
Netherlands	1	3
Ireland	2	2
Iceland	1	2
Norway	0	1
HBSC average (gender)	4	7
HBSC average (total)		5

15-year-olds who drink alcohol at least once a week

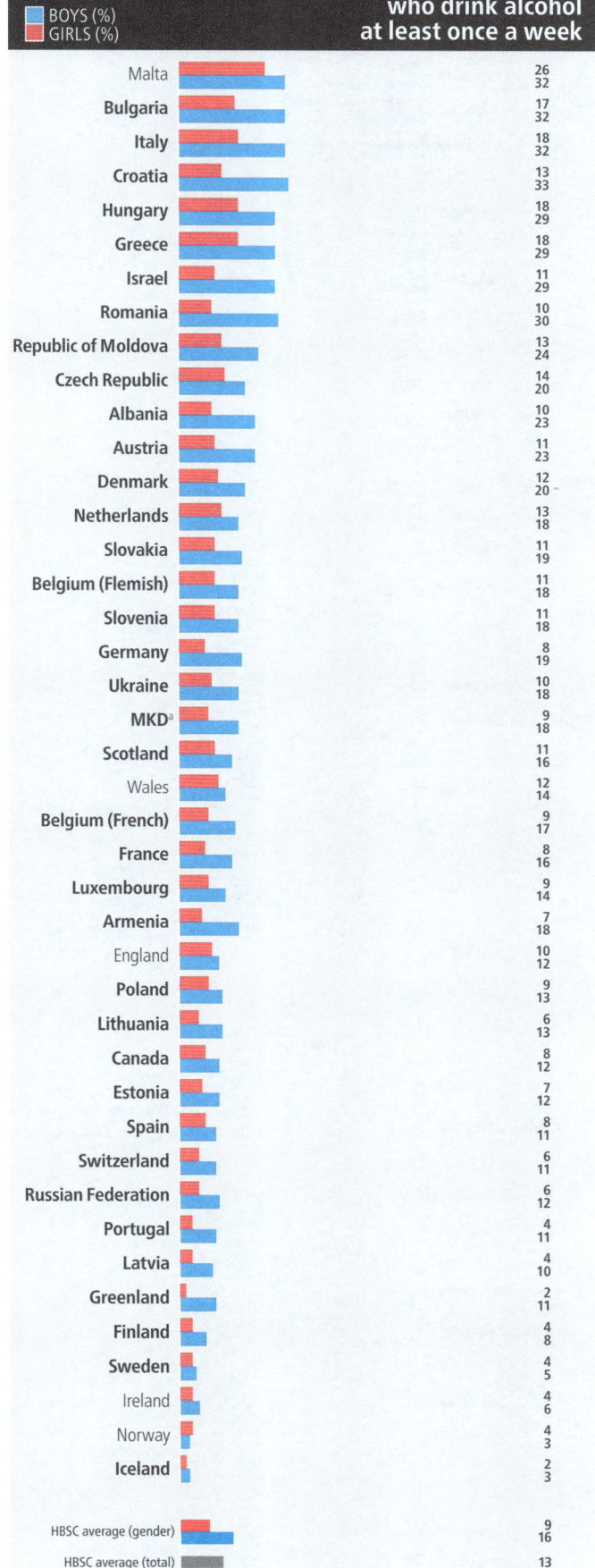

HBSC survey 2013/2014

- BOYS (%)
- GIRLS (%)

Country	Boys	Girls
Malta	26	32
Bulgaria	17	32
Italy	18	32
Croatia	13	33
Hungary	18	29
Greece	18	29
Israel	11	29
Romania	10	30
Republic of Moldova	13	24
Czech Republic	14	20
Albania	10	23
Austria	11	23
Denmark	12	20
Netherlands	13	18
Slovakia	11	19
Belgium (Flemish)	11	18
Slovenia	11	18
Germany	8	19
Ukraine	10	18
MKD[a]	9	18
Scotland	11	16
Wales	12	14
Belgium (French)	9	17
France	8	16
Luxembourg	9	14
Armenia	7	18
England	10	12
Poland	9	13
Lithuania	6	13
Canada	8	12
Estonia	7	12
Spain	8	11
Switzerland	6	11
Russian Federation	6	12
Portugal	4	11
Latvia	4	10
Greenland	2	11
Finland	4	8
Sweden	4	5
Ireland	4	6
Norway	4	3
Iceland	2	3
HBSC average (gender)	9	16
HBSC average (total)		13

Note: **indicates** significant gender difference (at p<0.05). 0 means less than +/-0.5%.
No data were received from Finland (11-year-olds) and Ukraine (11- and 13-year-olds).

15-year-olds who report first drunkenness at age 13 or younger

HBSC survey 2013/2014

Country	BOYS (%)	GIRLS (%)
Lithuania	15	25
Estonia	17	21
Bulgaria	13	19
Latvia	12	14
Finland	12	14
Scotland	12	12
Croatia	6	16
Slovakia	10	12
Czech Republic	9	12
Denmark	10	11
Wales	10	10
Hungary	9	11
Romania	4	16
England	10	9
Ukraine	6	13
Albania	6	13
Malta	9	9
Canada	8	10
Slovenia	6	11
Republic of Moldova	4	12
Germany	7	9
Poland	8	8
Austria	6	10
France	6	7
Spain	6	7
Greece	5	8
Armenia	4	8
Ireland	5	7
Portugal	5	6
Switzerland	4	7
Luxembourg	5	5
Belgium (French)	3	6
Sweden	5	5
Netherlands	4	4
Russian Federation	3	5
Israel	1	7
MKD[a]	2	6
Belgium (Flemish)	3	4
Italy	2	5
Norway	3	3
Iceland	2	3
HBSC average (gender)	7	10
HBSC average (total)		8

11-year-olds who have been drunk on two or more occasions

HBSC survey 2013/2014

Country	BOYS (%)	GIRLS (%)
Armenia	2	7
Bulgaria	1	3
Croatia	1	4
Albania	1	4
Ukraine	1	3
Hungary	2	2
Republic of Moldova	1	3
Romania	1	3
Lithuania	1	3
Belgium (French)	0	3
Poland	1	2
Israel	0	3
Greenland	2	1
Czech Republic	1	2
Slovenia	1	2
Slovakia	1	1
Latvia	0	2
Portugal	0	2
Ireland	0	2
Wales	1	1
Belgium (Flemish)	1	1
Italy	0	1
Luxembourg	0	1
Estonia	1	1
Russian Federation	1	1
Canada	1	1
England	0	1
Greece	0	1
Austria	0	1
France	0	1
Malta	0	1
Spain	1	0
Switzerland	0	1
Norway	0	1
Scotland	0	0
Sweden	0	0
Denmark	0	1
Netherlands	0	0
Germany	0	0
Iceland	0	0
HBSC average (gender)	1	2
HBSC average (total)		1

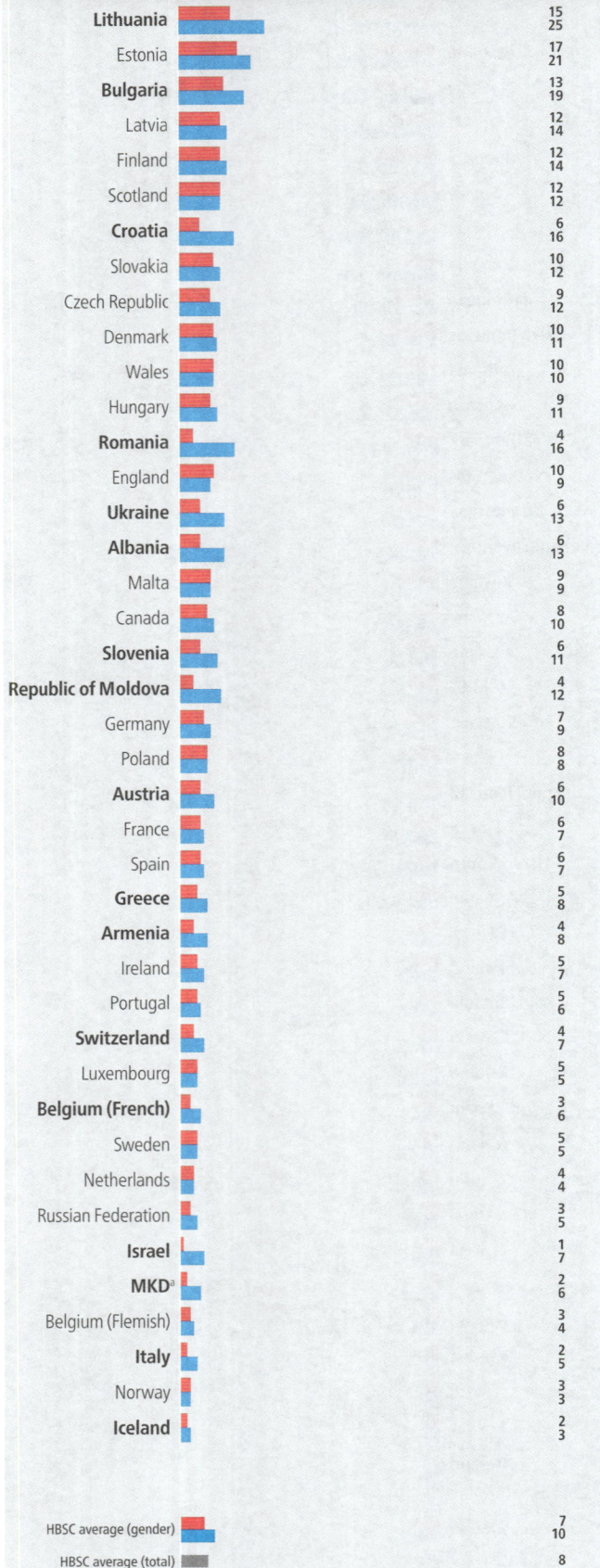

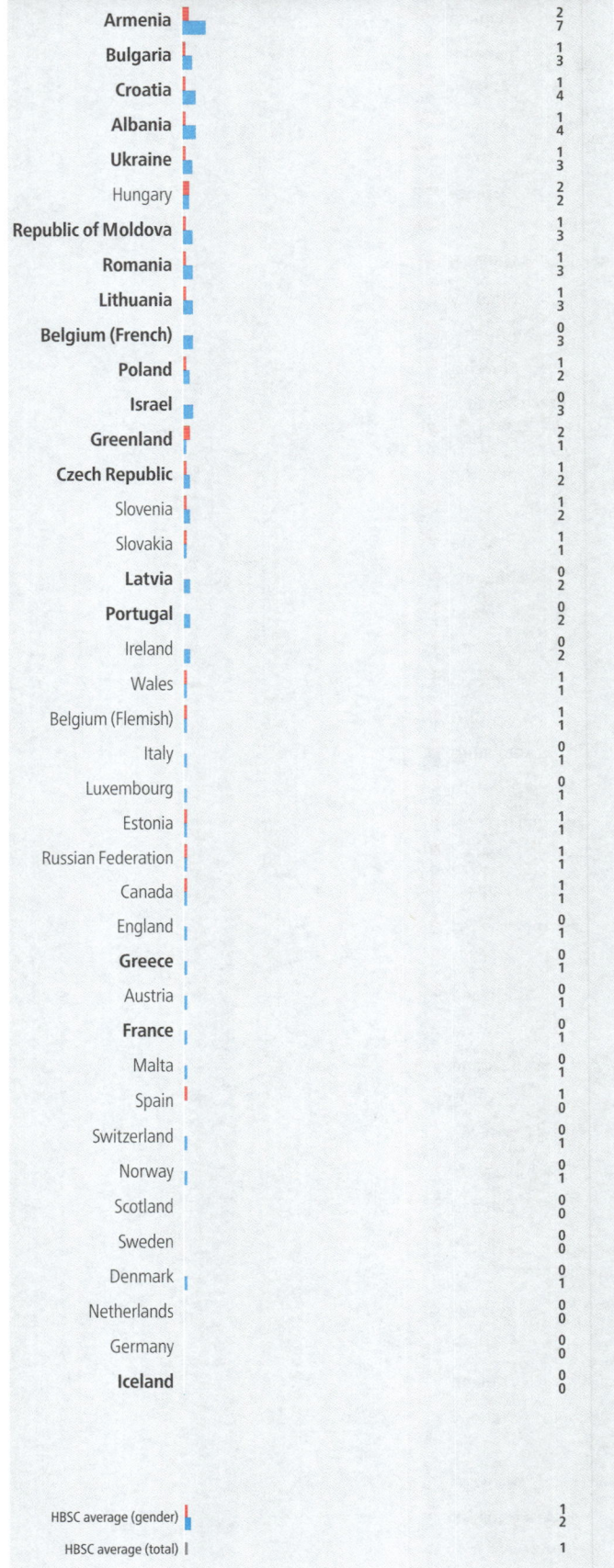

[a] The former Yugoslav Republic of Macedonia. No data were received from Greenland.

GROWING UP UNEQUAL: GENDER AND SOCIOECONOMIC
DIFFERENCES IN YOUNG PEOPLE'S HEALTH AND WELL-BEING
PART 2. KEY DATA | CHAPTER 5. RISK BEHAVIOURS
ALCOHOL USE

5

13-year-olds who have been drunk on two or more occasions

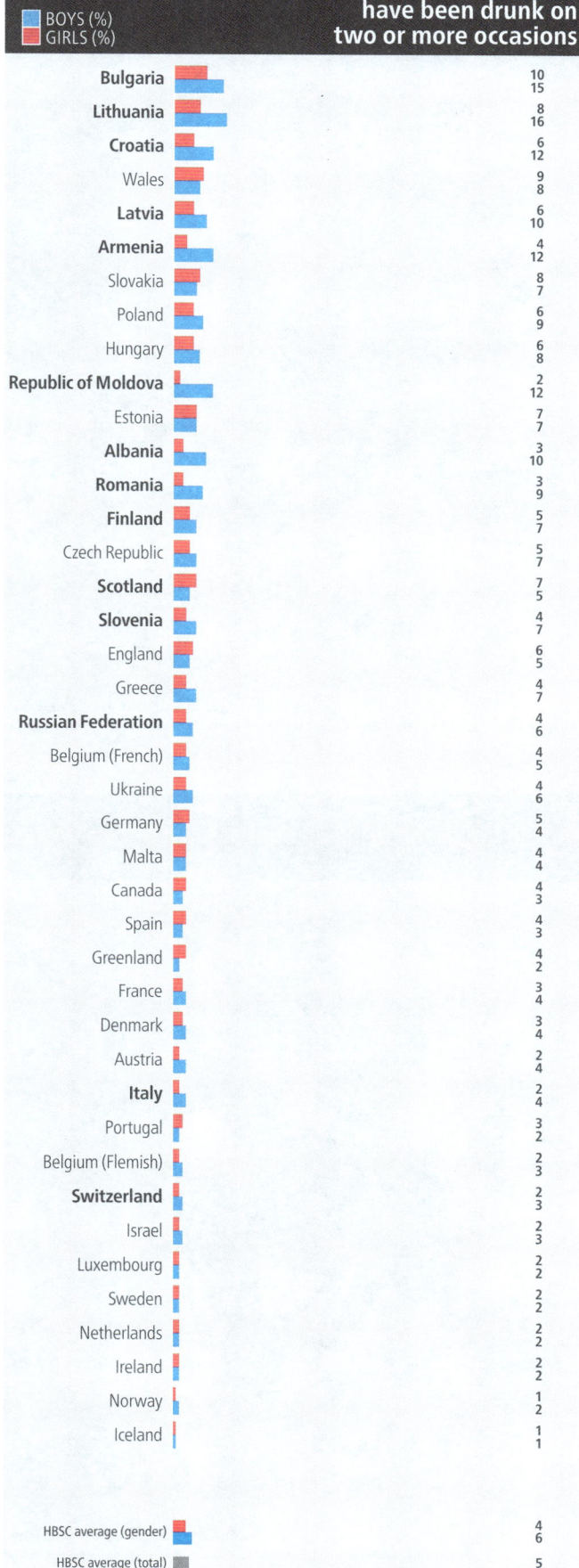

HBSC survey 2013/2014

BOYS (%) — blue
GIRLS (%) — red

Country	Girls (%)	Boys (%)
Bulgaria	10	15
Lithuania	8	16
Croatia	6	12
Wales	9	6
Latvia	6	10
Armenia	4	12
Slovakia	8	7
Poland	6	9
Hungary	6	8
Republic of Moldova	2	12
Estonia	7	7
Albania	3	10
Romania	3	9
Finland	5	7
Czech Republic	5	7
Scotland	7	5
Slovenia	4	7
England	6	5
Greece	4	7
Russian Federation	4	6
Belgium (French)	4	5
Ukraine	4	6
Germany	5	4
Malta	4	4
Canada	4	3
Spain	4	3
Greenland	4	2
France	3	4
Denmark	3	4
Austria	2	4
Italy	2	4
Portugal	3	2
Belgium (Flemish)	2	3
Switzerland	2	3
Israel	2	3
Luxembourg	2	2
Sweden	2	2
Netherlands	2	2
Ireland	2	2
Norway	1	2
Iceland	1	1
HBSC average (gender)	4	6
HBSC average (total)	5	

15-year-olds who have been drunk on two or more occasions

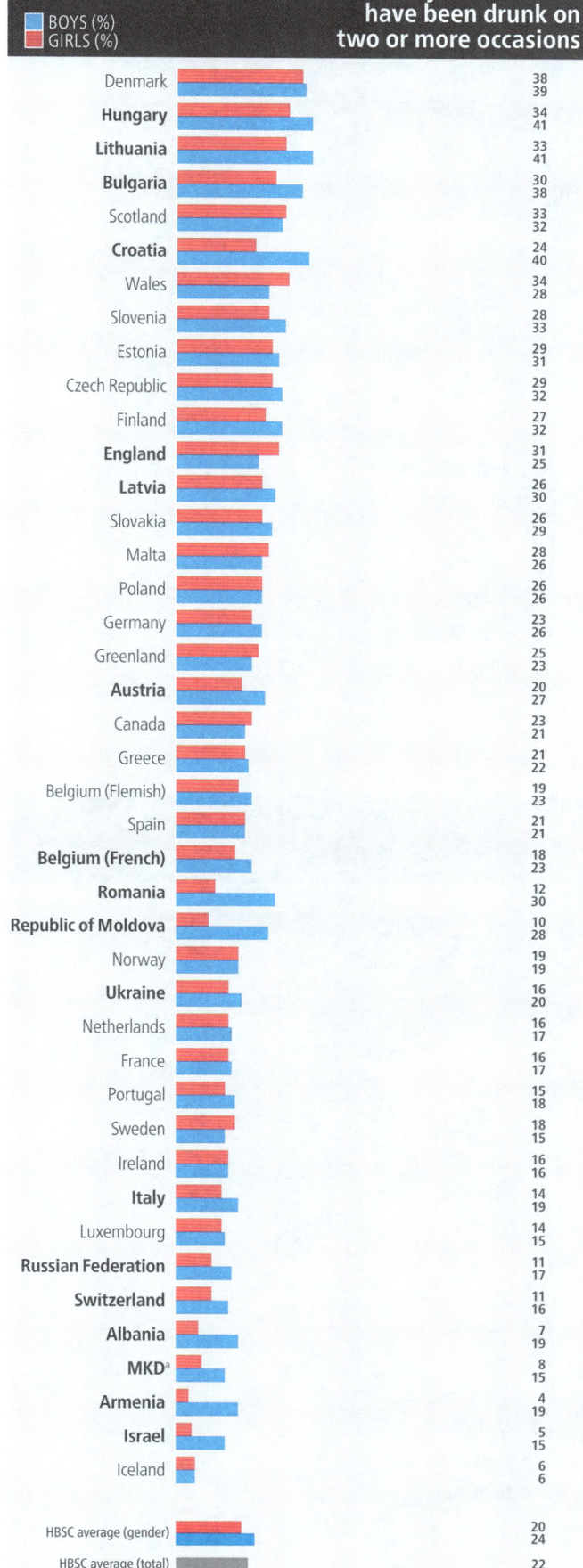

HBSC survey 2013/2014

BOYS (%) — blue
GIRLS (%) — red

Country	Girls (%)	Boys (%)
Denmark	38	39
Hungary	34	41
Lithuania	33	41
Bulgaria	30	38
Scotland	33	32
Croatia	24	40
Wales	34	28
Slovenia	28	33
Estonia	29	31
Czech Republic	29	32
Finland	27	32
England	31	25
Latvia	26	30
Slovakia	26	29
Malta	28	26
Poland	26	26
Germany	23	26
Greenland	25	23
Austria	20	27
Canada	23	21
Greece	21	22
Belgium (Flemish)	19	23
Spain	21	21
Belgium (French)	18	23
Romania	12	30
Republic of Moldova	10	28
Norway	19	19
Ukraine	16	20
Netherlands	16	17
France	16	17
Portugal	15	18
Sweden	18	15
Ireland	16	16
Italy	14	19
Luxembourg	14	15
Russian Federation	11	17
Switzerland	11	16
Albania	7	19
MKD[a]	8	15
Armenia	4	19
Israel	5	15
Iceland	6	6
HBSC average (gender)	20	24
HBSC average (total)	22	

Note: **indicates** significant gender difference (at p<0.05). 0 means less than +/-0.5%. No data were received from Finland (11-year-olds) and the former Yugoslav Republic of Macedonia (11- and 13-year-olds).

HBSC survey 2013/2014

15-year-old girls who drink alcohol at least once a week

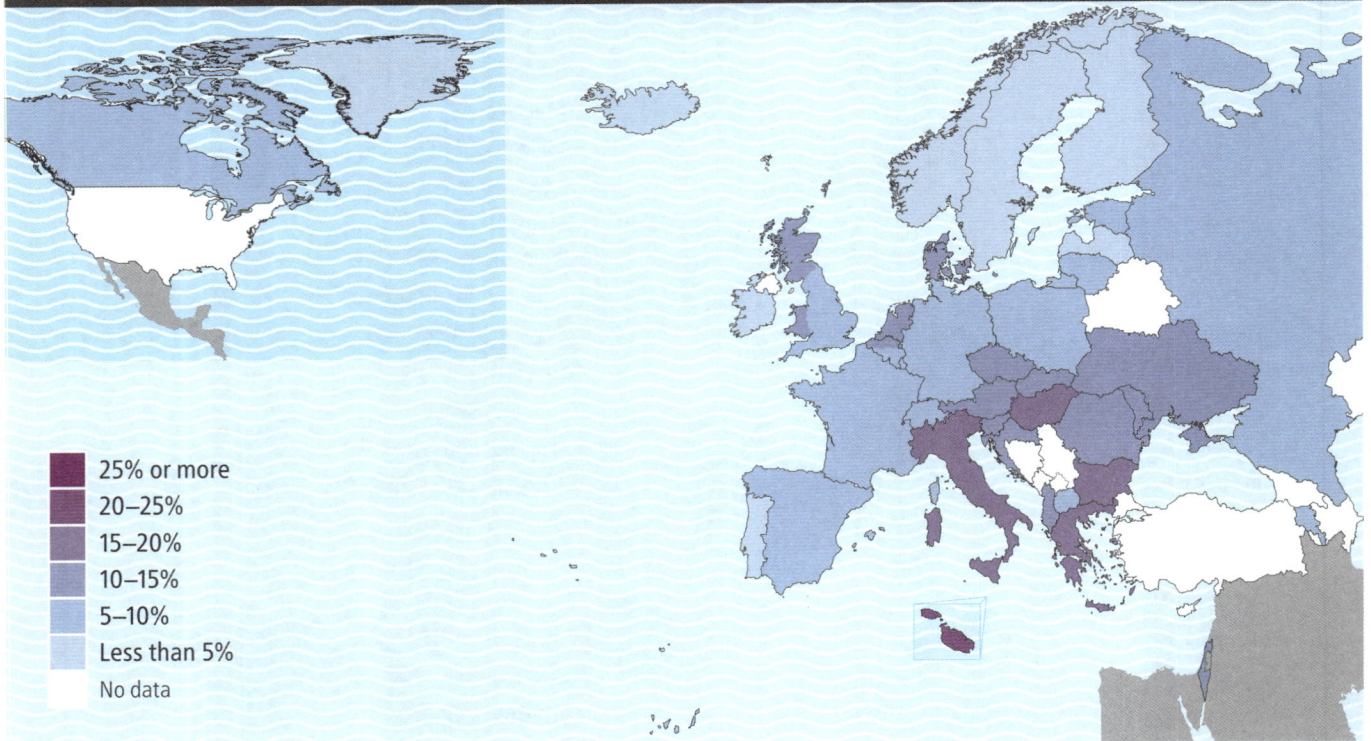

25% or more
20–25%
15–20%
10–15%
5–10%
Less than 5%
No data

Note: HBSC teams provided disaggregated data for Belgium and the United Kingdom; these data appear in the map above.

HBSC survey 2013/2014

15-year-old boys who drink alcohol at least once a week

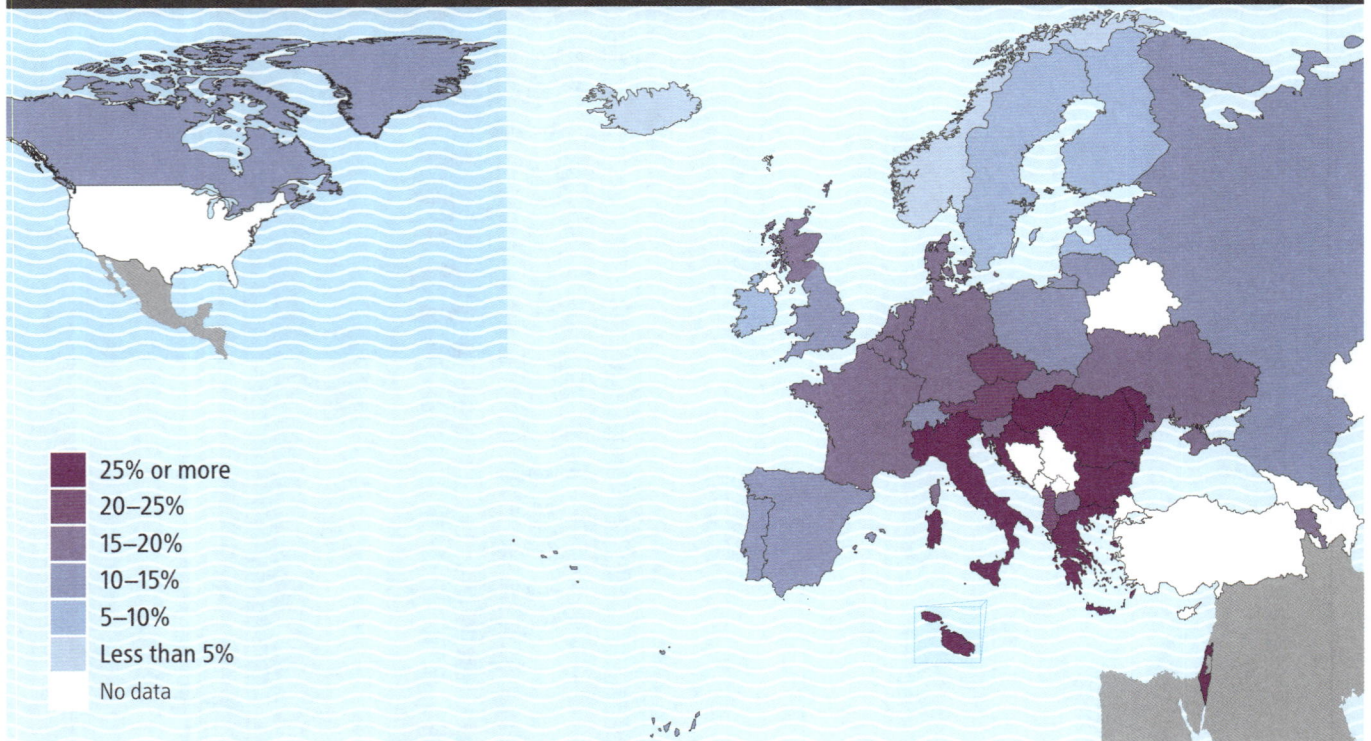

25% or more
20–25%
15–20%
10–15%
5–10%
Less than 5%
No data

Note: HBSC teams provided disaggregated data for Belgium and the United Kingdom; these data appear in the map above.

GROWING UP UNEQUAL: GENDER AND SOCIOECONOMIC
DIFFERENCES IN YOUNG PEOPLE'S HEALTH AND WELL-BEING
PART 2. KEY DATA | CHAPTER 5. RISK BEHAVIOURS
ALCOHOL USE

5

HBSC survey 2013/2014

15-year-old girls who report first drunkenness at age 13 or younger

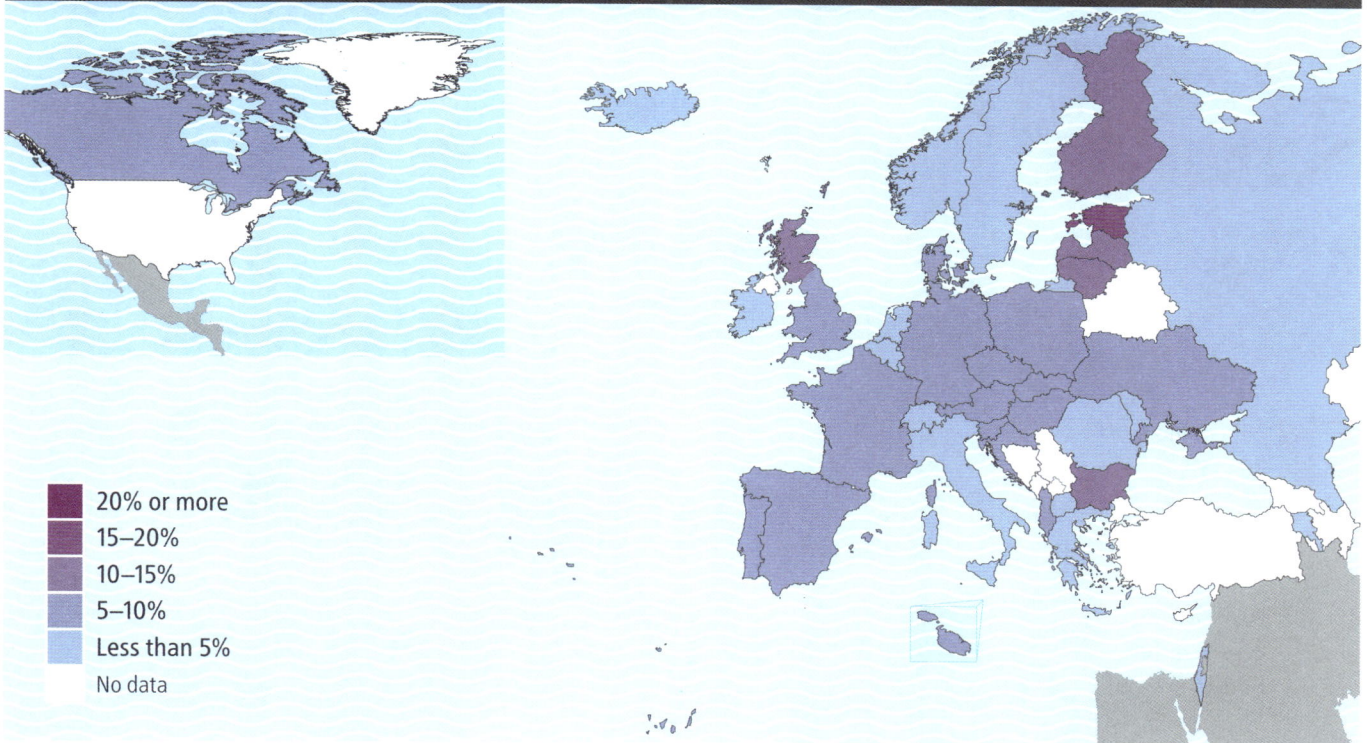

- 20% or more
- 15–20%
- 10–15%
- 5–10%
- Less than 5%
- No data

Note: HBSC teams provided disaggregated data for Belgium and the United Kingdom; these data appear in the map above.

HBSC survey 2013/2014

15-year-old boys who report first drunkenness at age 13 or younger

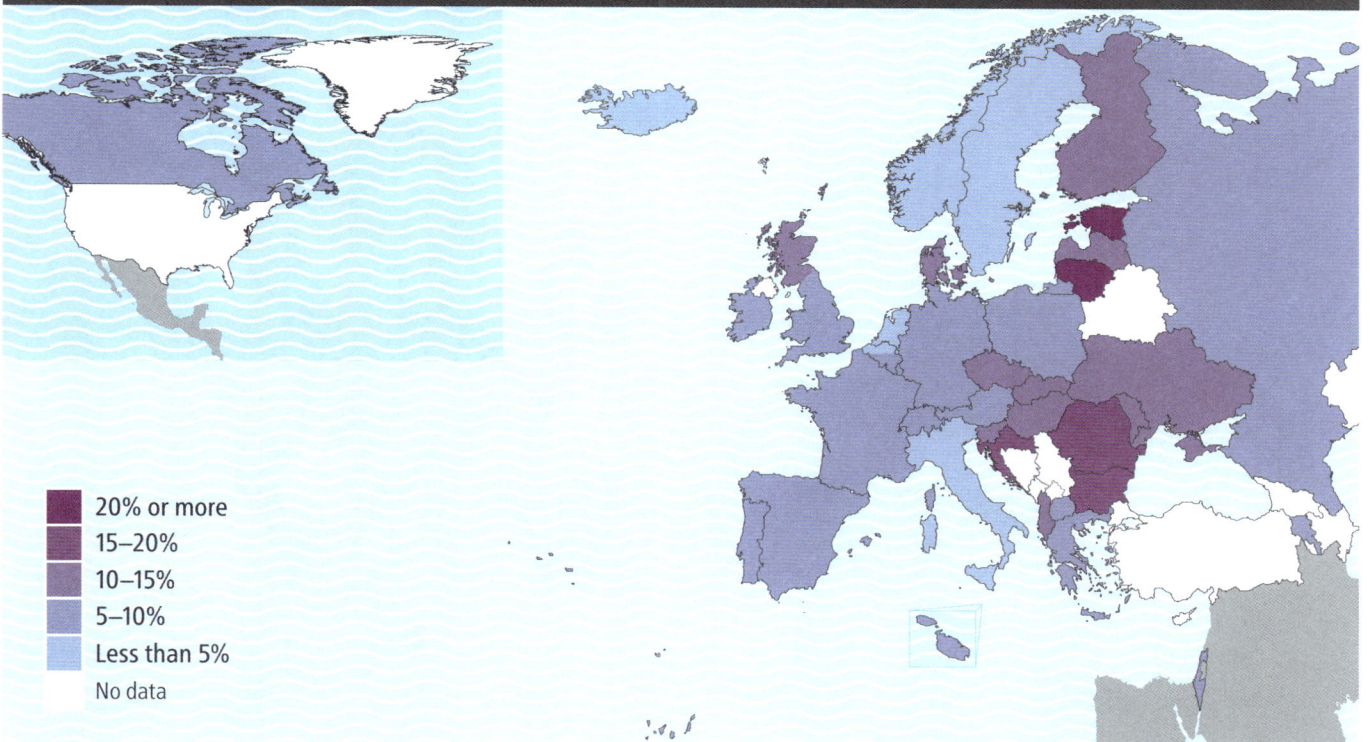

- 20% or more
- 15–20%
- 10–15%
- 5–10%
- Less than 5%
- No data

Note: HBSC teams provided disaggregated data for Belgium and the United Kingdom; these data appear in the map above.

HBSC survey 2013/2014

15-year-old girls who have been drunk on two or more occasions

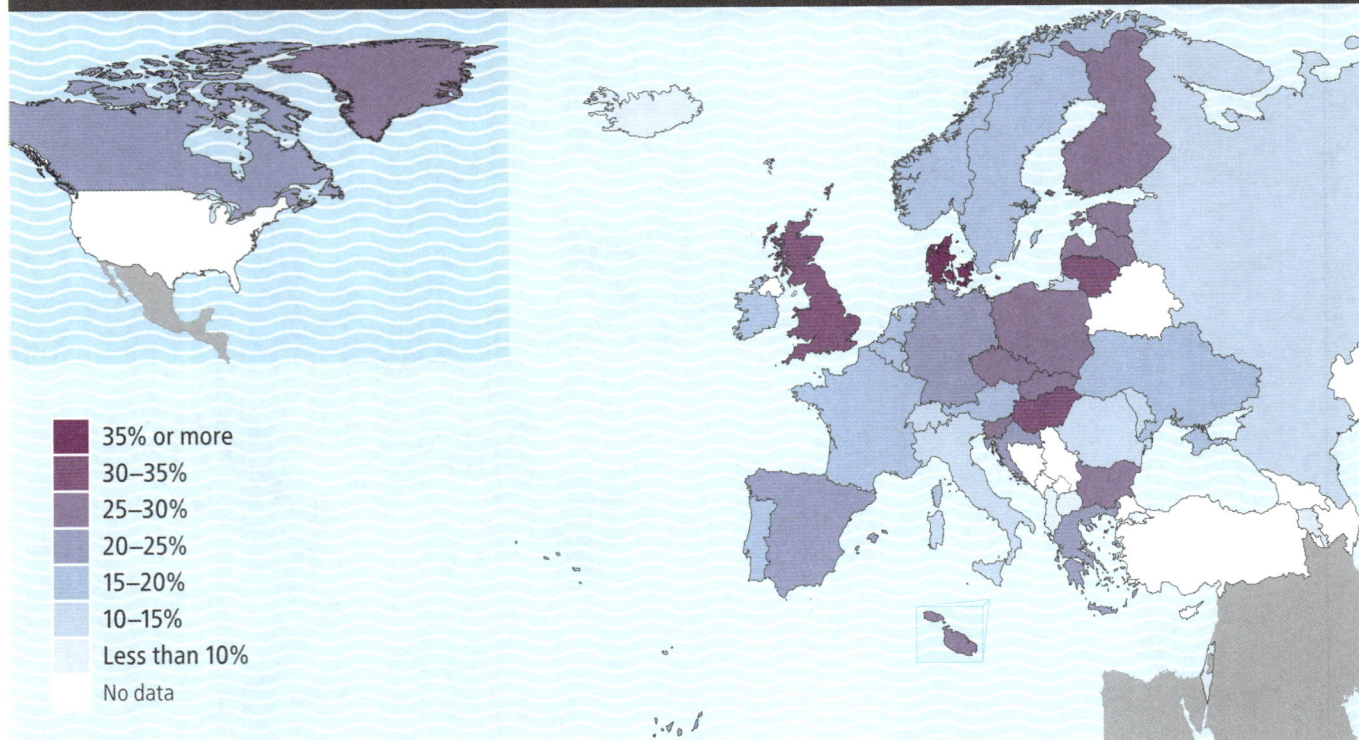

- 35% or more
- 30–35%
- 25–30%
- 20–25%
- 15–20%
- 10–15%
- Less than 10%
- No data

Note: HBSC teams provided disaggregated data for Belgium and the United Kingdom; these data appear in the map above.

HBSC survey 2013/2014

15-year-old boys who have been drunk on two or more occasions

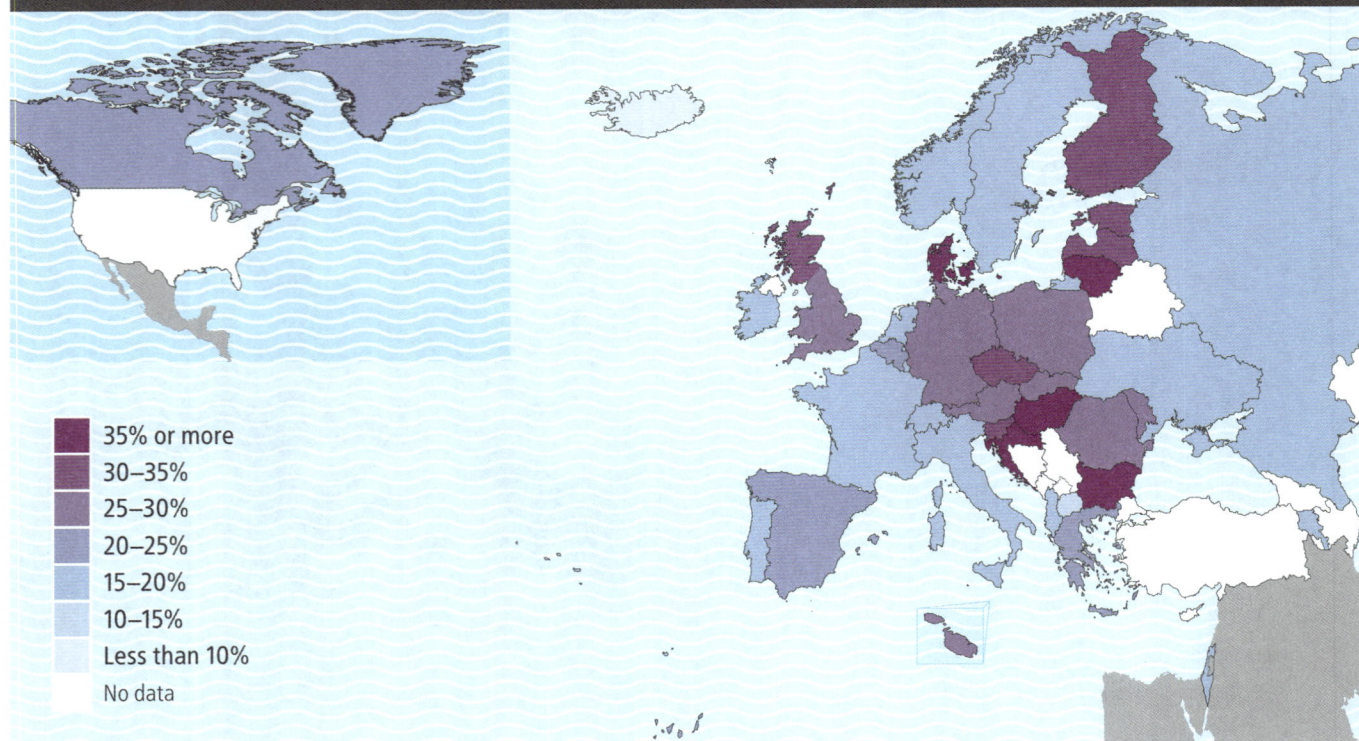

- 35% or more
- 30–35%
- 25–30%
- 20–25%
- 15–20%
- 10–15%
- Less than 10%
- No data

Note: HBSC teams provided disaggregated data for Belgium and the United Kingdom; these data appear in the map above.

GROWING UP UNEQUAL: GENDER AND SOCIOECONOMIC
DIFFERENCES IN YOUNG PEOPLE'S HEALTH AND WELL-BEING
PART 2. KEY DATA | CHAPTER 5. RISK BEHAVIOURS
ALCOHOL USE

5

ALCOHOL USE:
SCIENTIFIC DISCUSSION AND POLICY REFLECTIONS

SCIENTIFIC DISCUSSION

Adolescent alcohol use has decreased in most European and North American countries and regions since the beginning of the 21st century (6). The findings indicate that the decrease is ongoing in all age groups and among boys as well as girls.

The findings confirm previous HBSC data showing that prevalence rates of weekly alcohol use and (early) drunkenness increase substantially with age (especially between 13 and 15) for boys and girls in all countries and regions. It still tends to be more common among boys, but gender differences appear to be decreasing, particularly in relation to weekly drinking and drunkenness on more than one occasion. This finding is consistent with a pattern of gender convergence that has been observed since the beginning of the century (7,8): evidence has even emerged of girls in some northern European countries and regions reporting more alcohol use than boys.

Overall, family affluence is not found to have a large effect on adolescent use, a finding that is consistent with the literature (9). Parenting behaviours, such as providing support and monitoring adolescents' behaviour, and social position among peers may be more important than family SES in predicting adolescent alcohol use (10).

POLICY REFLECTIONS

A range of factors, including changes in disposable income, marketing, prevention approaches, changes in adult drinking behaviours and shifts in teen culture, may have influenced the general decrease in adolescent weekly drinking (6,8,11). Policies are in place in many countries and regions to limit underage access and restrict use among those of all ages (11,12), and stricter prevention policies are emerging (13). Changes in social norms, such as stronger societal disapproval of adolescent drinking, may also have contributed to the observed trends (6). More stringent policies and changing social norms may be related to greater insight into the potentially harmful effects of alcohol on adolescent brain development. Evidence suggests the need for more effort to address the increase in alcohol consumption between ages 13 and 15 that is evident across all countries and regions.

Evidence to support particular policies that contribute to reductions in adolescent use is growing. At country level, the absence of a minimum purchasing age and weak restrictions on alcohol availability and advertising are associated with adolescent use (11). Research on the effectiveness of school-based interventions is mixed (14), but programmes that target not only adolescents, but also their parents, can have considerable effects (15). Some generic psychosocial and developmental prevention programmes on life skills and healthy lifestyle may also be effective and can be considered as policy and practice options (16). Family interventions are effective in delaying alcohol initiation and reducing frequency of consumption among adolescents (16). Family treatments focused on change in maladaptive behaviours, multidimensional family therapy and group-administered cognitive behavioural therapies have received considerable empirical support (17).

REFERENCES

1. Anderson P, Baumberg B. Alcohol in Europe. A public health perspective. Brussels: European Commission; 2006 (http://ec.europa.eu/health/archive/ph_determinants/life_style/alcohol/documents/alcohol_europe_en.pdf, accessed 24 August 2015).

2. Johnston LD, O'Malley PM, Miech RA, Bachman JG, Schulenberg JE. Monitoring the future. National survey results on drug use, 1975–2014: overview, key findings on adolescent drug use. Ann Arbor (MI): Institute for Social Research, The University of Michigan; 2015 (http://www.monitoringthefuture.org/pubs/monographs/mtf-overview2014.pdf, accessed 24 August 2015).

3. Engels RCME, ter Bogt T. Influences of risk behaviours on the quality of peer relations in adolescence. J Youth Adolesc. 2001;30(6):675–95.

4. Boden JM, Fergusson DM. The short and long term consequences of adolescent alcohol use. In: Saunders J, Rey JM, editors. Young people and alcohol: impact, policy, prevention and treatment. Chichester: Wiley-Blackwell; 2011:32–46.

5. Feldstein Ewing SW, Sakhardande A, Blakemore S. The effect of alcohol consumption on the adolescent brain: a systematic review of MRI and fMRI studies of alcohol-using youth. Neuroimage Clin. 2014;5:420–37.

6. De Looze M, Raaijmakers Q, ter Bogt T, Bendtsen P, Farhat T, Ferreira M et al. Decreases in adolescent weekly alcohol use in Europe and North America: evidence from 28 countries from 2002 to 2010. Eur J Pub Health 2015;25:S69–72.

7. Kuntsche E, Kuntsche S, Knibbe R, Simons-Morton B, Farhat T, Hublet A et al. Cultural and gender convergence in adolescent drunkenness. Arch Pediatr Adolesc Med. 2011;165:152–8.

8. Simons-Morton B, Farhat T, ter Bogt T, Hublet A, Kuntsche E, NicGabhainn S. Gender specific trends in alcohol use: cross-cultural comparisons from 1998 to 2006 in 24 countries and regions. Int J Pub Health 2009;52:S199–208.

9. Hanson MD, Chen E. Socioeconomic status and health behaviors in adolescence: a review of the literature. J Behav Med. 2007;30:263–85.

10. Viner RM, Ozer EM, Denny S, Marmot M, Resnick M, Fatusi A et al. Adolescence and the social determinants of health. Lancet 2012;379(9826):1641–52.

11. Bendtsen P, Damsgaard MT, Huckle T, Casswell S, Kuntsche E, Arnold P et al. Adolescent alcohol use: a reflection of national drinking patterns and policy? Addiction 2014;109:1857–68.

12. Brand DA, Saisana M, Rynn LA, Lowenfelds AB. Comparative analysis of alcohol control policies in 30 countries. PLoS Med. 2007;4:e151.

13. Anderson P, Møller L, Galea G, editors. Alcohol in the European Union. Consumption, harm, and policy approaches. Copenhagen: WHO Regional Office for Europe; 2012 (http://www.euro.who.int/__data/assets/pdf_file/0003/160680/e96457.pdf, accessed 24 August 2015).

14. Carney T, Myers BJ, Louw J, Okwundu CI. Brief school-based interventions and behavioural outcomes for substance-using adolescents. Cochrane Database Syst Rev. 2014;2:CD008969.

15. Koning IM, Vollebergh WAM, Smit F, Verdurmen JE, Van den Eijnden, ter Bogt T et al. Preventing heavy alcohol use in adolescents (PAS): cluster randomized trial of a parent and student intervention offered separately and simultaneously. Addiction 2009;104(10):1669–78.

16. Foxcroft DR, Tsersvadze A. Universal school-based prevention programs for alcohol misuse in young people. Cochrane Database Syst Rev. 2011;5(5):CD009113.

17. Smit E, Verdurmen J, Monshouwer K, Smit F. Family interventions and their effect on adolescent alcohol use in general populations: a meta-analysis of randomized controlled trials. Drug Alcohol Depend. 2008;97(3):195–206.

GROWING UP UNEQUAL: GENDER AND SOCIOECONOMIC
DIFFERENCES IN YOUNG PEOPLE'S HEALTH AND WELL-BEING
PART 2. KEY DATA | CHAPTER 5. RISK BEHAVIOURS

5

CANNABIS USE

Cannabis is the most frequently used drug in Europe, with 14.6 million young adults using it in 2014 *(1)*. It was also the most commonly reported substance related to new admissions to drug treatment facilities across Europe in 2014 (37% cannabis, 28% heroin and 21% cocaine) *(1)*.

Cannabis, regarded as a so-called gateway drug *(2)*, is the illicit substance used most frequently by schoolchildren across Europe and North America, with a 12-month prevalence ranging from about 27% in Canada to around 3% in the former Yugoslav Republic of Macedonia. The HBSC median is in the region of 10% *(3–5)*. Adolescents use the drug for a variety of reasons, including experimentation, mood enhancement, social enhancement and peer conformity *(6)*.

Scientific evidence proves that cannabis is a dangerous and harmful substance, especially for children and young people who use it regularly *(7)*. Cannabis use is a risk factor for mental disorders and may trigger psychosis (particularly among those who are prone) *(8)*. Early onset and heavy and accelerating use are related to problems such as impairment in brain development, low height and weight, anxiety attacks, short-term memory loss and other cognitive disorders *(9)*, deteriorating school performance and dropout *(10)*, risk-taking, aggression and delinquency *(11)*, depression and anxiety *(11)*, and the development of the so-called lack-of-motivation syndrome *(12)*.

Young people in their teenage years are more likely to use cannabis if they have friends or older siblings who do so *(13–15)* and if they experience either low parental involvement and reinforcement or high levels of coercive discipline *(16)*.

Many countries have introduced new regulatory approaches and policies to enable the prescription of cannabis for medical purposes and public debate on legalization for recreational (non-medical) use is growing. Five states of the United States and two countries (the Netherlands and Uruguay) have implemented policies that legalize cannabis for recreational use for people over the age of 21 *(17)*. Population surveys show that the perception of cannabis-associated risk has declined significantly as a result of the ongoing debate, with some countries seeing an increase in use among adolescents and young adults *(18)*.

MEASURES

Lifetime use
Young people (15-year-olds only) were asked how often they had used cannabis in their lifetime.

Use in last 30 days
Young people (15-year-olds only) were asked how often they had used cannabis in the last 30 days.

Cannabis initiation
Young people (15-year-olds only) were asked how old they were when they used cannabis for the first time.

HBSC survey 2013/2014

BOYS GIRLS SIGNIFICANT TRENDS

Associations between family affluence and indicators of health, by country/region and gender: **lifetime cannabis use**

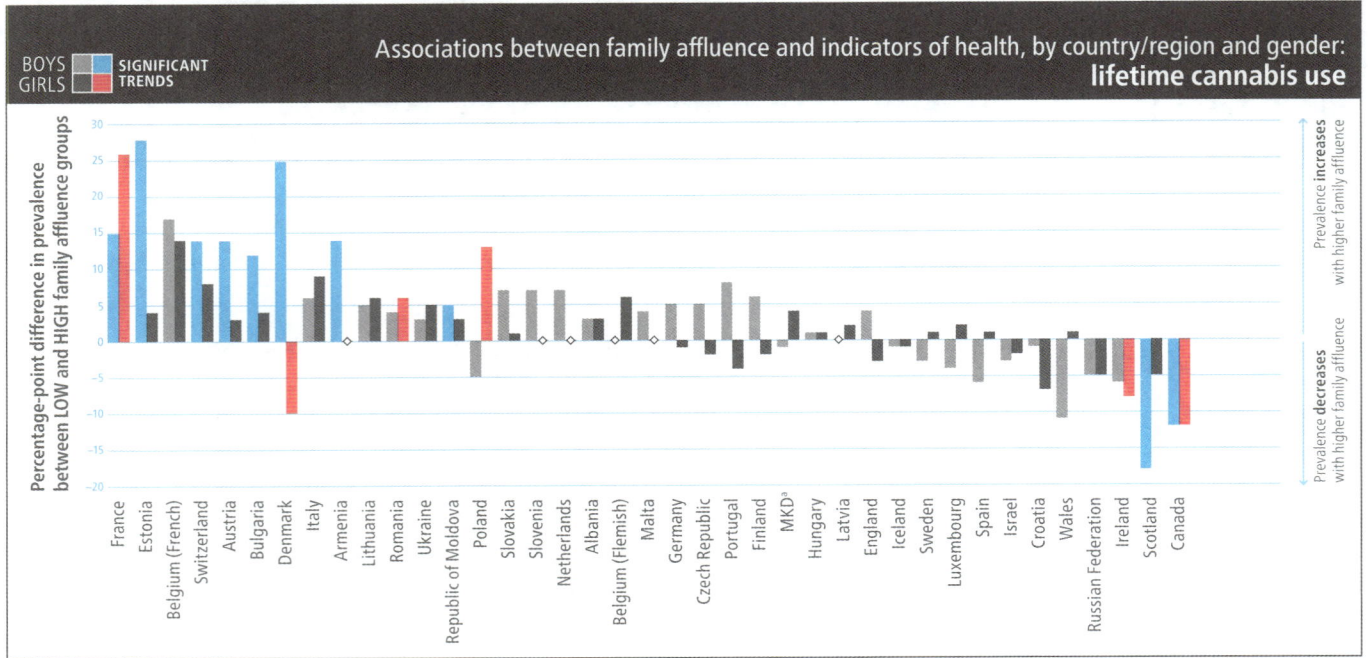

a The former Yugoslav Republic of Macedonia. *Note:* low- and high-affluence groups represent the lowest 20% and highest 20% in each country. ◇ means less than +/-0.5%. No data were received from Greece, Greenland and Norway.

BOYS GIRLS SIGNIFICANT TRENDS

Associations between family affluence and indicators of health, by country/region and gender: **cannabis use in the last 30 days**

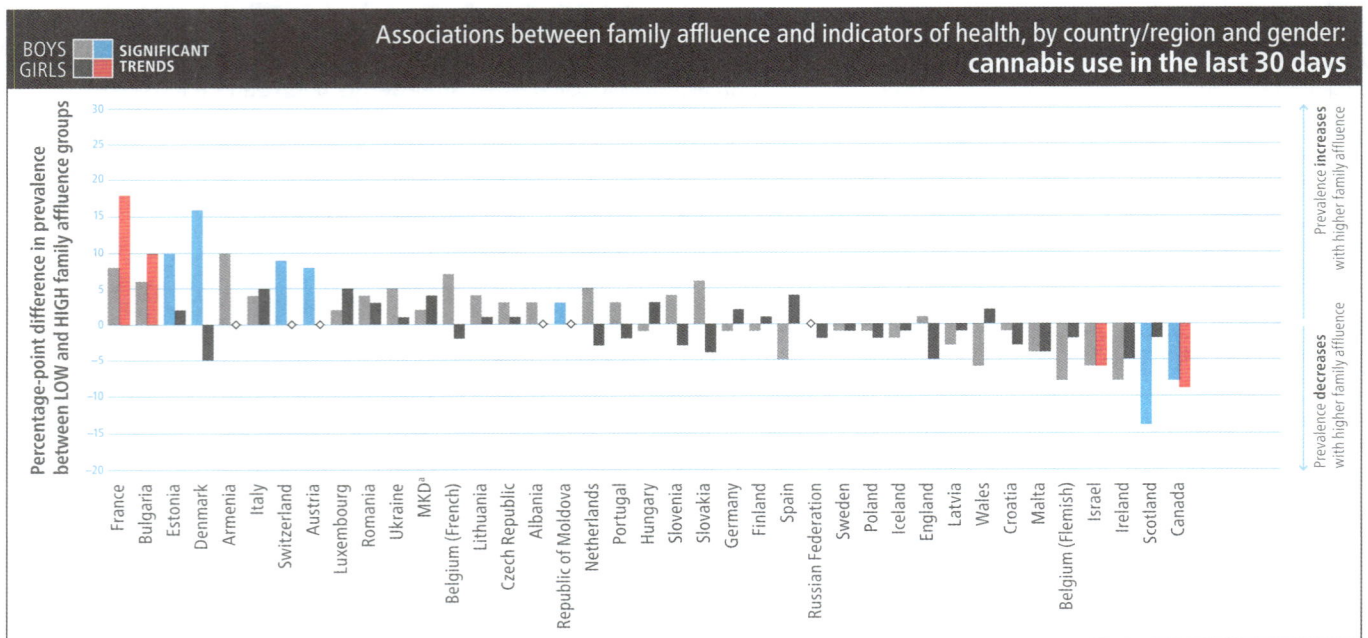

a The former Yugoslav Republic of Macedonia. *Note:* low- and high-affluence groups represent the lowest 20% and highest 20% in each country. ◇ means less than +/-0.5%. No data were received from Greece, Greenland and Norway.

GROWING UP UNEQUAL: GENDER AND SOCIOECONOMIC
DIFFERENCES IN YOUNG PEOPLE'S HEALTH AND WELL-BEING
PART 2. KEY DATA | CHAPTER 5. RISK BEHAVIOURS
CANNABIS USE

5

HBSC survey 2013/2014

BOYS GIRLS | **SIGNIFICANT TRENDS**

Associations between family affluence and indicators of health, by country/region and gender:
first cannabis use at age 13 or younger

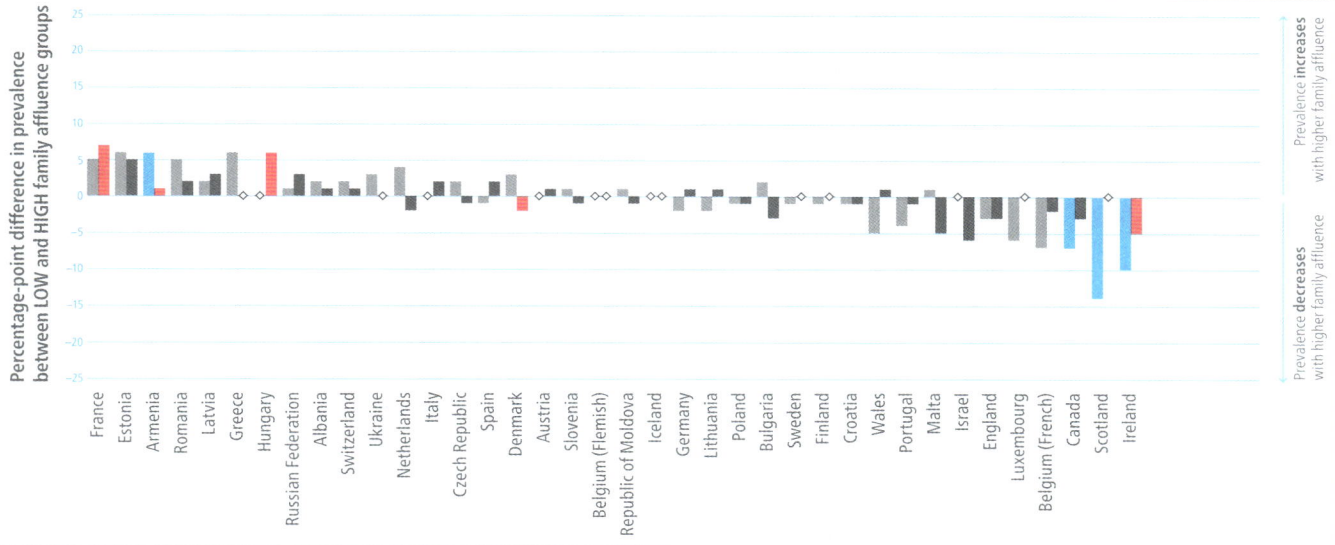

Note: low- and high-affluence groups represent the lowest 20% and highest 20% in each country. ◇ means less than +/-0.5%.
No data were received from Greenland, Norway, Slovakia and the former Yugoslav Republic of Macedonia.

RESULTS

Lifetime use

Findings presented here show the proportion of young people who had used cannabis at least once (lifetime use).

Age Data are presented for 15-year-olds only.

Gender Boys used cannabis more commonly in around half of countries and regions. A difference of 10 percentage points was seen in three (Estonia, Italy and Switzerland).

Family affluence No clear pattern was seen for boys and girls. Only a few countries and regions showed a significant relationship, but this was not uniform: higher prevalence was linked to high affluence in some and low affluence in others. Lifetime use was associated with high affluence in eight countries and regions for boys and three for girls. Prevalence was higher with low family affluence in four: Canada (boys and girls), Denmark (girls only), Ireland (girls only) and Scotland (boys only).

Use in last 30 days

Findings presented here show the proportion of young people using cannabis at least once during the last 30 days (recent use).

Age Data are presented for 15-year-olds only.

Gender Recent use was higher among boys in half of countries and regions. The largest difference between girls and boys was 6 percentage points.

Family affluence No clear association was found between recent cannabis use and family affluence in most countries and regions.

Cannabis initiation

Findings presented here show the proportion of young people who used cannabis for the first time when they were 13 years or younger (early age of initiation).

Age Data are presented for 15-year-olds only.

Gender The percentage of early initiators ranged from 1% to 8% in boys and 0% to 7% in girls. Prevalence was higher among boys in 17 countries and regions, although gender differences were small.

Family affluence No clear association with family affluence was found in most countries and regions. In those that had a significant association, the direction varied. The largest differences between high- and low-affluence groups were among boys in Ireland and Scotland, where early initiation was associated with lower affluence.

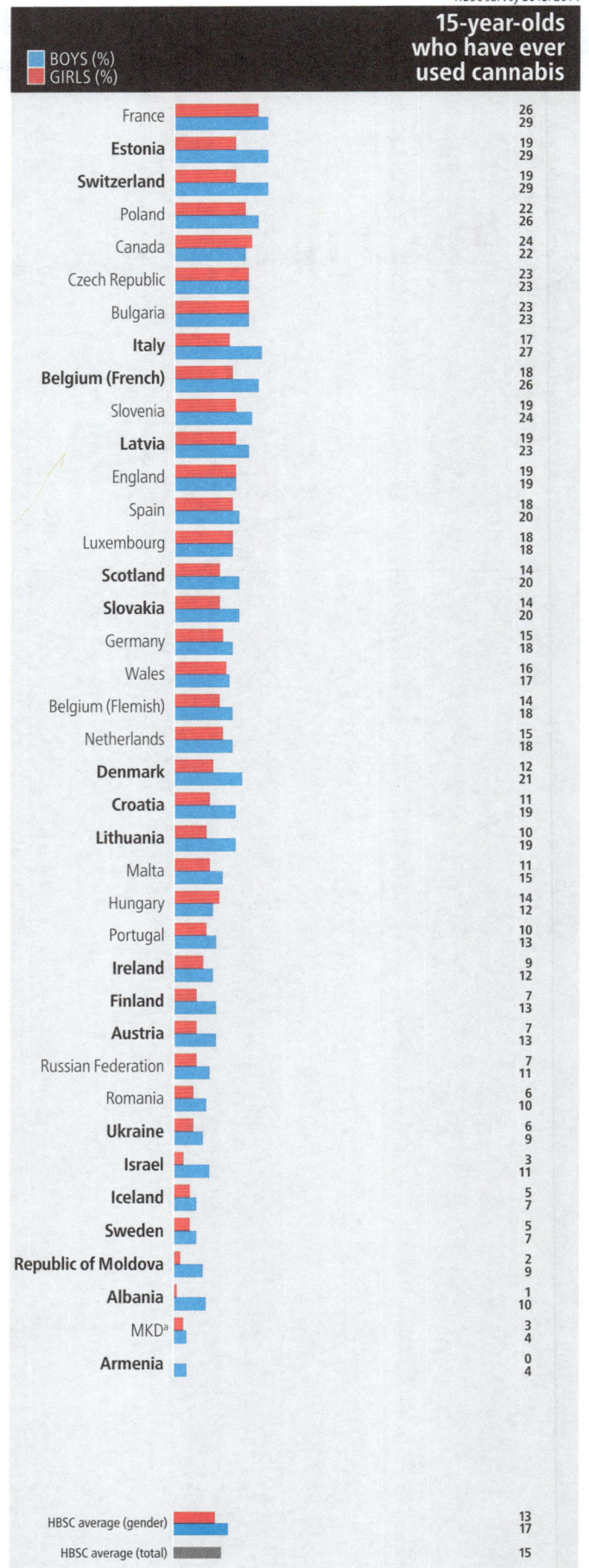

HBSC survey 2013/2014

15-year-olds who have ever used cannabis

	BOYS (%)	GIRLS (%)
France	26	29
Estonia	19	29
Switzerland	19	29
Poland	22	26
Canada	24	22
Czech Republic	23	23
Bulgaria	23	23
Italy	17	27
Belgium (French)	18	26
Slovenia	19	24
Latvia	19	23
England	19	19
Spain	18	20
Luxembourg	18	18
Scotland	14	20
Slovakia	14	20
Germany	15	18
Wales	16	17
Belgium (Flemish)	14	18
Netherlands	15	18
Denmark	12	21
Croatia	11	19
Lithuania	10	19
Malta	11	15
Hungary	14	12
Portugal	10	13
Ireland	9	12
Finland	7	13
Austria	7	13
Russian Federation	7	11
Romania	6	10
Ukraine	6	9
Israel	3	11
Iceland	5	7
Sweden	5	7
Republic of Moldova	2	9
Albania	1	10
MKD[a]	3	4
Armenia	0	4
HBSC average (gender)	13	17
HBSC average (total)		15

[a] The former Yugoslav Republic of Macedonia. *Note*: 0 means less than +/-0.5%. No data were received from Greece, Greenland and Norway. The question was asked only of a subset of 15-year-olds in Belgium (French).

GROWING UP UNEQUAL: GENDER AND SOCIOECONOMIC
DIFFERENCES IN YOUNG PEOPLE'S HEALTH AND WELL-BEING
PART 2. KEY DATA | CHAPTER 5. RISK BEHAVIOURS
CANNABIS USE

5

15-year-olds who have used cannabis in the last 30 days

HBSC survey 2013/2014

BOYS (%)
GIRLS (%)

Country	Boys	Girls
France	14	16
Canada	13	13
Italy	9	15
Switzerland	9	15
Bulgaria	10	12
Belgium (French)	9	13
Poland	8	13
Slovenia	9	12
Spain	9	11
Scotland	7	13
Luxembourg	7	11
Netherlands	8	9
England	8	9
Croatia	6	11
Belgium (Flemish)	7	9
Germany	7	9
Estonia	5	10
Malta	6	9
Czech Republic	7	8
Denmark	5	10
Wales	8	7
Ireland	6	8
Slovakia	5	8
Latvia	5	9
Lithuania	3	9
Israel	3	9
Portugal	4	7
Hungary	4	5
Russian Federation	3	4
Finland	2	5
Austria	2	5
Romania	2	4
Iceland	2	3
Ukraine	1	4
Albania	0	4
MKD[a]	1	3
Sweden	2	2
Armenia	0	3
Republic of Moldova	0	2
HBSC average (gender)	6	9
HBSC average (total)		7

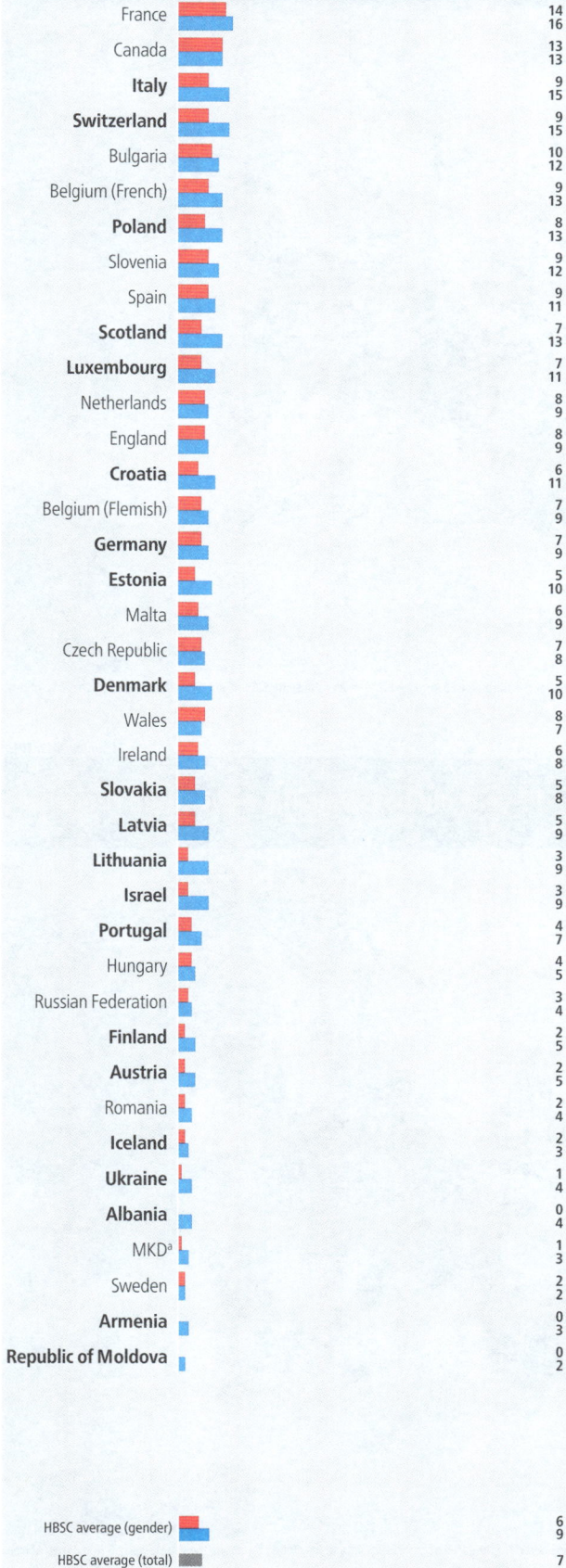

Note: 0 means less than +/-0.5%. No data were received from Greece, Greenland and Norway. The question was asked only of a subset of 15-year-olds in Belgium (French).

15-year-olds who report first cannabis use at age 13 or younger

HBSC survey 2013/2014

BOYS (%)
GIRLS (%)

Country	Boys	Girls
Canada	7	8
Czech Republic	6	7
Luxembourg	4	7
Bulgaria	4	7
Estonia	4	7
Scotland	3	7
France	4	6
Latvia	4	5
Poland	4	5
Switzerland	2	7
Belgium (French)	3	5
Croatia	2	6
England	3	5
Russian Federation	4	3
Netherlands	3	4
Germany	3	4
Wales	2	4
Ireland	3	3
Malta	3	3
Spain	2	3
Portugal	2	4
Slovenia	2	3
Lithuania	1	4
Denmark	1	3
Romania	1	4
Italy	1	3
Hungary	3	1
Belgium (Flemish)	0	3
Israel	1	3
Armenia	1	3
Sweden	1	2
Iceland	1	3
Finland	1	3
Ukraine	1	3
Albania	0	3
Austria	0	3
Republic of Moldova	0	1
Greece	0	2
HBSC average (gender)	3	4
HBSC average (total)		3

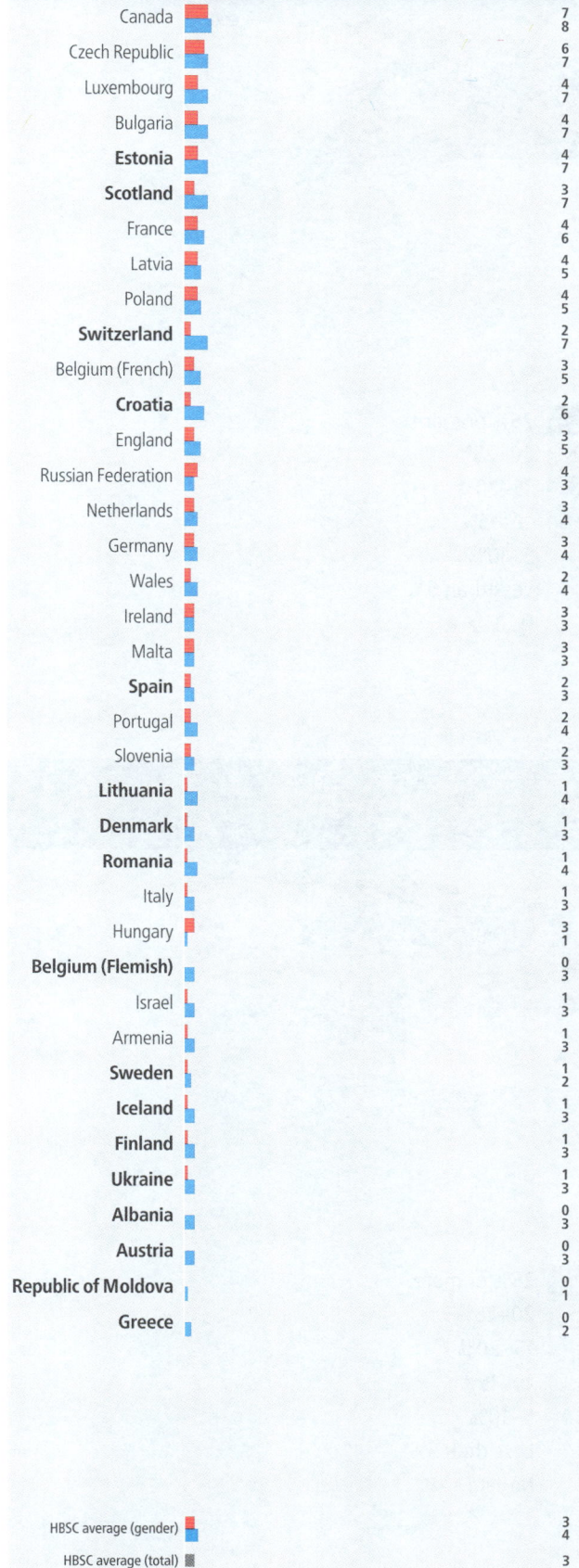

Note: **indicates** significant gender difference (at p<0.05). 0 means less than +/-0.5%. No data were received from Greenland, Norway, Slovakia and the former Yugoslav Republic of Macedonia. The question was asked only of a subset of 15-year-olds in Belgium (French).

HBSC survey 2013/2014

15-year-old girls who have ever used cannabis

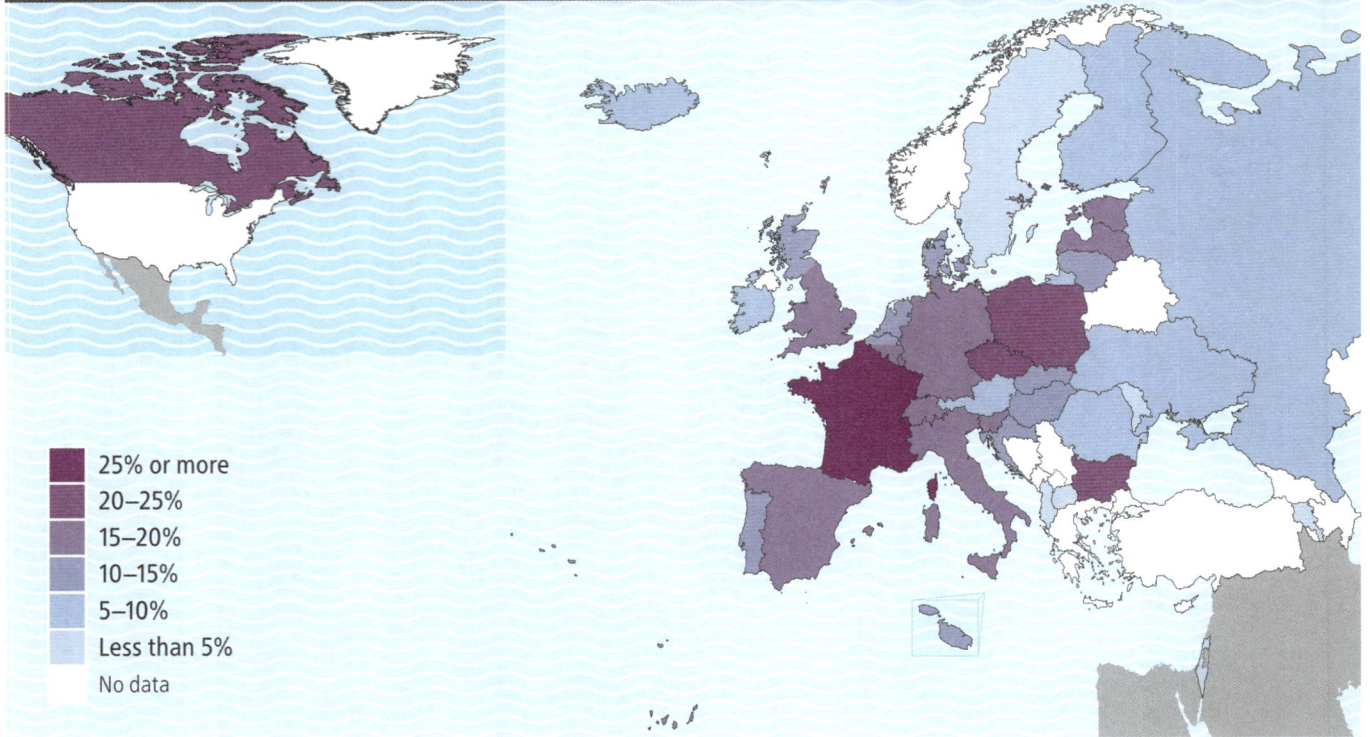

25% or more
20–25%
15–20%
10–15%
5–10%
Less than 5%
No data

Note: HBSC teams provided disaggregated data for Belgium and the United Kingdom; these data appear in the map above.

HBSC survey 2013/2014

15-year-old boys who have ever used cannabis

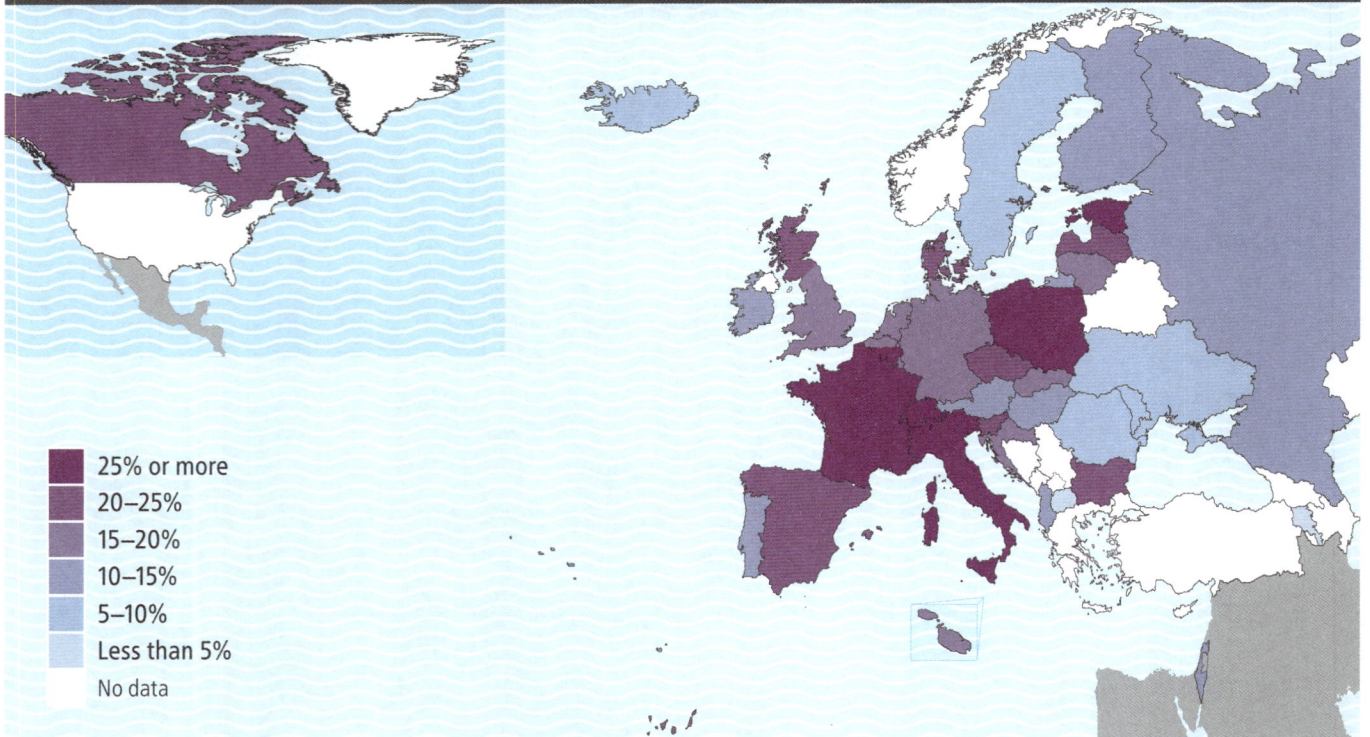

25% or more
20–25%
15–20%
10–15%
5–10%
Less than 5%
No data

Note: HBSC teams provided disaggregated data for Belgium and the United Kingdom; these data appear in the map above.

GROWING UP UNEQUAL: GENDER AND SOCIOECONOMIC
DIFFERENCES IN YOUNG PEOPLE'S HEALTH AND WELL-BEING
PART 2. KEY DATA | CHAPTER 5. RISK BEHAVIOURS
CANNABIS USE

5

HBSC survey 2013/2014

15-year-old girls who have used cannabis in the last 30 days

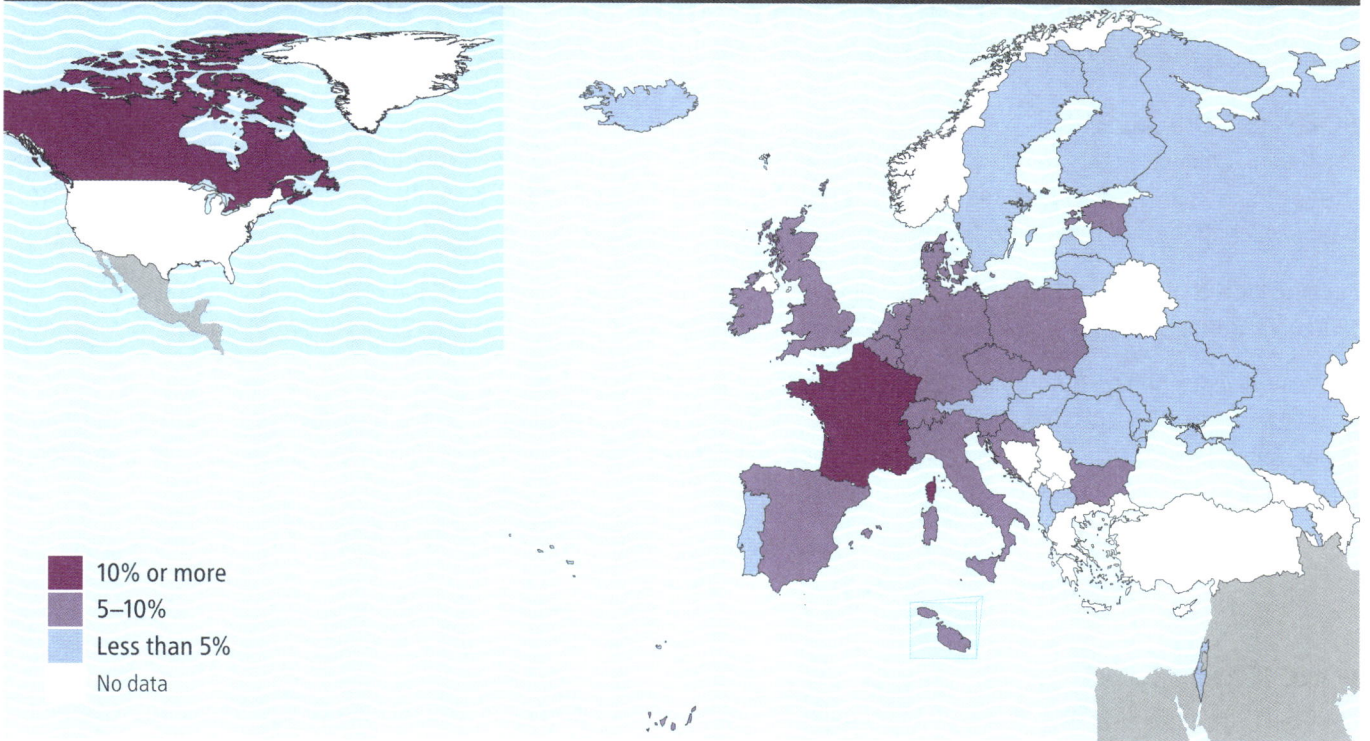

- 10% or more
- 5–10%
- Less than 5%
- No data

Note: HBSC teams provided disaggregated data for Belgium and the United Kingdom; these data appear in the map above.

HBSC survey 2013/2014

15-year-old boys who have used cannabis in the last 30 days

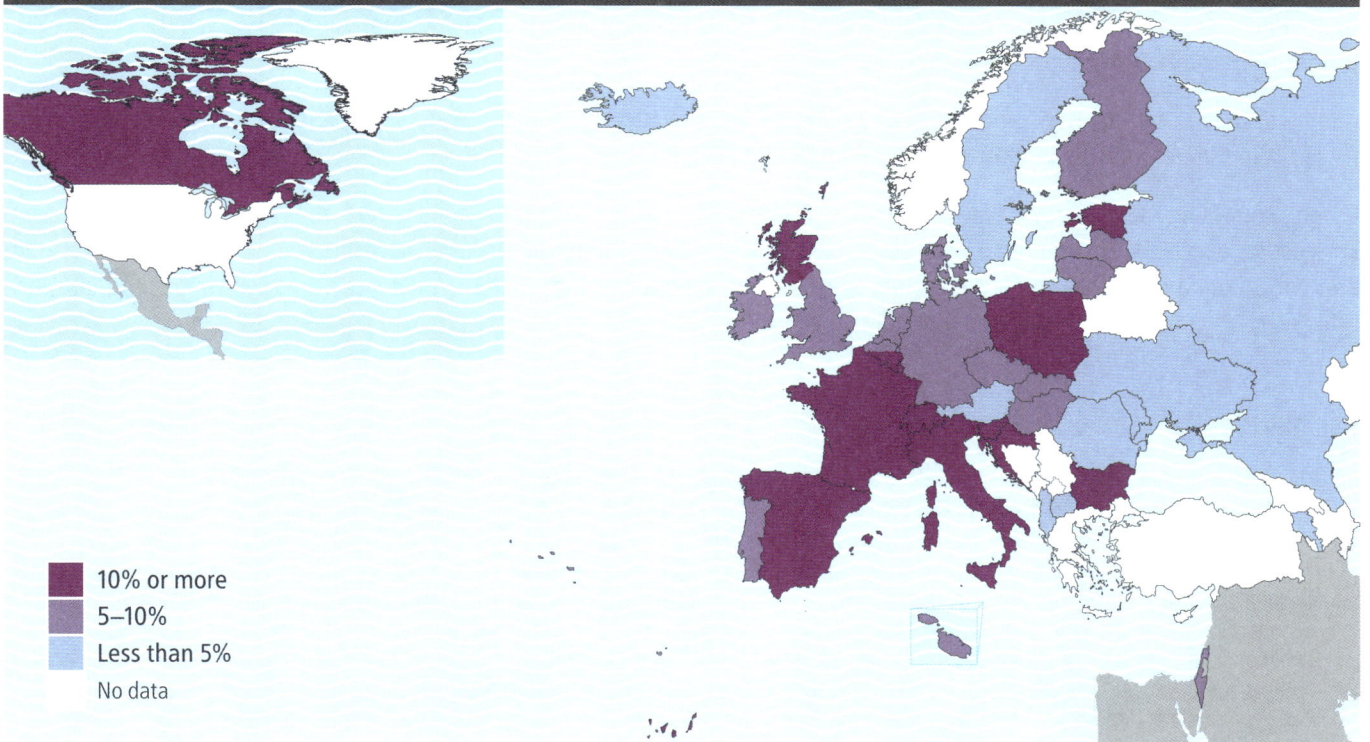

- 10% or more
- 5–10%
- Less than 5%
- No data

Note: HBSC teams provided disaggregated data for Belgium and the United Kingdom; these data appear in the map above.

CANNABIS USE:
SCIENTIFIC DISCUSSION AND POLICY REFLECTIONS

SCIENTIFIC DISCUSSION

The findings show that the prevalence of cannabis use varies substantially between countries and regions. Recent use in some, such as the Republic of Moldova and Sweden, is less than 2%, while it exceeds 13% in others (Canada and France). Some cross-national variations might be related to wealth, availability, perceived risk from cannabis or different peer cultures (15,18–20).

Findings also confirm that cannabis use is generally greater among boys. Early age of initiation is higher for boys in around a third of countries and regions, but findings on the association between use and family affluence are not consistent.

It is suggested that ongoing public debates and changes in national and state policies and regulations might explain future variations in trends across countries and regions as they affect perceptions of risk and availability and may encourage experimentation (18,21). More research into cross-national differences and trends in young people's cannabis use is needed to enable understanding of the mechanisms involved.

Debates on legalization may continue to exert a normalization effect on perceived risk and elevation rates that in turn might change the clustering effect of cannabis use with other risk behaviours.

POLICY REFLECTIONS

Recent debate and public pressure around cannabis has led to the introduction of decriminalization policies in most European countries that aim to focus enforcement efforts on drug dealers and allow recreational users to receive only a warning or symbolic penalty. It is still too early to determine whether this approach is effective, and the efficacy of various decriminalization models remains unsubstantiated.

Public debate and cannabis policy and regulation developments seem likely to intensify in coming years, so it is vital to continue to monitor and study changes in patterns of cannabis use among European and North American schoolchildren and investigate their effects on perceptions of risk and use. It is also important to study protective factors that might serve as buffers to prevent increases in cannabis use consequent to policy changes.

Adolescents who initiate substance use early and are frequent users are more likely to experience adverse consequences (11,13,14) and therefore warrant particular attention from policy-makers.

School, community and family-based interventions should be adapted to current policies and embrace a focus on increasing knowledge about the dangers and risks associated with cannabis, enhancing decision-making skills, promoting self-esteem and encouraging resistance to peer pressure. Evidence has shown that these intervention strategies can reduce cannabis use effectively (19,22).

REFERENCES

1. European drug report 2014: trends and developments. Lisbon: European Monitoring Centre for Drugs and Drug Addiction; 2014 (http://www.emcdda.europa.eu/publications/edr/trends-developments/2014, accessed 4 October 2015).

2. Kandel D. Stages in adolescent involvement in drug use. Science 1975;190:912–14.

3. Currie C, Zanotti C, Morgan A, Currie D, de Looze M, Roberts C et al., editors. Social determinants of health and well-being among young people. Health Behaviour in School-aged Children (HBSC) study: international report from the 2009/2010 survey. Copenhagen: WHO Regional Office for Europe; 2012 (Health Policy for Children and Adolescents, No. 6; http://www.euro.who.int/en/what-we-publish/abstracts/socialdeterminants-of-health-and-well-being-among-young-people.-health-behaviour-in-schoolaged-children-hbsc-study, accessed 24 August 2015).

4. Hibell B, Guttormsson U, Ahlström S, Balakireva O, Bjarnason T, Kokkevi A et al. The 2007 ESPAD report. Substance use among students in 35 European countries. Stockholm: Swedish Council for Information on Alcohol and Other Drugs; 2009 (http://www.espad.org/uploads/espad_reports/2007/the_2007_espad_report-full_091006.pdf, accessed 4 October 2015).

5. Johnston LD, O'Malley PM, Bachman JG, Schulenberg JE. Monitoring the future national survey results on drug use, 1975–2007. Vol. I. Secondary school students. Bethesda (MA): National Institute on Drug Abuse; 2008 (NIH Publication No. 08–6418A; http://monitoringthefuture.org/pubs/monographs/vol1_2007.pdf, accessed 4 October 2015).

GROWING UP UNEQUAL: GENDER AND SOCIOECONOMIC
DIFFERENCES IN YOUNG PEOPLE'S HEALTH AND WELL-BEING
PART 2. KEY DATA | CHAPTER 5. RISK BEHAVIOURS
CANNABIS USE

5

6. Lee CM, Woods BA. Marijuana motives; young adults' reasons for using marijuana. Addict Behav. 2007; 32(7):1384–94.

7. Volkow ND, Baler RD, Compton WM, Weiss SRB. Adverse health effects of marijuana use. N Eng J Med. 2014;370:2219–27.

8. Casadio P, Fernandes C, Murray RM, Di Forti M. Cannabis use in young people: the risk for schizophrenia. Neurosci Biobehav Rev. 2011;35(8):1779–87.

9. van Ours JC, Williams J. Why parents worry: initiation into cannabis use by youth and their educational attainment. J Health Econ. 2009;28(1):132–42.

10. Bachman J, O'Malley PM, Schulenberg JE, Johnston L, Freedman-Doan P, Messersmith EE. The education–drug use connection. How successes and failures in school relate to adolescent smoking, drinking, drug use, and delinquency. New York (NY): Lawrence Erlbaum Associates; 2008.

11. Giffith-Lendering MF, Huijbregts SC, Mooijaart A, Vollebergh WA, Swaab H. Cannabis use and development of externalizing and internalizing behavior problems in early adolescence: a TRAILS study. Drug Alcohol Depend. 2001;116(1–3):11–7.

12. Ding J, Gadit AM, Peer SB. School refusal in adolescent young men: could this be an idiopathic amotivational syndrome? BMJ Case Rep. 2014;doi:10.1136/bcr-2013-203508.

13. Kuntsche E, Simons-Morton B, Fotiou A, ter Bogt T, Kokkevi A. Decrease in adolescent cannabis use from 2002 to 2006 and links to evenings out with friends in 31 European and North America countries and regions. Arch Pediatr Adolesc Med. 2009;163(2):119–25.

14. Kokkevi A, Richardson C, Florescu S, Kuzman M, Stergar E. Psychosocial correlates of substance use in adolescence: a cross-national study in six European countries. Drug Alcohol Depend. 2007;86(1):67–74.

15. Bogot T, Schmid H, Gabhainn SN, Fotiou A, Vollebergh W. Economic and cultural correlates of cannabis use among mid-adolescents in 31 countries. Addiction 2006;101(2):241–51.

16. Anthony J, Chen C, Storr C. Influences of parenting practices on the risk of having a chance to try cannabis. Pediatrics 2005;115(6):1631–9.

17. Jonathan P, Caulkins BK, Kleiman MAR, MacCoun RJ, Midgette G, Oglesby P et al. Options and issues regarding marijuana legalization. Santa Monica (CA): RAND Corporation; 2015 (http://www.rand.org/pubs/perspectives/PE149.html, accessed 4 October 2015).

18. Harel-Fisch Y, Raiz Y, Lobel S, Shtinmiz N. Trend of substance use among Israeli youth: findings from the Israel HBSC survey 1994–2014. Jerusalem: Israel Anti-drug Authority; 2015.

19. Harel-Fisch Y. Country profile: Israel. In: The European Monitoring Centre for Drugs and Drug Addiction, neighbouring countries and Russia. Israel – country overview: country profile prepared by IADA [website]. Lisbon: European Monitoring Centre for Drugs and Drug Addiction; 2015 (http://www.emcdda.europa.eu/about/partners/nc, accessed 4 October 2015).

20. Sznitman S, Kolobov T, ter Bogt T, Kuntsche E, Walsh S, Boniel-Nissim M et al. Exploring substance use normalization among adolescents: a multilevel study in 35 countries. Soc Sci Med. 2013;97:143–51.

21. Simons-Morton BG, Pickett W, Boyce W, ter Bogt T, Vollebergh W. Cross-national comparison of adolescent drinking and cannabis use in the United States, Canada, and the Netherlands. Int J Drug Policy 2010;21(1):64–9.

22. Porath-Waller AJ, Beirness DJ. A meta-analytic review of school-based prevention for cannabis use. Health Educ Behav. 2010;37(5):709–23.

GROWING UP UNEQUAL: GENDER AND SOCIOECONOMIC
DIFFERENCES IN YOUNG PEOPLE'S HEALTH AND WELL-BEING
PART 2. KEY DATA | CHAPTER 5. RISK BEHAVIOURS

5

SEXUAL BEHAVIOUR:
EXPERIENCE OF SEXUAL INTERCOURSE

The emergence of romantic relationships is an important developmental marker of adolescence, and first intercourse often occurs at this time *(1)*. It is known that early sex has implications for self-perception, well-being, social status and future health behaviours, including sexual behaviours *(2,3)*. Early sexual initiation can be seen as part of broader risk-behaviour clusters that include substance use and unprotected sex *(4–7)*, with general genetic and environmental factors possibly being important mediators *(8)*.

Many young people rate their first sexual experience positively, but negative experiences are associated with first intercourse occurring outside of an established relationship or under pressure from the partner *(9)*. Having effective communication skills around sexual behaviour is therefore paramount at time of first intercourse.

Attitudes and expectations regarding adolescent sexuality and premarital sex in many countries and regions mean that young people may not receive adequate sex and relationships education prior to engaging in activity.

HBSC survey 2013/2014

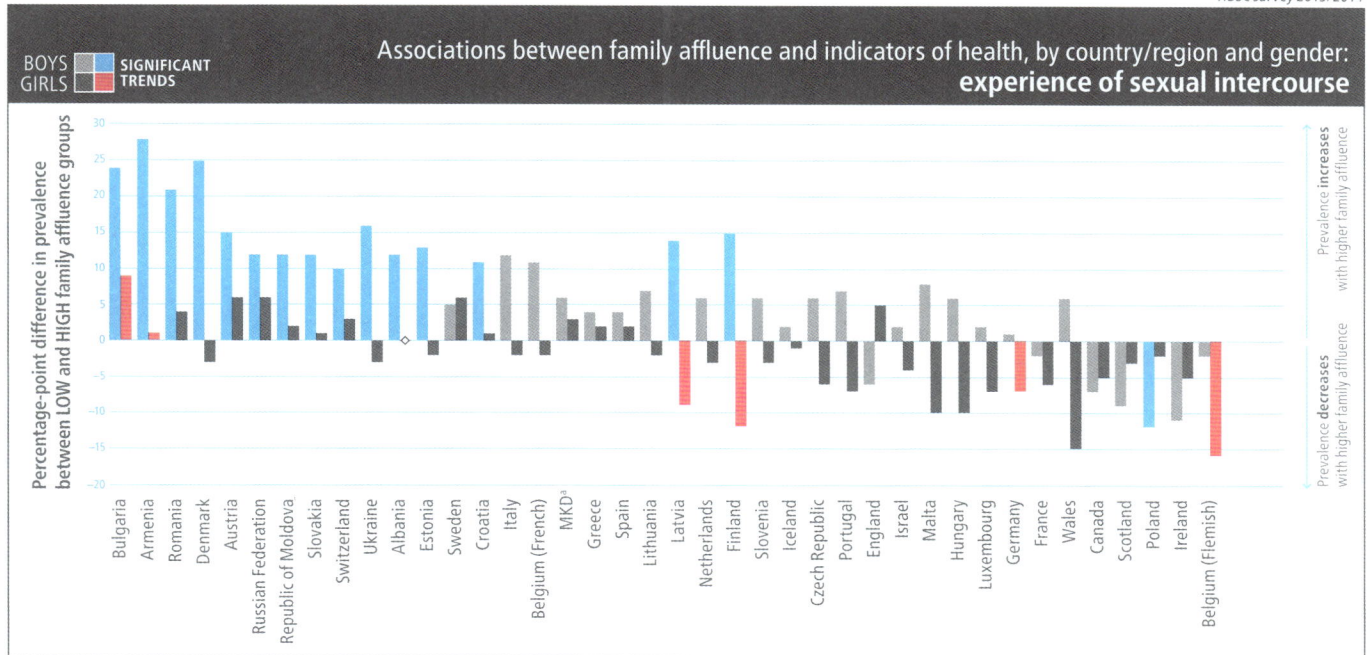

Associations between family affluence and indicators of health, by country/region and gender: **experience of sexual intercourse**

ᵃ The former Yugoslav Republic of Macedonia. *Note:* low- and high-affluence groups represent the lowest 20% and highest 20% in each country. ◇ means less than +/-0.5%. No data were received from Greenland and Norway.

MEASURES
Fifteen-year-olds only were asked whether they had ever had sexual intercourse. The question was presented using colloquial terminology (such as having sex or going all the way) to ensure respondents understood it was about full penetrative intercourse.

RESULTS

Findings presented here show the proportions who responded yes to having had sexual intercourse.

Age

Data are presented for 15-year-olds only.

Gender

Boys were more likely to report having had sexual intercourse in around half of countries and regions, with the greatest gender disparities being seen in eastern European countries. Higher prevalence among girls was reported in England and Wales.

Family affluence

Sexual intercourse was associated with family affluence in some countries and regions, but the direction of association varied. The relationship was stronger in boys, for whom the tendency was for higher prevalence among those in the highest-affluence group. For girls, the association was positive in two countries and regions and negative in four.

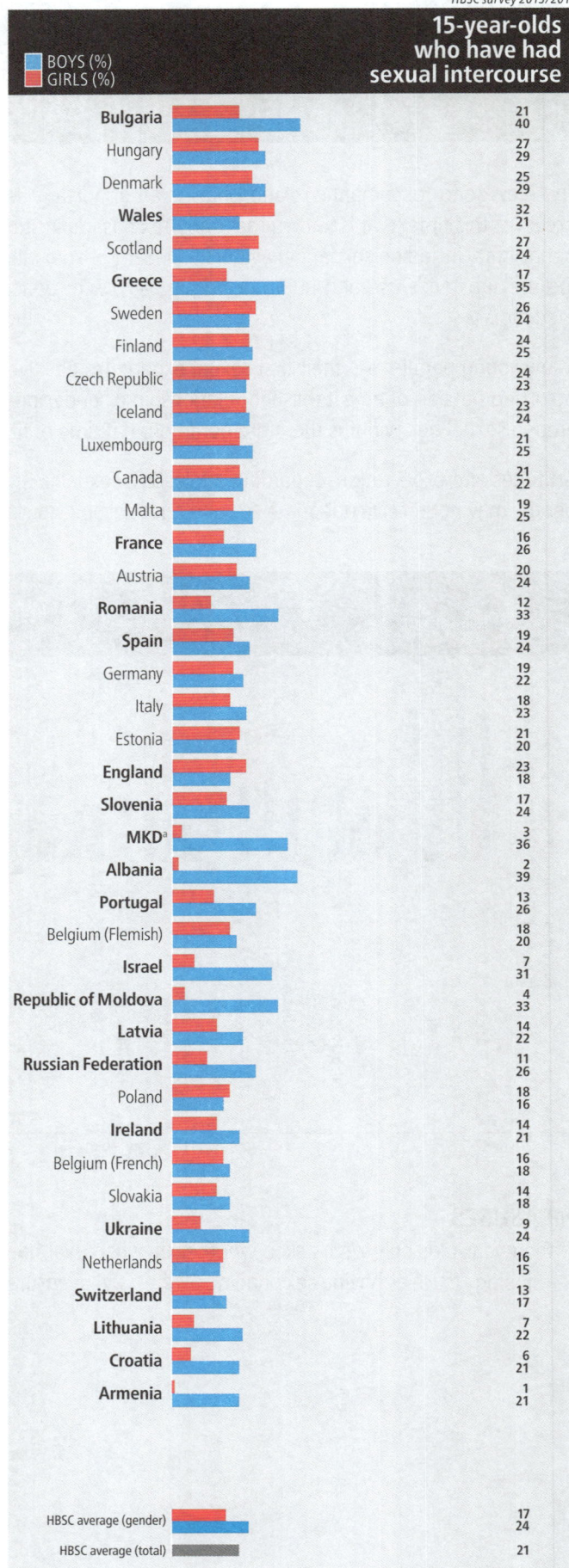

HBSC survey 2013/2014

15-year-olds who have had sexual intercourse

BOYS (%)
GIRLS (%)

Country	Boys	Girls
Bulgaria	21	40
Hungary	27	29
Denmark	25	29
Wales	32	21
Scotland	27	24
Greece	17	35
Sweden	26	24
Finland	24	25
Czech Republic	24	23
Iceland	23	24
Luxembourg	21	25
Canada	21	22
Malta	19	25
France	16	26
Austria	20	24
Romania	12	33
Spain	19	24
Germany	19	22
Italy	18	23
Estonia	21	20
England	23	18
Slovenia	17	24
MKD[a]	3	36
Albania	2	39
Portugal	13	26
Belgium (Flemish)	18	20
Israel	7	31
Republic of Moldova	4	33
Latvia	14	22
Russian Federation	11	26
Poland	18	16
Ireland	14	21
Belgium (French)	16	18
Slovakia	14	18
Ukraine	9	24
Netherlands	16	15
Switzerland	13	17
Lithuania	7	22
Croatia	6	21
Armenia	1	21
HBSC average (gender)	17	24
HBSC average (total)	21	

[a] The former Yugoslav Republic of Macedonia. *Note:* **indicates** significant gender difference (at p<0.05). No data were received from Greenland and Norway. The question was asked only of a subset of 15-year-olds in Belgium (French).

GROWING UP UNEQUAL: GENDER AND SOCIOECONOMIC
DIFFERENCES IN YOUNG PEOPLE'S HEALTH AND WELL-BEING
PART 2. KEY DATA | CHAPTER 5. RISK BEHAVIOURS
SEXUAL BEHAVIOUR: EXPERIENCE OF SEXUAL INTERCOURSE

5

HBSC survey 2013/2014

15-year-old girls who have had sexual intercourse

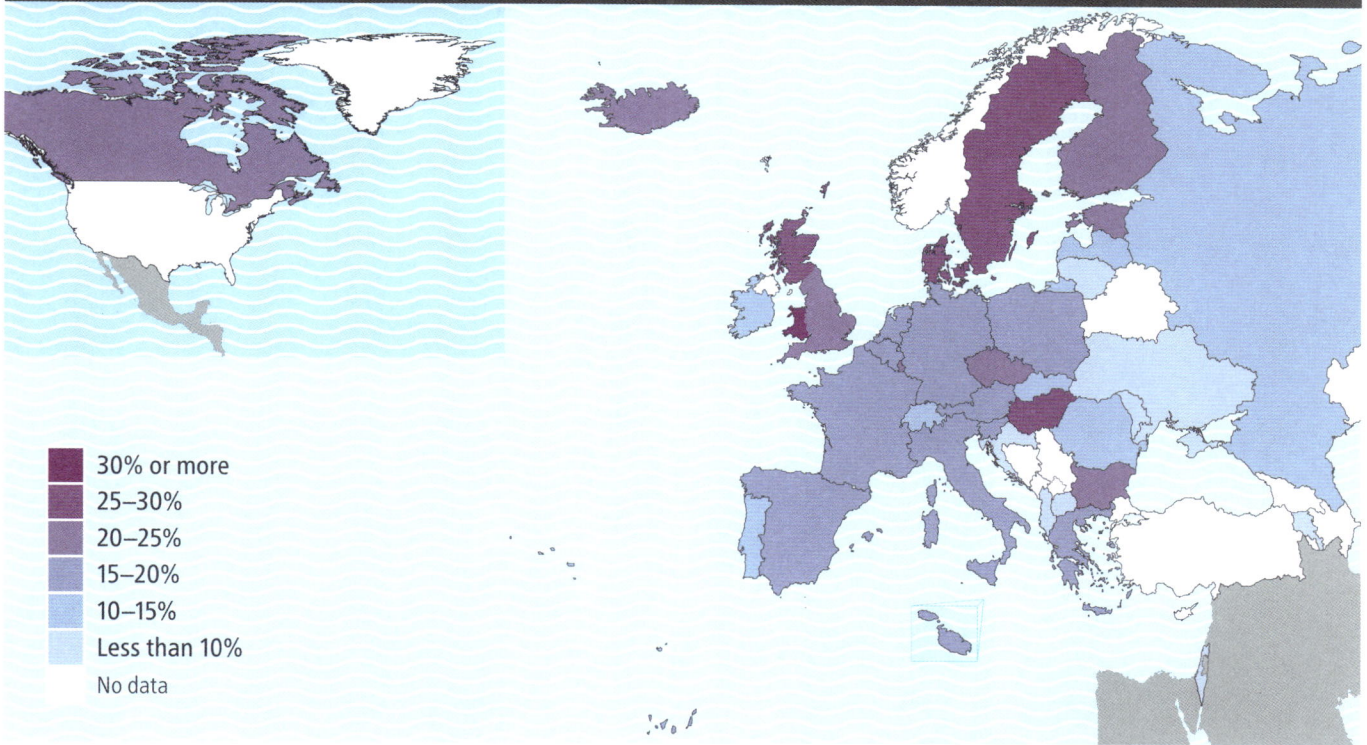

- 30% or more
- 25–30%
- 20–25%
- 15–20%
- 10–15%
- Less than 10%
- No data

Note: HBSC teams provided disaggregated data for Belgium and the United Kingdom; these data appear in the map above.

HBSC survey 2013/2014

15-year-old boys who have had sexual intercourse

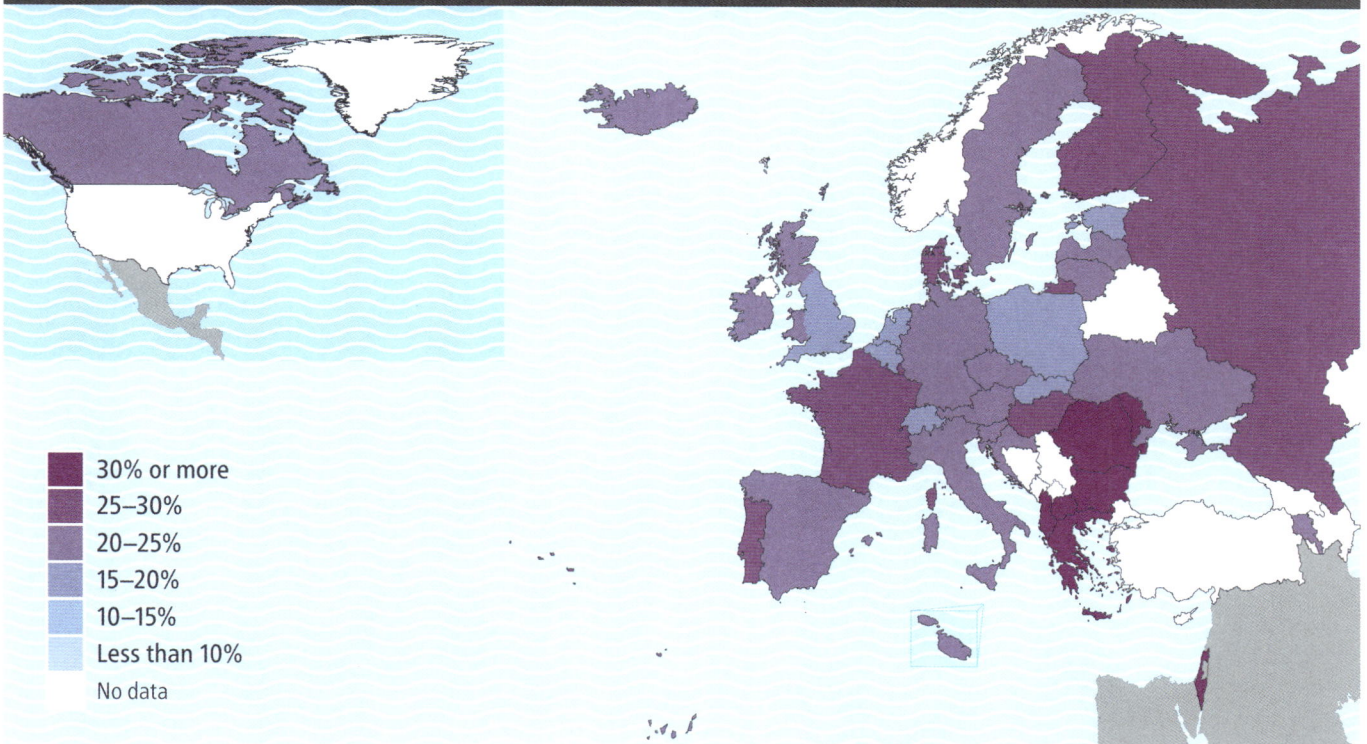

- 30% or more
- 25–30%
- 20–25%
- 15–20%
- 10–15%
- Less than 10%
- No data

Note: HBSC teams provided disaggregated data for Belgium and the United Kingdom; these data appear in the map above.

GROWING UP UNEQUAL: GENDER AND SOCIOECONOMIC
DIFFERENCES IN YOUNG PEOPLE'S HEALTH AND WELL-BEING
PART 2. KEY DATA | CHAPTER 5. RISK BEHAVIOURS

5

SEXUAL BEHAVIOUR: CONDOM AND PILL USE

Evidence suggests that sexually transmitted infections (STIs) are increasing among adolescents in many European countries and regions *(10)*, with adolescents being reported as having the highest incidence of some STIs of any age group *(11)*. Condoms are the only effective method of preventing STIs during sexual intercourse and can easily be accessed by adolescents.

The contraceptive pill is an effective method of preventing pregnancy and is frequently used by adolescents in some countries and regions *(12)*. Reducing adolescent pregnancies is an important goal in improving adolescent health and lowering maternal and child mortality *(13)*.

Use of contraceptive methods varies by country and region *(12)*.

HBSC survey 2013/2014

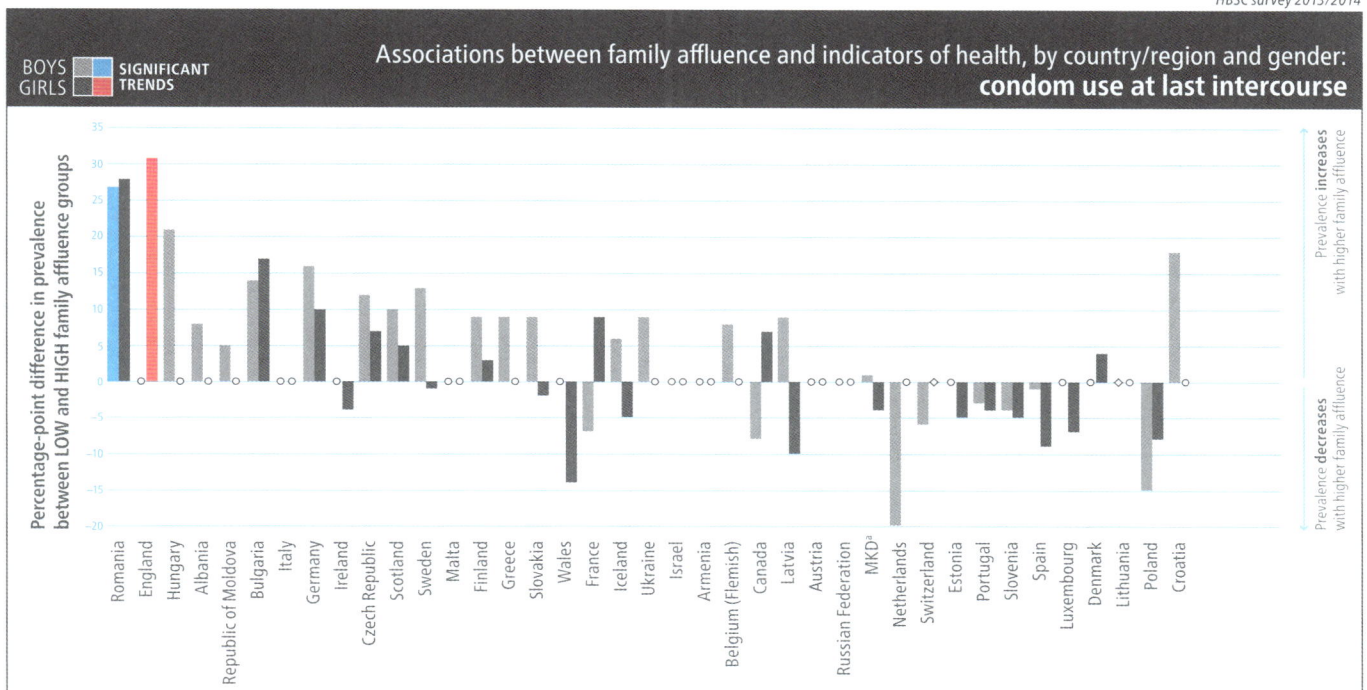

BOYS
GIRLS
SIGNIFICANT TRENDS

Associations between family affluence and indicators of health, by country/region and gender: condom use at last intercourse

Percentage-point difference in prevalence between LOW and HIGH family affluence groups

Prevalence *increases* with higher family affluence

Prevalence *decreases* with higher family affluence

Countries: Romania, England, Hungary, Albania, Republic of Moldova, Bulgaria, Italy, Germany, Ireland, Czech Republic, Scotland, Sweden, Malta, Finland, Greece, Slovakia, Wales, France, Iceland, Ukraine, Israel, Armenia, Belgium (Flemish), Canada, Latvia, Austria, Russian Federation, MKD[a], Netherlands, Switzerland, Estonia, Portugal, Slovenia, Spain, Luxembourg, Denmark, Lithuania, Poland, Croatia

[a] The former Yugoslav Republic of Macedonia. *Note:* low- and high-affluence groups represent the lowest 20% and highest 20% in each country. ◇ means less than +/-0.5%. ○ means no data are presented from the following countries and regions for boys and/or girls due to insufficient numbers of respondents: Albania (girls), Armenia (girls and boys), Austria (girls and boys), Belgium (Flemish) (girls), Croatia (girls), Denmark (boys), England (boys), Estonia (boys), Greece (girls), Hungary (girls), Ireland (girls), Israel (girls and boys), Italy (girls and boys), Lithuania (girls), Luxembourg (boys), Malta (girls and boys), Republic of Moldova (girls), Netherlands (girls), Russian Federation (girls and boys), Ukraine (girls) and Wales (boys). No data were received from Belgium (French), Greenland and Norway.

MEASURES

Fifteen-year-olds only were asked whether they or their partner had used a condom or birth control pills (two separate questions) the last time they had had intercourse.

This question was amended from the HBSC 2009/2010 survey, when pill and condom use for the purpose of contraception was measured by providing a list of methods of contraceptives and students were asked to mark those used at last intercourse. The question was changed in the 2013/2014 survey as the method was found to result in a large number of missing responses.

RESULTS

Findings presented here show the proportions of those who had had sexual intercourse who reported using a condom or the contraceptive pill at last intercourse, respectively.

Condom use

Age

Data are presented for 15-year-olds only.

Gender

Boys were more likely to report condom use in 13 countries and regions, with girls more likely in only one country (Spain). No major gender disparities were noted in most, however.

Family affluence

No clear association with family affluence emerged in most countries and regions. A significant association was observed in only one for boys and one for girls, where condom use was higher among high-affluence groups.

Pill use

Age

Data are presented for 15-year-olds only.

Gender

A significant gender difference was found in seven countries and regions, but no overall pattern of either boys or girls being more likely to report pill use emerged.

Family affluence

It was not possible to confirm significant relations between pill use at last intercourse and family affluence, as the numbers were too small to reliably identify statistical significance.

GROWING UP UNEQUAL: GENDER AND SOCIOECONOMIC
DIFFERENCES IN YOUNG PEOPLE'S HEALTH AND WELL-BEING
PART 2. KEY DATA | CHAPTER 5. RISK BEHAVIOURS
SEXUAL BEHAVIOUR: CONDOM AND PILL USE

5

15-year-olds who used a condom at last intercourse

HBSC survey 2013/2014

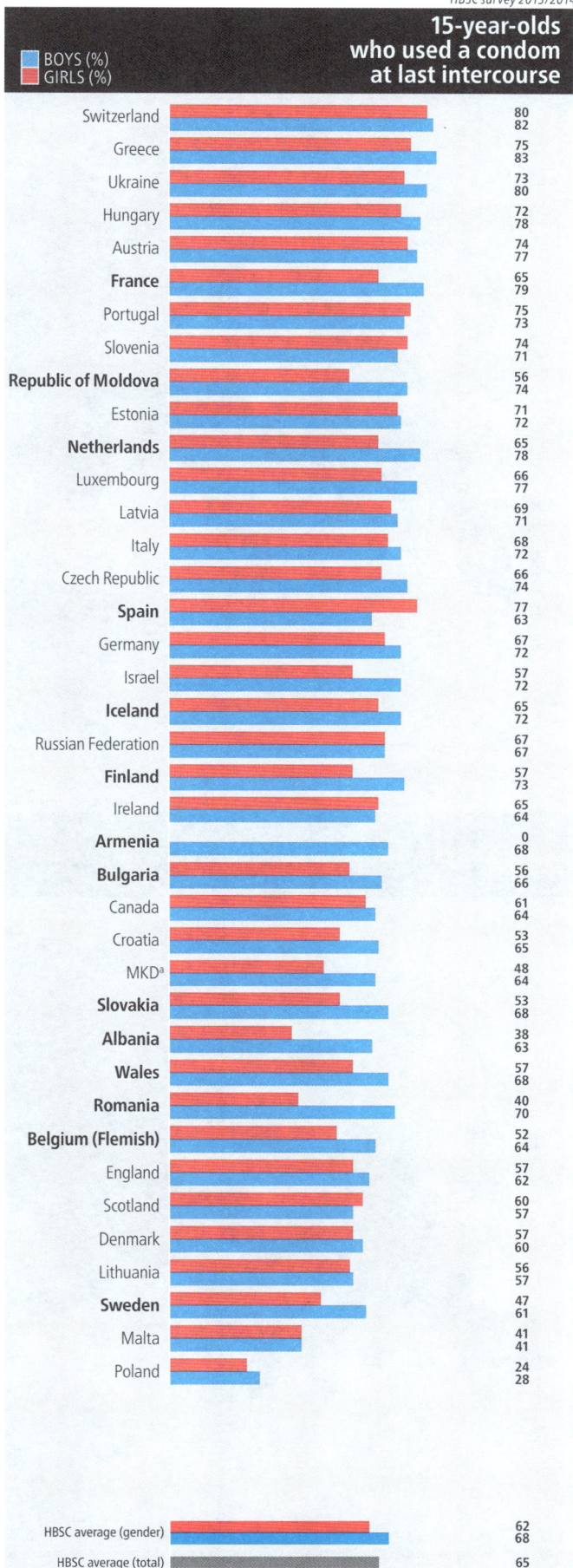

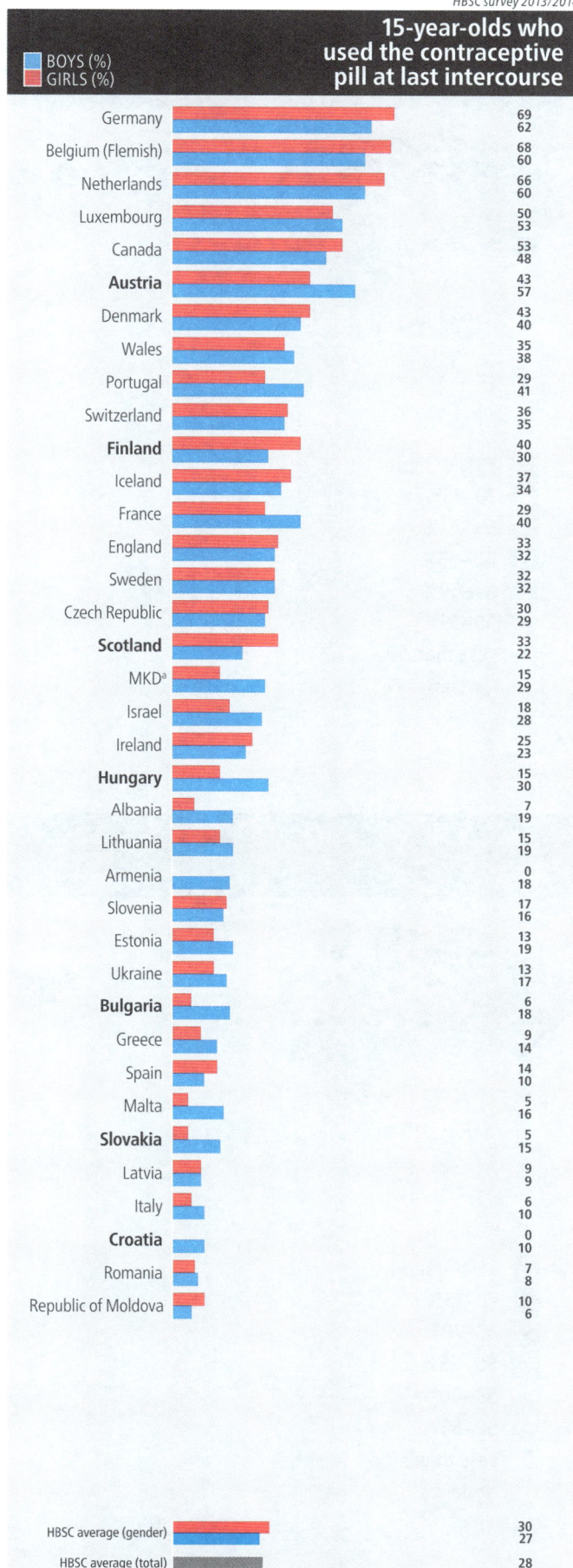

■ BOYS (%)
■ GIRLS (%)

Country	Girls	Boys
Switzerland	80	82
Greece	75	83
Ukraine	73	80
Hungary	72	78
Austria	74	77
France	65	79
Portugal	75	73
Slovenia	74	71
Republic of Moldova	56	74
Estonia	71	72
Netherlands	65	78
Luxembourg	66	77
Latvia	69	71
Italy	68	72
Czech Republic	66	74
Spain	77	63
Germany	67	72
Israel	57	72
Iceland	65	72
Russian Federation	67	67
Finland	57	73
Ireland	65	64
Armenia	0	68
Bulgaria	56	66
Canada	61	64
Croatia	53	65
MKD[a]	48	64
Slovakia	53	68
Albania	38	63
Wales	57	68
Romania	40	70
Belgium (Flemish)	52	64
England	57	62
Scotland	60	57
Denmark	57	60
Lithuania	56	57
Sweden	47	61
Malta	41	41
Poland	24	28

| HBSC average (gender) | 62 | 68 |
| HBSC average (total) | | 65 |

a The former Yugoslav Republic of Macedonia.
Note: no data were received from Armenia (girls), Belgium (French), Greenland and Norway.

15-year-olds who used the contraceptive pill at last intercourse

HBSC survey 2013/2014

■ BOYS (%)
■ GIRLS (%)

Country	Girls	Boys
Germany	69	62
Belgium (Flemish)	68	60
Netherlands	66	60
Luxembourg	50	53
Canada	53	48
Austria	43	57
Denmark	43	40
Wales	35	38
Portugal	29	41
Switzerland	36	35
Finland	40	30
Iceland	37	34
France	29	40
England	33	32
Sweden	32	32
Czech Republic	30	29
Scotland	33	22
MKD[a]	15	29
Israel	18	28
Ireland	25	23
Hungary	15	30
Albania	7	19
Lithuania	15	19
Armenia	0	18
Slovenia	17	16
Estonia	13	19
Ukraine	13	17
Bulgaria	6	18
Greece	9	14
Spain	14	10
Malta	5	16
Slovakia	5	15
Latvia	9	9
Italy	6	10
Croatia	0	10
Romania	7	8
Republic of Moldova	10	6

| HBSC average (gender) | 30 | 27 |
| HBSC average (total) | | 28 |

Note: **indicates** significant gender difference (at p<0.05). 0 means less than +/-0.5%. No data were received from Armenia (girls), Belgium (French), Croatia (girls), Greenland, Norway, Poland and the Russian Federation.

HBSC survey 2013/2014

15-year-old girls who used a condom at last intercourse

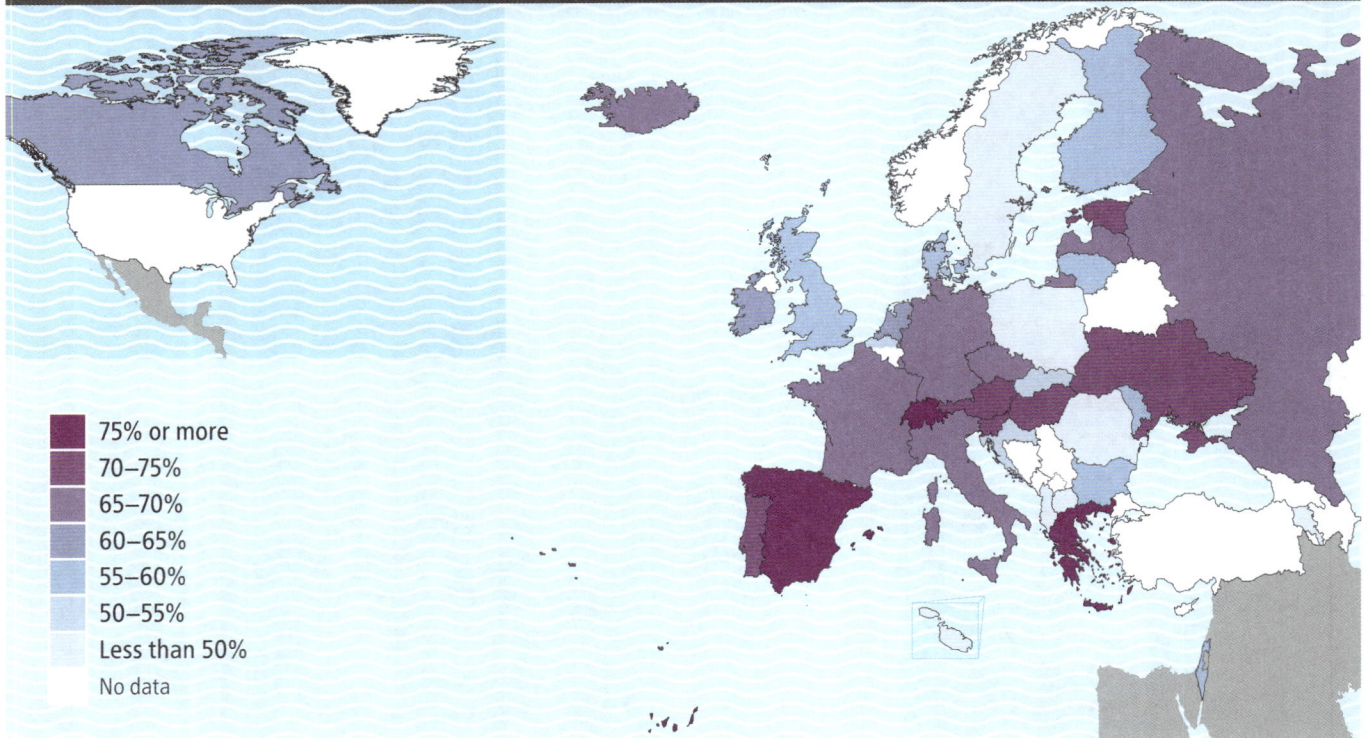

- 75% or more
- 70–75%
- 65–70%
- 60–65%
- 55–60%
- 50–55%
- Less than 50%
- No data

Note: HBSC teams provided disaggregated data for Belgium and the United Kingdom; these data appear in the map above.

HBSC survey 2013/2014

15-year-old boys who used a condom at last intercourse

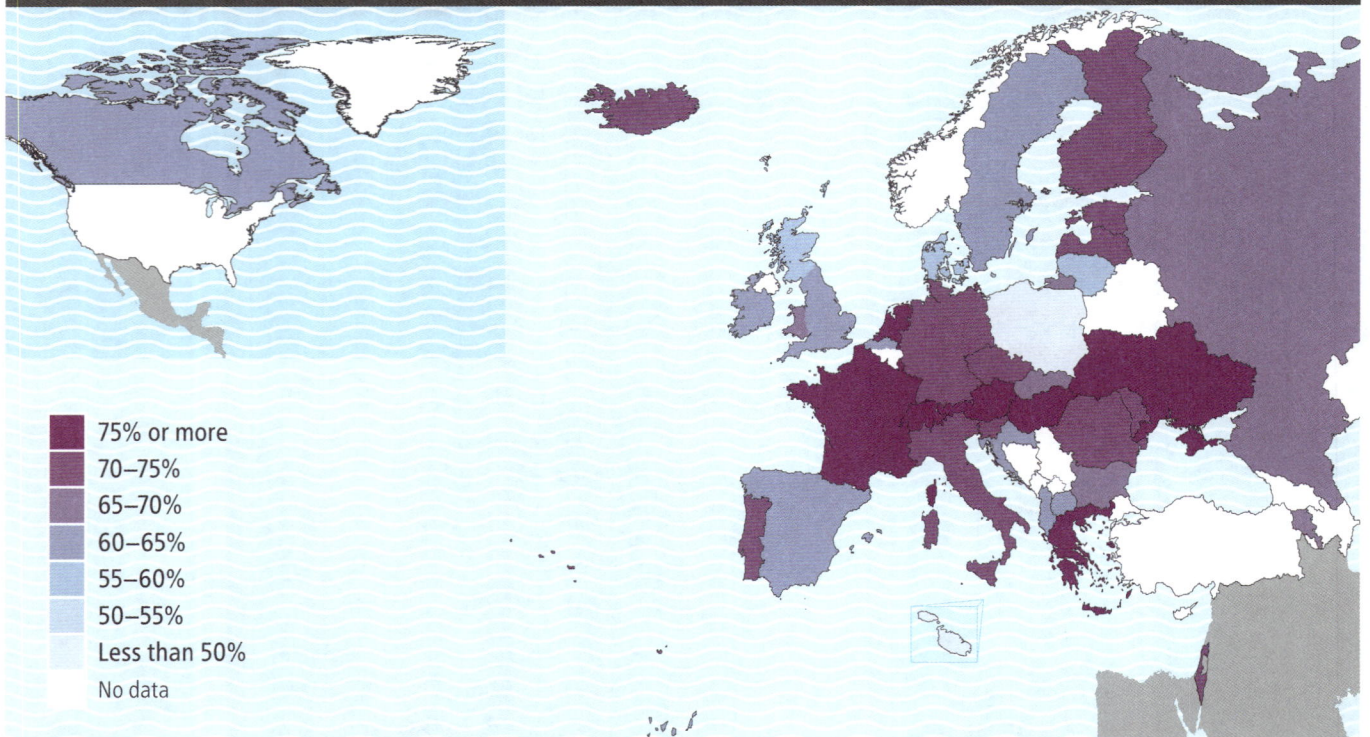

- 75% or more
- 70–75%
- 65–70%
- 60–65%
- 55–60%
- 50–55%
- Less than 50%
- No data

Note: HBSC teams provided disaggregated data for Belgium and the United Kingdom; these data appear in the map above.

GROWING UP UNEQUAL: GENDER AND SOCIOECONOMIC
DIFFERENCES IN YOUNG PEOPLE'S HEALTH AND WELL-BEING
PART 2. KEY DATA | CHAPTER 5. RISK BEHAVIOURS
SEXUAL BEHAVIOUR: CONDOM AND PILL USE

5

HBSC survey 2013/2014

15-year-old girls who used the contraceptive pill at last intercourse

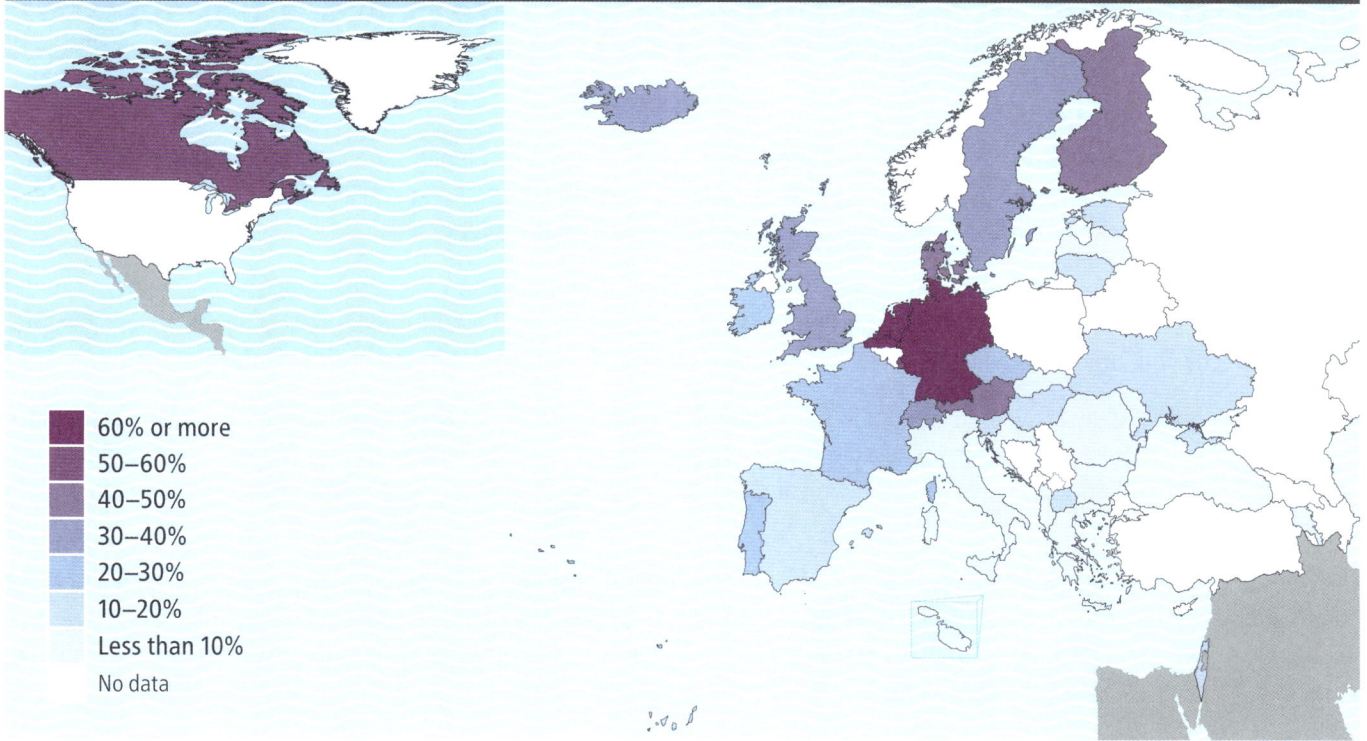

- 60% or more
- 50–60%
- 40–50%
- 30–40%
- 20–30%
- 10–20%
- Less than 10%
- No data

Note: HBSC teams provided disaggregated data for Belgium and the United Kingdom; these data appear in the map above.

HBSC survey 2013/2014

15-year-old boys who used the contraceptive pill at last intercourse

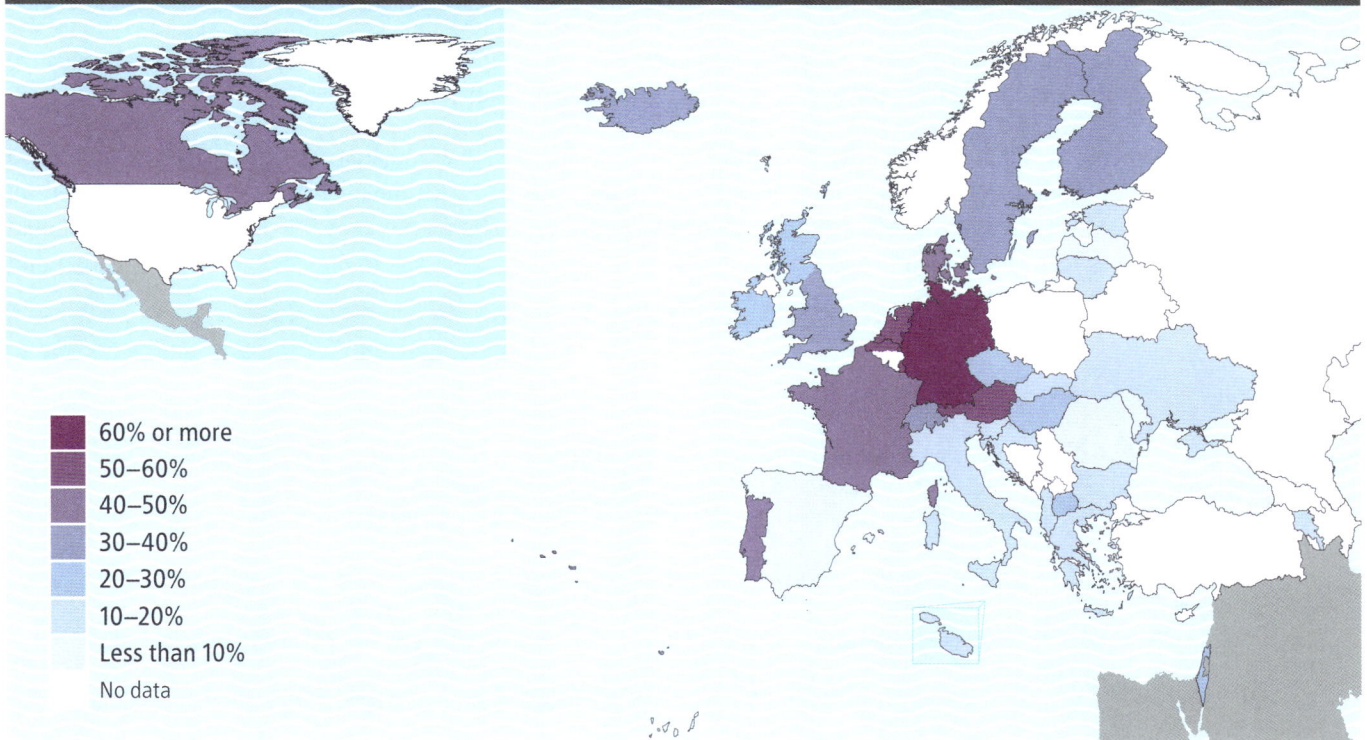

- 60% or more
- 50–60%
- 40–50%
- 30–40%
- 20–30%
- 10–20%
- Less than 10%
- No data

Note: HBSC teams provided disaggregated data for Belgium and the United Kingdom; these data appear in the map above.

SEXUAL BEHAVIOUR: SCIENTIFIC DISCUSSION AND POLICY REFLECTIONS

SCIENTIFIC DISCUSSION

Boys continue to be more likely to report sexual intercourse in most countries and regions, although there is evidence that the gender gap is reducing (14,15). The effect of family affluence on the likelihood of engaging in sexual intercourse varies by gender, but use of condoms and the contraceptive pill are not strongly associated with affluence.

Gender identity and norms determine expectations and behaviour (16) and are known to affect health outcomes (17). Gender identity solidifies in adolescence, so this is an important time period for addressing gender-based health inequalities (16). Working directly with boys to redefine gender roles may be a productive means of reducing health inequalities (18).

More than half of sexually active adolescents in most countries and regions report using a condom at last intercourse, but a significant minority leave themselves vulnerable to STIs. Use of contraceptive pills remains less frequent than condom use and is highest in northern and western European countries and regions. This may reflect a lack of access for young people elsewhere (19).

The decision to engage in sexual intercourse and the likelihood of using contraception during such encounters is influenced by young people's communication skills in relation to sex and relationships. Many young people in Europe still feel they receive inadequate information and advice on these matters, which they deem to be necessary before they become sexually active (9).

POLICY REFLECTIONS

Progress has been made at policy level in addressing adolescents' sexual and reproductive health through, for example, introducing comprehensive sex and relationships education and improving access to services in some countries and regions. Many young people, however, still lack access to modern contraceptives (10) and face barriers to using confidential services (20).

WHO has made it clear that it wishes to see an improvement in access to good health services for all young people, irrespective of ethnicity, religion or SES, but lack of practitioner skills may hinder policies (where they exist) from being implemented (20). Research shows that young people who have access to comprehensive sex and relationships education, confidential reproductive health services and appropriate methods of contraception have better sexual health (21).

The HBSC data show that a significant minority of adolescents are sexually active and that many risk STIs or unplanned pregnancy by not using condoms or effective methods of birth control. Access to such means of protection is hampered for many by restrictions due to religious or cultural attitudes to adolescent sexuality and premarital sex. Each young person should nevertheless have access to sexual health services (13), with the school setting being key to providing health education and nurturing lifestyle skills to promote personal health and well-being (13).

REFERENCES

1. Avery L, Lazdane G. What do we know about sexual and reproductive health of adolescents in Europe? Eur J Contracept Reprod Health Care 2010;15(S2):S54–S66.

2. Magnusson C, Trost K. Girls experiencing sexual intercourse early: could it play a part in reproductive health in middle adulthood? J Psychosom Obstet Gynaecol. 2006;27(4):237–44.

3. Fergus S, Zimmerman MA, Caldwell CA. Growth trajectories of sexual risk behavior in adolescence and young adulthood. Am J Public Health 2007;97(6):1096–101.

4. Cooper ML. Alcohol use and risky sexual behaviour among college students and youth: evaluating the evidence. J Stud Alcohol Drugs 2002;Suppl. 14:101–17.

5. Eaton DK, Kann L, Kinchen S, Ross J, Hawkins J, Harris WA et al. Youth risk behavior surveillance – United States, 2005. Morb Mortal Wkly Rep Surveill Summ. 2006;55(SS–5):1–108.

6. Parkes AP, Wight D, Henderson M, Hart G. Explaining association between adolescent substance use and condom use. J Adolesc Health 2007;40(2):e1–18.

GROWING UP UNEQUAL: GENDER AND SOCIOECONOMIC
DIFFERENCES IN YOUNG PEOPLE'S HEALTH AND WELL-BEING
PART 2. KEY DATA | CHAPTER 5. RISK BEHAVIOURS
SEXUAL BEHAVIOUR

5

7.   Poulin C, Graham L. The association between substance use, unplanned sexual intercourse and other sexual behaviours among adolescent students. Addiction 2001;96(4):607–21.

8.   Huibregtse BM, Bornovalova MA, Hicks BM, McGue M, Iacono W. Testing the role of adolescent sexual initiation in later-life sexual risk behavior: a longitudinal twin design. Psychol Sci. 2011;22(7):924–33.

9.   Increasing the knowledge base on young people's sexual and reproductive health and rights in Europe. Summary report of qualitative research conducted in five European countries under the SAFE II project. Brussels: IPPF European Network; 2012 (http://www.ippfen.org/sites/default/files/Summary%20research%20report.pdf, accessed 24 August 2015).

10. Laakkonen H. Adolescents' sexual and reproductive health (SRH): empowering young people to realize their full potential. Entre Nous 2014;80:3.

11. Dehne KL, Riedner G. Sexually transmitted infections among adolescents: the need for adequate health services. Geneva: World Health Organization; 2005 (http://www.who.int/reproductivehealth/publications/adolescence/9241562889/en/, accessed 24 August 2015).

12. Currie C, Zanotti C, Morgan A, Currie D, de Looze M, Roberts C et al., editors. Social determinants of health and well-being among young people. Health Behaviour in School-aged Children (HBSC) study: international report from the 2009/2010 survey. Copenhagen: WHO Regional Office for Europe; 2012 (Health Policy for Children and Adolescents, No. 6; http://www.euro.who.int/en/what-we-publish/abstracts/socialdeterminants-of-health-and-well-being-among-young-people.-health-behaviour-in-schoolaged-children-hbsc-study, accessed 24 August 2015).

13. Health for the world's adolescents. A second chance in the second decade. Geneva: World Health Organization; 2014 (http://apps.who.int/adolescent/second-decade/, accessed 24 August 2015).

14. Ramiro L, Windlin B, Reis M, Gabhainn SN, Jovic S, Matos MG et al. Gendered trends in early and very early sex and condom use in 20 European countries from 2002 to 2010. Eur J Public Health 2015;25(S2):65–8.

15. Godeau E, Nic Gabhainn S, Magnusson J, Zanotti C. A profile of young people's sexual behaviour: findings from the Health Behaviour in School-aged Children study. Entre Nous 2011;72:24–6.

16. Evidence for gender responsive actions for the prevention and management of HIV/AIDS and STIs. Copenhagen: WHO Regional Office for Europe; 2011 (http://www.euro.who.int/en/health-topics/health-determinants/gender/publications/2012/young-peoples-health-as-a-whole-of-society-response-series/evidence-for-gender-responsive-actions-for-the-prevention-and-management-of-hivaids-and-sti, accessed 24 August 2015).

17. Davidson KW, Trudeau KJ, van Roosmalen E, Stewart M, Kirkland S. Gender as a health determinant and implications for health education. Health Educ Behav. 2006;33(6):731–43.

18. Kaufman M. Engaging men, changing gender norms: directions for gender-transformative action. New York (NY): UNFPA/MenEngage; 2014 (http://www.unfpa.org/resources/brief-engaging-men-changing-gender-norms, accessed 24 August 2015).

19. Khomasuridze T, Seyidov T, Vasileva-Blazev M. Sexual and reproductive health (SRH) among adolescents and youth in eastern Europe and central Asia. Entre Nous 2014;80:12–3.

20. Baltag V, Mathieson A, editors. Youth friendly health policies and services in the European Region. Copenhagen: WHO Regional Office for Europe; 2010; (http://www.euro.who.int/__data/assets/pdf_file/0017/123128/E94322.pdf, accessed 24 August 2015).

21. Federal Centre for Health Education, United Nations Population Fund, WHO Regional Office for Europe. Sexuality education: what is its impact? Cologne: Federal Centre for Health Education (BZgA); 2015 (Sexuality Education Policy Brief No. 2; http://eeca.unfpa.org/sites/default/files/pub-pdf/GAKC_Policy_Brief_No_2_rz.pdf, accessed 24 August 2015).

GROWING UP UNEQUAL: GENDER AND SOCIOECONOMIC
DIFFERENCES IN YOUNG PEOPLE'S HEALTH AND WELL-BEING
PART 2. KEY DATA | CHAPTER 5. RISK BEHAVIOURS

5

FIGHTING

Despite the positive trend in reduction in levels over the past decade *(1)*, physical fighting remains a leading health concern and is the most common manifestation of youth violence. Involvement is known to be related to individual, family and school relationships: children who fight report lower life satisfaction, poorer family and peer relationships and worse perceptions of their school environments *(2,3)*.

Adolescents who fight are at risk of involvement in additional problem behaviours, such as alcohol and other substance use *(4–6)*. Research shows that levels of violence are related to socioeconomic factors: inequality intensifies social hierarchies, reduces social control over violence, increases feelings of dissatisfaction and resentment, and fosters a harsh social environment in which conflict is likely to occur *(7)*.

HBSC survey 2013/2014

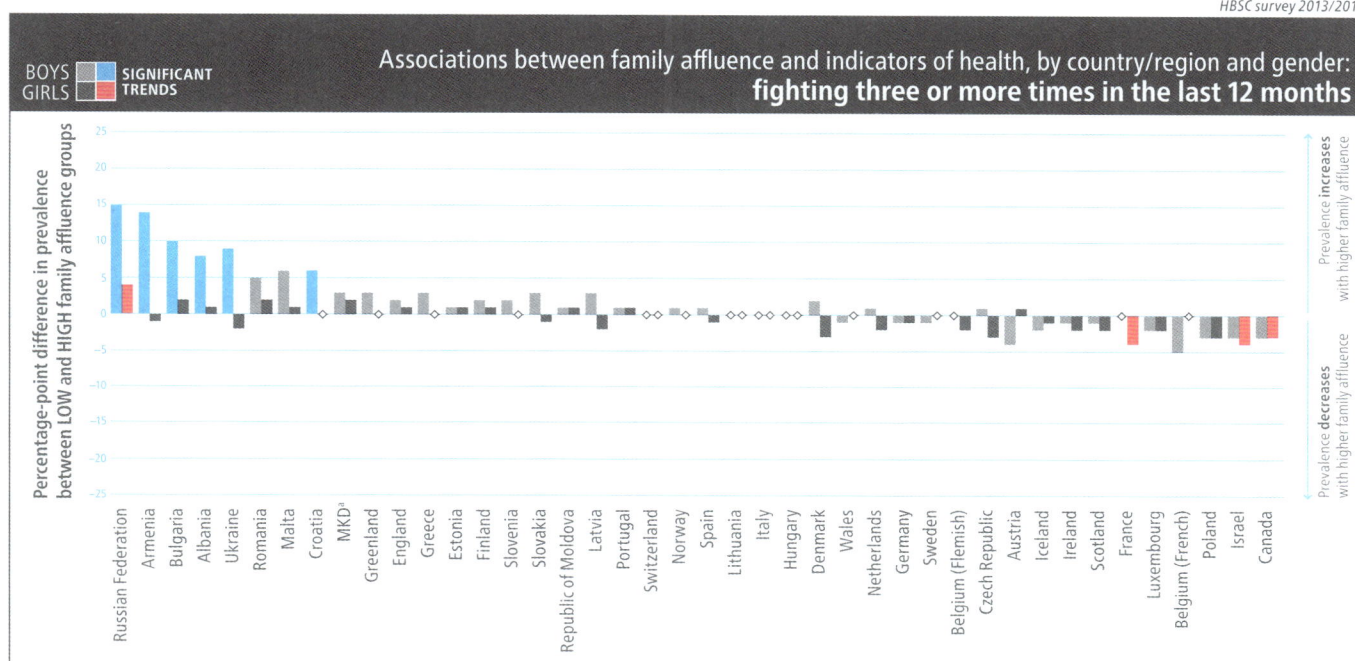

BOYS
GIRLS
SIGNIFICANT TRENDS

Associations between family affluence and indicators of health, by country/region and gender:
fighting three or more times in the last 12 months

Percentage-point difference in prevalence between LOW and HIGH family affluence groups

Prevalence **increases** with higher family affluence

Prevalence **decreases** with higher family affluence

ªThe former Yugoslav Republic of Macedonia. *Note:* low- and high-affluence groups represent the lowest 20% and highest 20% in each country. ◇ means less than +/-0.5%.

MEASURE

Young people were asked how many times in the past 12 months they had been involved in a physical fight. Response options ranged from none to four times or more.

Supplementary data on the proportion involved in a physical fight at least once in the past 12 months are provided in the Annex.

RESULTS

Findings presented here show the proportions who reported physical fighting three times or more in the past 12 months.

Age

Significant changes over age occurred for boys in most countries and regions, with fighting tending to decline with increasing age. Age-related patterns were less clear for girls. The cross-national range in prevalence was very large, especially for boys.

Gender

Boys were more likely to be involved at all ages and in all countries and regions except Malta (for 13-year-olds only).

Family affluence

Fighting differed according to family affluence in a few countries and regions, but no consistent pattern emerged for boys or girls. The largest difference was among boys in Armenia and the Russian Federation, where higher prevalence was associated with high affluence.

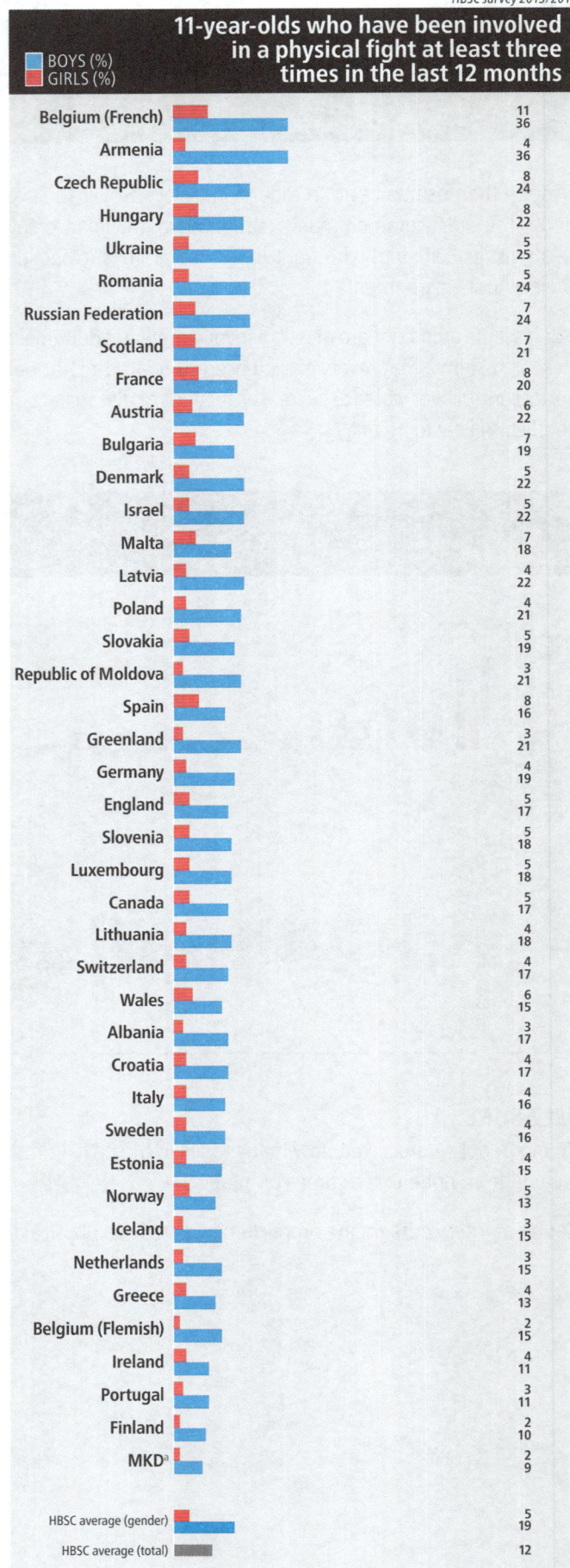

HBSC survey 2013/2014

11-year-olds who have been involved in a physical fight at least three times in the last 12 months

BOYS (%)
GIRLS (%)

Country	Boys (%)	Girls (%)
Belgium (French)	11	36
Armenia	4	36
Czech Republic	8	24
Hungary	8	22
Ukraine	5	25
Romania	5	24
Russian Federation	7	24
Scotland	7	21
France	8	20
Austria	6	22
Bulgaria	7	19
Denmark	5	22
Israel	5	22
Malta	7	18
Latvia	4	22
Poland	4	21
Slovakia	5	19
Republic of Moldova	3	21
Spain	8	16
Greenland	3	21
Germany	4	19
England	5	17
Slovenia	5	18
Luxembourg	5	18
Canada	5	17
Lithuania	4	18
Switzerland	4	17
Wales	6	15
Albania	3	17
Croatia	4	17
Italy	4	16
Sweden	4	16
Estonia	4	15
Norway	5	13
Iceland	3	15
Netherlands	3	15
Greece	4	13
Belgium (Flemish)	2	15
Ireland	4	11
Portugal	3	11
Finland	2	10
MKD[a]	2	9
HBSC average (gender)	5	19
HBSC average (total)	12	

[a] The former Yugoslav Republic of Macedonia.

GROWING UP UNEQUAL: GENDER AND SOCIOECONOMIC
DIFFERENCES IN YOUNG PEOPLE'S HEALTH AND WELL-BEING
PART 2. KEY DATA | CHAPTER 5. RISK BEHAVIOURS
FIGHTING

5

13-year-olds who have been involved in a physical fight at least three times in the last 12 months

HBSC survey 2013/2014

- BOYS (%)
- GIRLS (%)

Country	GIRLS	BOYS
Armenia	3	36
Belgium (French)	9	21
Slovakia	7	22
Czech Republic	6	23
Albania	7	21
Austria	4	24
Malta	10	16
Hungary	7	19
Romania	6	20
Poland	7	18
Republic of Moldova	5	19
Croatia	7	18
Bulgaria	6	17
Russian Federation	7	17
Slovenia	5	17
Latvia	4	19
Ukraine	4	18
Denmark	4	18
Germany	4	16
Canada	5	15
France	6	14
England	6	13
Wales	7	12
Greece	5	13
Israel	3	15
Luxembourg	5	14
Lithuania	3	14
Ireland	4	14
Italy	4	12
Spain	5	11
Norway	2	13
Scotland	5	10
MKD[a]	3	12
Netherlands	3	11
Estonia	3	11
Switzerland	3	12
Iceland	3	10
Sweden	3	10
Belgium (Flemish)	3	9
Finland	4	8
Portugal	2	9
Greenland	3	6
HBSC average (gender)	5	15
HBSC average (total)		10

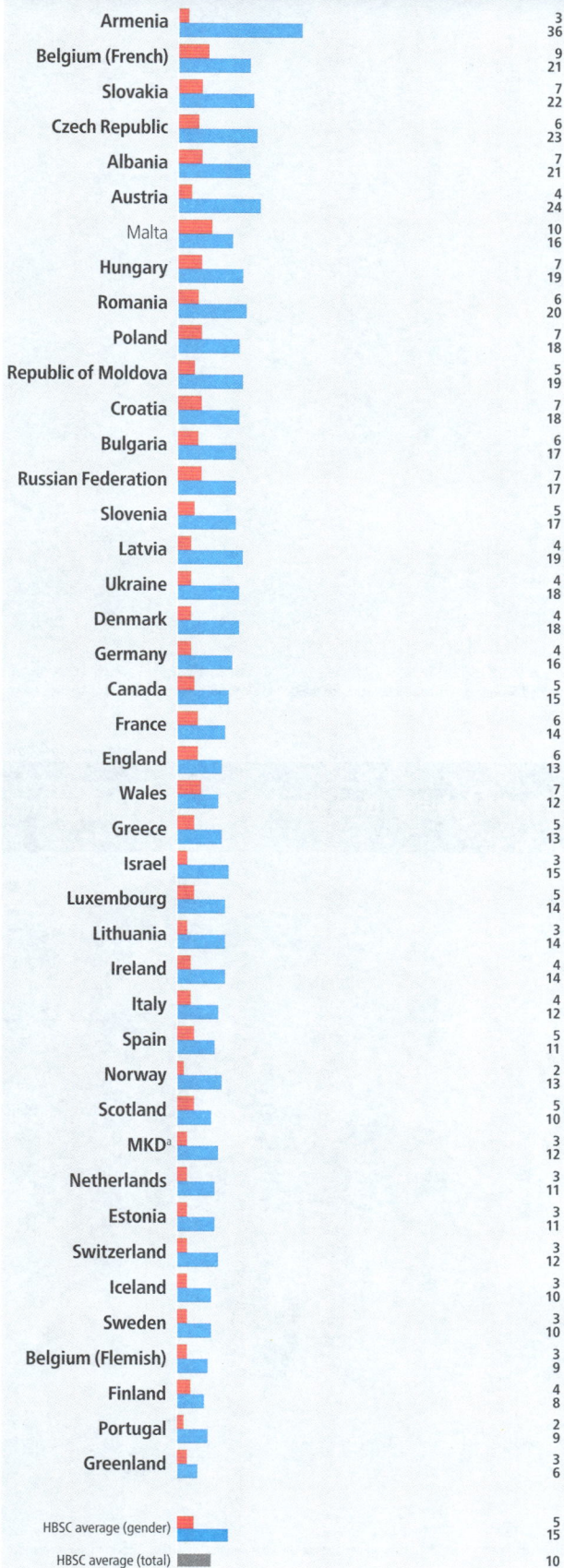

15-year-olds who have been involved in a physical fight at least three times in the last 12 months

HBSC survey 2013/2014

- BOYS (%)
- GIRLS (%)

Country	GIRLS	BOYS
Armenia	3	36
Albania	6	24
Bulgaria	6	20
Slovakia	6	19
Ukraine	4	20
Belgium (French)	7	14
Hungary	8	13
Republic of Moldova	4	17
Czech Republic	5	16
Russian Federation	5	16
Luxembourg	6	13
France	6	12
Malta	5	14
Romania	4	16
Croatia	3	14
Denmark	4	14
Ireland	5	15
Poland	4	14
Greece	4	14
Lithuania	3	13
Latvia	4	14
Austria	4	14
MKD[a]	3	13
England	4	11
Canada	5	10
Israel	3	13
Belgium (Flemish)	4	9
Germany	3	11
Slovenia	5	10
Wales	5	9
Scotland	3	11
Estonia	2	11
Norway	3	10
Netherlands	4	9
Italy	2	10
Spain	3	8
Iceland	3	7
Sweden	2	7
Portugal	2	8
Finland	2	7
Switzerland	2	7
Greenland	0	4
HBSC average (gender)	4	12
HBSC average (total)		8

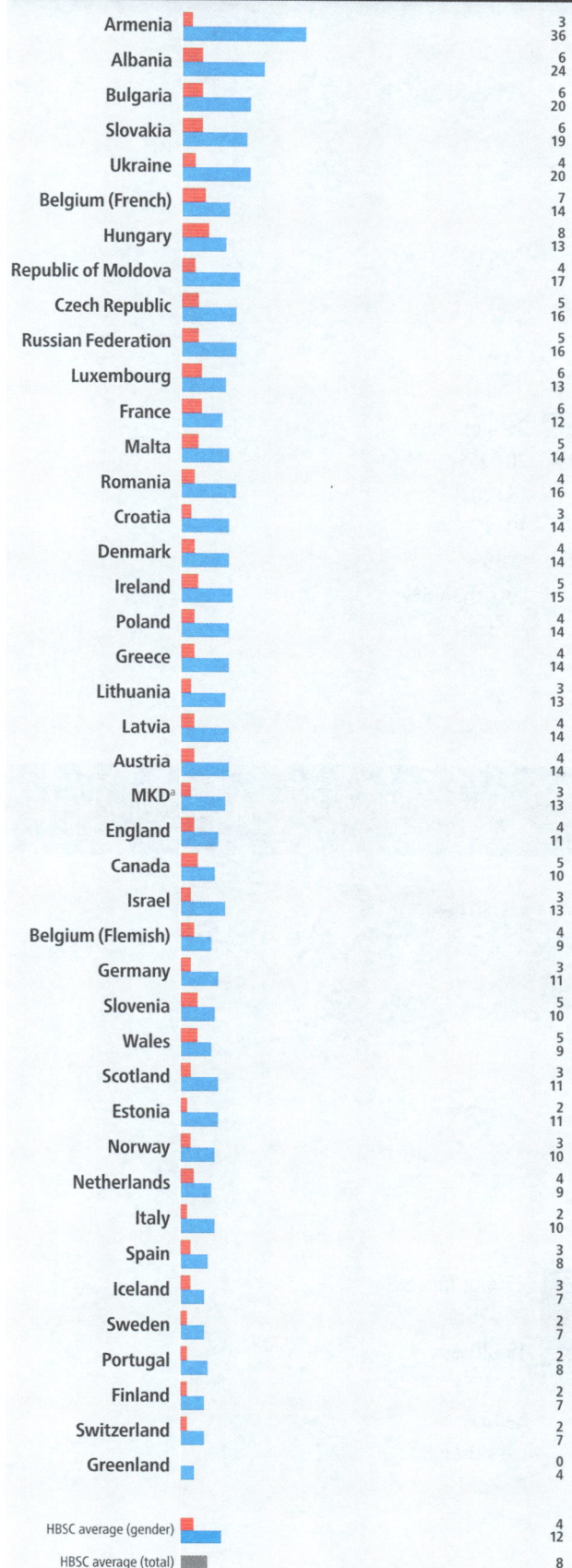

Note: **indicates** significant gender difference (at p<0.05).

HBSC survey 2013/2014

15-year-old girls who have been involved in a physical fight at least three times in the last 12 months

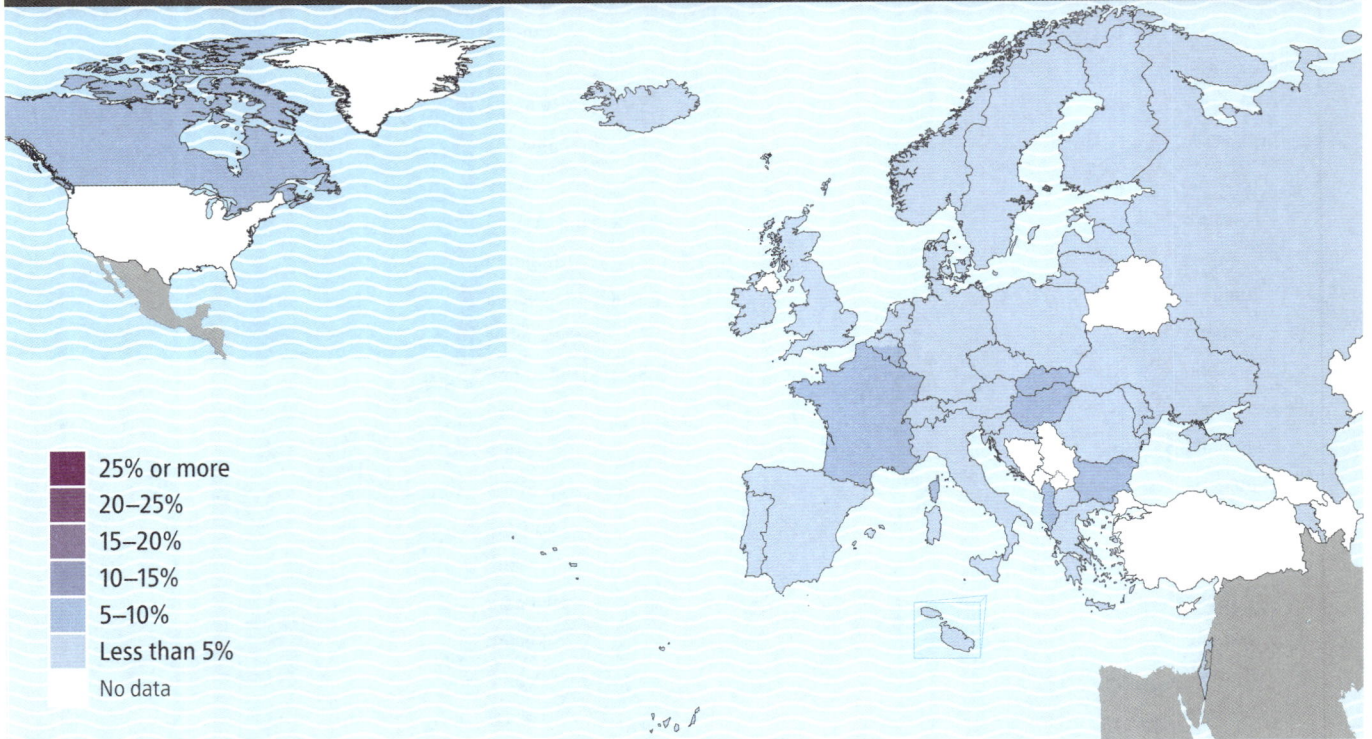

25% or more
20–25%
15–20%
10–15%
5–10%
Less than 5%
No data

Note: HBSC teams provided disaggregated data for Belgium and the United Kingdom; these data appear in the map above.

HBSC survey 2013/2014

15-year-old boys who have been involved in a physical fight at least three times in the last 12 months

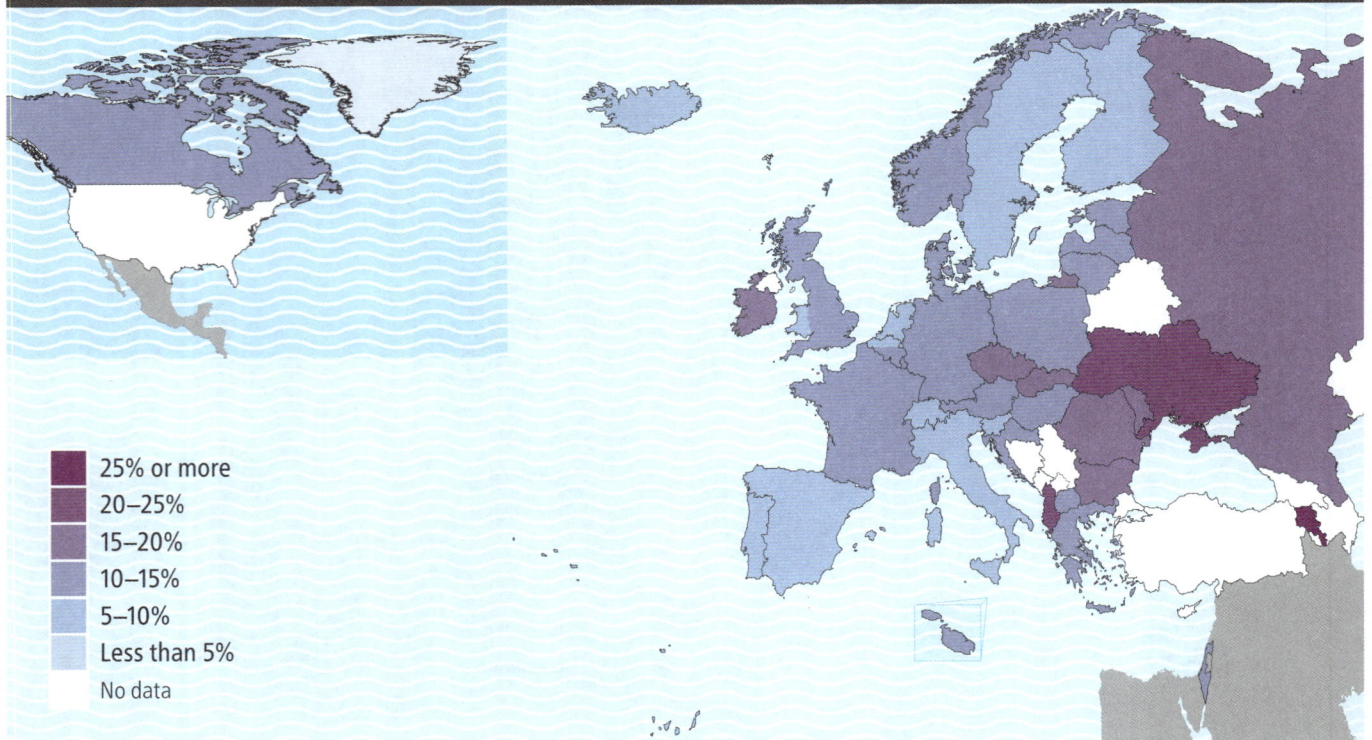

25% or more
20–25%
15–20%
10–15%
5–10%
Less than 5%
No data

Note: HBSC teams provided disaggregated data for Belgium and the United Kingdom; these data appear in the map above.

GROWING UP UNEQUAL: GENDER AND SOCIOECONOMIC
DIFFERENCES IN YOUNG PEOPLE'S HEALTH AND WELL-BEING
PART 2. KEY DATA | CHAPTER 5. RISK BEHAVIOURS
FIGHTING

5

FIGHTING:
SCIENTIFIC DISCUSSION AND POLICY REFLECTIONS

SCIENTIFIC DISCUSSION

The findings suggest a continuation of the positive downward trend in fighting among young people *(1)*. This may be a result of prevention initiatives in schools *(8)*, but prevalence rates differ dramatically across countries and regions, suggesting variations in cultural norms relating to fighting and the success of intervention programmes *(1)*.

As with previous findings, levels (notably among boys) decrease with age *(9)*. Adolescents may develop the cognitive, emotional, behavioural and verbal resources to cope with frustrations and conflicts in a more constructive and less physical manner as they become older.

Findings confirm previous research that shows boys are involved more than girls *(10)*, but there is no clear relationship with family affluence across countries and regions.

POLICY REFLECTIONS

Violence is a leading cause of death and physical injury for young people *(11)*. The main risk factors for involvement are male gender, younger age, bullying victimization, national homicide rates and poverty. In addition, multiple risk behaviours (such as alcohol use and smoking) are associated with violence *(1,12)*. Social and school support seem to act as protective factors *(12)*. Risk and protective factors may vary by race and ethnicity *(12)*.

Prevention programmes should begin early and be developed with a gendered lens *(1)*. Approaches that have proven effective include:

- universal school-based violence-prevention programmes, which provide students and school staff with information about violence, change how young people think and feel about it, and teach non-violent skills to resolve disputes;
- parenting-skill and family-relationship approaches, providing caregivers with support and teaching communication, problem-solving, monitoring and behaviour-management skills;
- intensive family-focused approaches that offer therapeutic services to high-risk chronic young offenders and their families to address individual, family, school and community factors that contribute to violence and delinquency;
- policy, environmental and structural approaches that create changes in community environments to enhance safety and affect risk and protective factors among young people; and
- early childhood education and care, which provides high-quality support to disadvantaged children and helps build a strong foundation for future learning and healthy development *(11)*.

REFERENCES

1. Pickett W, Molcho M, Elgar FJ, Brooks F, de Looze M, Rathmann K et al. Trends and socioeconomic correlates of adolescent physical fighting in 30 countries. Pediatrics 2013;131(1):e18–e26.
2. Walsh SD, Molcho M, Craig W, Harel-Fisch Y, Huynh Q, Kukaswadia A et al. Physical and emotional health problems experienced by youth engaged in physical fighting and weapon carrying. PloS ONE 2013;8(2):e56403.
3. Pickett W, Iannotti RJ, Simons-Morton B, Iannotti RJ. Social environments and physical aggression among 21,107 students in the United States and Canada. J Sch Health 2009;79(4):160–68.
4. Swahn MH, Donovan JE. Correlates and predictors of violent behavior among adolescent drinkers. J Adolesc Health 2004;34(6):480–92.
5. Sosin DM, Koepsell TD, Rivara FP, Mercy GA. Fighting as a marker for multiple problem behaviors in adolescents. J Adolesc Health 1995;16(3):209–15.
6. Resnick MD, Ireland M, Borowsky I. Youth violence perpetration: what protects? What predicts? Findings from the National Longitudinal Study of Adolescent Health. J Adolesc Health 2004;35(5):424.
7. Elgar FJ, Aitken N. Income inequality, trust and homicide in 33 countries. Eur J Public Health 2011;21(2):241–46.
8. Mytton JA, DiGuiseppi C, Gough D, Taylor R, Logan S. School-based secondary prevention programmes for preventing violence. Cochrane Database Syst Rev. 2006;3(3):CD004606.
9. Zahn-Waxler C, Park JH, Usher B, Belouad F, Cole P, Gruber R. Young children's representations of conflict and distress: a longitudinal study of boys and girls with disruptive behavior problems. Dev Psychopathol. 2008;20(1):99–119.

10. Dukes RL, Stein JA, Zane JI. Gender differences in the relative impact of physical and relational bullying on adolescent injury and weapon carrying. J Sch Psychol. 2010;48(6):511–32.

11. David-Ferdon C, Simon TR. Preventing youth violence: opportunities for action. Atlanta (GA): National Center for Injury Prevention and Control, Centers for Disease Control and Prevention; 2014 (http://www.cdc.gov/violenceprevention/youthviolence/pdf/opportunities-for-action.pdf, accessed 24 August 2015).

12. Shetgiri R, Kataoka S, Ponce N, Flores G, Chung PJ. Adolescent fighting: racial/ethnic disparities and the importance of families and schools. Acad Pediatr. 2010;10(5):323–9.

GROWING UP UNEQUAL: GENDER AND SOCIOECONOMIC
DIFFERENCES IN YOUNG PEOPLE'S HEALTH AND WELL-BEING
PART 2. KEY DATA | CHAPTER 5. RISK BEHAVIOURS

5

BULLYING:
BEING BULLIED AND BULLYING OTHERS

Short- and long-term effects of involvement in bullying, both as perpetrator and victim, have been documented. Involvement in bullying affects young people's physical health, resulting in somatic symptoms such as head, back and stomach aches *(1,2)*, psychological distress (depression, bad temper, nervousness, loneliness and suicidal ideation *(3–6)*) and long-term patterns of problem behaviour, including aggression, violence, problem drinking and substance use *(7–10)*. Young people involved in bullying report more negative school experiences *(11)*, reflected in poor relationships with peers and teachers.

Despite recent research showing positive trends towards a decrease in bullying victimization *(12)*, studies have particularly emphasized the negative mental health outcomes of being a victim, which include psychological maladjustment, psychosomatic health problems and suicide *(13,14)*. The risk for suicide is particularly high when harassment is prejudice-based, such as when related to race or sexual orientation *(15)*. Negative internalized emotions can also lead some young victims towards alcohol and/or substance misuse *(16)*.

MEASURES

Being bullied
Young people were asked how often they had been bullied at school in the past couple of months. The question was preceded by the following definition of bullying *(17)*:

We say a student is being bullied when another student, or a group of students, say or do nasty and unpleasant things to him or her. It is also bullying when a student is teased repeatedly in a way he or she does not like or when he or she is deliberately left out of things. But it is not bullying when two students of about the same strength or power argue or fight. It is also not bullying when a student is teased in a friendly and playful way.

Response options ranged from zero to several times a week.

Supplementary data on being bullied at school at least once in the past couple of months are provided in the Annex.

Bullying others
Young people were asked how often they had taken part in bullying (an)other student(s) at school in the past couple of months, using the same definition *(17)*. Response options ranged from zero to several times a week.

Supplementary data on bullying others at school at least once in the past couple of months are provided in the Annex.

HBSC survey 2013/2014

**Associations between family affluence and indicators of health, by country/region and gender:
being a victim of bullying at school at least two or three times
a month in the past couple of months**

BOYS
GIRLS

SIGNIFICANT
TRENDS

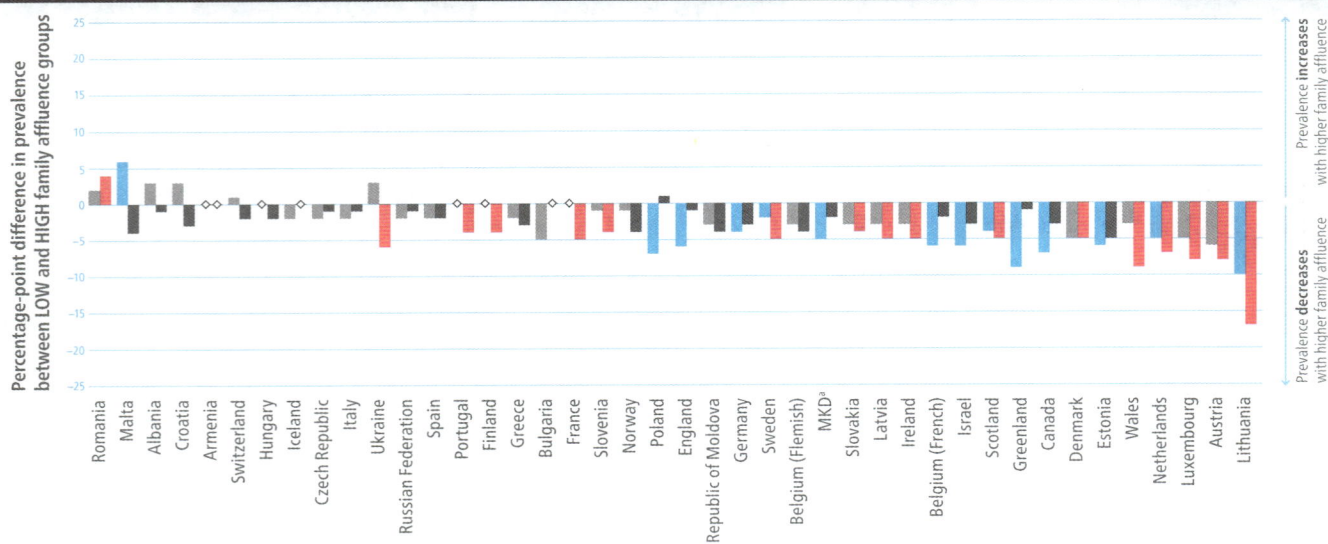

*The former Yugoslav Republic of Macedonia. *Note:* low- and high-affluence groups represent the lowest 20% and highest 20% in each country. ◇ means less than +/-0.5%.

GROWING UP UNEQUAL: GENDER AND SOCIOECONOMIC
DIFFERENCES IN YOUNG PEOPLE'S HEALTH AND WELL-BEING
PART 2. KEY DATA | CHAPTER 5. RISK BEHAVIOURS
BULLYING: BEING BULLIED AND BULLYING OTHERS

5

HBSC survey 2013/2014

Associations between family affluence and indicators of health, by country/region and gender:
**bullying others at school at least two or three times
a month in the past couple of months**

BOYS
GIRLS

SIGNIFICANT
TRENDS

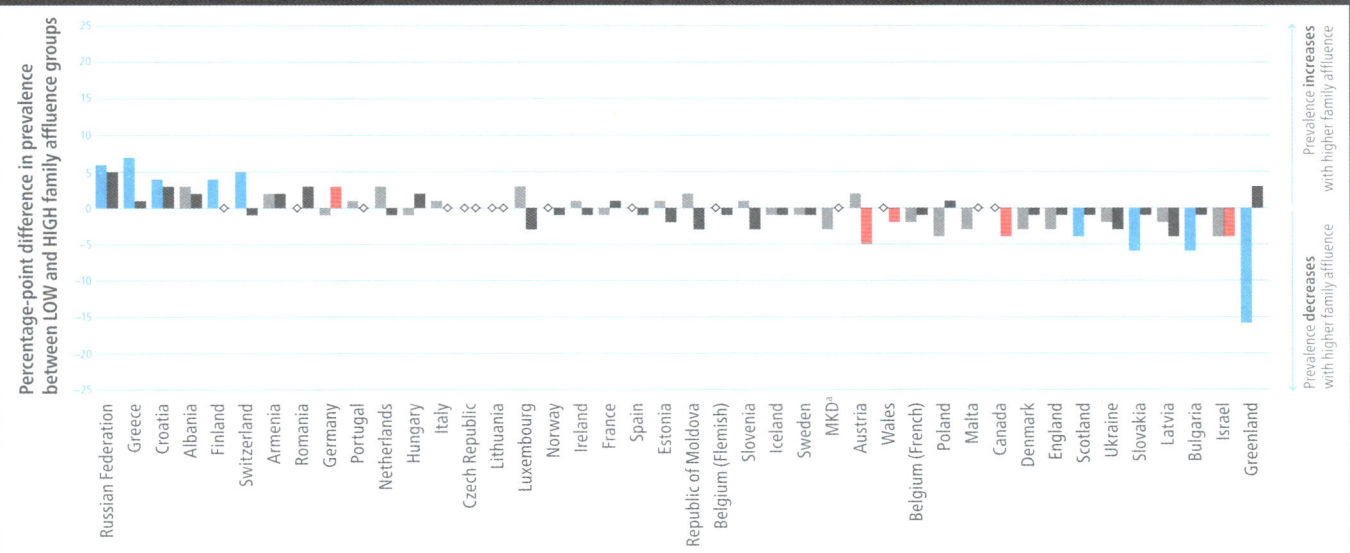

ᵃ The former Yugoslav Republic of Macedonia. *Note:* low- and high-affluence groups represent the lowest 20% and highest 20% in each country. ◇ means less than +/-0.5%.

RESULTS

Being bullied

Findings presented here show the proportions who reported being bullied at school at least two or three times a month in the past couple of months.

Age

Overall prevalence was around 12% for boys and 10% for girls. Significant changes across ages were seen in most countries and regions (almost all for boys). With very few exceptions, being bullied decreased as age increased, peaking for boys at 11 and dropping to the lowest levels at 15. Levels for girls were constant at ages 11 and 13 and dropped at 15. Very large cross-national differences were observed, with high prevalence in some countries and low in others.

Gender

Gender differences were seen in around a third of countries and regions. Generally, boys were bullied more, with findings suggesting different age-related patterns of victimization for boys and girls. Bullying peaked at age 13 for girls and 11 for boys.

Family affluence

Being bullied varied with family affluence in some countries and regions, involving lower bullying victimization with increasing affluence in virtually all cases.

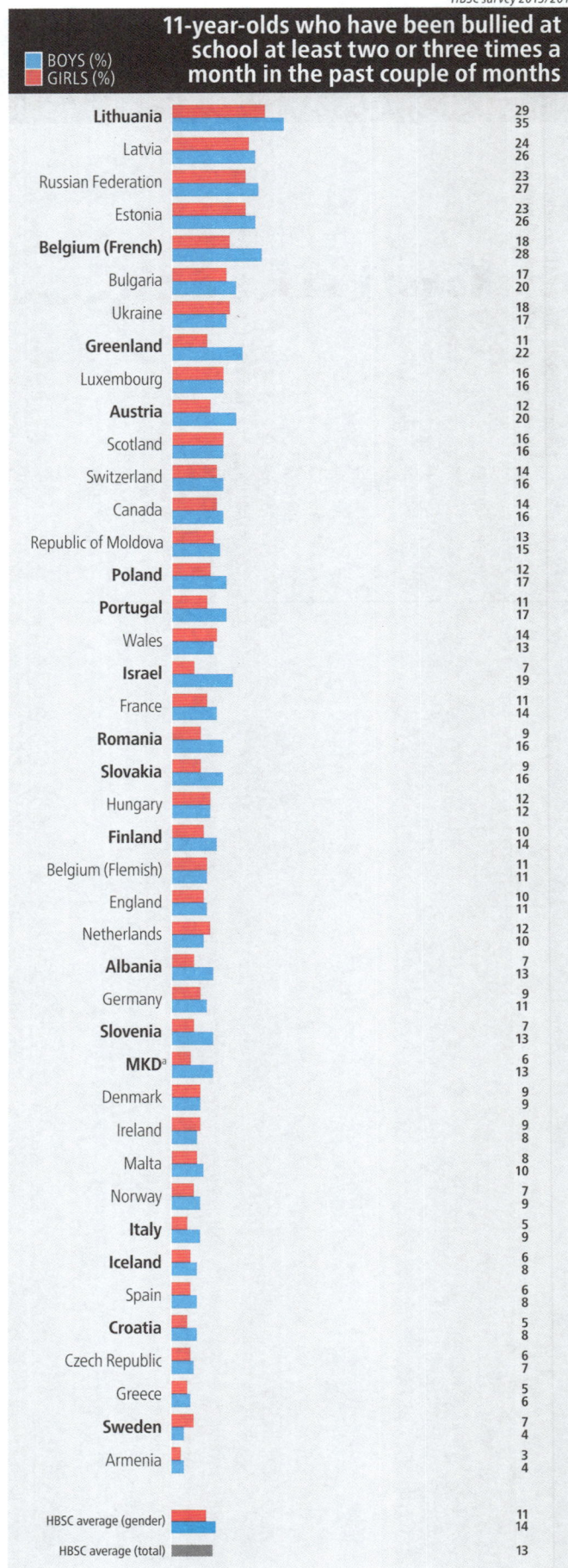

HBSC survey 2013/2014

11-year-olds who have been bullied at school at least two or three times a month in the past couple of months

BOYS (%)
GIRLS (%)

Country	Boys	Girls
Lithuania	35	29
Latvia	24	26
Russian Federation	23	27
Estonia	23	26
Belgium (French)	18	28
Bulgaria	17	20
Ukraine	18	17
Greenland	11	22
Luxembourg	16	16
Austria	12	20
Scotland	16	16
Switzerland	14	16
Canada	14	16
Republic of Moldova	13	15
Poland	12	17
Portugal	11	17
Wales	14	13
Israel	7	19
France	11	14
Romania	9	16
Slovakia	9	16
Hungary	12	12
Finland	10	14
Belgium (Flemish)	11	11
England	10	11
Netherlands	12	10
Albania	7	13
Germany	9	11
Slovenia	7	13
MKD[a]	6	13
Denmark	9	9
Ireland	9	8
Malta	8	10
Norway	7	9
Italy	5	9
Iceland	6	8
Spain	6	8
Croatia	5	8
Czech Republic	6	7
Greece	5	6
Sweden	7	4
Armenia	3	4
HBSC average (gender)	11	14
HBSC average (total)	13	

[a] The former Yugoslav Republic of Macedonia.

GROWING UP UNEQUAL: GENDER AND SOCIOECONOMIC
DIFFERENCES IN YOUNG PEOPLE'S HEALTH AND WELL-BEING
PART 2. KEY DATA | CHAPTER 5. RISK BEHAVIOURS
BULLYING: BEING BULLIED AND BULLYING OTHERS

5

HBSC survey 2013/2014

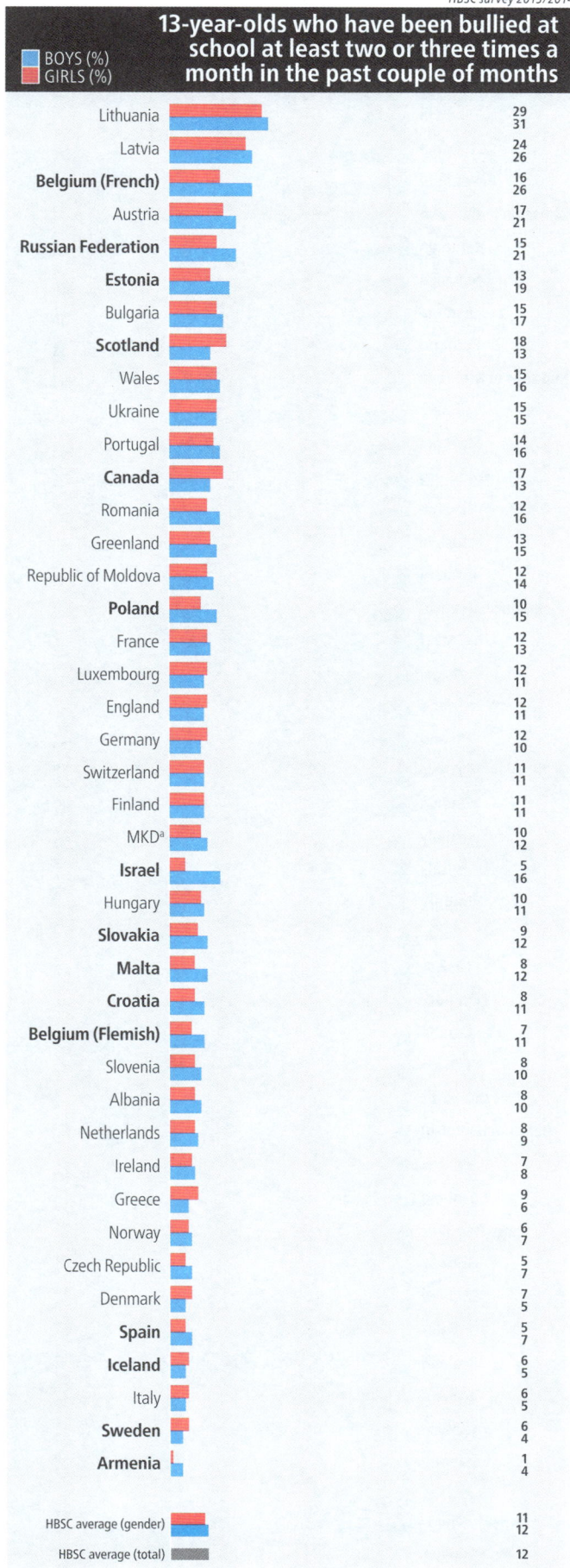

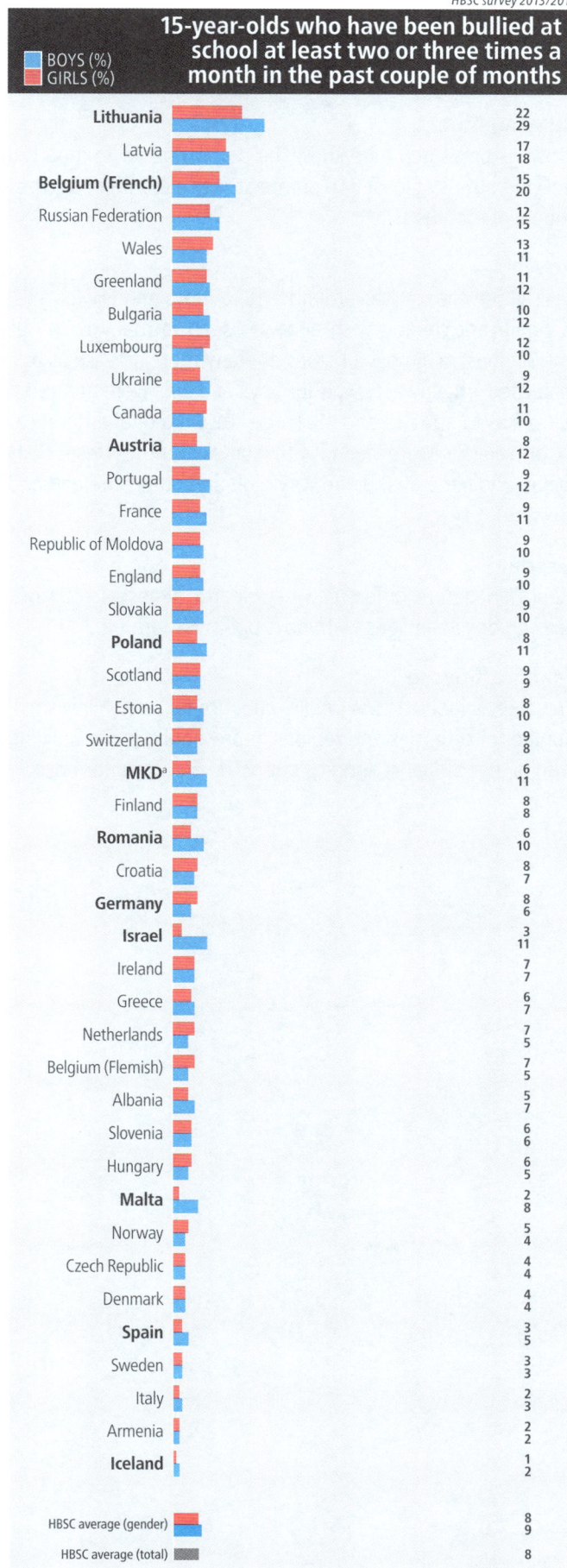

13-year-olds who have been bullied at school at least two or three times a month in the past couple of months

- BOYS (%)
- GIRLS (%)

Country	Girls	Boys
Lithuania	29	31
Latvia	24	26
Belgium (French)	16	26
Austria	17	21
Russian Federation	15	21
Estonia	13	19
Bulgaria	15	17
Scotland	18	13
Wales	15	16
Ukraine	15	15
Portugal	14	16
Canada	17	13
Romania	12	16
Greenland	13	15
Republic of Moldova	12	14
Poland	10	15
France	12	13
Luxembourg	12	11
England	12	11
Germany	12	10
Switzerland	11	11
Finland	11	11
MKD[a]	10	12
Israel	5	16
Hungary	10	11
Slovakia	9	12
Malta	8	12
Croatia	8	11
Belgium (Flemish)	7	11
Slovenia	8	10
Albania	8	10
Netherlands	8	9
Ireland	7	8
Greece	9	6
Norway	6	7
Czech Republic	5	7
Denmark	7	5
Spain	5	7
Iceland	6	5
Italy	6	5
Sweden	6	4
Armenia	1	4
HBSC average (gender)	11	12
HBSC average (total)		12

HBSC survey 2013/2014

15-year-olds who have been bullied at school at least two or three times a month in the past couple of months

- BOYS (%)
- GIRLS (%)

Country	Girls	Boys
Lithuania	22	29
Latvia	17	18
Belgium (French)	15	20
Russian Federation	12	15
Wales	13	11
Greenland	11	12
Bulgaria	10	12
Luxembourg	12	10
Ukraine	9	12
Canada	11	10
Austria	8	12
Portugal	9	12
France	9	11
Republic of Moldova	9	10
England	9	10
Slovakia	9	10
Poland	8	11
Scotland	9	9
Estonia	8	10
Switzerland	9	8
MKD[a]	6	11
Finland	8	8
Romania	6	10
Croatia	8	7
Germany	8	6
Israel	3	11
Ireland	7	7
Greece	6	7
Netherlands	7	5
Belgium (Flemish)	7	5
Albania	5	7
Slovenia	6	6
Hungary	6	5
Malta	2	8
Norway	5	4
Czech Republic	4	4
Denmark	4	4
Spain	3	5
Sweden	3	3
Italy	2	3
Armenia	2	2
Iceland	1	2
HBSC average (gender)	8	9
HBSC average (total)		8

Note: **indicates** significant gender difference (at p<0.05).

RESULTS

Bullying others

Findings presented here show the proportions who reported bullying others at least two or three times a month in the past couple of months.

Age

Overall prevalence was around 11% for boys and 6% for girls. A significant change with age was seen in many countries and regions; in almost all cases, there was an increase as age increased. The lowest levels for boys and girls were at age 11, with rises to ages 13 and 15. Large cross-national differences in prevalence were seen, with some countries (especially Latvia and Lithuania) being very high and others (Ireland and Sweden) very low.

Gender

Significant gender differences were seen in almost all countries and regions at all ages, with boys bullying more.

Family affluence

Prevalence varied across family affluence for a relatively small number of countries and regions, representing lower bullying with higher affluence for girls but no clear pattern for boys.

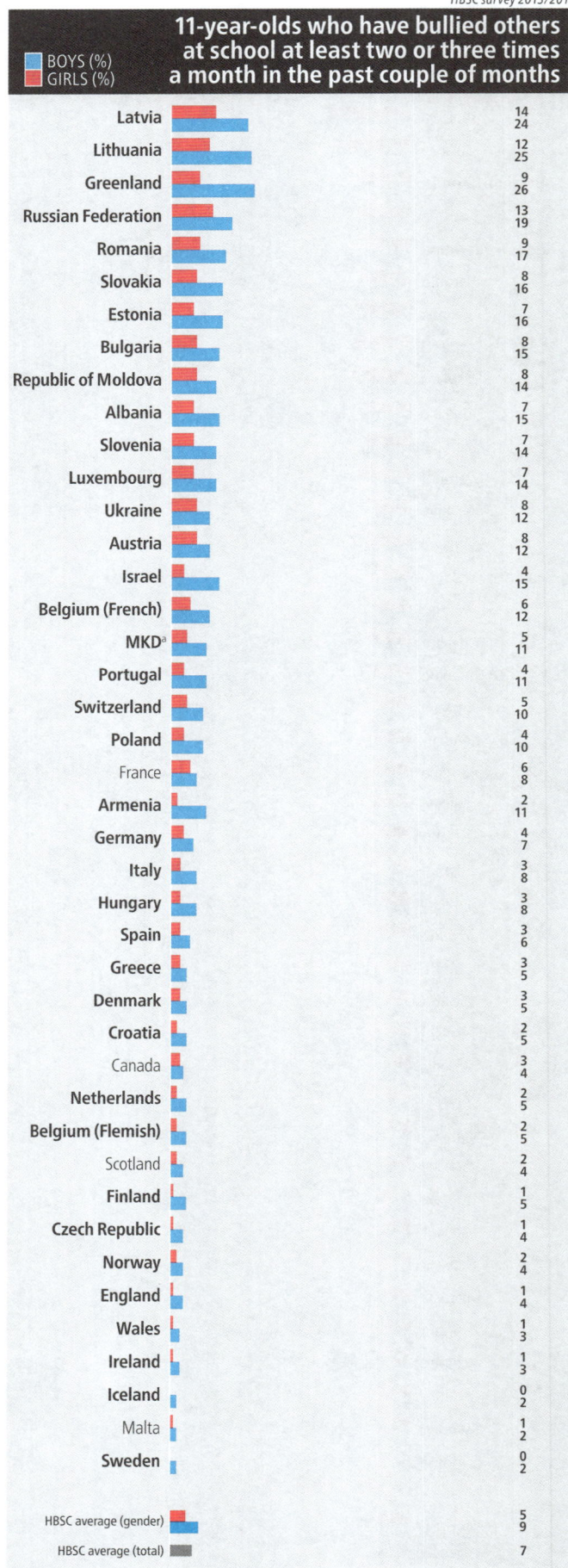

HBSC survey 2013/2014

11-year-olds who have bullied others at school at least two or three times a month in the past couple of months

BOYS (%)
GIRLS (%)

Country	Boys (%)	Girls (%)
Latvia	24	14
Lithuania	25	12
Greenland	26	9
Russian Federation	19	13
Romania	17	9
Slovakia	16	8
Estonia	16	7
Bulgaria	15	8
Republic of Moldova	14	8
Albania	15	7
Slovenia	14	7
Luxembourg	14	7
Ukraine	12	8
Austria	12	8
Israel	15	4
Belgium (French)	12	6
MKD[a]	11	5
Portugal	11	4
Switzerland	10	5
Poland	10	4
France	8	6
Armenia	11	2
Germany	7	4
Italy	8	3
Hungary	8	3
Spain	6	3
Greece	5	3
Denmark	5	3
Croatia	5	2
Canada	4	3
Netherlands	5	2
Belgium (Flemish)	5	2
Scotland	4	2
Finland	5	1
Czech Republic	4	1
Norway	4	2
England	4	1
Wales	3	1
Ireland	3	1
Iceland	2	0
Malta	2	1
Sweden	2	0
HBSC average (gender)	9	5
HBSC average (total)	7	

[a] The former Yugoslav Republic of Macedonia.

GROWING UP UNEQUAL: GENDER AND SOCIOECONOMIC
DIFFERENCES IN YOUNG PEOPLE'S HEALTH AND WELL-BEING
PART 2. KEY DATA | CHAPTER 5. RISK BEHAVIOURS
BULLYING: BEING BULLIED AND BULLYING OTHERS

5

13-year-olds who have bullied others at school at least two or three times a month in the past couple of months

HBSC survey 2013/2014

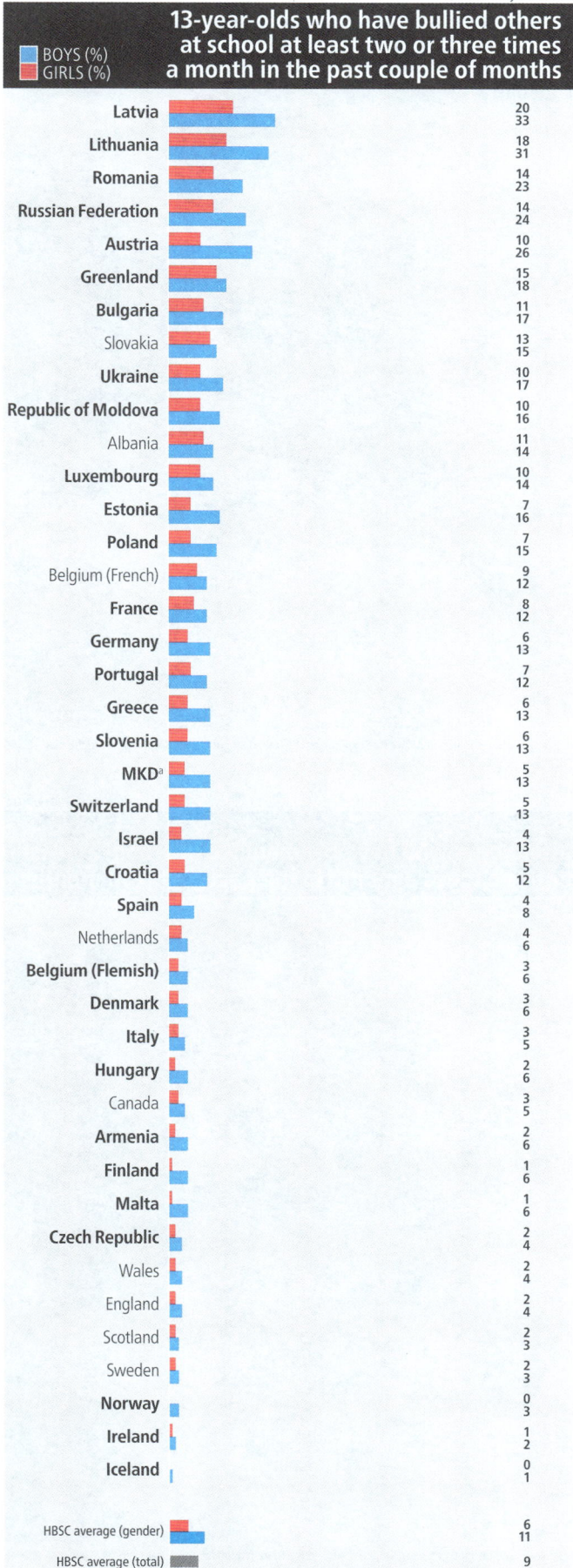

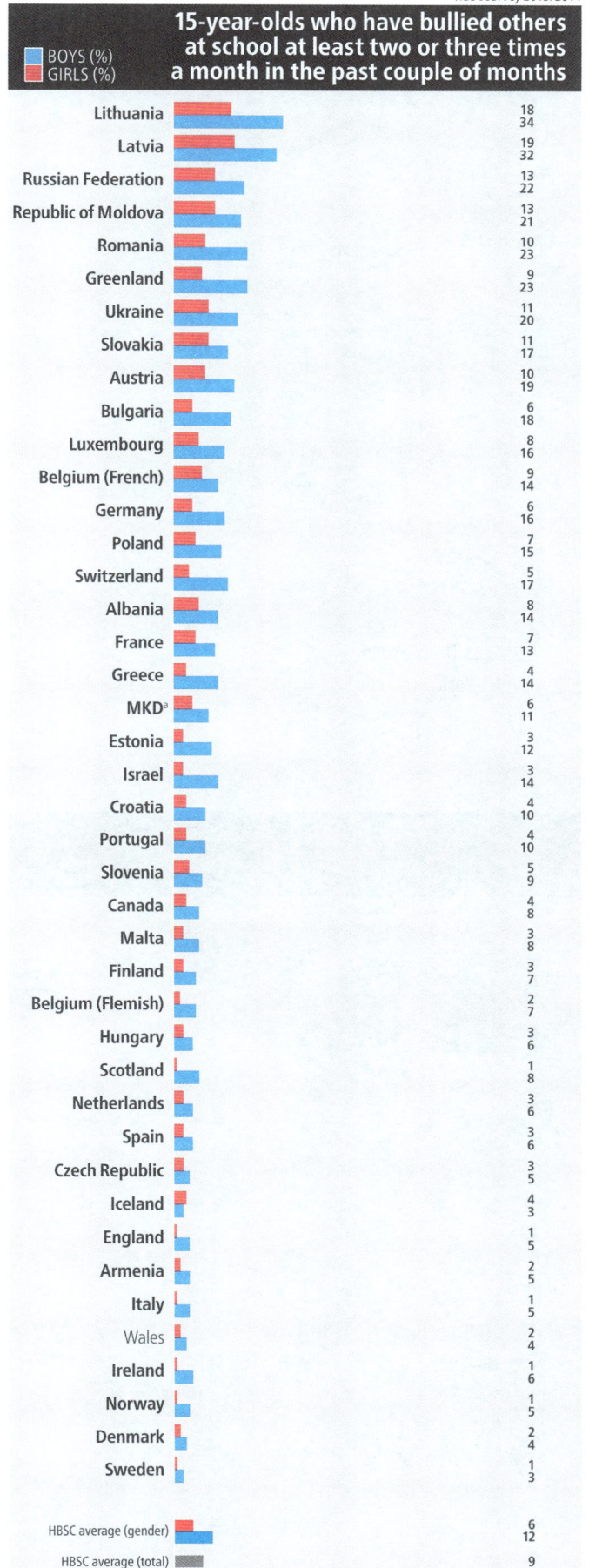

Legend: BOYS (%) / GIRLS (%)

Country	Boys (%)	Girls (%)
Latvia	20	33
Lithuania	18	31
Romania	14	23
Russian Federation	14	24
Austria	10	26
Greenland	15	18
Bulgaria	11	17
Slovakia	13	15
Ukraine	10	17
Republic of Moldova	10	16
Albania	11	14
Luxembourg	10	14
Estonia	7	16
Poland	7	15
Belgium (French)	9	12
France	8	12
Germany	6	13
Portugal	7	12
Greece	6	13
Slovenia	6	13
MKD[a]	5	13
Switzerland	5	13
Israel	4	13
Croatia	5	12
Spain	4	8
Netherlands	4	6
Belgium (Flemish)	3	6
Denmark	3	6
Italy	3	5
Hungary	2	6
Canada	3	5
Armenia	2	6
Finland	1	6
Malta	1	6
Czech Republic	2	4
Wales	2	4
England	2	4
Scotland	2	3
Sweden	2	3
Norway	0	3
Ireland	1	2
Iceland	0	1
HBSC average (gender)	6	11
HBSC average (total)	9	

15-year-olds who have bullied others at school at least two or three times a month in the past couple of months

HBSC survey 2013/2014

Legend: BOYS (%) / GIRLS (%)

Country	Boys (%)	Girls (%)
Lithuania	18	34
Latvia	19	32
Russian Federation	13	22
Republic of Moldova	13	21
Romania	10	23
Greenland	9	23
Ukraine	11	20
Slovakia	11	17
Austria	10	19
Bulgaria	6	18
Luxembourg	8	16
Belgium (French)	9	14
Germany	6	16
Poland	7	15
Switzerland	5	17
Albania	8	14
France	7	13
Greece	4	14
MKD[a]	6	11
Estonia	3	12
Israel	3	14
Croatia	4	10
Portugal	4	10
Slovenia	5	9
Canada	4	8
Malta	3	8
Finland	3	7
Belgium (Flemish)	2	7
Hungary	3	6
Scotland	1	8
Netherlands	3	6
Spain	3	6
Czech Republic	3	5
Iceland	4	3
England	1	5
Armenia	2	5
Italy	1	5
Wales	2	4
Ireland	1	6
Norway	1	5
Denmark	2	4
Sweden	1	3
HBSC average (gender)	6	12
HBSC average (total)	9	

Note: indicates significant gender difference (at p<0.05). 0 means less than +/-0.5%.

HBSC survey 2013/2014

15-year-old girls who have been bullied at school at least two or three times a month in the past couple of months

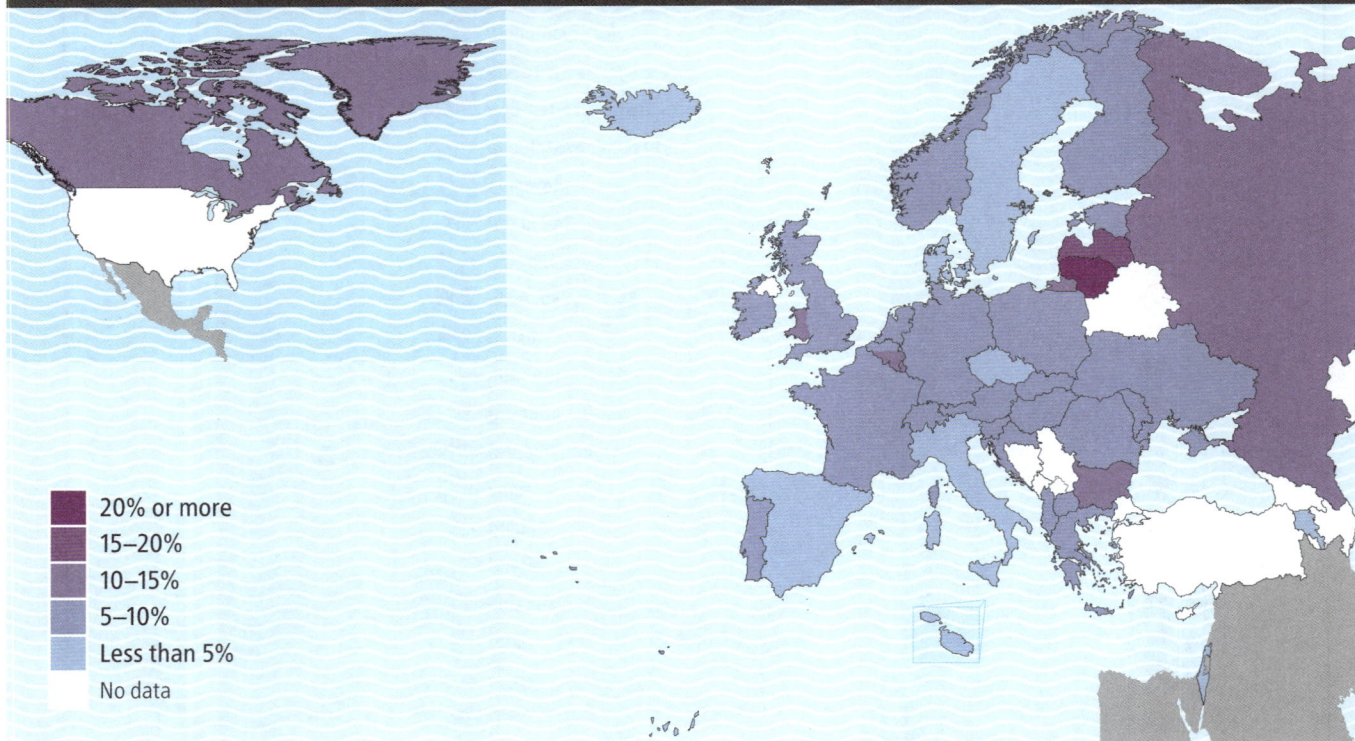

- 20% or more
- 15–20%
- 10–15%
- 5–10%
- Less than 5%
- No data

Note: HBSC teams provided disaggregated data for Belgium and the United Kingdom; these data appear in the map above.

HBSC survey 2013/2014

15-year-old boys who have been bullied at school at least two or three times a month in the past couple of months

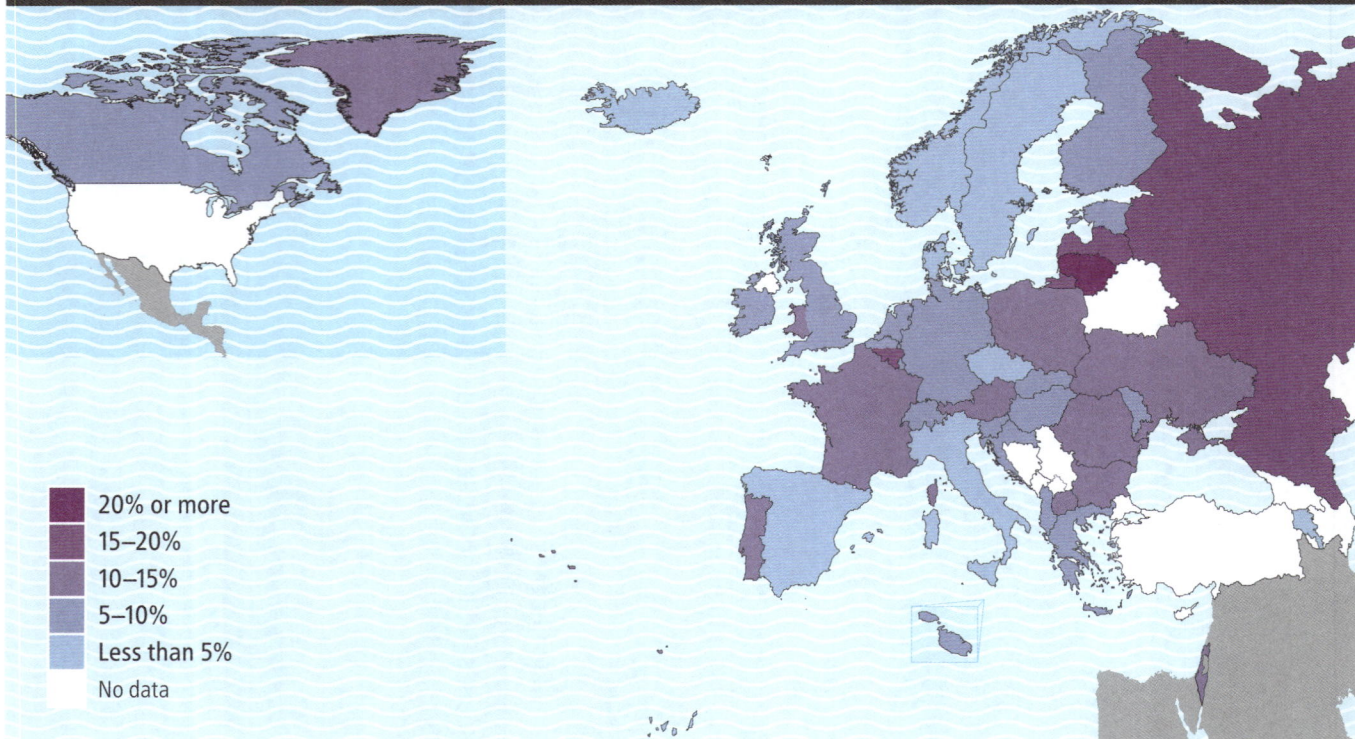

- 20% or more
- 15–20%
- 10–15%
- 5–10%
- Less than 5%
- No data

Note: HBSC teams provided disaggregated data for Belgium and the United Kingdom; these data appear in the map above.

GROWING UP UNEQUAL: GENDER AND SOCIOECONOMIC
DIFFERENCES IN YOUNG PEOPLE'S HEALTH AND WELL-BEING
PART 2. KEY DATA | CHAPTER 5. RISK BEHAVIOURS
BULLYING: BEING BULLIED AND BULLYING OTHERS

5

HBSC survey 2013/2014

15-year-old girls who have bullied others at school at least two or three times a month in the past couple of months

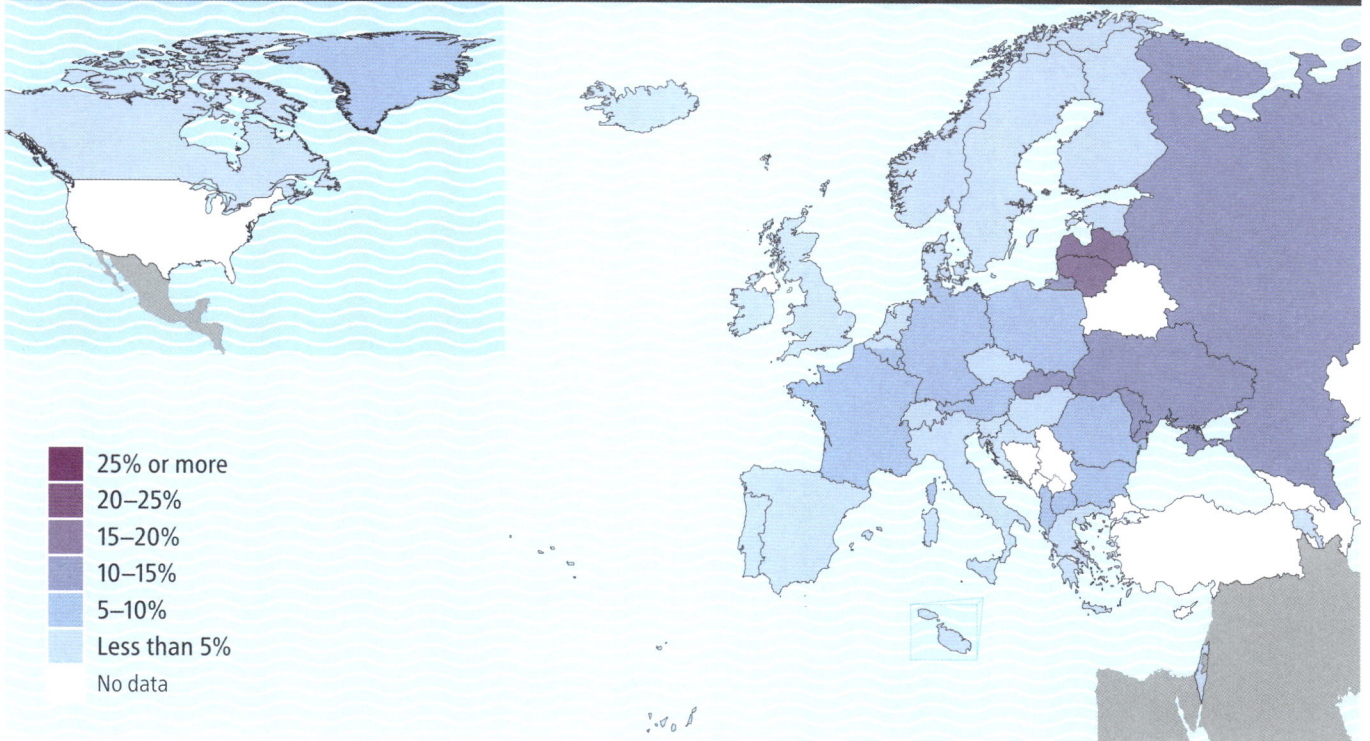

25% or more
20–25%
15–20%
10–15%
5–10%
Less than 5%
No data

Note: HBSC teams provided disaggregated data for Belgium and the United Kingdom; these data appear in the map above.

HBSC survey 2013/2014

15-year-old boys who have bullied others at school at least two or three times a month in the past couple of months

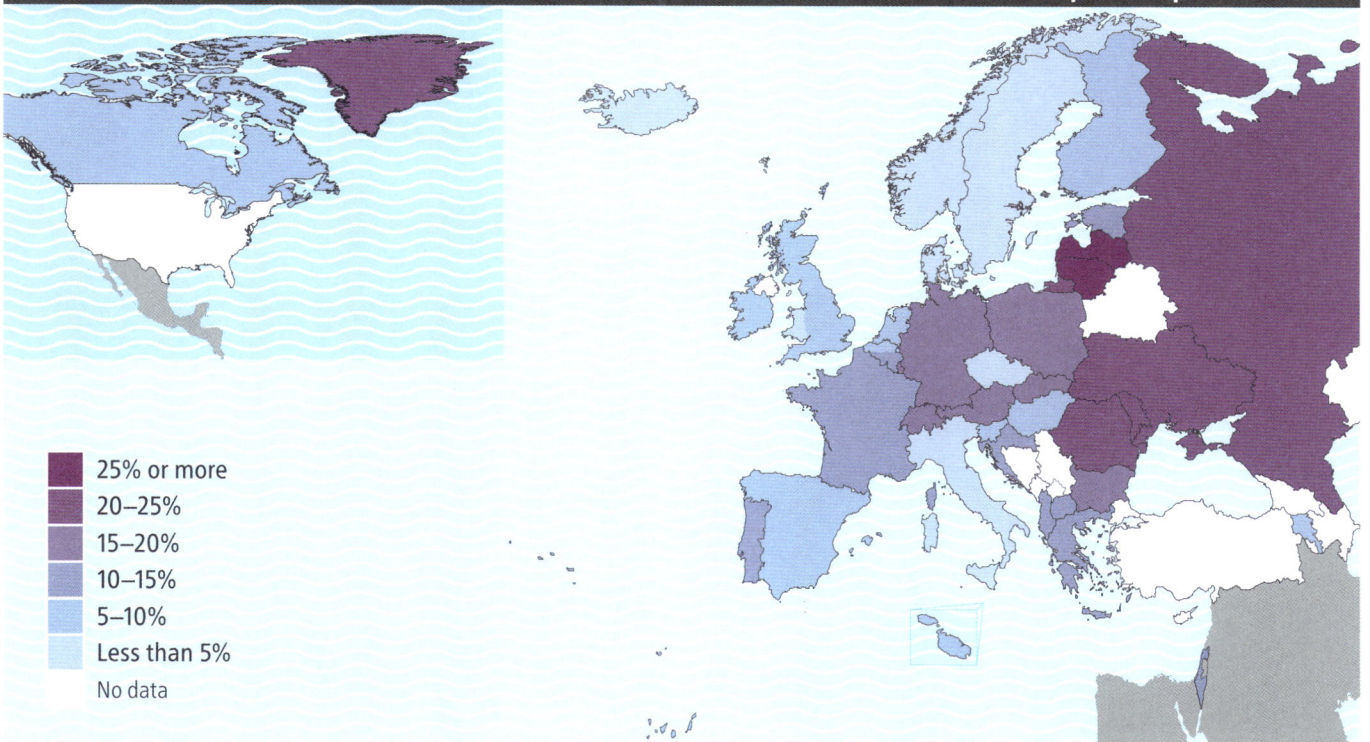

25% or more
20–25%
15–20%
10–15%
5–10%
Less than 5%
No data

Note: HBSC teams provided disaggregated data for Belgium and the United Kingdom; these data appear in the map above.

GROWING UP UNEQUAL: GENDER AND SOCIOECONOMIC
DIFFERENCES IN YOUNG PEOPLE'S HEALTH AND WELL-BEING
PART 2. KEY DATA | CHAPTER 5. RISK BEHAVIOURS

5

BULLYING:
CYBERBULLYING

Although research into cyberbullying is relatively nascent, clear and worrying relations have consistently been found between being a victim of cyberbullying and negative mental health outcomes such as depression, self-harm and suicidal ideation and attempts *(18,19)*.

Cyberbullying has also been related to negative academic achievement and school difficulties, violent behaviour, difficulties with peers, unsafe sex practices and involvement in substance use *(20–23)*.

HBSC survey 2013/2014

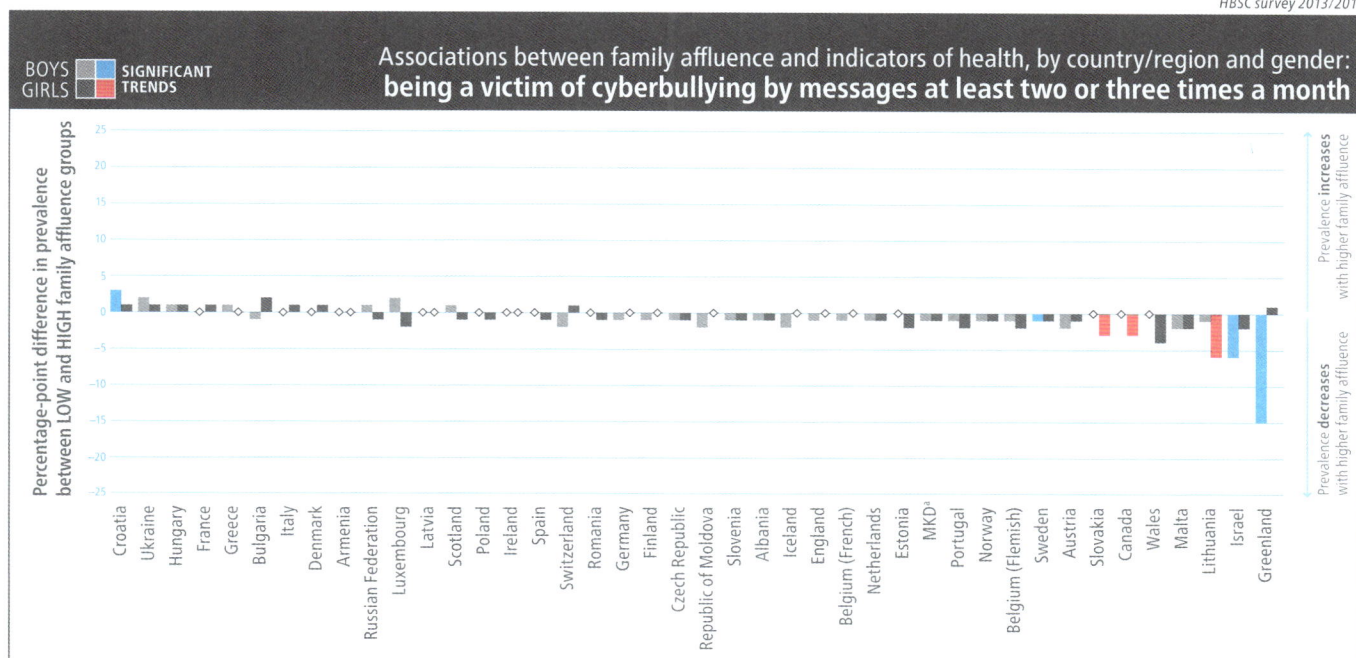

Associations between family affluence and indicators of health, by country/region and gender:
being a victim of cyberbullying by messages at least two or three times a month

ᵃThe former Yugoslav Republic of Macedonia. *Note:* low- and high-affluence groups represent the lowest 20% and highest 20% in each country. ◇ means less than +/-0.5%.

MEASURE

Young people were asked how often they had been bullied through someone sending mean instant messages, wall-postings, emails and text messages, or had created a website that made fun of them. Options ranged from not at all in the past couple of months to several times a week.

An additional item on whether someone had taken unflattering or inappropriate pictures of the young person without permission and posted them online was included in the HBSC 2013/2014 survey. A summary table of the results and supplementary data on being cyberbullied by messages at least once can be found in the Annex.

RESULTS

Findings presented here show the proportions who reported being a victim of cyberbullying at least two or three times a month.

Age

Prevalence was similar for boys and girls. The age effect was significant in a minority of countries and regions, in which levels were slightly higher at age 11 for boys and peaked for girls at 13. This generally represented a decrease over age for boys, but the pattern was less clear for girls. Some cross-national differences in prevalence were observed, but these were less marked than for more traditional forms of bullying.

Gender

Gender differences were seen in less than half of countries and regions, with no clear pattern emerging: some showed boys being cyberbullied more and others girls.

Family affluence

Differences according to family affluence were evident in very few countries and regions, in which cyberbullying was generally associated with lower affluence.

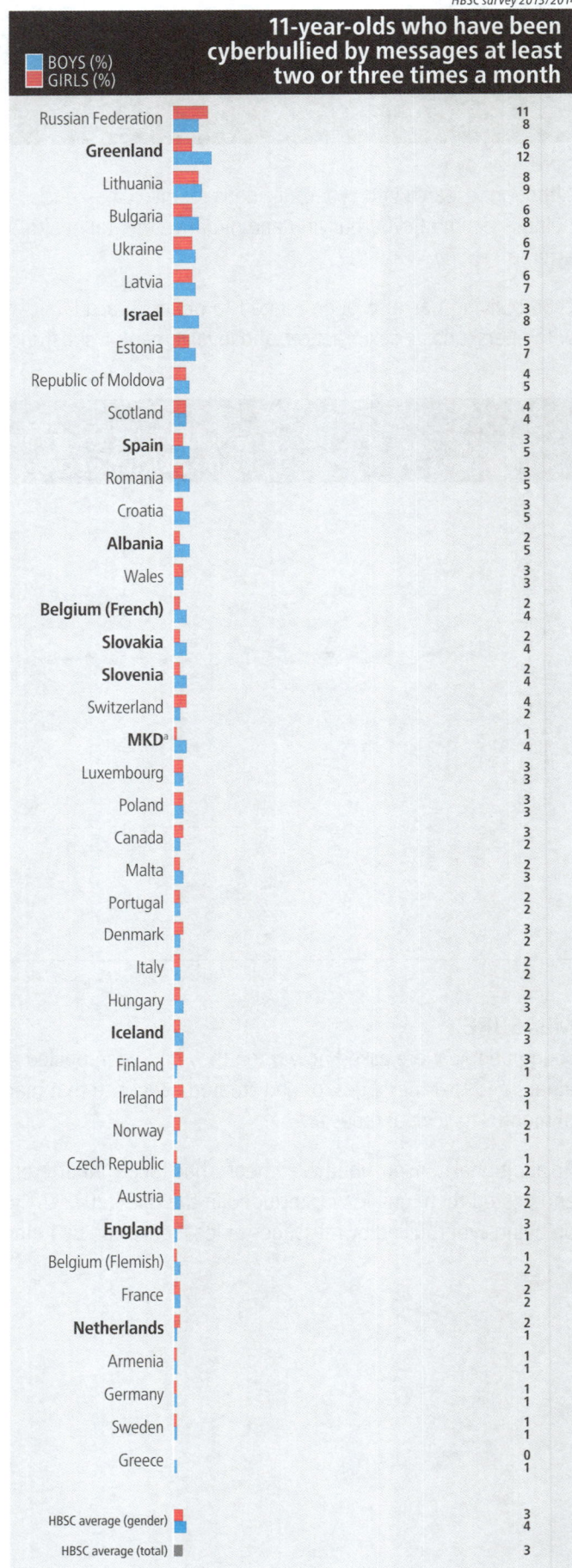

HBSC survey 2013/2014

11-year-olds who have been cyberbullied by messages at least two or three times a month

	BOYS (%)	GIRLS (%)
Russian Federation	11	8
Greenland	6	12
Lithuania	8	9
Bulgaria	6	8
Ukraine	6	7
Latvia	6	7
Israel	3	8
Estonia	5	7
Republic of Moldova	4	5
Scotland	4	4
Spain	3	5
Romania	3	5
Croatia	3	5
Albania	2	5
Wales	3	3
Belgium (French)	2	4
Slovakia	2	4
Slovenia	2	4
Switzerland	4	2
MKD[a]	1	4
Luxembourg	3	3
Poland	3	3
Canada	3	2
Malta	2	3
Portugal	2	2
Denmark	3	2
Italy	2	2
Hungary	2	3
Iceland	2	3
Finland	3	1
Ireland	3	1
Norway	2	1
Czech Republic	1	2
Austria	2	2
England	3	1
Belgium (Flemish)	1	2
France	2	2
Netherlands	2	1
Armenia	1	1
Germany	1	1
Sweden	1	1
Greece	0	1
HBSC average (gender)	3	4
HBSC average (total)	3	

[a] The former Yugoslav Republic of Macedonia.

GROWING UP UNEQUAL: GENDER AND SOCIOECONOMIC
DIFFERENCES IN YOUNG PEOPLE'S HEALTH AND WELL-BEING
PART 2. KEY DATA | CHAPTER 5. RISK BEHAVIOURS
BULLYING: CYBERBULLYING

5

HBSC survey 2013/2014

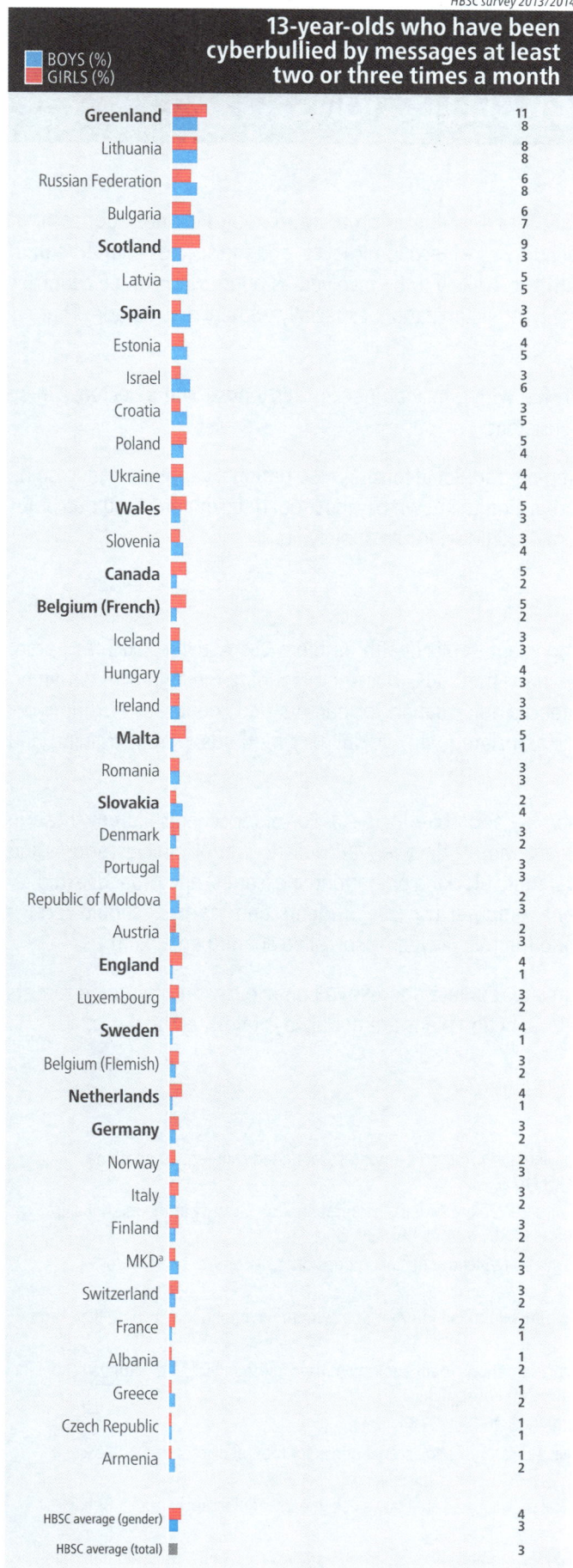

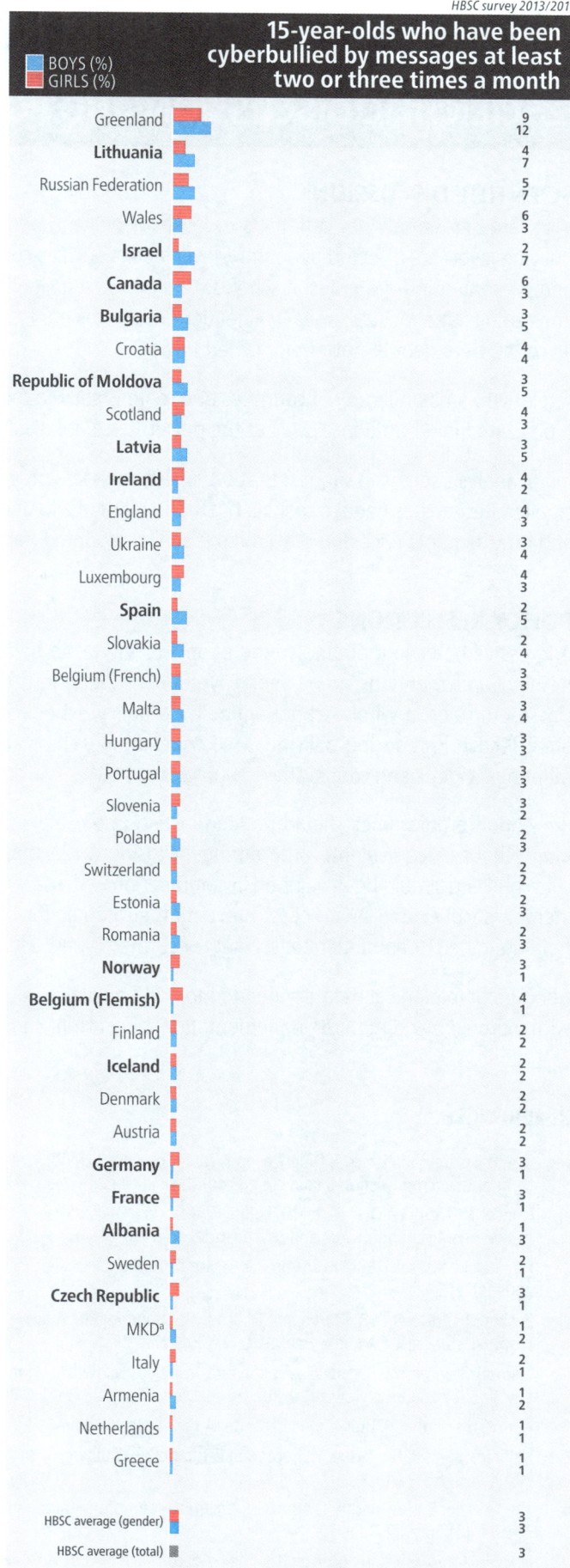

13-year-olds who have been cyberbullied by messages at least two or three times a month

- BOYS (%)
- GIRLS (%)

	Boys	Girls
Greenland		11 / 8
Lithuania		8 / 8
Russian Federation		6 / 8
Bulgaria		6 / 7
Scotland		9 / 3
Latvia		5 / 5
Spain		3 / 6
Estonia		4 / 5
Israel		3 / 6
Croatia		3 / 5
Poland		5 / 4
Ukraine		4 / 4
Wales		5 / 3
Slovenia		3 / 4
Canada		5 / 2
Belgium (French)		5 / 2
Iceland		3 / 3
Hungary		4 / 3
Ireland		3 / 3
Malta		5 / 1
Romania		3 / 3
Slovakia		2 / 4
Denmark		3 / 2
Portugal		3 / 3
Republic of Moldova		2 / 3
Austria		2 / 3
England		4 / 1
Luxembourg		3 / 2
Sweden		4 / 1
Belgium (Flemish)		3 / 2
Netherlands		4 / 1
Germany		3 / 2
Norway		2 / 3
Italy		3 / 2
Finland		3 / 2
MKD[a]		2 / 3
Switzerland		3 / 2
France		2 / 1
Albania		1 / 2
Greece		1 / 2
Czech Republic		1 / 1
Armenia		1 / 2
HBSC average (gender)		4 / 3
HBSC average (total)		3

HBSC survey 2013/2014

15-year-olds who have been cyberbullied by messages at least two or three times a month

- BOYS (%)
- GIRLS (%)

	Boys	Girls
Greenland		9 / 12
Lithuania		4 / 7
Russian Federation		5 / 7
Wales		6 / 3
Israel		2 / 7
Canada		6 / 3
Bulgaria		3 / 5
Croatia		4 / 4
Republic of Moldova		3 / 5
Scotland		4 / 3
Latvia		3 / 5
Ireland		4 / 2
England		4 / 3
Ukraine		3 / 4
Luxembourg		4 / 3
Spain		2 / 5
Slovakia		2 / 4
Belgium (French)		3 / 3
Malta		3 / 4
Hungary		3 / 3
Portugal		3 / 3
Slovenia		3 / 2
Poland		2 / 3
Switzerland		2 / 2
Estonia		2 / 3
Romania		2 / 3
Norway		3 / 1
Belgium (Flemish)		4 / 1
Finland		2 / 2
Iceland		2 / 2
Denmark		2 / 2
Austria		2 / 2
Germany		3 / 1
France		3 / 1
Albania		1 / 3
Sweden		2 / 1
Czech Republic		3 / 1
MKD[a]		1 / 2
Italy		2 / 1
Armenia		1 / 2
Netherlands		1 / 1
Greece		1 / 1
HBSC average (gender)		3 / 3
HBSC average (total)		3

Note: **indicates** significant gender difference (at p<0.05). 0 means less than +/-0.5%.

BULLYING:
SCIENTIFIC DISCUSSION AND POLICY REFLECTIONS

SCIENTIFIC DISCUSSION

Very large cross-national variations in levels of bullying perpetration and victimization are apparent. Findings suggest that bullying levels are affected by country-level factors such as cultural norms, socioeconomic levels and the success of intervention and prevention programmes in schools. While boys are significantly more likely to be involved as perpetrators in all countries and regions at almost all ages (24), gender differences are less strong for victimization, especially with increasing age. There is as yet no clear gender pattern for cyberbullying.

A relatively small minority of countries and regions show a relationship with family affluence. This tends to be a decrease in all types with higher affluence (25), but the patterns are not always consistent.

Initial analysis seems to suggest that cyberbullying is less prevalent than traditional forms. Cross-national variations may also be smaller. Research is needed to investigate the relationship of cyberbullying to known psychosocial determinants and outcomes and how its prevalence and patterning is similar to, and differs from, traditional forms of bullying.

POLICY REFLECTIONS

Aggressive behaviour among young people continues to be an important public health problem (26). Activities such as parent training and meetings, improved playground supervision, disciplinary methods, classroom management, teacher training, classroom rules, a whole-school antibullying policy, school conferences, information for parents and cooperative group work are effective in reducing bullying (27). Reduction in victimization is associated with disciplinary methods, parent training and meetings, videos and cooperative group work (27).

Prevention programmes should be long-lasting (more than six months) and accredited (27). For older schoolchildren (those in high school or equivalent), programmes focusing on bystanders are more effective (28). Holistic school policies addressing cyberbullying should be developed in combination with reactive (deleting, blocking or ignoring messages) and proactive (digital literacy, security and awareness) prevention strategies for student computer use (29). Students and teachers should receive training to help them understand what constitutes cyberbullying and the role played by so-called sharing and liking.

Good epidemiological data are needed to build realistic action plans to regulate aggressive behaviours, set quantified targets with a timeline and monitor implementation, but current country-level action plans are not always informed by data (27).

REFERENCES

1. Due P, Holstein BE, Lynch J, Diderichsen F, Nic Gabhain S, Scheidt P et al. Bullying and symptoms among school-aged children: international comparative cross sectional study in 28 countries. Eur J Public Health 2005;15(2):128–32.

2. Nansel TR, Craig W, Overpeck MD, Saluja G, Ruan WJ, the HBSC Bullying Analyses Working Group. Cross-national consistency in the relationship between bullying behaviors and psychosocial adjustment. Arch Pediatr Adolesc Med. 2004;158(8):730–36.

3. Haynie DL, Nansel T, Eitel P, Crump AD, Saylor K, Yu K et al. Bullies, victims, and bully/victims: distinct groups of at-risk youth. J Early Adolesc. 2001;21(1):29.

4. Peskin MF, Tortolero SR, Markham CM, Addy RC, Baumier ER. Bullying and victimization and internalizing symptoms among low-income Black and Hispanic students. J Adolesc Health 2007;40(4):372–75.

5. Salmon G, James A, Cassidy EL, Auxiliadora Javaloyes M. Bullying a review: presentations to an adolescent psychiatric service and within a school for emotionally and behaviourally disturbed children. Clin Child Psychol Psychiatry 2000;5(4):563.

6. Kim YS, Leventhal B. Bullying and suicide. A review. Int J Adolesc Med Health 2008;20(2):133–54.

7. Kaltiala-Heino R, Rimpelae M, Rantanen P, Rimpelä A. Bullying at school – an indicator of adolescents at risk for mental disorders. J Adolesc. 2000;23(6):661–74.

8. Tharp-Taylor S, Haviland A, D'Amico EJ. Victimization from mental and physical bullying and substance use in early adolescence. Addict Behav. 2009;34(6):561–67.

9. Luk JW, Wang J, Simons-Morton BG. The co-occurrence of substance use and bullying behaviors among US adolescents: understanding demographic characteristics and social influences. J Adolesc. 2012;35:1351–60.

GROWING UP UNEQUAL: GENDER AND SOCIOECONOMIC
DIFFERENCES IN YOUNG PEOPLE'S HEALTH AND WELL-BEING
PART 2. KEY DATA | CHAPTER 5. RISK BEHAVIOURS
BULLYING

5

10. Radliff KM, Wheaton JE, Robinson K, Morris J. Illuminating the relationship between bullying and substance use among middle and high school youth. Addict Behav. 2012;37(4):569–72.

11. Harel-Fisch Y, Walsh SD, Grinvald-Fogel H, Amitai G, Molcho M, Due P et al. Negative school perceptions and involvement in school bullying: a universal relationship across 40 countries. J Adolesc. 2011;34:369–52.

12. Chester KL, Callaghan M, Cosma A, Donnelly P, Craig W, Walsh S et al. Cross-national time trends in bullying victimization in 33 countries among children aged 11, 13 and 15 from 2002 to 2010. Eur J Public Health 2015;25(Suppl. 2):61–4.

13. Brunstein K. Bullying, depression, and suicidality in adolescents. J Am Acad Child Adolesc Psychiatry 2007;46(1):40.

14. Brunstein KA, Sourander A, Gould M. The association of suicide and bullying in childhood to young adulthood: a review of cross-sectional and longitudinal research findings. Can J Psychiatry 2010;55(5):282–8.

15. Russell ST, Sinclair KO, Poteat VP, Koenig BW. Adolescent health and harassment based on discriminatory bias. Am J Public Health 2012;102(3):493–5.

16. Luk JW, Wang J, Simons-Morton BG. Bullying victimization and substance use among US adolescents: mediation by depression. Prev Sci. 2010;11(4):355–59.

17. Olweus D. The revised Olweus bully/victim questionnaire. Bergen: University of Bergen; 1996.

18. Hinduja S, Patchin JW. Bullying, cyberbullying, and suicide. Arch Suicide Res. 2010;14(3):206–21.

19. Bauman S, Toomey RB, Walker JL. Associations among bullying, cyberbullying, and suicide in high school students. J Adolesc. 2013;36(2):341–50.

20. Sinclair KO, Bauman S, Poteat VP, Koenig B, Russell ST. Cyber and bias-based harassment: associations with academic, substance use, and mental health problems. J Adolesc Health 2012;50(5):521–3.

21. Litwiller BJ, Brausch AM. Cyber bullying and physical bullying in adolescent suicide: the role of violent behavior and substance use. J Youth Adolesc. 2013;42(5):675–84.

22. Hinduja S, Patchin JW. Cyberbullying: an exploratory analysis of factors related to offending and victimization. Deviant Behav. 2008;29(2):129–56.

23. Sourander A, Klomek AB, Ikonen M, Lindroos J, Luntamo T, Koskelainen M et al. Psychosocial risk factors associated with cyberbullying among adolescents: a population-based study. Arch Gen Psychiatry 2010;67(7):720–8.

24. Wang J, Iannotti RJ, Nansel TR. School bullying among adolescents in the United States: physical, verbal, relational, and cyber. J Adolesc Health 2009;45(4):368–75.

25. Due P, Merlo J, Harel-Fisch Y, Damsgaard MT, Holstein PE, Hetland J et al. Socioeconomic inequality in exposure to bullying during adolescence: a comparative, cross-sectional, multilevel study in 35 countries. Am J Public Health 2009;99(5):907.

26. Global status report on violence prevention 2014. Geneva: World Health Organization; 2014 (http://www.who.int/violence_injury_prevention/violence/status_report/2014/en/, accessed 24 August 2015).

27. Ttofi MM, Farrington DP. Effectiveness of school-based programs to reduce bullying: a systematic and meta-analytic review. J Exp Criminol. 2011;7(1):27–56.

28. Polanin JR, Espelage DL, Pigott TD. A meta-analysis of school-based bullying prevention programs' effects on bystander intervention behavior. School Psych Rev. 2012;41(1):47–65.

29. Cassidy W, Faucher C, Jackson M. Cyberbullying among youth: a comprehensive review of current international research and its implications and application to policy and practice. Sch Psychol Int. 2013;34:575–612.

GROWING UP UNEQUAL: GENDER AND SOCIOECONOMIC
DIFFERENCES IN YOUNG PEOPLE'S HEALTH AND WELL-BEING
PART 3. DISCUSSION | CHAPTER 6. AGE

6

AGE

AGE

The three age groups included in the HBSC study – 11-, 13- and 15-year-olds – represent the entry point to, and early years of, adolescence and adolescent development. Young people experience rapid changes to their physical, emotional and psychological state and health throughout adolescence. Changes relate to important developmental trajectories across this age span in relation to formation of identity and values, transformations in relationships with parents and peers, and establishment of health and risk behaviours (1). It is therefore vital to understand age differences in relation to perceived social context, health behaviour and risk behaviours to facilitate a developmental trajectory that promotes young people's health and well-being during adolescence.

SOCIAL CONTEXT

Findings from the HBSC 2013/2014 survey show that young people's perceptions of their social context tend to have a negative developmental trajectory from age 11 through 13 to 15 in families and at school, while the role of peers has a more stable or even positive developmental trajectory. The quality of communication with mother and father (how easy it is to talk to them) reduces from 11 to 13 and declines further at age 15. The same pattern is observed for liking school and perceived school performance, with perceived school pressure increasing throughout the age span and adding to the observed negative development.

A somewhat less negative age trajectory from 11 to 15 is reflected in a stable level of perceived support from classmates in half of the countries and regions, although a reduction is reported for the other half. Stability in perceived peer support outside of school from 11 through 15 is observed in most countries and regions. The same applies to spending time with friends in the afternoon and early evening (in about half) which increases from age 11 to 15 in a quarter. An increase with age is seen for communication via social media.

HEALTH OUTCOMES

Negative development across age is also seen for health outcomes, with increasing reports of poor health from 11 to 15 in three quarters of countries and regions and a substantial drop in life satisfaction over the same age period. Added to this is an extensive increase in reported multiple health complaints for girls from 11 to 15, although the situation is stable for boys.

In relation to overweight and obesity, a change across age groups is seen for boys and girls, with 15-year-olds reporting lower BMIs than those of 11. A girls-only age-related change is seen for body image, with 15-year-olds reporting poorer body image than those who are 11 and 13. The change across age for weight-reduction behaviours goes in opposite directions for girls and boys: there is an increase in weight-reduction behaviours for girls in most countries and regions, but a reduction for boys from 11 to 15 in a quarter and stability in the rest.

HEALTH BEHAVIOURS

Overall, a negative drop in healthy behaviours is seen with increasing age. This pattern is observed for boys and girls in relation to breakfast and fruit consumption, although the decrease in fruit consumption is lower for girls. Soft-drink consumption increases from age 11 to 15 in half of the countries and regions, adding to the pattern of negative developmental trajectory for health-promoting behaviours. There is nevertheless a positive age-related drop in the prevalence of medically attended injuries between ages 11 and 15.

A positive age trend is also seen for girls' oral health, with an increase in toothbrushing behaviours from age 11 to 15, but a drop with increasing age is observed for boys.

Eleven-year-olds are more likely to meet physical activity guidelines of at least 60 minutes of MVPA daily than 15-year-olds in almost all countries and regions, which represents a negative developmental age trajectory. The same negative trend is seen for watching television, with an increase from age 11 to 15.

GROWING UP UNEQUAL: GENDER AND SOCIOECONOMIC
DIFFERENCES IN YOUNG PEOPLE'S HEALTH AND WELL-BEING
PART 3. DISCUSSION | CHAPTER 6. AGE

6

RISK BEHAVIOURS

Some of the risk behaviours measured in the survey (tobacco initiation, cannabis use and sexual behaviours) are only reported for 15-year-olds, so it is not possible to comment on age trends in relation to these behaviours. Weekly smoking, alcohol use and drunkenness increase with age. The same applies to bullying others, but being bullied and (for boys) cyberbullying and fighting decrease. Cyberbullying and fighting are more stable during the adolescent years for girls, but with a peak at age 13 for cyberbullying.

DISCUSSION

Overall, a negative developmental trajectory with an increasing burden of negative health perceptions and health-compromising behaviours with advancing age is evident. A relevant question to raise is how much of this negative development is related to individual-level pubertal trajectories and the change process of increasing autonomy and responsibility from childhood to adolescence, and how much to influences from the settings in which young people live and participate, such as home, school and leisure facilities?

The age span from 11 to 15 years represents for most young people the prepubertal or pubertal periods. These are characterized by biological changes, conscious establishment of self-identity and exploration of risk behaviours such as tobacco and alcohol use, and sexual behaviour. Early entrance to puberty is associated with increased levels of health-compromising behaviours (2), possibly through seeking older friends who have already started exploring risk behaviours. A healthy developmental trajectory involves increasing possibilities for autonomous decision-making to stimulate the establishment of self-identity and self-management.

Findings show that despite the overall pattern of a negative developmental trajectory for health and health behaviours with increasing age, variation across countries and regions is substantial. This might be related to variation in cultural norms in relation to what is considered appropriate exploration of behaviours and levels of autonomy. It could also be explained by differences in policy in areas such as regulation of smoking in schools and the legal age for purchasing cigarettes and alcohol. The behaviour effect of policy regulations might influence role-modelling of parents and peers' smoking behaviours and provide another explanation for observed country/region differences.

Few children at age 11 have entered puberty, which may explain why there is less variation in health perceptions and health behaviours across countries and regions for this group. The number of adolescents exploring new behaviours and experiences is likely to rise as young people enter the pubertal phase. The exploration of risk behaviours can be explained by young people's inclination to sensation-seek, which may be related to a biological drive to achieve rewards (3). The drive for sensation-seeking and its acceptance in cultural norms is likely to represent a prominent effect of cultural norms on variations seen within and across countries and regions.

The influence of social relations and determinants may also help to explain variations in young people's health behaviours and perceptions (4,5). It is likely that parents have a stronger effect than peers on the health-related behaviours of the youngest age group (6). The parents of 11-year-olds have a strong structural influence on behaviours by being providers of daily meals and encouraging and facilitating participation in leisure activities. They are also more likely to set norms and regulations on where and with whom the children can spend their time and when they go to bed. Similarity across countries and regions in parental structuring of the youngest age group's day in relation to meals and regulation of behaviour is expected, but some variation in children's autonomy and influence is likely to develop because of cultural norms.

Increasing age typically involves increased maturation; with this, parents tend to give children room to influence or even make their own decisions on how to fill their time and with whom it is spent. Cultural variation is still to be expected, particularly in norms set for girls, but also in relation to a country or region's wealth and the priority it gives to health interventions (5).

Parental norms and role-modelling continue to be influential in preventing health-compromising behaviours in 13- and 15-year-olds (7), but the influence of peers' norms and behaviours becomes increasingly important (6,8). A major mechanism in this change of influence from parents to peers is the increasing time spent with friends. The influence of peer norms and role-modelling is communicated through in-group behaviour – that is, behaviour considered relevant and important to the group of friends, which may include smoking or experimenting with alcohol, or abstaining from using any substances. Friends may also take over the role of confidant, particularly in relation to situations of stress, frustration and insecurity that may include family-related conflicts (6).

Entry into adolescence therefore marks an increase in autonomy at home, with peers and in school. Escalation of autonomy in relation to the home and with peers is reflected in decisions around which activities and behaviours to pursue and with whom to spend time. At school, adolescents are allowed greater influence with increasing age on tasks and effort around tasks. With increased autonomy comes higher levels of responsibility and greater expectations of having the capacity to take care of self in relation to, for example, eating adequately, doing homework and getting enough sleep. Increased responsibility in the school setting is reflected in more and more of the learning process being left to the students, with them assuming responsibility for ensuring they make progress and use the resources available to them. Although most adolescents are likely to enjoy their increased autonomy and freedom, increased responsibility, in which more depends on the individual's choices and efforts, can create perceptions of greater stress (9).

The age-related developmental trajectory identified in the HBSC survey may be explained through the interplay between young people going through the developmental pubertal process and their experiences in different social contexts, such as family, leisure and school (10). Better understanding of this interplay and how it evolves during adolescence is important in identifying unique and shared individual and social correlates of different health behaviours and perceived health (4).

Age trajectories in adolescent health behaviours not only affect health during the adolescent years, but may also track into adulthood (5,11). Young people who are physically active during the adolescent years, for example, are more likely to continue to be physically active in adulthood (12,13). This activity pattern, particularly if combined with healthy eating, may prevent the development of cardiovascular disease and cancer. Stimulation of healthy behaviours from an early age is therefore an important health-promotion initiative.

The same principle holds for preventing the development of risk behaviours such as smoking and excessive alcohol use to avoid their tracking into adulthood. Psychosomatic complaints established in adolescence are also likely to persist into adulthood, so preventing stress experiences in school, at home and with peers by providing young people with opportunities for autonomy and perceived control is vital in promoting healthy development.

CONCLUSION

A notable finding from the survey is that health-compromising behaviours are less frequent and relatively stable across countries and regions for the youngest age group (11-year-olds). The situation is somewhat different for 13- and 15-year-olds, in that health-compromising behaviours increase with age and more variation in the pattern of increase is seen.

The age-related increase may be explained by the escalation of peer influence during adolescence, with possibly greater experimentation with risk behaviours and less prioritization of healthy behaviours such as physical activity and healthy eating. The variation across countries and regions is likely to relate to differences in cultural and economic contexts, and individual developmental growth trajectories are likely to interact with contextual influences. Better understanding of the interplay between individual and contextual contexts and how they change with age is needed.

Specifically, the findings underscore the need to develop age-differentiated interventions that address the interplay between the individual and the context in which he or she lives to promote young people's health and well-being. The school setting has

GROWING UP UNEQUAL: GENDER AND SOCIOECONOMIC
DIFFERENCES IN YOUNG PEOPLE'S HEALTH AND WELL-BEING
PART 3. DISCUSSION | CHAPTER 6. AGE

6

been identified as a particularly powerful arena for such interventions, providing an opportunity to combine the knowledge and skills of teachers and health support staff *(14–16)*.

REFERENCES

1. Rice P, Dolgin K. The adolescent: development, relationships and culture, 10th edition. Boston (MA): Allyn and Bacon; 2002.

2. Golub MS, Collman GW, Foster PMD, Kimmel CA, Rajpert-De Meyts E, Reiter EO et al. Public health implications of altered puberty timing. Pediatrics 2008;121:S218. doi:10.1542/peds.2007-1813G.

3. Steinberg L. A social neuroscience perspective on adolescent risk-taking. Dev Rev. 2008;8:78–106.

4. Peters LWH, Wiefferink CH, Hoekstra F, Buijs GJ, ten Dam GTM, Paulussen TGWM. A review of similarities between domain-specific determinants of four health behaviors among adolescents. Health Educ Res. 2009;24(2):198–223.

5. Viner RM, Ozer EM, Denny S, Marmot M, Resnick M, Fatusi A et al. Adolescence and the social determinants of health. Lancet 2012;379(9826):1641–52.

6. Ciairano S, Rabaglietti E, Roggero A, Bonino S, Beyers W. Patterns of adolescent friendships, psychological adjustment and antisocial behavior: the moderating role of family stress and friendship reciprocity. Int J Behav Dev. 2007;31(6):539–48. doi:10.1177/0165025407080573.

7. DiClemente RJ, Wingood GM, Crosby R, Sionean C, Cobb BK, Harrington K et al. Monitoring: association with adolescents' risk behaviors. Pediatrics 2001;107(6):1363–8. doi:10.1542/peds.107.6.1363.

8. Cauce AM, Srebnik DS. Returning to social support systems: a morphological analysis of social networks. Am J Community Psychol. 1990;18(4)609–16.

9. Samdal O, Torsheim T. School as a resource or risk to students' subjective health and well-being In: Wold B, Samdal O, editors. An ecological perspective on health promotion: systems, settings and social processes. London: Bentham; 2012:48–59.

10. Bronfenbrenner U. Making human beings human: bioecological perspectives on human development. Thousand Oaks (CA): Sage; 2005.

11. Due P, Krølner R, Rasmussen M, Andersen A, Damsgaard MT, Graham H et al. Pathways and mechanisms in adolescence contribute to adult health inequalities Scand J Public Health 2011;39:62. doi:10.1177/1403494810395989.

12. Kjønniksen L, Torsheim T, Wold B. Tracking of leisure-time physical activity during adolescence and young adulthood: a 10-year longitudinal study. Int J Behav Nutr Phys Act. 2008;5:69.

13. Wiium N, Breivik K, Wold B. Growth trajectories of health behaviours from adolescence through young adulthood. Int J Environ Res Public Health 2015;2(11):13711–29. doi:10.3390/ijerph121113711.

14. Eccles JS, Roeser RW. Schools as developmental contexts during adolescence. J Res Adolesc. 2011;21(1)225–41.

15. Danielsen AG. Supportive and motivating environments in school: main factors to make well-being and learning a reality. Nor Epidemiol. 2010;20(1):33–9.

16. Ward NL, Linke LH. Commentary: understanding adolescent health-risk behaviors from a prevention science perspective. J Am Acad Psychiatry Law 2011;39(1):53–6.

GROWING UP UNEQUAL: GENDER AND SOCIOECONOMIC
DIFFERENCES IN YOUNG PEOPLE'S HEALTH AND WELL-BEING
PART 3. DISCUSSION | CHAPTER 7. GENDER

7

GENDER

GENDER

Young women and men take on adult gender roles (social expectations of what is regarded as male or female) in all spheres – personal, family and work – during adolescence. These gender roles are shaped by society, so are likely to differ across countries and regions (1).

National political and economic opportunities for women and cultural and religious gender norms affect young people's conceptions of gender roles and may influence their exposure to health risks and protective factors (2). Cross-national differences in adolescent health may therefore be understood as a reflection of cross-national variation in gender roles. Awareness of gender differences and similarities and understanding of their origins are prerequisites for designing successful and targeted interventions.

SOCIAL CONTEXT

The HBSC study gathers information on key social contexts for adolescent health, such as family, peers and school environment. These contexts have been found to strongly affect adolescent health (2–5), so it is relevant to identify and explain gender differences within them.

Some clear gender differences emerge in relation to family life, with boys generally reporting more positive relationships. When asked about ease of communication with parents, for example, boys are more likely to report finding it easy to talk to their fathers about things that really bother them. No clear gender differences exist for communication with mothers, but they arise in older age groups in relation to perceived family support, with boys reporting higher levels.

Girls tend to report higher levels of perceived peer support, with gender differences becoming more pronounced in the older age group. Meeting friends every day is more common among boys, while girls tend to have more contact with friends via social media, although this is not the case in all countries and regions.

Girls (especially in the younger age group) are more likely to report high satisfaction with school and high perceived academic achievement, indicating that they have more positive school experiences. Eleven-year-old girls also perceive less school-related pressure, but this changes with age: at 15, girls report more school-related pressure than boys. Classmate support shows no clear patterning by gender.

HEALTH OUTCOMES

Some of the most persistent gender differences relate to adolescent health outcomes. Specifically, girls are more likely to report fair or poor health and multiple health complaints, and also to describe lower life satisfaction. Each of these gender differences increases with age.

Boys have a higher prevalence of medically attended injuries, which may be due to greater participation in physical activities. While boys are more likely to be overweight or obese, girls report perceiving their body to be too fat and being engaged in weight-reduction behaviour more commonly. The size of these gender differences tends to increase with age.

HEALTH BEHAVIOURS

Clear gender differences in young people's health behaviours are evident. Girls are less likely to have breakfast every weekday, but also report eating fruit more frequently. Boys generally report higher consumption of soft drinks. Regular toothbrushing (more than once a day) is more common among girls. Boys take part in MVPA more often, but are also more likely to report screen-time behaviour (watching television, videos, DVDs and other entertainment on a screen on weekdays).

GROWING UP UNEQUAL: GENDER AND SOCIOECONOMIC
DIFFERENCES IN YOUNG PEOPLE'S HEALTH AND WELL-BEING
PART 3. DISCUSSION | CHAPTER 7. GENDER

7

RISK BEHAVIOURS

Risk behaviours in the HBSC study include substance use, sexual behaviour, fighting and bullying. Overall, boys tend to engage more in these behaviours.

Boys in general report early and weekly smoking more often. Weekly drinking and (early) drunkenness also tend to be more common among boys, as is use of cannabis. Although not significant, a pattern in which girls appear to be catching up with boys in relation to substance use seems to be developing in some countries and regions with, for instance, different forms of alcohol use becoming more common among girls.

In most countries and regions, boys are more likely to report having had sexual intercourse, although the opposite pattern is found in some. Boys are also more likely to report condom use, but no clear gender pattern emerges regarding contraceptive pill use.

Boys are involved in fighting more often at all ages and are significantly more likely to be perpetrators of bullying, but gender differences are less strong for bullying victimization. No clear gender pattern has yet emerged for cyberbullying.

DISCUSSION

The current HBSC data reflect gender-specific social relationships shaped by gender socialization, the process by which boys and girls learn feminine and masculine identities. They also appear to be influenced by societal expectations, which may differ across countries and regions (6). Boys' social networks are typically based on activities, with higher levels of physical activity and sports, while girls' networks and friendships are based more on personal communication. This gendered pattern is also reflected in boys and girls' use of screen devices, with girls tending to use them primarily for homework and social purposes and boys for gaming and watching television (7).

Girls in many countries and regions perform better at school. Boys are lagging behind: they dislike school more and rate their achievements lower. School-based factors, such as teaching practices and examination systems, and conceptions of masculinity in peer cultures at school may make schools less appealing to boys (8,9).

Persistent gendered patterns in self-rated health are identified, with girls reporting lower subjective health. These may reflect girls' higher expectations for daily life or a gender bias in measuring self-rated health. HBSC questions may focus on female-specific reactions to stress (internalizing – headache, stomach ache and feeling nervous) rather than anger-based reactions (externalizing) seen more frequently among boys (10).

While boys are more likely to be overweight or obese, girls more commonly report that they perceive their body to be too fat and that they are engaged in weight-reduction behaviour. This gender difference in body dissatisfaction can be attributed to physical changes in puberty, combined with societal standards for ideal appearances. Boys' bodies change in the desired direction, becoming more muscular and strong, while girls lose their so-called ideal appearance through gaining body fat.

A notable process of gender equalization in some risk behaviours has been observed over the past decade (11–13). The findings confirm this tendency. Specifically, equalizing of traditional gender differences in tobacco use through increased prevalence of smoking among girls has been seen in some countries and regions. Alcohol use still tends to be more common among boys, but a pattern of gender convergence is emerging (12,13): there is even evidence of girls reporting more excessive alcohol use than boys in some countries, particularly in the United Kingdom. These equalizing trends may reflect men and women's changing social positions and gender identities. Heavy drinking, for example, may now be considered to be less in accordance with dominant norms of masculinity, consequently becoming more acceptable among girls and challenging traditional codes of femininity (14).

Boys are more likely to report sexual intercourse in most countries and regions, with the differences being largest in those in eastern Europe. Specific features of national contexts may withhold girls (especially) from engaging in sexual intercourse at an early age: country/region-level age norms appear to affect the timing of sexual initiation in girls to a greater extent than in boys *(15)*. Physical and psychological symptoms are associated with early sexual initiation in girls – but not boys – in countries with more traditional gender norms *(16)*. National features that might generate these differences should be explored further.

Fighting, bullying and getting injured remain more common for boys. These health-compromising behaviours can be considered gendered, with young boys being pushed to perform more risky behaviours to fulfil notions of masculinity *(17,18)*. The higher prevalence of injuries among boys may also reflect the fact that they engage more in injury-producing sports *(19,20)*.

Overall, the extent to which structural factors reinforce the gendered nature of health during adolescence needs greater exploration. The United Nations Sex Inequality Index provides an opportunity to assess associations between gender inequality and health outcomes across countries and regions. It shows that those with greater gender inequality have poorer health outcomes for both sexes, after adjustment for national wealth. This suggests that gender inequality is detrimental to both young men and young women, and supports the need for policies to actively address gender inequalities *(2)*.

CONCLUSION

HBSC findings highlight systematic and international gender differences in adolescent health. The magnitude of the differences tends to vary across countries and regions, which suggests that more research into the potential influence on adolescent health of (national) social structures and cultural factors (such as gender norms and roles) is needed. The observed differences also suggest that strategies for health promotion and disease prevention may need to be tailored differently for boys and girls.

Special attention may need to be paid to boys' well-being at school, as they score systematically lower than girls in relation to school experiences. Many risk behaviours are still more common among boys, so health-promotion activities that specifically target boys may be needed. Potential increases in girls' risk behaviours, resulting in gender equalization of health-compromising behaviours, should be monitored carefully.

Persistent gendered patterns in self-rated health and well-being, with girls reporting lower subjective health, require attention. Boys and girls may react differently to mental health interventions *(21)*, so they may need to be tailored. Girls' relatively low self-perceptions call for mental health promotion to give stronger emphasis to strengthening their self-esteem and preventing them from developing negative ideas about their bodies.

REFERENCES

1. Rudman LA, Glick P. The social psychology of gender: how power and intimacy shape gender relations. New York (NY): Guilford Press; 2008.

2. Viner RM, Ozer EM, Denny S, Marmot M, Resnick M, Fatusi A et al. Adolescence and the social determinants of health. Lancet 2012;379(9826):1641–52.

3. Freeman J, King M, Kuntsche E, Pickett W. Protective roles of home and school environments for the health of young Canadians. J Epidemiol Community Health 2011;65:438–44.

4. Molcho M, Nic Gabhainn S, Kelleher CC. Interpersonal relationships as predictors of positive health among Irish youth: the more the merrier? Ir Med J. 2007;100(8):33–6.

5. Morgan A, Currie C, Due P, Nic Gabhain S, Rasmussen M, Samdal O et al. Mental well-being in school-aged children in Europe: associations with social cohesion and socioeconomic circumstances. In: Social cohesion for mental well-being among adolescents. Copenhagen: WHO Regional Office for Europe; 2008 (http://www.euro.who.int/__data/assets/pdf_file/0005/84623/E91921.pdf, accessed 16 November 2015).

6. Martin CL, Ruble DN. Children's search for gender cues: cognitive perspectives on gender development. Curr Dir Psychol Sci. 2004;13:67–70.

7. Leech RM, McNaughton SA, Timperio A. The clustering of diet, physical activity and sedentary behavior in children and adolescents: a review. Int J Behav Nutr Act. 2014;11(1):4.

8. Legewie J, DiPreta TA. School context and the gender gap in educational achievement. Am Sociol Rev. 2012;77(3):463–85.

9. Machin S, McNally S. Gender and student achievement in English schools. London: Centre for the Economics of Education, London School of Economics and Political Science; 2006.

GROWING UP UNEQUAL: GENDER AND SOCIOECONOMIC
DIFFERENCES IN YOUNG PEOPLE'S HEALTH AND WELL-BEING
PART 3. DISCUSSION | CHAPTER 7. GENDER

7

10. Ruiz-Cantero M, Vives-Cases C, Artazcoz L, Delgado A, del Mar García Calvente M, Miqueo C et al. A framework to analyse gender bias in epidemiological research. J Epidemiol Com Health 2007;61(Suppl. II):ii46–53.

11. Pitel L, Geckova AM, van Dijk JP, Reijneveld SA. Gender differences in adolescent health-related behaviour diminished between 1998 and 2006. Public Health 2010;124:512–18.

12. Kuntsche E, Kuntsche S, Knibbe R, Simons-Morton B, Farhat T, Hublet A et al. Cultural and gender convergence in adolescent drunkenness: evidence from 23 European and North American countries. Arch Pedriatr Adolesc Med. 2001;165(2):152–8.

13. Simons-Morton B, Farhat T, ter Bogt T, Hublet A, Kuntsche E, NicGabhainn S. Gender specific trends in alcohol use: cross-cultural comparisons from 1998 to 2006 in 24 countries and regions. Int J Pub Health 2009;52:S199–208.

14. Lyons AC, Willot SA. Alcohol consumption, gender identities and women's changing social positions. Sex Roles 2008;59(9):694–712.

15. Madkour AS, de Looze M, Ma P, Halpern CT, Farhat T, ter Bogt TFM et al. Macro-level age norms for the timing of sexual initiation and adolescents' early sexual initiation in 17 European countries. J Adolesc Health 2014;55(1):114–21.

16. Madkour AS, Farhat T, Halpern CT, Godeau E, Nic Gabhainn S. Early adolescent sexual initiation and physical/psychological symptoms: a comparative analysis of five nations. J Youth Adolsc. 2010;39(10):1211–25.

17. Courtenay WH. Constructions of masculinity and their influence on men's well-being: a theory of gender and health. Soc Sc Med. 2000;50:1385–1401.

18. Fleming PJ, Lee JGL, Dworkin SL. "Real mem don't": constructions of masculinity and inadvertent harm in public health interventions. Am J Public Health 2014;104(6):1029–35.

19. De Looze M, Pickett W, Raaijmakers Q, Kuntsche E, Hublet A, Nic Gabhainn S et al. Early risk behaviours and adolescent injury in 25 European and North American countries: a cross-national consistent relationship. J Early Adolesc. 2012;32(1):104–25.

20. Pickett W, Molcho M, Simpson K, Janssen I, Kuntsche E, Mazur J et al. Cross-national study of injury and social determinants in adolescents. Inj Prev. 2005;11:213–18.

21. Merry SN, Hetrick SE, Cox GR, Brudevold-Iversen T, Bir JJ, McDowell H. Psychological and educational interventions for preventing depression in children and adolescents. Cochrane Database Syst Rev. 2011;12:CD003380.

GROWING UP UNEQUAL: GENDER AND SOCIOECONOMIC
DIFFERENCES IN YOUNG PEOPLE'S HEALTH AND WELL-BEING
PART 3. DISCUSSION | CHAPTER 8. FAMILY AFFLUENCE

8

FAMILY AFFLUENCE

FAMILY AFFLUENCE

Socioeconomic differences are found in many areas of health and health behaviours and the social relationships that support them. In general, young people with higher affluence tend to get along better with their families and peers, do better in school and report better health outcomes. The pattern is less clear in relation to some risk behaviours and in spending time with peers.

SOCIAL CONTEXT
Young people with higher affluence have better communication with parents, although the association is stronger for communication with fathers and among girls. Family affluence positively relates to perceived family support in over half the countries and regions and to peer support in about two thirds. It is also related to school performance, despite having no consistent association with liking school or school pressure.

HEALTH OUTCOMES
Inequalities related to family affluence exist across a range of health outcomes. Higher family affluence relates to better self-rated health and higher life satisfaction. It is also associated with frequency of multiple health complaints in around a third of countries and regions for boys and about half for girls. Low affluence relates to excess body mass and perceptions of being too fat, although this is not observed across all countries and regions. Medically attended injuries increase with higher family affluence, which might reflect differences in accessing health services or participation in sports in some countries and regions.

HEALTH BEHAVIOURS
Higher affluence relates to more frequent physical activity, more regular toothbrushing, higher fruit intake and more frequent breakfast consumption in most countries and regions. Inequalities in soft-drink consumption vary, with higher affluence relating to higher consumption in some countries and regions but lower in others. Higher television-watching is associated with lower affluence, largely in western Europe, but the opposite relationship is observed in some eastern European countries.

RISK BEHAVIOURS
No clear pattern of inequalities is found in risk behaviours. Low affluence relates to weekly smoking in most countries and regions, but not to age of smoking onset, drinking initiation or cannabis use. Young people from low-affluence families are more likely to have been bullied, but there is no consistent relationship for fighting, bullying others and cyberbullying.

DISCUSSION
Adolescent health and health behaviours share a complex association with family affluence. Longitudinal research in this area has found that the effects are bidirectional in nature. Obesity in adolescence, for example, predicts less education and lower incomes in adulthood (1); conversely, low adolescent SES increases the risk for adult obesity after differences in adult SES are taken into account (2,3). Research has also found that international differences in income inequality determine the size of health inequalities in adolescents (4). Health, SES and social mobility are intricately linked from an early age, which helps explain why health inequalities endure throughout the life-course.

The mechanisms that underlie these inequalities involve multiple causal pathways (5). First, family affluence affects adolescent health by limiting access to material resources that support health, such as good-quality schools, healthy food options and access to parks and playgrounds that facilitate physical activity (6).

Second, low family affluence levies the psychosocial effects of low socioeconomic rank and the stress and anxieties of living in relative poverty (7). This psychosocial path explains why the socioeconomic gradient in health extends through the full range of family affluence and why socioeconomic differences are observed in all HBSC countries and regions regardless of their

GROWING UP UNEQUAL: GENDER AND SOCIOECONOMIC
DIFFERENCES IN YOUNG PEOPLE'S HEALTH AND WELL-BEING
PART 3. DISCUSSION | CHAPTER 8. FAMILY AFFLUENCE

8

national wealth. Material and psychosocial pathways work in tandem: inequalities in food choices, for example, are determined by affordability of healthy food options and the stressors of relative deprivation, which disinhibit dietary restraint and drive preferences for high-fat, high-caloric foods *(8–10)*.

Third, family affluence indirectly affects adolescent health though social stratification. Lower-affluence adolescents have less structured mealtimes and poorer communication with parents, perceive less social support from their families and peers, and do less well in school. Research has found that antisocial behaviour, school dropout and exposure to crime-ridden neighbourhoods are more common experiences for lower-affluence adolescents *(11)*. Health inequalities are created and then reinforced by multiple social contexts.

Fourth, observed differences in health outcomes are also a consequence of socially patterned differences in early life experiences and the cumulative effects of psychological stress on the development of neuroregulatory centres of the brain that govern emotion, attention and social functioning *(12)*.

CONCLUSION

The likelihood that adolescents are healthy, happy and doing well in school becomes significantly and progressively stronger as family affluence rises *(11)*. Early socioeconomic exposures have lasting effects on lifelong health and well-being *(13,14)*. The HBSC study provides valuable information about the magnitude of these differences across multiple health behaviours and health outcomes.

REFERENCES

1. Gortmaker SL, Must A, Perrin JM, Sobol AM, Dietz WH. Social and economic consequences of overweight in adolescence and young adulthood. N Engl J Med. 1993;329:1008–12.

2. Power C, Graham H, Due P, Hallqvist J, Joung I, Kuh D et al. The contribution of childhood and adult socioeconomic position to adult obesity and smoking behaviour: an international comparison. Int J Epidemiol. 2005;34:335–44.

3. Senese LC, Almeida ND, Fath AK, Smith BT, Loucks EB. Associations between childhood socioeconomic position and adulthood obesity. Epidemiol Rev. 2009;31:21–51.

4. Elgar FJ, Pförtner TK, Moor I, De Clercq B, Stevens GW, Currie C. Socioeconomic inequalities in adolescent health 2002–2010: a time-series analysis of 34 countries participating in the Health Behaviour in School-aged Children study. Lancet 2015;385(9982):2088–95.

5. Adler NE, Ostrove JM. Socioeconomic status and health: what we know and what we don't. Ann NY Acad Sci. 1999;896:3–15.

6. Conrad D, Capewell S. Associations between deprivation and rates of childhood overweight and obesity in England, 2007–2010: an ecological study. BMJ Open 2012;2(2):e000463.

7. Wilkinson RG, Pickett KE. The problems of relative deprivation: why some societies do better than others. Soc Sci Med. 2007;65(9):1965–78.

8. Oliver G, Wardle J. Perceived effects of stress on food choice. Physiol Behav. 1999;66(3):511–5.

9. Roemmich JN, Wright SM, Epstein LH. Dietary restraint and stress-induced snacking in youth. Obes Res. 2002;10(11):1120–6.

10. Torres SJ, Nowson CA. Relationship between stress, eating behavior, and obesity. Nutrition 2007;23(11–12):887–94.

11. Repetti RL, Taylor SE, Seeman T. Risky families: family social environments and the mental and physical health of offspring. Psychol Bull. 2002;128(2):330–66.

12. Richter M, Erhart M, Vereecken CA, Zambon A, Boyce W, Nic Gabhainn S. The role of behavioural factors in explaining socio-economic differences in adolescent health: a multilevel study in 33 countries. Soc Sci Med. 2009;69(3):396–403.

13. Shonkoff JP, Boyce WT, McEwen BS. Neuroscience, molecular biology, and the childhood roots of health disparities: building a new framework for health promotion and disease prevention. JAMA 2009;301(21):2252–9.

14. Galobardes B, Smith GD, Lynch JW. Systematic review of the influence of childhood socioeconomic circumstances on risk for cardiovascular disease in adulthood. Ann Epidemiol. 2006;16(2):91–104.

GROWING UP UNEQUAL: GENDER AND SOCIOECONOMIC
DIFFERENCES IN YOUNG PEOPLE'S HEALTH AND WELL-BEING
PART 3. DISCUSSION | CHAPTER 9. CONCLUSION

9

CONCLUSION

CONCLUSION

SCIENTIFIC CONCLUSIONS

Young people are regarded as being healthy relative to other population groups, but adolescence is now recognized as a critical stage of the life-course during which many behavioural patterns that help determine current health status and future health outcomes are established. Emerging evidence suggests that adolescents are particularly sensitive to environmental influences, which emphasizes the importance of adopting a social determinants approach to understanding adolescent health and well-being.

The HBSC study provides a unique insight into the lives of young people across Europe and North America. This latest report presents key findings from the 2013/2014 survey in relation to health behaviours, risk behaviours and health outcomes, and the social context in which young people live.

The data show that family relationships change during the adolescent years, especially for girls, and that the role of family as a protective factor may diminish during this time. In contrast, perceived support from friends remains relatively stable, potentially providing an important resource at a time when many changes are taking place. The quotes from young people featured throughout the report demonstrate the essential role that friendships play in supporting young people through the challenges they face.

The way young people interact and communicate has changed in recent years, with the growth of social and other forms of electronic media. Technological developments over past decades present benefits and risks for young people. Most of the adolescents surveyed engage in daily EMC with their peers, with an increasing trend compared to previous years [1].

Increased use of mobile devices and media technology has the potential to facilitate the development of online/electronic aggression, so questions on cyberbullying were included for the first time in the 2013/2014 survey. Interest in this new phenomenon is growing, as exposure to cyberbullying has been associated with a wide range of negative outcomes for those victimized. Overall, young people reported being victims of cyberbullying less often than traditional bullying, but this balance may shift in the future.

Evidence that electronic media use can have positive and negative effects on young people's health highlights the importance of continuing to monitor the changing nature of peer relations to better understand their impact. Large variation in prevalence of face-to-face contact time and use of social media exists between countries and regions, highlighting the role of wider cultural factors in determining social norms and practices.

School has an important influence on young people's lives, and health and learning are closely linked. There is considerable cross-national variation in young people's experiences at school, particularly in relation to how much they like school and feel pressured by schoolwork. This is not surprising, given the diversity of school systems across countries and regions and differences in the way the school day is organized. Younger children tend to have more positive experiences, although younger boys are more likely than girls to experience school-related stress. The opposite relationship is seen for older students, where stress is higher among girls. This may be a contributing factor to the lower levels of mental well-being experienced by girls of this age.

The findings show a marked decline in subjective well-being among girls during the adolescent years. On average, one in five girls reports fair or poor health by age 15 and half experience multiple health complaints more than once a week. Body dissatisfaction also increases significantly during this period for girls, particularly in western and central European countries, despite actual levels of overweight and obesity remaining stable. Indeed, the data indicate that older female adolescents have a different trajectory in relation to the main health and well-being indicators. In addition to poorer mental health, 15-year-old girls also report the lowest levels of life satisfaction, daily breakfast consumption and physical activity.

Many positive behaviours appear to be influenced by gender. Girls are more likely to include fruit and vegetables in their diet and brush their teeth, while boys are more likely to be physically active. Negative health outcomes and risk behaviours are also

GROWING UP UNEQUAL: GENDER AND SOCIOECONOMIC
DIFFERENCES IN YOUNG PEOPLE'S HEALTH AND WELL-BEING
PART 3. DISCUSSION | CHAPTER 9. CONCLUSION

9

strongly gendered. Boys, for example, are more likely to experience injury and be involved in physical fights. They drink alcohol and smoke tobacco more often, although the gender gap has been closing in some countries in recent years as girls adopt behaviours typically regarded as masculine. Despite this, encouraging trends in risk behaviour are seen compared with previous surveys, with substantial reductions in substance use, fighting [2] and bullying victimization [3] among boys and girls in many countries and regions [4,5].

Differences in family affluence continue to have a strong effect on young people's health and well-being. The findings show that adolescents from low-affluence families tend to have poorer health, lower life satisfaction, higher levels of obesity and sedentary behaviours, poorer communication with their parents, less social interaction via social media and lower levels of support from friends and family. In contrast, those from high-affluence families tend to report better outcomes. Many of these inequalities are persistent and evidence suggests they may be increasing, with widening gaps in several key domains of adolescent health [6]. Socioeconomic patterning of behaviours is less evident for risk behaviours and school experience, which suggests that schools can provide a supportive environment for young people's health and development regardless of family circumstances.

Health-related behaviours in adolescence are affected by structural determinants of health (such as national wealth and income inequality, and employment opportunities) and proximal or intermediate determinants (including the connectedness of adolescents to family and school) [7]. The large variation in prevalence between countries and regions observed for many indicators reinforces the importance of country-level factors and cultural norms in determining young people's health and well-being. As Sawyer et al. [7] note:

> The complex interaction of social determinants of health and risk and protective factors with the biological and social-role transitions of adolescence explains the growing disparities between the health of adolescents in different regions and countries. These same factors also affect the experience of growing up within the same country, where adolescents can have highly heterogeneous life experiences and diverse health outcomes.

HBSC is in a unique position to be able to describe and explain patterning of health among this age group within and between countries and regions, and to identify the main influences on young people's engagement in health-related behaviours within a risk- and protective-factors framework. The findings in this report should be addressed through a positive youth-development approach [8] in which the focus is adolescents' assets and developmental strengths, whether internal to the young person (resilience, for example) or external (such as peers and school).

POLICY CONCLUSIONS

This report reflects on international efforts towards meeting the overall priority of the WHO European child and adolescent health strategy to make children's lives more visible [9]. The HBSC study raises the profile of adolescence as a critical period in the life-course, shedding light on adolescents' health behaviours and social and developmental context over time. It is a unique instrument for understanding new challenges to adolescent health [10] and provides a common voice that speaks to the national and international realities of young people's lives. The report highlights priority areas for action and identifies modifiable risk and protective factors that can be used to inform the development and implementation of intervention and prevention programmes.

Findings show that young people increasingly use digital social media to interact and become informed. Innovative interventions should be designed to make use of new communication technologies to disseminate health-promoting messages. Frequent use of electronic media highlights the need to address young people's health literacy to ensure they know how to assess the quality of information and validity of sources. Measurement and evaluation of interventions that make use of new communication technologies are critical to building a knowledge base that can enhance the ability to improve opportunities and outcomes in this age group.

The breadth of the HBSC study can support a range of policy actions to improve young people's health and well-being. It cannot directly identify the causes of observed trends in adolescents' health, but can reflect on changes in policies that coincide with alterations in reported behaviours. For example, some of the positive changes in young people's lives reflected in the report could be attributable to international and national efforts to promote healthy eating, increase physical activity, encourage positive oral health and reduce risk behaviours. Room for improvement remains, however.

Prevention programmes should begin early and be developed with a gendered lens for issues such as fighting, sexual behaviour, subjective health, toothbrushing and school perception. The burden of deterioration in adolescent subjective health is a major health problem that calls for structural changes through a HiAP approach (11). Oral health promotion should be integrated with general health promotion: further investment in oral health promotion to help prevent oral disease could generate sizeable savings in treatment costs later in life (12).

Access to modern contraceptives and confidential sexual and reproductive health services is critical, especially for boys from low-affluence backgrounds, but lack of skilled practitioners may hinder policies to improve sexual health in this age group.

Greater insight into the harmful effects of alcohol on the brains of adolescents has supported the introduction of more stringent policies to curb teenage drinking and changes in social norms. Interventions that focus on preventing experimentation among young people and preventing those who have experimented from adopting a regular habit, and policies to restrict their access to tobacco products through commercial sources (13), should be scaled-up to delay onset as much as possible.

A systemic approach to addressing obesity and overweight rates that includes the provision of healthy and nutritious food, safe neighbourhoods and opportunities for physical activity and sports participation should be adopted. School fruit schemes and food-based guidelines and labelling have proven effective in improving eating habits, but data suggest that the school food environment is also of importance in shaping children's diet.

Injury prevention is an important public health area in which small investments could realize big gains. Common macro approaches, such as the use of legislation, product and environmental modifications to promote children's safety, supportive home visits, promoting the use of safety devices (such as helmets, seat belts and smoke alarms) and educational programmes, are supported (14).

Relationships are critical during adolescence, with peers and parents having a key role as protective assets in young people's lives. Policies should support the establishment and maintenance of supportive social relationships among adolescents through, for example, opportunities to interact with peers in safe and structured settings. It is also important to change misleading discourses which imply that time spent alone with peers leads to risk-taking and offending; this very much depends on the conditions under which the interactions take place (15). Increased attention to, and more investment in, programmes that promote positive parenting during adolescence are necessary.

The overall health and behaviours described in this report are quite positive, but the need to address existing social, age and gender inequities persists. Members of the HBSC network have been working closely with WHO in monitoring the European child and adolescent health strategy, which aims to address the social determinants of health and bridge the equality gap for young people (9). HBSC data will play an important role in ensuring that the strategy's commitments are realized.

The adoption of supportive environments for the whole community, rather than just for at-risk populations, is necessary. Supportive environments include schools and communities, but also cyberspace. Investment is needed for programmes that contribute to young people being informed online users, foster healthy and responsible online interactions with peers and include educational messages about the potentially negative consequences of online activities.

Comprehensive, integrated, flexible and sustainable policies to achieve positive health outcomes in this age group are only possible with the necessary political will to ensure sufficient resources are allocated for implementation and evaluation.

GROWING UP UNEQUAL: GENDER AND SOCIOECONOMIC
DIFFERENCES IN YOUNG PEOPLE'S HEALTH AND WELL-BEING
PART 3. DISCUSSION | CHAPTER 9. CONCLUSION

9

The knowledge generated from these activities can provide valuable insights into what works in promoting young people's health.

The HBSC study has now been active for over 30 years. It is well positioned to provide solid evidence on children and young people's needs and strengths and relevant data to enhance understanding of health inequalities. The study's efforts to increase young people's participation in the production of science and policy results in data that better reflects their lifestyles and priorities *(16)*, while also being of significant value to programme and policy design.

The report underscores the importance of giving young people a stronger voice and offering them more opportunities for engagement in activities related to their health and well-being. Young people should play an active role in identifying their social and health problems and challenges and contribute to the development of solutions and interventions that target them as a group.

REFERENCES

1. Boniel-Nissim M, Lenzi M, Zsiros E, Gaspar de Matos M, Gommans R, Harel-Fisch Y et al. International trends in electronic media communication among 11- to 15-year-olds in 30 countries from 2002 to 2010: association with ease of communication with friends of the opposite sex. Eur J Public Health 2015;25(Suppl. 2):41–5.

2. Pickett W, Craig W, Harel-Fisch Y, Cunningham J, Simpson K, Molcho M et al. Cross-national study of fighting and weapon carrying as determinants of adolescent injury. Pediatrics 2005;116(6):e855–63.

3. Chester KL, Callaghan M, Cosma A, Donnelly P, Craig W, Walsh S et al. Cross-national time trends in bullying victimization in 33 countries among children aged 11, 13 and 15 from 2002 to 2010. Eur J Public Health 2015;25(Suppl. 2):61–4.

4. de Looze M, Vermeulen-Smit E, ter Bogt TF, van Dorsselaer SA, Verdurmen J, Schulten I et al. Trends in alcohol-specific parenting practices and adolescent alcohol use between 2007 and 2011 in the Netherlands. Int J Drug Policy 2014;25(1):133–41. doi:10.1016/j.drugpo.2013.09.007.

5. Hublet A, Bendtsen P, de Looze M, Fotiou A, Donnelly P, Vilhjalmsson R et al. Trends in the co-occurrence of tobacco and cannabis use in 15-year-olds from 2002 to 2010 in 28 countries of Europe and North America. Eur J Public Health 2015;25(Suppl. 2):73–5.

6. Elgar FJ, Pförtner T-K, Moor I, De Clercq B, Stevens GWJM, Currie C. Socioeconomic inequalities in adolescent health 2002–2010: a time-series analysis of 34 countries participating in the Health Behaviour in School-aged Children study. Lancet 2015;385(9982):2088–95.

7. Sawyer SM, Afifi RA, Bearinger LH, Blakemore S-J, Dick B, Ezeh AC et al. Adolescence: a foundation for future health. Lancet 2012;379(9826): 1630–40.

8. Lerner RM, Almerigi JB, Theokas C, Lerner JV. Positive youth development: a view of the issues. J Early Adolesc. 2005;25(1):10–6.

9. Investing in children: the European child and adolescent health strategy 2015–2020. Copenhagen: WHO Regional Office for Europe; 2014 (http://www.euro.who.int/en/health-topics/Life-stages/child-and-adolescent-health/policy/investing-in-children-the-european-child-and-adolescent-health-strategy-20152020, accessed 17 November 2015).

10. Currie C, Aleman-Diaz AY. The importance of large-scale (cross-national) data collection on early adolescents (10–15 years old): shedding light on socioeconomic and gender inequalities in health [website]. Florence: UNICEF Innocenti Research Centre; 2015 (UNICEF Research Watch; http://www.unicef-irc.org/research-watch/are-we-failing-adolescent-girls/1157/, accessed 17 November 2015).

11. Woolf SH, Purnell JQ, Simon SM, Zimmerman EB, Camberos GJ, Haley A et al. Translating evidence into population health improvement: strategies and barriers. Annu Rev Public Health 2015;36:463–82.

12. Schwendicke F, Dörfer CE, Schlattmann P, Page LF, Thomson WM, Paris S. Socioeconomic inequality and caries: a systematic review and meta-analysis. J Dent Res. 2015;94(1):10–8.

13. Gendall P, Hoek J, Marsh L, Edwards R, Healey B. Youth tobacco access: trends and policy implications. BMJ Open 2014;4:e004631. doi:10.1136/bmjopen-2013-004631.

14. Sleet DA, Ballesteros MF, Borse NN. A review of unintentional injuries in adolescents. Annu Rev Public Health 2010;31:195–212.

15. Rubin KH, Bukowski W, Parker J. Peer interactions, relationships, and groups. In: Damon W, Lerner RM, editors. Handbook of child psychology. New York (NY): John Wiley & Sons Inc.; 2007:571–645.

16. Daniels N, Burke L, O'Donnell A, McGovern O, Kelly C, D'Eath M et al. Expanding the role of young people in research: towards a better understanding of their lives. Zdrowie Publiczne i Zarządzanie [Public Health and Management] 2014;12(1):36–44.

SOCIAL DETERMINANTS OF
HEALTH AND WELL-BEING
AMONG YOUNG PEOPLE

ANNEX.
METHODOLOGY AND
SUPPLEMENTARY
DATA TABLES

METHODOLOGY AND SUPPLEMENTARY DATA TABLES

HBSC METHODOLOGY FOR THE 2013/2014 SURVEY

Detailed information on the research methods used by the HBSC network during the 2013/2014 survey can be accessed by registering online for a copy of the 2013/2014 HBSC international study protocol [1] or referring to Schnohr et al. [2].

Sample design

The aim was to ensure that the sample was nationally representative for the age groups of 11-, 13- and 15-year-olds attending school in each country and region. At least 95% of children within these age groups should have been included in the sample frame. The minor proportion not included would represent young people who for different reasons were not in school or who attended schools for children with special needs.

Cluster probability sampling (systematic or random) of school classes was carried out in each country and region. Sampling of schools (proportional to size) was carried out where lists of classes were not available, followed by sampling of classes within school. Samples in some countries and regions were first stratified (by, for example, geopolitical unit or language group). Countries and regions timed their data collection to meet the target ages of 11.5, 13.5 and 15.5 years.

The recommended sample size was 1500 in each age group in each country and region, based on an expected design factor (deft=1.2) that takes into account the effect of clustering, stratification and weighting on the precision of estimates. Compared to random sampling, cluster sampling decreases precision for the same number of individual students. A larger sample must therefore be taken when using cluster sampling than with simple random sampling to maintain a desired level of precision. Previous analyses of HBSC data indicate that a sample size of 1500 will ensure a 95% confidence interval in each age group of ±3% around an estimated proportion of 50%. This level of precision is adequate for the purposes of the study.

In practice, many countries and regions chose to sample more than the minimum sample size in each age group to increase precision of estimates in subpopulations. A census survey approach was considered appropriate in Greenland, Iceland, Luxembourg and Malta owing to the small populations of young people in these countries.

Survey administration

Self-report anonymous questionnaires were administered in school classes between September 2013 and January 2015. This period was longer than in previous HBSC surveys, as a few countries and regions did not compete fieldwork by June 2014 due to individual circumstances. The fieldwork period was six months or less in 34 countries. Table A1 indicates the data collection period for each country and region included in the report. Administration of questionnaires was completed by researchers or teachers using a standard protocol provided by country teams.

Appropriate ethical approval was gained in all countries and regions. Standardized information about the study was provided to parents and students with the invitation to participate. Where possible, special adjustments were made to accommodate students who could not complete the questionnaire under standard conditions (through provision of, for instance, large-print versions or a reader).

GROWING UP UNEQUAL: GENDER AND SOCIOECONOMIC
DIFFERENCES IN YOUNG PEOPLE'S HEALTH AND WELL-BEING
ANNEX. METHODOLOGY AND SUPPLEMENTARY DATA TABLES

A

TABLE A1. FIELDWORK DATES IN THE HBSC 2013/2014 SURVEY

Country/region	Fieldwork period	Country/region	Fieldwork period
Albania	April–May 2014	Italy	April–June 2014
Armenia	November 2013–May 2014	Latvia	January–March 2014
Austria	January–June 2014	Lithuania	March–June 2014
Belgium (Flemish)	January–May 2014	Luxembourg	April–July 2014
Belgium (French)	April–June 2014	Malta	March 2014
Bulgaria	May–June 2014	Netherlands	September–December 2013
Canada	November 2013–June 2014	Norway	March 2014–January 2015
Croatia	March–April 2014	Poland	October 2013–June 2014
Czech Republic	April–June 2014	Portugal	January–March 2014
Denmark	January–March 2014	Republic of Moldova	April 2014
England	September 2013–April 2014	Romania	May–June 2014
Estonia	February–April 2014	Russian Federation	March–October 2014
Finland	March–May 2014	Scotland	February–June 2014
France	April–June 2014	Slovakia	May–June 2014
Germany	October 2013–August 2014	Slovenia	February 2014
Greece	January–April 2014	Spain	March 2014–December 2014
Greenland	April–May 2014	Sweden	January 2014
Hungary	April–May 2014	Switzerland	January–April 2014
Iceland	February 2014	MKD[a]	May 2014
Ireland	April–June 2014	Ukraine	April–May 2014
Israel	May–June 2014	Wales	November 2013–March 2014

[a] The former Yugoslav Republic of Macedonia.

Survey response, achieved sample size and mean ages

Preliminary calculation indicates that student-level response rates were over 60% in most countries and regions. Complete tabulation will be made available on the HBSC website (3). The achieved sample size in each age group was at or above the study aim of 1500 students in most countries and regions (with the exception of those carrying out a census) (Table A2). Nine achieved less than 90% of the desired sample size, resulting in larger confidence intervals.

TABLE A2. NUMBER OF RESPONDENTS IN THE HBSC 2013/2014 SURVEY

Country/region	Gender		Age group			Total
	Boys	Girls	11-year-olds	13-year-olds	15-year-olds	
Albania	2 463	2 561	1 593	1 629	1 699	5 024
Armenia	1 759	1 920	1 471	1 163	1 044	3 679
Austria	1 613	1 845	1 072	1 084	1 264	3 458
Belgium (French)	2 929	2 963	1 977	1 983	1 932	5 892
Belgium (Flemish)	2 407	1 986	1 453	1 177	1 717	4 393
Bulgaria	2 523	2 273	1 592	1 554	1 650	4 796
Canada	6 412	6 519	3 134	4 824	4 973	12 931
Croatia	2 884	2 857	1 792	2 002	1 946	5 741
Czech Republic	2 420	2 662	1 574	1 721	1 760	5 082
Denmark	1 815	2 076	1 223	1 357	1 263	3 891
England	2 768	2 567	2 116	1 593	1 608	5 335
Estonia	2 041	2 016	1 354	1 428	1 269	4 057
Finland	2 914	3 011	1 983	1 887	1 965	5 925
France	2 868	2 823	1 716	2 180	1 740	5 691
Germany	3 035	2 926	1 736	2 070	2 104	5 961
Greece	2 064	2 077	1 357	1 436	1 320	4 141
Greenland	488	532	315	369	320	1 020
Hungary	1 958	1 977	1 424	1 352	1 100	3 935
Iceland	5 312	5 290	3 437	3 686	3 316	10 602
Ireland	1 595	2 503	1 050	1 508	1 520	4 098
Israel	3 018	3 175	2 466	1 863	1 864	6 193
Italy	2 050	2 022	1 337	1 410	1 262	4 072
Latvia	2 653	2 904	1 854	1 955	1 726	5 557
Lithuania	2 910	2 820	2 015	2 017	1 698	5 730
Luxembourg	1 566	1 752	906	1 126	1 079	3 318
Malta	1 165	1 100	809	802	645	2 265
Netherlands	2 114	2 187	1 353	1 524	1 357	4 301
Norway	1 507	1 565	1 233	942	874	3 072
Poland	2 263	2 282	1 507	1 525	1 484	4 545
Portugal	2 371	2 618	1 646	1 983	1 360	4 989
Republic of Moldova	2 348	2 300	1 543	1 549	1 556	4 648
Romania	1 880	2 100	1 259	1 240	1 442	3 980
Russian Federation	2 067	2 649	1 380	1 749	1 445	4 716
Scotland	2 973	2 959	1 867	2 061	1 869	5 932
Slovakia	3 066	3 033	1 772	2 407	1 835	6 099
Slovenia	2 449	2 548	1 633	1 734	1 615	4 997
Spain	5 474	5 662	3 049	4 328	3 759	11 136
Sweden	3 838	3 862	2 621	2 267	2 766	7 700
Switzerland	3 277	3 357	1 972	2 346	2 212	6 634
MKD[a]	2 114	2 104	1 395	1 307	1 457	4 218
Ukraine	2 159	2 393	1 474	1 384	1 694	4 552
Wales	2 631	2 523	1 833	1 863	1 432	5 154
Total	**108 161**	**111 299**	**70 293**	**75 385**	**71 941**	**219 460**

[a] The former Yugoslav Republic of Macedonia.

GROWING UP UNEQUAL: GENDER AND SOCIOECONOMIC
DIFFERENCES IN YOUNG PEOPLE'S HEALTH AND WELL-BEING
ANNEX. METHODOLOGY AND SUPPLEMENTARY DATA TABLES

A

The mean ages across the whole sample were 11.6, 13.5 and 15.5 years (Table A3). Deviations ranged from 11.1 to 11.8 in the youngest age group. The patterns were similar among those aged 13 and 15. The age range is largely explained by countries and regions being unable to undertake data collection around the date determining school entry. In some, the number of children repeating a school year was substantial, resulting in an unbalanced age composition within classes.

TABLE A3. MEAN AGES IN THE HBSC 2013/2014 SURVEY

Country/region	Age group			Total
	11-year-olds	13-year-olds	15-year-olds	
Albania	11.5	13.5	15.5	13.5
Armenia	11.5	13.3	15.3	13.1
Austria	11.3	13.3	15.3	13.4
Belgium (Flemish)	11.5	13.5	15.5	13.6
Belgium (French)	11.5	13.5	15.5	13.5
Bulgaria	11.6	13.7	15.7	13.7
Canada	11.8	13.5	15.4	13.8
Croatia	11.6	13.6	15.6	13.6
Czech Republic	11.4	13.4	15.4	13.4
Denmark	11.7	13.7	15.7	13.7
England	11.7	13.7	15.7	13.5
Estonia	11.8	13.8	15.8	13.8
Finland	11.8	13.8	15.8	13.8
France	11.5	13.5	15.5	13.5
Germany	11.3	13.3	15.3	13.5
Greece	11.7	13.6	15.6	13.6
Greenland	11.5	13.5	15.4	13.5
Hungary	11.6	13.6	15.6	13.4
Iceland	11.6	13.6	15.6	13.6
Ireland	11.6	13.5	15.5	13.7
Israel	12.0	13.8	15.8	13.7
Italy	11.7	13.7	15.7	13.7
Latvia	11.7	13.6	15.6	13.6
Lithuania	11.7	13.7	15.6	13.6
Luxembourg	11.5	13.4	15.4	13.6
Malta	11.7	13.7	15.7	13.5
Netherlands	11.6	13.5	15.4	13.5
Norway	11.6	13.6	15.6	13.3
Poland	11.6	13.6	15.6	13.6
Portugal	11.7	13.6	15.6	13.5
Republic of Moldova	11.6	13.6	15.5	13.6
Romania	11.1	13.1	15.1	13.2
Russian Federation	11.5	13.5	15.4	13.5
Scotland	11.7	13.7	15.7	13.7
Slovakia	11.6	13.5	15.3	13.5
Slovenia	11.7	13.6	15.6	13.6
Spain	11.4	13.4	15.5	13.6
Sweden	11.6	13.5	15.6	13.6
Switzerland	11.5	13.5	15.3	13.5
MKD[a]	11.8	13.6	15.6	13.7
Ukraine	11.6	13.5	15.6	13.7
Wales	11.8	13.8	15.8	13.6
HBSC total	**11.6**	**13.5**	**15.5**	**13.6**

[a] The former Yugoslav Republic of Macedonia.

Table A4 provides an overview of family affluence according to Family Affluence Scale (FAS) scores across countries and regions (for further information about FAS, refer to the HBSC international study protocol *(1)*). In this table, countries and regions' mean level of affluence is expressed through an index. The possible index score ranges from 0 to 100, where a value of 100 is the maximum possible affluence score and 0 is the minimum possible score. HBSC countries and regions differ on this index, with values ranging from 38 (Albania) to 76 (Luxembourg).

TABLE A4. FAMILY AFFLUENCE ACCORDING TO FAS COMPOSITE SCORES (ALL AGES)

Country/region	Mean FAS index score (0 to 100)	Country/region	Mean FAS index score (0 to 100)
Albania	38	Canada	65
Republic of Moldova	40	Finland	65
Ukraine	41	Iceland	65
Armenia[a]	41	Belgium (French)	65
Romania	43	Portugal	66
Greenland	45	Netherlands	66
Russian Federation	48	Ireland	67
Hungary	49	Scotland	68
Latvia	50	England	68
Greece	51	France	68
Bulgaria	52	Germany	69
MKD[b]	53	Belgium (Flemish)	69
Poland	53	Austria	69
Slovakia	55	Slovenia	69
Croatia	56	Wales	70
Estonia	58	Sweden	71
Italy	58	Malta	71
Israel	59	Denmark	71
Czech Republic	61	Switzerland	74
Lithuania[a]	62	Norway	76
Spain	63	Luxembourg	76

[a] The index for Armenia and Lithuania was based on a subset of family affluence items. [b] The former Yugoslav Republic of Macedonia.

Analyses

Results for some indicators are presented only for a subset of countries and regions, either due to the relevant indicator not being included or deviations at country/region level. Tables for some indicators from the report are presented in this Annex with different cut-offs (such as daily smoking in addition to the weekly smoking cut-off used in the main report), along with some additional indicators that do not appear in the main text.

Analyses for age and gender take account of the effect of the survey design (including stratification, clustering and weighting) on the precision of estimates presented. The significance level was set at 5%.

Design-adjusted analyses were completed using the Complex Samples module IBM® SPSS® Statistics 22.0 (Armonk (NY): IBM Corp.; 2013). Gender differences were tested for statistical significance using design-adjusted chi-square tests for independence. Statistical significance of linear trends across age groups and across family affluence were tested using design-adjusted chi-square test. To avoid overinterpretation of small differences, only statistically significant and consistent patterns between individual variables and family affluence are discussed in the text.

GROWING UP UNEQUAL: GENDER AND SOCIOECONOMIC
DIFFERENCES IN YOUNG PEOPLE'S HEALTH AND WELL-BEING
ANNEX. METHODOLOGY AND SUPPLEMENTARY DATA TABLES

A

SUPPLEMENTARY DATA TABLES

The following tables are supplementary to data presented in Chapters 2–5.

1. Social context:
- family structure: young people living in different family types
- immigrant status
- high quality of family communication
- spending time with friends after 8 pm (20:00) daily
- contacting friends using texting/SMS daily.

2. Health outcomes:
- overweight and obesity, using International Obesity Task Force cut-off points
- overweight and obesity: rates of missing BMI data
- most serious injury requiring medical treatment
- reporting difficulties getting to sleep more than once a week
- reporting stomach ache more than once a week
- reporting feeling nervous more than once a week
- reporting a headache more than once a week
- reporting feeling low more than once a week.

3. Health behaviours:
- participating in vigorous physical activity for two or more hours per week
- daily vegetable consumption
- daily sweets consumption
- having breakfast with mother or father every day
- using a computer for email, internet or homework for two or more hours on weekdays
- playing games on a computer or games console for two or more hours on weekdays.

4. Risk behaviour:
- drinking beer at least once a week
- drinking alcopops at least once a week
- drinking wine at least once a week
- drinking spirits at least once a week
- first alcohol use at age 13 or younger
- ever smoked tobacco
- daily smoking
- involved in a physical fight at least once in the past 12 months
- been bullied at school at least once in the past couple of months
- bullying others at school at least once in the past couple of months
- been cyberbullied by messages at least once
- been cyberbullied by pictures at least once
- been cyberbullied by pictures at least 2–3 times a month.

SOCIAL CONTEXT
FAMILY STRUCTURE: YOUNG PEOPLE LIVING IN DIFFERENT FAMILY TYPES

Country/region	Both parents (%)	Single parent (%)	Stepfamily (%)	Other (%)
Albania	93	6	1	0
Armenia	89	9	0	1
MKD[a]	87	10	1	2
Malta	85	11	1	3
Israel	84	11	4	1
Croatia	84	10	4	2
Greece	84	12	3	1
Italy	82	13	3	2
Slovenia	79	13	6	2
Spain	79	14	6	2
Poland	78	14	6	2
Switzerland	77	14	8	1
Ireland	77	16	6	1
Republic of Moldova	77	14	5	5
Slovakia	76	22	1	1
Netherlands	76	15	9	1
Austria	75	16	7	2
Romania	75	17	4	5
Norway	75	14	10	1
Bulgaria	74	16	5	5
Germany	74	15	10	2
Portugal	73	16	9	2
Ukraine	73	17	8	2
Denmark	72	17	10	1
Belgium (Flemish)	71	14	14	1
Luxembourg	71	15	12	3
Lithuania	70	18	9	3
Finland	70	14	14	1
England	70	18	11	2
France	69	16	13	2
Hungary	69	18	10	3
Iceland	69	16	13	1
Sweden	69	18	10	3
Canada	68	17	10	5
Czech Republic	68	18	12	2
Russian Federation	67	20	10	2
Belgium (French)	66	15	17	2
Estonia	66	19	14	2
Scotland	65	21	12	3
Latvia	64	21	11	4
Wales	61	24	11	4
Greenland	52	23	14	11

MEASURE Young people were asked about their family living arrangements and who they lived with most of the time. Findings presented here show the proportions who reported living primarily with both parents, within a stepfamily, single-parent family or some other arrangement (for instance, a foster home or cared for by non-parental family members).

[a] The former Yugoslav Republic of Macedonia.

GROWING UP UNEQUAL: GENDER AND SOCIOECONOMIC
DIFFERENCES IN YOUNG PEOPLE'S HEALTH AND WELL-BEING
ANNEX. METHODOLOGY AND SUPPLEMENTARY DATA TABLES

A

SOCIAL CONTEXT
IMMIGRANT STATUS

Country/region	First-generation (%)	Second-generation (%)	Non-immigrant (%)
Albania	6	0	94
Austria[a]	5	17	77
Belgium (Flemish)	8	18	75
Belgium (French)	11	27	62
Bulgaria	1	2	96
Croatia	4	21	76
Czech Republic[a]	2	7	91
Denmark	6	21	74
Estonia	2	15	82
Finland	4	7	89
Germany	5	23	72
Greece	5	18	77
Iceland	7	6	88
Ireland	14	17	69
Israel	7	29	65
Italy	5	9	87
Luxembourg	20	47	33
Malta	5	16	79
Netherlands	4	19	77
Norway	7	15	78
Portugal[a]	6	16	78
Republic of Moldova	2	6	92
Romania	3	2	95
Russian Federation	7	13	80
Scotland[b]	5	10	85
Slovenia	5	12	83
Spain	10	11	79
Sweden	10	21	69
Switzerland	10	39	51
Ukraine	2	11	88
Wales[c]	4	8	88

Note: no data were received from Armenia, Canada, England, France, Greenland, Hungary, Latvia, Lithuania, Poland, Slovakia and the former Yugoslav Republic of Macedonia.

MEASURE Young people were asked if both they and their parents were born in their country of residence or in another country. First-generation immigrant means that the child was born abroad; second-generation immigrant means the child was born in the country of residence, but at least one of the parents was born abroad; and non-immigrant means the child and both parents were born in the country of residence.

[a] Data were available only for 15-year-olds. [b] Adolescents or parents born in England or Wales are not considered immigrants. [c] Adolescents or parents born in England or Scotland are not considered immigrants.

SOCIAL CONTEXT
HIGH QUALITY OF FAMILY COMMUNICATION

11-year-olds (%)				13-year-olds (%)				15-year-olds (%)			
Country/region	Boys	Girls	Total	Country/region	Boys	Girls	Total	Country/region	Boys	Girls	Total
Romania	68	72	70	Albania	60	67	64	Albania	64	68	66
Israel	62	69	66	Republic of Moldova	58	62	60	Republic of Moldova	52	55	53
Croatia	68	64	66	Romania	54	61	58	Greenland	59	46	52
Albania	62	68	65	Israel	51	57	54	Romania	51	52	52
Republic of Moldova	61	63	62	Iceland	51	56	54	Iceland	48	54	51
Iceland	57	65	61	MKDª	52	52	52	Israel	46	51	49
Spain	59	61	60	Switzerland	52	50	51	Switzerland	49	45	47
Malta	54	65	59	Croatia	47	51	49	Norway	41	48	44
MKDª	58	59	59	Luxembourg	51	45	48	Sweden	42	46	44
Germany	56	59	58	Sweden	47	48	48	MKDª	44	45	44
Switzerland	56	56	56	Malta	45	49	47	Finland	40	43	42
Sweden	54	58	56	Germany	49	45	47	Germany	44	39	42
Finland	53	56	55	Spain	48	43	46	Malta	43	40	41
Slovenia	54	54	54	Hungary	44	43	44	Croatia	42	39	40
Denmark	58	48	52	Norway	41	45	43	Hungary	37	42	39
Norway	50	54	52	Finland	40	45	42	Armenia	41	37	38
Portugal	52	52	52	Armenia	42	42	42	Luxembourg	44	33	38
Luxembourg	50	53	51	Portugal	42	40	41	Portugal	38	37	37
Greece	49	52	50	Denmark	46	37	41	Denmark	38	34	36
Wales	49	50	50	Greenland	45	37	41	Spain	37	34	35
Scotland	47	51	49	Slovenia	38	40	39	Russian Federation	34	33	34
England	48	50	49	Greece	39	38	38	Estonia	30	35	33
Lithuania	46	48	47	Estonia	36	37	37	Greece	31	33	32
Hungary	46	47	46	Lithuania	38	35	36	Ukraine	29	35	32
Bulgaria	47	45	46	France	40	32	36	Austria	30	33	32
Greenland	49	43	46	Ukraine	32	40	36	Bulgaria	31	32	32
Latvia	42	47	45	Italy	37	34	36	Netherlands	32	32	32
Estonia	39	50	45	Canada	37	33	35	Latvia	33	29	31
Poland	43	46	45	Russian Federation	32	37	35	Slovenia	30	30	30
France	46	42	44	Scotland	34	34	34	France	33	26	29
Ireland	39	43	42	Poland	35	33	34	Lithuania	30	27	29
Armenia	40	42	41	Bulgaria	36	31	33	Italy	28	26	27
Italy	39	42	41	Netherlands	32	35	33	Canada	28	27	27
Austria	35	43	39	England	32	33	33	Wales	27	24	25
Canada	38	40	39	Latvia	35	31	33	Belgium (Flemish)	26	24	25
Belgium (Flemish)	38	37	38	Ireland	32	33	33	Czech Republic	25	23	24
Belgium (French)	37	36	37	Austria	33	32	33	Scotland	25	23	24
Slovakia	39	35	37	Belgium (Flemish)	33	31	32	Belgium (French)	25	23	24
Russian Federation	36	37	36	Wales	32	31	31	England	25	22	24
Ukraine	36	36	36	Czech Republic	31	28	29	Ireland	23	24	23
Czech Republic	33	34	34	Slovakia	30	27	28	Poland	23	23	23
Netherlands	28	37	33	Belgium (French)	31	24	28	Slovakia	19	22	20
HBSC average	**49**	**51**	**50**	**HBSC average**	**41**	**41**	**41**	**HBSC average**	**35**	**36**	**36**

MEASURE Young people were asked several questions about the quality of their family communication, including whether important things are talked about, if someone listens, and whether misunderstandings are clarified. Responses options ranged from strongly agree to strongly disagree. Findings presented here show the proportions with a mean score of 4.5 or higher, indicating high quality of family communication.

ª The former Yugoslav Republic of Macedonia.

GROWING UP UNEQUAL: GENDER AND SOCIOECONOMIC
DIFFERENCES IN YOUNG PEOPLE'S HEALTH AND WELL-BEING
ANNEX. METHODOLOGY AND SUPPLEMENTARY DATA TABLES

A

SOCIAL CONTEXT
SPENDING TIME WITH FRIENDS AFTER 8 PM (20:00) DAILY

11-year-olds (%) Country/region	Boys	Girls	Total	13-year-olds (%) Country/region	Boys	Girls	Total	15-year-olds (%) Country/region	Boys	Girls	Total
Bulgaria	30	20	25	Bulgaria	39	28	34	Bulgaria	46	37	42
Lithuania	18	11	15	MKD[a]	28	15	21	MKD[a]	41	21	31
Norway	16	13	15	Lithuania	23	14	19	Romania	26	22	24
MKD[a]	20	7	13	Albania	25	8	16	Hungary	23	17	20
Albania	21	6	13	Greece	20	9	14	Greece	26	14	20
Armenia	15	8	12	Romania	15	13	14	Lithuania	25	13	19
Russian Federation	12	9	10	Iceland	14	13	14	Albania	30	7	18
Romania	12	7	10	Armenia	19	8	13	Russian Federation	20	16	18
Scotland	12	6	9	Scotland	14	12	13	Iceland	20	15	18
Croatia	11	6	9	Hungary	17	8	12	Israel	20	15	17
Luxembourg	11	7	9	Russian Federation	13	11	12	Croatia	22	12	17
Hungary	11	6	8	Croatia	14	8	11	Ukraine	19	13	16
Canada	11	6	8	Luxembourg	14	9	11	Armenia	29	6	15
Ukraine	11	4	7	Ukraine	12	8	10	Luxembourg	19	10	14
Greece	9	4	7	Norway	10	9	10	Scotland	16	12	14
Wales	8	4	6	Wales	8	9	9	Slovakia	15	12	14
Republic of Moldova	8	4	6	Slovakia	10	8	9	Republic of Moldova	15	9	12
Iceland	5	5	5	Canada	11	6	8	Finland	17	7	12
Slovakia	7	3	5	Republic of Moldova	10	6	8	Poland	13	9	11
Finland	6	4	5	Israel	9	5	7	Norway	11	9	10
Poland	5	4	4	Finland	9	4	6	Wales	13	8	10
Denmark	5	4	4	Italy	9	4	6	Italy	11	10	10
Malta	7	1	4	Latvia	6	6	6	Latvia	11	8	9
Latvia	5	3	4	Poland	6	5	6	Canada	11	6	9
Belgium (French)	6	2	4	France	7	3	5	Estonia	9	6	7
France	6	2	4	Estonia	6	4	5	Sweden	9	5	7
Italy	6	2	4	Sweden	6	3	5	Netherlands	8	6	7
Germany	4	2	3	England	6	3	4	France	9	5	7
Czech Republic	3	2	3	Denmark	4	4	4	England	8	5	6
Israel	3	2	3	Netherlands	5	3	4	Malta	8	5	6
England	3	2	3	Malta	6	1	4	Germany	7	5	6
Estonia	3	1	2	Belgium (French)	6	2	4	Austria	8	4	6
Sweden	3	1	2	Germany	4	3	4	Belgium (French)	7	3	5
Netherlands	3	1	2	Czech Republic	5	2	3	Czech Republic	5	4	5
Slovenia	3	1	2	Austria	4	2	3	Denmark	6	3	4
Austria	3	1	2	Switzerland	4	2	3	Belgium (Flemish)	6	2	4
Portugal	2	2	2	Slovenia	4	2	3	Slovenia	5	3	4
Switzerland	2	2	2	Belgium (Flemish)	3	2	3	Switzerland	5	3	4
Belgium (Flemish)	2	1	2	Portugal	2	1	2	Portugal	4	3	3
HBSC average	**8**	**5**	**6**	**HBSC average**	**11**	**7**	**9**	**HBSC average**	**15**	**9**	**12**

Note: no data were received from Greenland, Ireland and Spain.

MEASURE Young people were asked how often they meet friends outside school time after 8 o'clock in the evening. Response options ranged from hardly ever or never to daily. Findings presented here show the proportions who reported spending time with friends daily.

[a] The former Yugoslav Republic of Macedonia.

SOCIAL CONTEXT
CONTACTING FRIENDS USING TEXTING/SMS DAILY

11-year-olds (%)				13-year-olds (%)				15-year-olds (%)			
Country/region	Boys	Girls	Total	Country/region	Boys	Girls	Total	Country/region	Boys	Girls	Total
Italy	51	63	57	Italy	77	83	80	Italy	83	91	87
Israel	38	58	49	Netherlands	59	74	66	Netherlands	67	82	74
Lithuania	33	48	40	Sweden	45	74	59	France	64	79	71
England	30	46	37	Luxembourg	52	63	58	Austria	58	78	70
Sweden	26	47	36	Israel	53	60	57	Luxembourg	62	76	69
Germany	29	38	33	Belgium (Flemish)	47	68	57	Belgium (Flemish)	62	77	68
Wales	27	38	33	Lithuania	42	67	55	Sweden	58	78	68
Ireland	27	37	33	Germany	47	61	54	Israel	62	69	66
Denmark	22	35	29	England	41	65	53	Lithuania	51	78	64
Luxembourg	23	33	28	Ireland	44	58	52	England	53	67	60
Netherlands	22	35	28	Wales	34	61	47	Wales	48	72	60
Canada	21	34	28	Finland	40	51	45	Germany	54	65	60
Greenland	19	33	26	Latvia	31	58	45	Latvia	44	72	59
Latvia	18	29	24	Belgium (French)	33	54	44	Ireland	48	66	59
Scotland	16	29	23	Scotland	33	54	43	Belgium (French)	46	66	56
Russian Federation	15	27	22	Denmark	33	52	43	Canada	46	66	56
Belgium (Flemish)	18	24	21	Canada	30	51	41	Scotland	44	66	55
Albania	26	14	20	Poland	24	45	35	Denmark	43	65	55
Bulgaria	17	21	19	Russian Federation	23	41	33	Poland	38	61	50
Armenia	21	17	19	Albania	36	30	33	Switzerland	46	52	49
Croatia	12	22	17	Greenland	21	42	32	Slovenia	34	60	48
MKD[a]	15	17	16	Slovenia	20	36	28	Finland	46	42	44
Norway	12	20	16	Norway	20	33	27	Albania	48	38	42
Poland	10	20	15	Croatia	20	33	27	Russian Federation	35	48	42
Malta	14	14	14	Armenia	19	31	25	Iceland	33	50	41
Portugal	7	17	13	Greece	18	32	25	Portugal	28	54	41
Republic of Moldova	12	13	12	Iceland	18	32	25	Romania	26	51	40
Slovenia	9	15	12	Bulgaria	19	31	25	Malta	33	43	38
Ukraine	8	14	11	MKD[a]	19	28	24	Norway	26	46	36
Iceland	8	13	10	Romania	16	31	23	Greenland	26	44	35
Romania	9	11	10	Portugal	15	31	23	MKD[a]	30	38	34
Estonia	7	11	9	Malta	15	26	20	Armenia	27	35	32
Czech Republic	6	12	9	Ukraine	10	24	17	Bulgaria	26	39	32
Greece	7	9	8	Republic of Moldova	13	21	17	Croatia	22	35	29
Hungary	4	9	6	Estonia	10	20	15	Greece	20	34	27
Austria	–	–	–	Czech Republic	11	14	12	Ukraine	18	35	27
Belgium (French)	–	–	–	Hungary	6	11	8	Republic of Moldova	18	25	22
Finland	–	–	–	Austria	–	–	–	Czech Republic	11	24	17
France	–	–	–	France	–	–	–	Estonia	12	19	15
Switzerland	–	–	–	Switzerland	–	–	–	Hungary	9	12	10
HBSC average	**19**	**27**	**23**	**HBSC average**	**30**	**45**	**38**	**HBSC average**	**41**	**56**	**49**

Note: no data were received from Austria (11- and 13-year-olds), Belgium (French) (11-year-olds), Finland (11-year-olds), France (11-year-olds), Slovakia, Spain and Switzerland (11- and 13-year-olds).

MEASURE Young people were asked how often they contact friends using texting/SMS. Response options ranged from hardly ever or never to daily. Findings presented here show the proportions who reported texting with their friends every day.

[a] The former Yugoslav Republic of Macedonia.

GROWING UP UNEQUAL: GENDER AND SOCIOECONOMIC
DIFFERENCES IN YOUNG PEOPLE'S HEALTH AND WELL-BEING
ANNEX. METHODOLOGY AND SUPPLEMENTARY DATA TABLES

A

HEALTH OUTCOMES
OVERWEIGHT AND OBESITY, USING INTERNATIONAL OBESITY TASK FORCE CUT-OFF POINTS

11-year-olds (%)

Country/region	Boys	Girls	Total
Malta[a]	28	28	28
Greece	25	22	23
MKD[b]	29	14	22
Canada[a]	23	18	21
Bulgaria	25	16	20
Wales[a]	20	20	20
Greenland[a]	24	15	20
Italy	22	17	20
Spain	22	16	19
Poland	21	16	19
Armenia[a]	20	16	18
Croatia	23	14	18
Portugal	22	15	18
Slovenia	20	17	18
Romania[a]	24	11	18
Latvia	20	15	17
Ireland[a]	5	29	17
Slovakia	20	14	17
Russian Federation	20	14	17
England[a]	17	15	16
Hungary	21	11	16
Estonia	19	13	16
Czech Republic	19	12	15
Finland	16	13	14
Lithuania[a]	17	11	14
Israel[a]	17	11	14
Scotland[a]	15	13	14
Albania	17	10	14
Austria	14	13	13
France	12	13	12
Luxembourg	13	11	12
Iceland	14	11	12
Belgium (French)[a]	13	12	12
Sweden	12	10	11
Belgium (Flemish)	11	11	11
Ukraine	12	8	10
Germany	11	8	10
Republic of Moldova	10	9	9
Switzerland	10	9	9
Norway	11	7	9
Netherlands	10	7	8
Denmark	9	7	8
HBSC average	**18**	**13**	**15**

13-year-olds (%)

Country/region	Boys	Girls	Total
Malta[a]	26	27	27
Canada	24	21	22
Portugal	21	18	19
Italy	23	15	19
Greece	22	15	18
MKD[b]	23	14	18
Slovenia	22	12	17
Greenland[a]	16	19	17
Scotland[a]	18	15	17
Spain	20	14	17
Bulgaria	21	12	17
Wales[a]	19	13	16
Hungary	19	12	16
Latvia	17	14	16
Finland	20	11	15
Croatia	20	11	15
Austria	18	12	15
England[a]	21	9	15
Armenia	20	10	15
Iceland	17	12	15
Poland	19	10	15
Luxembourg	18	11	15
Belgium (French)[a]	16	13	14
Czech Republic	20	10	14
Slovakia	19	10	14
Estonia	15	13	14
Ireland[a]	12	15	14
Israel	16	11	13
Romania[a]	18	8	13
Sweden	15	11	13
Russian Federation	17	10	13
Germany	15	10	13
Belgium (Flemish)	13	11	12
Republic of Moldova	13	11	12
France	14	9	11
Norway	14	8	11
Ukraine	14	8	11
Lithuania[a]	14	7	10
Netherlands	11	9	10
Switzerland	13	7	10
Albania	12	5	8
Denmark	8	8	8
HBSC average	**18**	**12**	**15**

15-year-olds (%)

Country/region	Boys	Girls	Total
Malta[a]	29	25	27
Greenland[a]	23	26	25
Canada	30	19	24
Greece	28	15	21
Wales[a]	23	16	20
Bulgaria	24	11	18
Iceland	20	16	18
Israel	21	13	17
Finland	20	14	17
Slovenia	21	13	17
Sweden	20	13	16
Spain	20	13	16
MKD[b]	21	12	16
Hungary	20	12	16
Germany	20	12	16
Portugal	17	14	16
Ireland[a]	18	13	15
Italy	22	9	15
Luxembourg	17	13	15
Czech Republic	19	11	15
Belgium (French)	17	13	15
Croatia	21	8	15
Scotland[a]	16	11	14
England[a]	16	12	14
Estonia	19	9	14
Romania	18	9	13
Belgium (Flemish)	15	11	13
Slovakia	17	9	13
Norway	18	7	13
Russian Federation	20	6	12
Latvia	16	9	12
Poland	19	6	12
France	14	10	12
Netherlands	13	12	12
Switzerland	15	9	12
Austria	16	9	12
Lithuania	14	7	11
Republic of Moldova	13	7	10
Denmark	10	9	10
Armenia	14	6	9
Ukraine	13	6	9
Albania	11	4	7
HBSC average	**19**	**11**	**15**

MEASURE Young people were asked how much they weigh without clothes and how tall they are without shoes, and to record these in country-appropriate units (centimetres versus inches, pounds versus kilograms). These data were (re)coded in centimetres and kilograms respectively to compute the body mass index (BMI) as weight (kg) divided by height (m²). The analysis presented here uses the international BMI standards for young people adopted by the International Obesity Task Force (IOTF), called the IOTF BMI cut-off points.

[a] BMI is missing for more than 30% of the age-group sample. [b] The former Yugoslav Republic of Macedonia.

HEALTH OUTCOMES
OVERWEIGHT AND OBESITY: RATES OF MISSING BMI DATA

11-year-olds (%)				13-year-olds (%)				15-year-olds (%)			
Country/region	Boys	Girls	Total	Country/region	Boys	Girls	Total	Country/region	Boys	Girls	Total
Ireland	82	88	85	Ireland	68	75	72	Ireland	55	65	61
Scotland	78	79	79	Scotland	70	73	72	Scotland	58	64	61
Wales	72	79	76	England	55	63	59	Wales	38	44	41
England	62	72	66	Wales	57	58	57	England	31	47	39
Malta	58	56	57	Greenland	40	57	49	Malta	35	35	35
Greenland	44	56	50	Malta	44	39	42	Greenland	35	30	33
Romania	46	54	50	Belgium (French)	40	40	40	Belgium (French)	31	29	30
Israel	39	44	42	Romania	35	42	38	Romania	25	33	29
Lithuania	37	41	39	Lithuania	32	34	33	Lithuania	21	22	22
Belgium (French)	38	40	39	Israel	27	27	27	Israel	19	20	20
Armenia	32	42	37	Canada	23	29	26	MKD[a]	19	19	19
Canada	32	40	37	Armenia	20	25	22	Canada	15	16	16
Iceland	28	30	29	Netherlands	22	18	20	Armenia	13	17	15
Germany	25	30	27	Sweden	19	17	18	Sweden	14	12	13
MKD[a]	21	23	22	Iceland	18	17	18	Netherlands	13	10	11
Sweden	21	20	20	France	16	19	17	Spain	11	11	11
Netherlands	19	21	20	Germany	16	18	17	Germany	9	12	11
Belgium (Flemish)	18	21	19	Spain	17	15	16	Belgium (Flemish)	11	10	10
Italy	16	22	19	MKD[a]	15	16	16	Russian Federation	10	10	10
Norway	16	20	18	Switzerland	10	16	13	Iceland	10	9	10
Estonia	21	12	17	Luxembourg	12	13	12	Norway	7	13	10
France	16	17	17	Italy	10	14	12	Switzerland	8	10	9
Hungary	15	16	16	Hungary	11	12	11	Italy	8	10	9
Finland	15	16	16	Belgium (Flemish)	11	11	11	Luxembourg	9	9	9
Spain	16	14	15	Norway	9	12	11	Slovakia	8	8	8
Denmark	11	18	15	Slovakia	11	11	11	France	7	8	7
Switzerland	12	17	14	Russian Federation	11	10	11	Hungary	6	9	7
Luxembourg	12	14	13	Albania	9	10	10	Bulgaria	6	8	7
Albania	13	13	13	Austria	9	10	10	Austria	7	7	7
Slovakia	12	13	13	Finland	9	9	9	Estonia	8	6	7
Russian Federation	15	10	12	Estonia	9	8	8	Albania	7	6	6
Austria	11	12	12	Denmark	7	9	8	Ukraine	6	6	6
Poland	11	9	10	Bulgaria	6	10	8	Poland	4	8	6
Ukraine	12	9	10	Poland	8	8	8	Czech Republic	6	6	6
Bulgaria	9	9	9	Ukraine	8	6	7	Finland	5	5	5
Czech Republic	9	9	9	Slovenia	5	5	5	Denmark	3	5	4
Slovenia	9	7	8	Czech Republic	5	5	5	Croatia	4	4	4
Croatia	5	6	5	Croatia	5	5	5	Latvia	3	2	3
Greece	5	5	5	Latvia	4	3	4	Slovenia	3	3	3
Latvia	6	3	4	Greece	2	4	3	Greece	2	2	2
Portugal	4	3	3	Portugal	2	2	2	Portugal	2	1	1
Republic of Moldova	0	0	0	Republic of Moldova	0	0	0	Republic of Moldova	0	0	0
HBSC average	**24**	**26**	**25**	**HBSC average**	**19**	**21**	**20**	**HBSC average**	**13**	**15**	**14**

MEASURE Young people were asked to give their height (without shoes) and weight (without clothes). BMI was calculated from this information and cut-offs for overweight and obesity allocated. Findings presented here show the levels of missing data across all countries and regions.

[a] The former Yugoslav Republic of Macedonia.

GROWING UP UNEQUAL: GENDER AND SOCIOECONOMIC
DIFFERENCES IN YOUNG PEOPLE'S HEALTH AND WELL-BEING
ANNEX. METHODOLOGY AND SUPPLEMENTARY DATA TABLES

A

HEALTH OUTCOMES
MOST SERIOUS INJURY REQUIRING MEDICAL TREATMENT

11-year-olds (%)				13-year-olds (%)				15-year-olds (%)			
Country/region	Boys	Girls	Total	Country/region	Boys	Girls	Total	Country/region	Boys	Girls	Total
France	34	26	30	France	32	29	31	France	34	26	30
Latvia	28	21	24	Italy	32	21	26	Latvia	30	22	25
Lithuania	28	20	24	Latvia	31	21	26	Czech Republic	25	24	25
Russian Federation	27	21	23	Lithuania	28	22	25	Italy	27	18	23
Italy	28	18	23	Germany	27	22	25	Germany	26	19	23
Romania	26	18	22	Czech Republic	23	23	23	Austria	25	19	22
Ukraine	26	18	22	Croatia	26	18	22	Lithuania	24	19	22
Belgium (French)	27	17	22	Denmark	25	19	22	Denmark	24	20	22
Germany	24	19	22	Belgium (French)	25	16	21	Russian Federation	25	18	21
Armenia	28	15	21	Greece	23	17	20	Croatia	24	15	19
Croatia	24	18	21	Iceland	23	17	20	Slovenia	25	14	19
Luxembourg	25	17	21	Estonia	22	18	20	Estonia	23	15	19
Scotland	25	16	20	Luxembourg	26	15	20	Canada	22	16	19
Estonia	23	17	20	Russian Federation	22	18	20	Scotland	24	14	19
Republic of Moldova	22	16	19	Republic of Moldova	24	15	20	Luxembourg	23	15	19
Belgium (Flemish)	21	17	19	Wales	24	15	20	Ukraine	21	16	19
Greece	23	15	19	Ukraine	25	15	20	Switzerland	22	15	19
Denmark	23	15	19	Slovenia	25	14	20	Ireland	23	16	18
Iceland	19	17	18	Armenia	26	12	19	Sweden	22	15	18
Israel	23	14	18	Sweden	25	14	19	Belgium (Flemish)	19	15	18
Bulgaria	22	14	18	Ireland	22	17	19	Iceland	20	15	18
Slovenia	18	16	17	Bulgaria	24	13	19	Wales	21	14	17
Wales	17	16	17	Romania	20	16	18	Poland	20	15	17
England	19	13	17	Norway	22	14	18	Belgium (French)	22	13	17
Ireland	16	17	16	Scotland	22	14	18	Hungary	17	15	16
Canada	18	15	16	Canada	20	15	18	Romania	18	15	16
Poland	18	14	16	Poland	21	13	17	Republic of Moldova	20	13	16
Malta	22	9	16	Belgium (Flemish)	16	18	17	Bulgaria	20	10	16
Sweden	20	12	16	Israel	19	12	16	Portugal	18	13	15
Norway	20	10	15	Portugal	20	11	15	Norway	17	14	15
Netherlands	17	12	15	Netherlands	16	14	15	Greece	19	12	15
Finland	17	12	15	Finland	19	12	15	Malta	20	10	15
Portugal	18	10	13	England	17	13	15	Finland	20	10	15
Hungary	15	11	13	Hungary	18	12	15	Armenia	19	11	14
Albania	14	6	10	Malta	16	12	14	England	18	10	14
Austria	–	–	–	Albania	14	10	12	Netherlands	17	12	14
Czech Republic	–	–	–	Austria	–	–	–	Israel	18	11	14
Switzerland	–	–	–	Switzerland	–	–	–	Albania	14	8	11
HBSC average	**22**	**16**	**19**	**HBSC average**	**23**	**16**	**20**	**HBSC average**	**22**	**15**	**18**

Note: no data were received from Austria (11- and 13-year-olds), Czech Republic (11-year-olds), Greenland, the former Yugoslav Republic of Macedonia, Slovakia, Spain and Switzerland (11- and 13-year-olds).

MEASURE Young people were asked if the most serious injury required medical treatment such as the placement of a cast, stitches, surgery or staying in a hospital overnight. Findings presented here show the proportions who responded yes.

HEALTH OUTCOMES
REPORTING DIFFICULTIES GETTING TO SLEEP MORE THAN ONCE A WEEK

11-year-olds (%)				13-year-olds (%)				15-year-olds (%)			
Country/region	Boys	Girls	Total	Country/region	Boys	Girls	Total	Country/region	Boys	Girls	Total
France	37	40	38	France	33	43	38	France	30	45	37
Belgium (French)	27	35	31	Sweden	26	38	32	Sweden	28	39	33
Netherlands	27	30	29	Belgium (French)	24	38	31	Greenland	30	34	32
Iceland	26	28	27	Greenland	21	35	29	Canada	25	38	31
Sweden	25	29	27	Netherlands	23	32	27	Belgium (French)	25	36	31
Switzerland	23	30	27	Iceland	24	29	27	Luxembourg	25	34	30
Denmark	24	28	26	Wales	22	31	26	Scotland	22	36	29
Luxembourg	24	25	25	Canada	19	32	26	Wales	21	35	28
Canada	24	25	24	Denmark	19	31	26	Ireland	17	34	28
Greenland	19	28	24	Switzerland	20	29	25	Israel	25	28	27
Wales	21	23	22	Luxembourg	18	29	24	England	20	33	26
Czech Republic	22	21	22	Bulgaria	21	28	24	Iceland	20	31	26
Israel	21	22	21	Israel	23	25	24	Denmark	22	29	26
Belgium (Flemish)	18	23	21	Slovenia	17	30	24	Slovenia	18	31	25
Scotland	21	20	21	Belgium (Flemish)	21	26	23	Bulgaria	20	31	25
Bulgaria	19	21	20	England	18	27	23	Netherlands	17	32	25
England	19	20	19	Czech Republic	18	27	23	Poland	17	31	24
Germany	19	19	19	Scotland	17	26	21	Belgium (Flemish)	17	33	23
Italy	17	21	19	Ireland	17	24	21	Switzerland	17	29	23
Slovenia	16	21	19	Austria	18	22	20	Romania	15	29	23
Estonia	16	19	18	Germany	16	25	20	Czech Republic	17	27	22
Austria	17	18	18	Finland	16	24	20	Malta	18	27	22
Norway	15	19	17	Italy	16	24	20	Germany	14	28	21
Finland	14	20	17	Poland	17	22	20	Italy	16	26	21
Latvia	17	17	17	Romania	13	25	19	MKD[a]	16	25	21
Romania	15	18	16	Lithuania	13	24	19	Lithuania	15	26	20
Ireland	15	17	16	Latvia	15	21	18	Latvia	17	23	20
Hungary	13	18	16	Slovakia	15	21	18	Estonia	18	22	20
Malta	17	14	16	Hungary	13	23	18	Hungary	14	25	20
Poland	14	17	15	Malta	14	22	18	Finland	15	23	19
Lithuania	15	16	15	Estonia	15	20	18	Norway	13	24	19
Armenia	15	15	15	MKD[a]	12	21	16	Portugal	11	25	18
Russian Federation	15	14	14	Norway	11	21	16	Greece	13	21	17
Republic of Moldova	14	14	14	Greece	11	18	15	Slovakia	12	22	17
Spain	13	13	13	Portugal	11	17	14	Austria	15	18	17
MKD[a]	12	13	12	Croatia	12	16	14	Albania	11	20	16
Croatia	12	12	12	Spain	11	16	14	Croatia	12	20	16
Slovakia	13	12	12	Republic of Moldova	12	14	13	Spain	12	18	15
Portugal	8	13	11	Armenia	13	13	13	Republic of Moldova	12	17	14
Ukraine	11	10	10	Russian Federation	11	14	12	Armenia	9	15	13
Greece	8	12	10	Albania	9	8	9	Russian Federation	11	14	13
Albania	8	9	9	Ukraine	8	8	8	Ukraine	10	13	12
HBSC average	**18**	**20**	**19**	**HBSC average**	**17**	**25**	**21**	**HBSC average**	**18**	**28**	**23**

MEASURE Young people were asked how often they had experienced the following symptoms in the last six months: headache; stomach ache; feeling low, irritable or bad tempered; feeling nervous; difficulties in getting to sleep; and feeling dizzy. Response options for each symptom ranged from about every day to rarely or never. Findings presented here show the proportions who reported experiencing difficulties getting to sleep more than once a week.

[a] The former Yugoslav Republic of Macedonia.

GROWING UP UNEQUAL: GENDER AND SOCIOECONOMIC
DIFFERENCES IN YOUNG PEOPLE'S HEALTH AND WELL-BEING
ANNEX: METHODOLOGY AND SUPPLEMENTARY DATA TABLES

A

HEALTH OUTCOMES
REPORTING STOMACH ACHE MORE THAN ONCE A WEEK

11-year-olds (%)				13-year-olds (%)				15-year-olds (%)			
Country/region	Boys	Girls	Total	Country/region	Boys	Girls	Total	Country/region	Boys	Girls	Total
Israel	20	23	21	Israel	16	21	19	Malta	15	25	20
Armenia	16	18	17	Poland	13	24	18	Israel	15	24	20
Romania	13	19	16	France	10	21	15	Poland	13	21	17
Italy	13	19	16	Hungary	10	20	15	Sweden	9	22	15
Poland	10	22	16	Republic of Moldova	11	18	15	Luxembourg	9	20	15
France	11	20	15	Slovakia	9	19	14	Hungary	7	21	14
Greenland	8	21	15	Luxembourg	8	19	14	France	8	21	14
MKD[a]	11	18	14	Belgium (French)	10	16	13	Greenland	7	20	14
Iceland	11	17	14	Iceland	11	16	13	Iceland	8	21	14
Bulgaria	12	16	14	Malta	11	15	13	Italy	8	20	14
Russian Federation	13	15	14	Romania	10	15	13	Slovakia	11	17	14
Malta	12	16	14	Sweden	7	18	13	Bulgaria	8	18	12
Hungary	10	17	13	Armenia	13	12	12	Latvia	7	17	12
Republic of Moldova	12	15	13	Italy	6	19	12	Belgium (Flemish)	8	19	12
Slovakia	10	15	13	Russian Federation	10	14	12	Lithuania	8	17	12
Latvia	11	13	12	Bulgaria	9	16	12	Republic of Moldova	8	16	12
Croatia	9	15	12	Spain	8	15	12	Russian Federation	10	13	12
Ukraine	9	14	12	Belgium (Flemish)	10	13	12	Belgium (French)	9	14	12
Luxembourg	7	15	11	Lithuania	8	14	11	Scotland	6	16	11
Spain	9	13	11	Greenland	9	13	11	Romania	7	14	11
Lithuania	10	12	11	Latvia	8	14	11	Wales	6	16	11
Sweden	8	14	11	Wales	5	16	10	England	5	17	11
Belgium (French)	8	13	11	Croatia	7	14	10	Ireland	5	14	11
Belgium (Flemish)	8	12	10	MKD[a]	8	12	10	Canada	5	16	10
Switzerland	6	14	10	England	6	14	10	Norway	7	13	10
Norway	7	12	9	Switzerland	5	14	10	Spain	6	13	10
Netherlands	7	11	9	Canada	6	13	10	Greece	6	14	10
Estonia	7	11	9	Netherlands	7	12	9	Albania	5	12	9
Denmark	5	12	9	Scotland	5	13	9	Netherlands	4	15	9
Wales	5	12	9	Slovenia	6	12	9	Slovenia	5	12	9
Canada	8	9	9	Ukraine	6	11	8	Armenia	7	10	9
England	6	11	8	Germany	5	12	8	Croatia	4	14	9
Greece	6	9	8	Austria	3	13	8	Germany	4	13	9
Germany	6	10	8	Norway	5	11	8	Ukraine	6	11	8
Slovenia	6	10	8	Greece	6	10	8	MKD[a]	6	10	8
Czech Republic	7	8	7	Ireland	5	10	8	Austria	4	11	8
Scotland	5	9	7	Finland	5	10	8	Switzerland	4	12	8
Albania	6	8	7	Denmark	3	10	7	Finland	4	11	8
Ireland	5	8	7	Czech Republic	4	10	7	Czech Republic	3	11	7
Austria	5	7	6	Portugal	5	9	7	Portugal	5	9	7
Finland	4	8	6	Estonia	5	8	7	Denmark	3	9	6
Portugal	3	7	5	Albania	6	7	6	Estonia	4	7	6
HBSC average	**9**	**13**	**11**	**HBSC average**	**8**	**14**	**11**	**HBSC average**	**7**	**15**	**11**

MEASURE Young people were asked how often they had experienced the following symptoms in the last six months: headache; stomach ache; feeling low, irritable or bad tempered; feeling nervous; difficulties in getting to sleep; and feeling dizzy. Response options for each symptom ranged from about every day to rarely or never. Findings presented here show the proportions who reported experiencing stomach ache more than once a week.

[a] The former Yugoslav Republic of Macedonia.

HEALTH OUTCOMES
REPORTING FEELING NERVOUS MORE THAN ONCE A WEEK

11-year-olds (%)				13-year-olds (%)				15-year-olds (%)			
Country/region	Boys	Girls	Total	Country/region	Boys	Girls	Total	Country/region	Boys	Girls	Total
Bulgaria	26	32	29	Bulgaria	33	46	39	Italy	34	57	45
Israel	28	30	29	Italy	28	48	38	MKD[a]	33	52	43
Czech Republic	25	28	26	MKD[a]	30	44	37	Bulgaria	33	53	42
MKD[a]	23	29	26	Israel	27	39	33	Poland	31	46	39
Italy	24	28	26	Slovakia	27	36	32	Malta	30	44	37
Malta	23	27	25	Czech Republic	24	38	31	Israel	33	40	36
Poland	23	26	24	Greece	24	36	30	Greece	25	44	35
Croatia	22	25	24	Croatia	23	36	30	Belgium (French)	26	38	32
Slovakia	23	21	22	Poland	24	35	29	Albania	22	39	31
Belgium (French)	20	22	21	Belgium (French)	22	32	27	Czech Republic	24	37	31
Ukraine	16	25	21	Malta	21	33	27	France	23	37	30
France	17	22	20	Hungary	19	33	26	Hungary	25	34	30
Hungary	19	20	19	Spain	20	31	26	Slovakia	24	36	30
Romania	18	20	19	Luxembourg	20	30	25	Croatia	22	38	30
Spain	18	20	19	France	19	28	23	Luxembourg	20	37	29
Greece	16	20	18	Romania	15	30	23	Ireland	19	34	28
Lithuania	16	19	17	Lithuania	16	29	22	Ukraine	19	35	28
Russian Federation	15	18	17	Canada	13	30	21	Scotland	17	39	28
Luxembourg	17	16	16	Scotland	15	28	21	Latvia	19	34	27
Estonia	16	16	16	Slovenia	14	28	21	Slovenia	18	35	27
Canada	13	18	16	Albania	16	26	21	Canada	16	38	27
Armenia	17	15	16	Ukraine	16	26	21	Spain	19	34	27
Switzerland	15	16	15	Russian Federation	16	25	21	Lithuania	17	38	27
Latvia	15	16	15	Ireland	14	25	21	Romania	16	35	27
Republic of Moldova	15	16	15	Armenia	16	25	20	Portugal	14	37	26
Finland	12	18	15	Latvia	15	24	20	Estonia	19	32	26
Greenland	10	18	14	Sweden	12	26	19	Russian Federation	18	32	26
Belgium (Flemish)	12	17	14	Finland	13	24	19	Armenia	19	27	24
Wales	11	17	14	Belgium (Flemish)	15	22	18	Sweden	16	31	24
Scotland	12	15	13	Republic of Moldova	13	23	18	England	15	29	22
Albania	12	15	13	Estonia	12	23	18	Wales	13	30	22
Portugal	9	16	13	Wales	11	24	17	Republic of Moldova	14	29	21
Netherlands	13	13	13	Portugal	12	23	17	Iceland	11	31	21
Slovenia	11	16	13	England	11	23	17	Finland	13	27	20
Sweden	9	14	12	Netherlands	14	21	17	Belgium (Flemish)	15	26	20
Denmark	10	13	12	Switzerland	14	19	17	Norway	9	25	17
England	8	14	11	Greenland	10	20	15	Denmark	9	22	16
Ireland	8	11	10	Denmark	10	19	15	Switzerland	12	19	16
Norway	7	12	10	Iceland	11	19	15	Greenland	13	16	15
Austria	8	11	9	Austria	11	16	14	Netherlands	10	19	14
Iceland	8	9	9	Norway	7	17	12	Austria	10	13	12
Germany	9	9	9	Germany	8	10	9	Germany	7	15	11
HBSC average	**15**	**18**	**17**	**HBSC average**	**17**	**28**	**22**	**HBSC average**	**19**	**34**	**26**

MEASURE Young people were asked how often they had experienced the following symptoms in the last six months: headache; stomach ache; feeling low, irritable or bad tempered; feeling nervous; difficulties in getting to sleep; and feeling dizzy. Response options for each symptom ranged from about every day to rarely or never. Findings presented here show the proportions who reported being nervous more than once a week.

[a] The former Yugoslav Republic of Macedonia.

GROWING UP UNEQUAL: GENDER AND SOCIOECONOMIC
DIFFERENCES IN YOUNG PEOPLE'S HEALTH AND WELL-BEING
ANNEX. METHODOLOGY AND SUPPLEMENTARY DATA TABLES

A

HEALTH OUTCOMES
REPORTING A HEADACHE MORE THAN ONCE A WEEK

11-year-olds (%)				13-year-olds (%)				15-year-olds (%)			
Country/region	Boys	Girls	Total	Country/region	Boys	Girls	Total	Country/region	Boys	Girls	Total
Israel	23	25	24	Poland	20	31	26	Malta	28	40	34
Republic of Moldova	21	24	22	Israel	18	33	26	Israel	21	37	30
Romania	17	26	22	Italy	15	32	23	Albania	16	40	28
Russian Federation	21	21	21	Greenland	17	28	23	Poland	20	36	28
Greenland	13	28	21	Republic of Moldova	16	29	22	Greenland	17	36	27
Italy	16	24	20	Malta	19	26	22	Republic of Moldova	16	36	26
Malta	19	20	19	Russian Federation	17	26	22	Italy	14	38	26
Poland	15	24	19	Romania	15	28	21	Hungary	13	35	25
Armenia	19	19	19	Armenia	17	25	21	Armenia	17	29	24
Belgium (French)	14	20	17	Slovakia	16	25	21	Bulgaria	15	35	24
Iceland	14	20	17	Belgium (French)	15	26	21	Romania	13	32	24
Latvia	14	19	17	Hungary	13	27	20	Slovakia	15	32	23
Hungary	13	19	16	Latvia	13	26	19	Belgium (French)	15	31	23
Slovakia	15	17	16	Bulgaria	14	25	19	Ireland	11	30	23
France	14	18	16	Albania	12	25	19	Latvia	12	31	22
Bulgaria	15	17	16	Wales	12	25	18	Luxembourg	14	29	22
Albania	13	19	16	Lithuania	13	23	18	Russian Federation	17	26	22
Netherlands	13	18	15	Netherlands	12	24	18	Wales	11	32	21
Czech Republic	11	19	15	Iceland	14	21	18	Sweden	13	29	21
Ukraine	14	15	15	France	15	21	18	Canada	12	31	21
Lithuania	12	17	14	Belgium (Flemish)	14	21	17	MKD[a]	13	29	21
Wales	11	16	13	Spain	13	22	17	Greece	12	30	21
Estonia	11	15	13	Sweden	12	23	17	Scotland	11	30	21
Spain	11	15	13	Finland	12	21	17	Netherlands	10	33	21
MKD[a]	11	14	13	Luxembourg	12	21	17	England	11	31	21
Canada	11	14	12	England	11	22	17	Spain	12	26	20
Sweden	11	13	12	Czech Republic	11	22	17	Belgium (Flemish)	14	28	20
Switzerland	9	15	12	Greece	11	22	17	Iceland	12	26	19
Denmark	10	14	12	Estonia	11	22	16	France	11	28	19
Germany	10	13	11	Scotland	9	22	16	Lithuania	10	28	19
Greece	8	14	11	Portugal	10	19	14	Czech Republic	10	27	18
England	10	12	11	MKD[a]	10	18	14	Portugal	9	26	18
Belgium (Flemish)	10	12	11	Canada	9	19	14	Finland	11	24	18
Croatia	9	11	10	Ireland	10	17	14	Germany	8	26	17
Portugal	7	13	10	Croatia	9	19	14	Slovenia	10	23	17
Luxembourg	8	12	10	Ukraine	8	18	13	Estonia	9	25	17
Finland	7	13	10	Denmark	8	17	13	Ukraine	10	22	17
Scotland	9	10	10	Switzerland	10	16	13	Switzerland	9	23	16
Slovenia	7	11	9	Norway	9	17	13	Croatia	7	26	16
Ireland	5	11	9	Slovenia	9	16	13	Austria	7	22	16
Austria	7	10	8	Germany	8	18	13	Norway	7	22	15
Norway	5	10	8	Austria	6	13	10	Denmark	7	19	13
HBSC average	**12**	**16**	**14**	**HBSC average**	**12**	**22**	**17**	**HBSC average**	**12**	**29**	**21**

MEASURE Young people were asked how often they had experienced the following symptoms in the last six months: headache; stomach ache; feeling low, irritable or bad tempered; feeling nervous; difficulties in getting to sleep; and feeling dizzy. Response options for each symptom ranged from about every day to rarely or never. Findings presented here show the proportions who reported experiencing a headache more than once a week.

[a] The former Yugoslav Republic of Macedonia.

HEALTH OUTCOMES
REPORTING FEELING LOW MORE THAN ONCE A WEEK

11-year-olds (%)				13-year-olds (%)				15-year-olds (%)			
Country/region	Boys	Girls	Total	Country/region	Boys	Girls	Total	Country/region	Boys	Girls	Total
Italy	21	31	26	Italy	24	48	36	Italy	28	52	40
Romania	23	29	26	Romania	19	39	29	Armenia	24	37	32
Republic of Moldova	20	25	22	Armenia	20	33	27	Romania	19	40	31
Greenland	11	31	21	Hungary	19	32	26	MKD[a]	21	39	30
Armenia	20	21	21	MKD[a]	20	29	25	Malta	20	36	28
Luxembourg	17	23	20	Republic of Moldova	19	30	24	Albania	18	38	28
Israel	18	20	19	Israel	18	27	23	Republic of Moldova	21	35	28
Estonia	15	22	18	Greece	15	30	23	Hungary	21	32	27
Malta	15	21	18	Slovakia	13	30	22	Poland	17	35	27
Hungary	15	18	17	Malta	14	30	22	Luxembourg	16	34	26
Slovakia	13	19	16	Luxembourg	12	29	21	Scotland	15	37	26
Lithuania	12	19	16	Poland	15	27	21	Israel	21	30	26
MKD[a]	13	17	15	Greenland	8	31	20	Sweden	14	36	25
Switzerland	10	19	15	Estonia	11	29	20	Greece	15	34	25
Iceland	13	17	15	Sweden	10	29	19	Latvia	14	34	25
Russian Federation	11	17	14	Albania	14	24	19	Greenland	15	32	24
France	13	15	14	Lithuania	11	26	18	England	14	33	23
Denmark	8	19	14	Czech Republic	10	24	17	Ireland	13	29	23
Poland	11	16	14	Croatia	10	24	17	Wales	15	32	23
Croatia	11	15	13	Scotland	10	24	17	Belgium (French)	17	28	23
Belgium (French)	12	15	13	France	12	23	17	Estonia	12	33	23
Latvia	11	15	13	Slovenia	8	25	17	Slovenia	10	33	22
Albania	12	12	12	Russian Federation	11	20	16	Iceland	13	31	22
Bulgaria	10	13	12	Latvia	10	22	16	Lithuania	12	32	21
Czech Republic	10	14	12	Wales	8	24	16	France	13	29	21
Ukraine	9	14	12	Iceland	11	21	16	Slovakia	14	28	21
Greece	10	13	11	Switzerland	8	23	16	Russian Federation	14	26	20
Canada	10	12	11	Belgium (French)	12	19	15	Czech Republic	12	28	20
Sweden	7	13	10	England	9	21	15	Spain	13	24	19
Norway	8	12	10	Ireland	10	18	15	Canada	11	27	19
Wales	7	11	10	Canada	8	21	15	Croatia	8	30	19
Slovenia	7	11	9	Netherlands	10	17	13	Bulgaria	11	25	17
Scotland	9	10	9	Spain	9	18	13	Switzerland	8	25	17
Netherlands	8	10	9	Denmark	5	20	13	Norway	7	25	16
Spain	8	10	9	Norway	7	19	13	Ukraine	10	21	16
Finland	8	8	8	Bulgaria	8	19	13	Portugal	8	22	15
England	6	8	7	Portugal	7	15	11	Denmark	5	21	14
Portugal	5	8	7	Ukraine	7	14	11	Netherlands	7	21	14
Austria	6	6	6	Finland	7	14	11	Germany	8	19	13
Germany	5	6	6	Belgium (Flemish)	8	13	10	Austria	7	17	13
Ireland	3	7	6	Germany	6	14	10	Belgium (Flemish)	7	21	13
Belgium (Flemish)	4	7	6	Austria	6	12	9	Finland	7	16	12
HBSC average	**11**	**15**	**13**	**HBSC average**	**11**	**23**	**17**	**HBSC average**	**13**	**29**	**21**

MEASURE Young people were asked how often they had experienced the following symptoms in the last six months: headache; stomach ache; feeling low, irritable or bad tempered; feeling nervous; difficulties in getting to sleep; and feeling dizzy. Response options for each symptom ranged from about every day to rarely or never. Findings presented here show the proportions who reported feeling low more than once a week.

[a] The former Yugoslav Republic of Macedonia.

GROWING UP UNEQUAL: GENDER AND SOCIOECONOMIC
DIFFERENCES IN YOUNG PEOPLE'S HEALTH AND WELL-BEING
ANNEX. METHODOLOGY AND SUPPLEMENTARY DATA TABLES

A

HEALTH BEHAVIOURS
PARTICIPATING IN VIGOROUS PHYSICAL ACTIVITY FOR TWO OR MORE HOURS PER WEEK

11-year-olds (%)				13-year-olds (%)				15-year-olds (%)			
Country/region	Boys	Girls	Total	Country/region	Boys	Girls	Total	Country/region	Boys	Girls	Total
Netherlands	83	80	82	Netherlands	83	73	78	Denmark	79	73	76
Luxembourg	78	67	72	Norway	73	76	75	Netherlands	79	68	74
Switzerland	77	67	72	Denmark	81	69	74	Norway	72	75	74
Belgium (Flemish)	75	68	71	Switzerland	84	62	73	Belgium (Flemish)	74	62	69
Norway	72	65	69	Luxembourg	77	62	69	Finland	68	69	68
Denmark	75	62	68	Finland	70	68	69	Switzerland	76	60	68
Finland	69	66	68	Austria	74	62	68	Luxembourg	75	56	65
Austria	70	64	67	Belgium (Flemish)	73	58	66	Germany	73	55	64
Scotland	67	60	63	Germany	68	60	64	Sweden	66	59	62
Germany	66	58	62	Belgium (French)	70	52	61	Austria	74	54	62
Belgium (French)	69	53	61	Scotland	66	53	59	Belgium (French)	70	52	60
Sweden	61	58	59	Sweden	62	56	59	Lithuania	67	50	59
Canada	63	56	59	Iceland	58	58	58	Canada	64	51	58
Greece	64	52	58	Canada	63	53	58	Scotland	63	53	58
France	63	44	54	Greece	62	51	57	Spain	68	44	55
Ireland	58	49	52	France	65	46	56	Ireland	62	47	53
Slovakia	57	46	51	Spain	66	43	54	Czech Republic	58	47	52
Poland	57	41	49	Lithuania	61	45	53	Estonia	60	44	52
Slovenia	55	43	49	Ireland	61	47	53	Latvia	58	47	52
Spain	58	38	48	Italy	60	43	52	Italy	62	41	52
Iceland	50	46	48	Czech Republic	56	48	52	France	62	40	51
Italy	54	39	47	Slovenia	60	43	51	England	62	40	51
Hungary	51	39	45	Wales	57	44	51	Greece	60	41	50
Israel	53	37	45	Estonia	51	48	50	Wales	59	41	50
England	51	38	45	England	58	41	49	Hungary	58	41	49
Bulgaria	51	38	44	Hungary	58	37	47	Slovenia	57	40	48
Wales	51	37	44	Israel	58	37	47	Slovakia	56	37	47
Malta	50	36	43	Slovakia	55	38	46	Israel	54	37	45
Latvia	48	38	43	Latvia	53	39	46	Greenland	46	43	44
Estonia	45	40	43	Malta	53	36	45	Russian Federation	49	39	44
Lithuania	47	36	42	Croatia	54	35	44	Croatia	55	29	43
Czech Republic	46	37	41	Poland	53	32	43	Poland	53	32	42
Romania	50	32	41	Bulgaria	49	35	42	Bulgaria	50	32	42
Croatia	45	33	39	Russian Federation	46	39	42	Portugal	53	29	40
MKD[a]	42	28	35	MKD[a]	48	36	42	Ukraine	47	33	40
Portugal	45	27	35	Romania	48	32	40	MKD[a]	47	27	37
Russian Federation	39	32	35	Greenland	48	32	39	Romania	49	27	37
Greenland	33	36	34	Portugal	54	25	39	Republic of Moldova	47	25	36
Ukraine	41	27	34	Ukraine	42	30	36	Malta	47	24	35
Armenia	40	23	31	Armenia	45	26	36	Armenia	50	22	34
Republic of Moldova	39	24	31	Republic of Moldova	39	26	33	Albania	41	21	30
Albania	30	18	24	Albania	35	23	28	Iceland	19	23	21
HBSC average	**56**	**45**	**50**	**HBSC average**	**60**	**46**	**53**	**HBSC average**	**59**	**44**	**51**

MEASURE Young people were asked to report the number of hours per week that they were usually physically active in their free time (outside school hours), so much so that they got out of breath or sweated. Findings presented here show the proportions who participated in vigorous physical activity for two or more hours per week.

[a] The former Yugoslav Republic of Macedonia.

HEALTH BEHAVIOURS
DAILY VEGETABLE CONSUMPTION

11-year-olds (%) Country/region	Boys	Girls	Total	13-year-olds (%) Country/region	Boys	Girls	Total	15-year-olds (%) Country/region	Boys	Girls	Total
Ukraine	52	61	57	Belgium (French)	50	60	55	Belgium (French)	53	65	59
Belgium (Flemish)	50	62	56	Ukraine	49	59	54	Belgium (Flemish)	50	57	53
Belgium (French)	49	61	55	Belgium (Flemish)	46	59	52	Ukraine	44	54	50
Israel	48	56	52	Israel	42	58	49	Israel	38	52	46
Canada	45	57	51	Netherlands	45	50	48	Switzerland	37	52	45
Netherlands	46	55	50	Canada	42	52	47	Canada	39	49	44
Denmark	43	53	48	Switzerland	40	47	44	Ireland	41	45	44
Ireland	44	50	48	MKD[a]	39	47	43	Netherlands	38	49	43
Switzerland	45	50	47	Ireland	37	47	43	Denmark	34	48	41
Bulgaria	41	52	47	Denmark	37	48	43	England	36	44	40
France	44	49	46	England	40	45	43	Republic of Moldova	37	40	39
Sweden	40	50	45	Greenland	38	46	42	Sweden	33	44	39
England	42	46	44	Bulgaria	36	44	40	Greenland	35	41	38
Greenland	36	50	43	Scotland	35	42	39	France	37	39	38
MKD[a]	36	50	43	France	36	41	39	Bulgaria	32	43	37
Republic of Moldova	39	46	42	Albania	36	41	38	MKD[a]	31	43	37
Norway	40	43	41	Republic of Moldova	36	40	38	Albania	32	41	37
Luxembourg	38	44	41	Sweden	32	42	37	Malta	38	32	35
Scotland	37	44	41	Russian Federation	33	39	37	Scotland	32	38	35
Romania	38	42	40	Romania	33	38	36	Armenia	29	38	35
Albania	37	42	40	Greece	33	36	34	Iceland	29	39	34
Greece	32	42	37	Wales	33	35	34	Russian Federation	33	34	33
Russian Federation	35	36	36	Norway	33	34	33	Norway	29	35	32
Hungary	33	37	35	Armenia	29	37	33	Greece	26	35	31
Austria	31	37	34	Hungary	31	31	31	Luxembourg	29	32	31
Poland	29	39	34	Luxembourg	28	33	31	Italy	21	37	29
Croatia	34	34	34	Malta	35	23	29	Lithuania	26	32	29
Lithuania	30	37	33	Lithuania	24	34	29	Romania	25	30	28
Slovenia	32	34	33	Portugal	26	32	29	Wales	28	28	28
Armenia	29	36	33	Austria	24	32	28	Poland	26	28	27
Portugal	26	38	32	Croatia	26	30	28	Austria	22	30	27
Iceland	31	33	32	Slovakia	25	30	27	Finland	15	36	26
Wales	30	34	32	Poland	25	30	27	Latvia	20	30	26
Finland	29	33	31	Czech Republic	24	30	27	Hungary	22	29	25
Czech Republic	27	33	31	Iceland	23	29	26	Croatia	22	28	25
Slovakia	27	30	29	Finland	18	32	25	Czech Republic	20	29	24
Estonia	26	30	28	Italy	20	31	25	Slovenia	19	29	24
Latvia	25	31	28	Germany	19	29	24	Slovakia	19	29	24
Germany	23	32	28	Latvia	19	27	23	Germany	16	31	24
Malta	35	18	27	Slovenia	20	27	23	Portugal	21	25	23
Spain	24	28	26	Spain	20	24	22	Estonia	20	25	22
Italy	23	28	25	Estonia	21	22	22	Spain	17	22	20
HBSC average	**35**	**42**	**39**	**HBSC average**	**31**	**38**	**35**	**HBSC average**	**30**	**38**	**34**

MEASURE Young people were asked how often they eat vegetables. Response options ranged from never to more than once a day. Findings presented here show the proportions who reported eating vegetables every day or more than once a day.

[a] The former Yugoslav Republic of Macedonia.

GROWING UP UNEQUAL: GENDER AND SOCIOECONOMIC
DIFFERENCES IN YOUNG PEOPLE'S HEALTH AND WELL-BEING
ANNEX. METHODOLOGY AND SUPPLEMENTARY DATA TABLES

A

HEALTH BEHAVIOURS
DAILY SWEETS CONSUMPTION

11-year-olds (%)				13-year-olds (%)				15-year-olds (%)			
Country/region	Boys	Girls	Total	Country/region	Boys	Girls	Total	Country/region	Boys	Girls	Total
Armenia	47	48	47	Armenia	50	58	54	Armenia	52	63	59
Bulgaria	44	43	44	Bulgaria	42	50	46	MKD[a]	40	48	44
Ukraine	36	39	37	Romania	38	49	43	Belgium (French)	42	46	44
Belgium (French)	34	41	37	Ukraine	36	45	41	Bulgaria	37	47	42
Scotland	33	39	36	Belgium (French)	37	43	40	Ukraine	34	45	40
Slovakia	33	36	34	Albania	38	38	38	Romania	36	42	40
Romania	32	35	34	Slovakia	34	40	37	Albania	36	43	39
Israel	31	35	33	MKD[a]	32	42	37	Scotland	34	36	35
Russian Federation	26	35	31	Hungary	32	40	36	Slovakia	30	39	35
Hungary	30	31	31	Israel	28	42	35	Republic of Moldova	30	35	33
Netherlands	30	32	31	Scotland	33	35	34	Croatia	26	38	32
Albania	30	31	31	Croatia	32	35	34	Hungary	30	34	32
Germany	28	30	29	Russian Federation	30	36	34	Israel	27	35	32
Republic of Moldova	27	30	28	Austria	29	36	33	Latvia	24	36	31
Austria	28	29	28	Netherlands	32	31	31	Russian Federation	23	37	31
Italy	27	27	27	Poland	28	34	31	Switzerland	27	33	30
Croatia	26	27	27	Italy	31	31	31	Ireland	27	32	30
Switzerland	25	28	26	Switzerland	29	32	30	Greenland	31	28	30
Luxembourg	27	24	25	Latvia	23	36	30	Netherlands	27	31	29
MKD[a]	25	25	25	Republic of Moldova	26	33	30	Austria	29	29	29
Malta	25	25	25	Greenland	26	31	29	Poland	25	31	28
Estonia	21	29	25	Germany	24	29	27	Italy	28	26	27
Poland	23	26	25	Wales	24	28	26	France	24	29	26
Greenland	30	19	24	Ireland	23	28	26	Germany	24	27	26
Latvia	20	27	24	England	22	29	25	Luxembourg	23	26	24
Lithuania	22	23	23	Estonia	23	28	25	England	24	24	24
Wales	21	23	22	France	23	27	25	Belgium (Flemish)	25	21	24
Belgium (Flemish)	20	22	21	Luxembourg	24	24	24	Wales	23	22	23
Czech Republic	22	19	20	Lithuania	22	24	23	Estonia	20	24	22
England	21	20	20	Czech Republic	22	23	23	Malta	15	26	21
Ireland	18	21	20	Belgium (Flemish)	22	21	21	Czech Republic	19	21	20
France	21	19	20	Malta	19	24	21	Lithuania	18	21	19
Slovenia	14	14	14	Greece	17	19	18	Portugal	17	19	18
Canada	14	14	14	Slovenia	15	19	17	Greece	16	20	18
Portugal	13	10	12	Portugal	16	16	16	Slovenia	14	18	16
Greece	10	10	10	Canada	15	15	15	Canada	16	14	15
Spain	8	10	9	Spain	13	15	14	Spain	13	15	14
Denmark	4	5	4	Denmark	7	9	8	Denmark	8	7	8
Norway	4	2	3	Norway	7	5	6	Norway	9	5	7
Iceland	2	2	2	Sweden	5	4	4	Sweden	5	4	5
Sweden	3	2	2	Finland	3	3	3	Finland	3	3	3
Finland	2	1	2	Iceland	3	2	2	Iceland	3	2	3
HBSC average	**21**	**23**	**22**	**HBSC average**	**23**	**27**	**25**	**HBSC average**	**23**	**26**	**24**

MEASURE Young people were asked how often they eat sweets. Response options ranged from never to more than once a day. Findings presented here show the proportions who reported eating sweets every day or more than once a day.

[a] The former Yugoslav Republic of Macedonia.

HEALTH BEHAVIOURS
HAVING BREAKFAST WITH MOTHER OR FATHER EVERY DAY

11-year-olds (%) Country/region	Boys	Girls	Total	13-year-olds (%) Country/region	Boys	Girls	Total	15-year-olds (%) Country/region	Boys	Girls	Total
Republic of Moldova	64	68	66	Republic of Moldova	59	58	59	Republic of Moldova	55	46	50
Ukraine	60	66	63	Ukraine	57	58	57	MKD[a]	46	42	44
Armenia	49	54	51	Armenia	43	48	45	Ukraine	43	40	42
Portugal	51	51	51	Albania	43	44	44	Armenia	39	39	39
Albania	47	53	50	Portugal	43	34	39	Lithuania	34	24	29
Lithuania	48	49	49	Lithuania	41	34	38	Albania	28	27	27
Spain	47	48	48	Russian Federation	39	33	35	Russian Federation	31	23	26
Russian Federation	48	47	48	Switzerland	33	29	31	Portugal	27	21	24
Netherlands	46	46	46	Spain	36	25	31	Belgium (French)	24	21	22
Switzerland	48	42	45	Luxembourg	31	29	30	Luxembourg	24	18	21
Latvia	45	45	45	Belgium (French)	31	28	30	Switzerland	22	19	21
Luxembourg	46	42	44	Netherlands	31	28	29	Italy	22	18	20
Germany	44	42	43	Belgium (Flemish)	31	28	29	Belgium (Flemish)	23	15	20
Belgium (French)	43	41	42	Germany	32	27	29	Latvia	22	18	20
France	43	40	41	Italy	34	24	29	Germany	21	19	20
Belgium (Flemish)	41	41	41	Latvia	30	26	28	Spain	22	15	18
Sweden	41	38	39	France	30	23	26	Bulgaria	17	16	17
Romania	39	39	39	Croatia	27	24	25	Croatia	18	15	17
Austria	40	36	38	Bulgaria	28	20	24	Netherlands	21	12	16
Denmark	41	35	38	Austria	28	21	24	France	19	13	16
Norway	41	32	36	Romania	25	23	24	Malta	19	12	16
Italy	37	34	35	Iceland	26	20	23	Denmark	17	12	14
Iceland	37	34	35	Denmark	26	19	22	Israel	14	14	14
Croatia	38	33	35	Malta	27	16	21	Norway	17	10	13
Bulgaria	33	36	34	Norway	24	18	21	Ireland	18	10	13
Estonia	35	30	33	Estonia	27	14	21	Austria	15	11	12
Ireland	33	30	31	Sweden	25	16	21	Estonia	16	9	12
Israel	34	28	31	Poland	23	16	20	Iceland	15	9	12
Poland	33	28	30	Israel	19	20	19	Canada	13	10	12
Malta	31	29	30	Hungary	21	17	19	Greece	14	8	11
Hungary	28	27	27	Ireland	20	18	19	Romania	12	10	11
Canada	27	25	26	Canada	21	15	18	Sweden	15	7	11
Greece	25	25	25	Greece	18	15	17	Slovakia	12	8	10
Czech Republic	25	23	24	Czech Republic	15	15	15	Hungary	11	8	9
Scotland	24	23	23	Wales	17	12	14	Poland	12	6	9
Slovenia	22	21	22	Scotland	16	10	13	Wales	10	7	9
Wales	22	20	21	Slovenia	11	11	11	Scotland	10	7	8
England	22	19	21	England	13	9	11	England	8	7	7
Finland	17	12	14	Finland	9	6	8	Czech Republic	9	5	7
MKD[a]	–	–	–	MKD[a]	–	–	–	Slovenia	9	5	7
Slovakia	–	–	–	Slovakia	–	–	–	Finland	5	3	4
HBSC average	**38**	**36**	**37**	**HBSC average**	**28**	**23**	**26**	**HBSC average**	**19**	**15**	**17**

Note: no data were received from Greenland, the former Yugoslav Republic of Macedonia (11- and 13-year-olds) and Slovakia (11- and 13-year-olds).

MEASURE Young people were asked how often they eat breakfast with their family. Findings presented here show the proportions who eat breakfast with at least one of their parents every day.

[a] The former Yugoslav Republic of Macedonia.

GROWING UP UNEQUAL: GENDER AND SOCIOECONOMIC
DIFFERENCES IN YOUNG PEOPLE'S HEALTH AND WELL-BEING
ANNEX. METHODOLOGY AND SUPPLEMENTARY DATA TABLES

A

HEALTH BEHAVIOURS
USING A COMPUTER FOR EMAIL, INTERNET OR HOMEWORK FOR TWO OR MORE HOURS ON WEEKDAYS

11-year-olds (%)				13-year-olds (%)				15-year-olds (%)			
Country/region	Boys	Girls	Total	Country/region	Boys	Girls	Total	Country/region	Boys	Girls	Total
Israel	51	57	54	Bulgaria	64	72	68	Scotland	74	82	78
Bulgaria	52	48	50	Scotland	63	72	67	Netherlands	72	85	78
Wales	53	47	50	Wales	65	68	66	Norway	70	78	74
Scotland	42	45	44	Netherlands	62	70	66	Sweden	69	78	74
Russian Federation	43	42	42	Sweden	60	70	65	Wales	69	76	72
Netherlands	41	44	42	England	59	69	64	England	68	76	72
England	39	43	41	Russian Federation	55	67	61	Estonia	65	78	72
Slovakia	45	36	40	Norway	55	67	61	Poland	65	75	70
Denmark	44	37	40	Israel	55	67	61	Russian Federation	63	76	70
Sweden	44	36	40	Poland	51	68	59	Bulgaria	67	72	69
Canada	39	38	38	Estonia	54	64	59	Malta	66	71	69
Latvia	40	35	38	Slovakia	55	58	57	Slovakia	64	72	68
Estonia	39	35	37	Denmark	56	57	57	Spain	61	73	67
MKDª	40	31	36	Canada	50	60	55	Israel	66	68	67
Malta	37	33	35	Iceland	52	56	54	Denmark	64	70	67
Czech Republic	44	27	35	Germany	54	54	54	Luxembourg	66	67	67
Poland	36	34	35	Malta	50	57	54	Republic of Moldova	63	70	66
Romania	36	33	35	Finland	44	63	54	Germany	64	68	66
Norway	35	33	34	Latvia	51	55	53	Czech Republic	62	68	65
Finland	32	35	33	MKDª	51	52	52	Latvia	58	71	65
Ukraine	37	29	33	Greece	49	52	51	Canada	59	71	65
Belgium (Flemish)	33	32	32	France	49	52	50	France	61	68	64
Iceland	35	28	31	Belgium (Flemish)	47	54	50	Ukraine	60	68	64
Republic of Moldova	30	31	31	Romania	48	52	50	Iceland	57	64	61
France	30	28	29	Ireland	45	52	50	Ireland	53	65	61
Ireland	30	28	29	Czech Republic	50	49	50	Belgium (French)	56	64	60
Belgium (French)	30	26	28	Luxembourg	50	49	49	Belgium (Flemish)	56	64	60
Armenia	34	20	27	Ukraine	49	49	49	Finland	50	68	59
Germany	32	22	27	Belgium (French)	44	53	48	Romania	58	60	59
Hungary	30	24	27	Italy	46	50	48	Greece	59	59	59
Luxembourg	31	23	27	Spain	42	53	48	Slovenia	56	61	58
Italy	27	26	27	Republic of Moldova	44	51	47	Hungary	50	65	58
Croatia	32	22	26	Croatia	46	45	46	Croatia	56	59	57
Austria	29	24	26	Slovenia	44	44	44	MKDª	52	58	55
Lithuania	31	20	26	Austria	48	41	44	Italy	50	60	55
Greece	28	22	25	Portugal	42	44	43	Austria	48	57	53
Slovenia	31	18	25	Hungary	40	44	42	Switzerland	48	58	53
Portugal	27	22	24	Lithuania	40	42	41	Albania	53	46	50
Spain	28	16	22	Albania	47	33	40	Portugal	48	49	49
Albania	27	14	20	Armenia	43	32	38	Armenia	53	45	48
Switzerland	18	17	18	Switzerland	33	40	37	Lithuania	43	50	46
HBSC average	**36**	**31**	**33**	**HBSC average**	**50**	**55**	**52**	**HBSC average**	**59**	**67**	**63**

Note: no data were received from Greenland.

MEASURE Young people were asked how many hours per day they use a computer for email, internet or homework in their spare time on weekdays and at weekends. Findings presented here show the proportions who reported using a computer in these ways for two or more hours every weekday.

ª The former Yugoslav Republic of Macedonia.

HEALTH BEHAVIOURS
PLAYING GAMES ON A COMPUTER OR GAMES CONSOLE FOR TWO OR MORE HOURS ON WEEKDAYS

11-year-olds (%)				13-year-olds (%)				15-year-olds (%)			
Country/region	Boys	Girls	Total	Country/region	Boys	Girls	Total	Country/region	Boys	Girls	Total
Bulgaria	62	50	56	Bulgaria	71	51	61	Malta	62	53	57
Denmark	68	39	53	Scotland	70	52	61	Netherlands	66	46	56
Israel	55	48	51	Netherlands	67	52	60	Scotland	64	44	54
Scotland	61	42	51	Wales	70	44	58	Bulgaria	65	37	53
Netherlands	55	43	49	Denmark	73	39	54	Canada	59	44	52
Wales	61	38	49	Israel	56	50	53	Wales	63	37	50
Romania	53	36	44	Malta	60	45	53	Germany	58	41	50
Sweden	57	30	44	Canada	59	46	52	Israel	58	42	49
Canada	50	37	43	England	60	45	52	Belgium (French)	55	44	49
Estonia	58	29	43	Lithuania	63	40	51	Norway	67	32	48
Slovakia	56	31	43	Sweden	67	36	51	Lithuania	60	34	48
Russian Federation	51	36	42	Romania	61	37	49	Slovakia	62	31	47
Malta	48	35	42	Iceland	62	34	48	Romania	62	34	46
England	45	36	41	Estonia	70	26	48	Sweden	65	29	46
Lithuania	52	28	40	Austria	58	38	48	England	55	35	45
Iceland	51	27	39	Latvia	64	31	47	Luxembourg	53	36	44
Latvia	52	27	39	Belgium (French)	51	44	47	Hungary	58	30	44
Czech Republic	55	22	37	Slovakia	61	34	47	Ukraine	57	31	43
Republic of Moldova	43	28	36	Russian Federation	58	37	46	Russian Federation	55	32	42
Hungary	43	26	34	Norway	56	38	46	Denmark	63	25	42
MKD[a]	42	26	34	France	55	35	46	Czech Republic	64	21	42
France	40	26	33	Germany	50	39	45	Estonia	63	19	41
Belgium (French)	40	25	33	Czech Republic	62	29	45	Republic of Moldova	54	28	41
Poland	43	22	33	Greece	54	33	44	Italy	46	36	41
Ukraine	41	25	33	Hungary	52	35	43	Iceland	56	24	40
Belgium (Flemish)	40	25	33	Italy	49	38	43	Albania	51	29	40
Italy	39	25	32	Republic of Moldova	52	34	43	Spain	43	36	39
Ireland	38	27	31	Albania	54	31	42	Latvia	58	24	39
Austria	39	25	31	Ukraine	55	30	42	Greece	52	25	38
Norway	37	25	31	MKD[a]	51	31	41	France	48	27	38
Finland	44	16	30	Luxembourg	49	33	40	Austria	47	28	36
Luxembourg	35	23	29	Ireland	44	36	39	MKD[a]	46	25	36
Greece	38	19	28	Belgium (Flemish)	48	28	39	Armenia	47	26	35
Albania	37	19	28	Spain	39	36	37	Poland	50	17	32
Portugal	34	18	25	Poland	50	23	37	Belgium (Flemish)	42	18	32
Croatia	34	18	25	Croatia	50	22	36	Portugal	45	21	32
Germany	32	19	25	Portugal	42	26	34	Croatia	46	17	32
Slovenia	34	14	24	Finland	56	10	33	Switzerland	39	23	31
Armenia	29	17	23	Armenia	38	27	32	Ireland	32	29	30
Spain	29	16	23	Slovenia	48	17	32	Finland	51	8	29
Switzerland	25	16	20	Switzerland	32	24	28	Slovenia	42	14	27
HBSC average	**46**	**28**	**37**	**HBSC average**	**56**	**35**	**45**	**HBSC average**	**54**	**30**	**42**

Note: no data were received from Greenland.

MEASURE Young people were asked how many hours per day they played games on a computer or a games console in their spare time on weekdays and at weekends. Findings presented here show the proportions who reported computer/games console use for two or more hours every weekday.

[a] The former Yugoslav Republic of Macedonia.

GROWING UP UNEQUAL: GENDER AND SOCIOECONOMIC
DIFFERENCES IN YOUNG PEOPLE'S HEALTH AND WELL-BEING
ANNEX. METHODOLOGY AND SUPPLEMENTARY DATA TABLES

A

RISK BEHAVIOURS
DRINKING BEER AT LEAST ONCE A WEEK

11-year-olds (%)				13-year-olds (%)				15-year-olds (%)			
Country/region	Boys	Girls	Total	Country/region	Boys	Girls	Total	Country/region	Boys	Girls	Total
Israel	10	4	7	Bulgaria	16	9	13	Bulgaria	27	12	20
Armenia	8	2	5	Croatia	11	4	7	Croatia	25	5	16
Bulgaria	6	2	4	Israel	10	5	7	Italy	21	9	15
Slovenia	5	3	4	Romania	11	4	7	Israel	23	6	14
Croatia	4	2	3	Italy	6	4	5	Malta	19	9	14
Czech Republic	3	3	3	Greece	7	3	5	Hungary	20	7	13
Lithuania	3	2	3	Hungary	6	3	5	Greece	18	10	13
Romania	4	1	3	Albania	6	2	4	Czech Republic	17	8	13
Austria	2	3	3	Slovakia	6	2	4	Romania	22	4	12
Albania	3	1	2	Czech Republic	6	2	4	Belgium (Flemish)	14	7	11
Portugal	2	2	2	Slovenia	5	3	4	Slovakia	15	5	11
Hungary	2	1	2	Poland	4	2	3	Austria	19	3	10
Luxembourg	3	1	2	Russian Federation	4	3	3	Belgium (French)	13	6	9
Canada	3	1	2	Armenia	5	1	3	Germany	16	3	9
Slovakia	3	0	2	Lithuania	5	1	3	MKD[a]	15	3	9
Poland	2	1	2	MKD[a]	5	1	3	Netherlands	16	2	9
Republic of Moldova	2	0	1	Portugal	3	2	3	Denmark	15	4	9
MKD[a]	3	0	1	Republic of Moldova	4	1	3	Ukraine	13	5	9
Russian Federation	1	1	1	Austria	3	2	3	Poland	10	7	8
Italy	2	1	1	Malta	4	1	3	Luxembourg	11	5	8
Switzerland	1	1	1	Canada	3	2	3	Albania	12	3	7
Iceland	1	1	1	Luxembourg	3	2	2	Slovenia	11	3	7
Wales	2	0	1	Wales	4	1	2	Canada	9	3	6
Latvia	1	1	1	Germany	2	2	2	France	9	4	6
Belgium (French)	2	0	1	Finland	4	1	2	Wales	9	3	6
Malta	1	1	1	Switzerland	3	1	2	Lithuania	10	2	6
Estonia	1	0	1	England	3	1	2	Switzerland	8	4	6
Sweden	1	1	1	France	2	1	2	Republic of Moldova	10	2	6
Scotland	1	0	1	Belgium (French)	2	1	2	Scotland	9	2	5
France	1	0	1	Latvia	2	1	1	Armenia	9	2	5
England	1	0	1	Sweden	2	0	1	Portugal	9	2	5
Greece	1	0	1	Belgium (Flemish)	2	1	1	Spain	6	4	5
Denmark	1	0	0	Estonia	2	0	1	England	8	2	5
Germany	1	0	0	Iceland	1	1	1	Russian Federation	6	3	5
Belgium (Flemish)	1	0	0	Scotland	1	1	1	Latvia	6	1	4
Ireland	0	0	0	Denmark	1	1	1	Greenland	5	2	4
Greenland	1	0	0	Spain	1	1	1	Finland	6	1	3
Norway	1	0	0	Netherlands	1	0	1	Estonia	6	0	3
Spain	0	0	0	Ireland	1	0	1	Norway	3	2	3
Netherlands	0	0	0	Greenland	1	1	1	Sweden	3	1	2
Finland	–	–	–	Norway	1	0	0	Ireland	3	1	2
Ukraine	–	–	–	Ukraine	–	–	–	Iceland	3	1	2
HBSC average	**2**	**1**	**2**	**HBSC average**	**4**	**2**	**3**	**HBSC average**	**12**	**4**	**8**

Note: no data were received from Finland (11-year-olds) and Ukraine (11- and 13-year-olds).

MEASURE Young people were asked how often they drink any alcoholic beverage and were given a list of drinks: beer, wine, spirits, alcopops or any other drink that contains alcohol. Response options ranged from never to every day. Findings presented here show the proportions who reported drinking beer at least every week.

[a] The former Yugoslav Republic of Macedonia.

RISK BEHAVIOURS
DRINKING ALCOPOPS AT LEAST ONCE A WEEK

11-year-olds (%) Country/region	Boys	Girls	Total	13-year-olds (%) Country/region	Boys	Girls	Total	15-year-olds (%) Country/region	Boys	Girls	Total
Israel	8	3	5	Croatia	7	4	6	Malta	16	14	15
Slovenia	5	3	4	Italy	7	2	5	Denmark	11	10	11
Croatia	5	3	4	Israel	6	3	5	Hungary	9	9	9
Lithuania	4	2	3	Lithuania	6	2	4	Israel	11	6	8
Italy	4	2	3	Slovenia	6	3	4	Croatia	10	7	8
Portugal	2	3	2	Greece	4	2	3	Ukraine	10	6	7
Austria	2	3	2	Bulgaria	4	2	3	Slovenia	10	5	7
Luxembourg	3	1	2	Wales	3	3	3	Netherlands	6	8	7
Bulgaria	2	1	2	Austria	4	2	3	Italy	8	5	7
Romania	2	1	2	Russian Federation	3	3	3	Austria	7	6	7
Hungary	2	1	2	Portugal	3	2	3	Canada	5	6	6
Poland	2	1	2	Hungary	4	2	3	Estonia	6	5	5
Canada	2	1	1	Malta	3	1	2	Greenland	10	1	5
Greenland	1	1	1	Romania	4	1	2	Germany	7	4	5
MKD[a]	2	0	1	Canada	3	2	2	Lithuania	6	4	5
Republic of Moldova	2	1	1	Republic of Moldova	3	2	2	Greece	7	3	5
Czech Republic	1	1	1	Greenland	2	2	2	Bulgaria	5	4	5
Russian Federation	1	1	1	Luxembourg	3	2	2	Belgium (French)	6	3	4
Iceland	1	1	1	Albania	3	1	2	Scotland	4	5	4
Albania	1	1	1	Scotland	1	2	2	Wales	4	4	4
Latvia	1	1	1	Poland	3	1	2	Czech Republic	4	3	3
Sweden	1	1	1	Estonia	2	1	2	Luxembourg	4	3	3
Belgium (French)	1	0	1	Belgium (French)	2	1	2	Switzerland	4	2	3
Estonia	1	0	1	Switzerland	2	1	2	Republic of Moldova	4	2	3
Wales	1	0	1	France	2	1	2	England	3	3	3
Scotland	1	1	1	Finland	2	1	2	Romania	5	2	3
France	1	0	1	Latvia	2	1	1	Latvia	4	2	3
Greece	1	0	1	Sweden	2	1	1	Belgium (Flemish)	3	3	3
Switzerland	0	1	1	Czech Republic	2	1	1	Poland	4	2	3
Malta	0	1	1	Germany	1	1	1	Spain	3	2	3
Netherlands	1	0	0	England	2	1	1	France	3	2	3
Germany	1	0	0	Ireland	2	1	1	Portugal	4	1	2
Slovakia	0	0	0	MKD[a]	1	1	1	MKD[a]	3	2	2
Ireland	0	0	0	Belgium (Flemish)	1	1	1	Sweden	3	2	2
England	0	0	0	Denmark	1	1	1	Finland	3	1	2
Belgium (Flemish)	0	0	0	Iceland	1	1	1	Russian Federation	3	1	2
Norway	1	0	0	Spain	1	1	1	Norway	2	2	2
Spain	0	0	0	Slovakia	1	1	1	Slovakia	3	1	2
Denmark	0	0	0	Netherlands	1	1	1	Albania	3	1	2
Finland	–	–	–	Norway	1	0	0	Ireland	2	1	2
Ukraine	–	–	–	Ukraine	–	–	–	Iceland	2	1	2
HBSC average	**2**	**1**	**1**	**HBSC average**	**3**	**2**	**2**	**HBSC average**	**5**	**4**	**4**

Note: no data were received from Armenia, Finland (11-year-olds) and Ukraine (11- and 13-year-olds).

MEASURE Young people were asked how often they drink any alcoholic beverage and were given a list of drinks: beer, wine, spirits, alcopops or any other drink that contains alcohol. Response options ranged from never to every day. Findings presented here show the proportions who reported drinking alcopops at least every week.

[a] The former Yugoslav Republic of Macedonia.

GROWING UP UNEQUAL: GENDER AND SOCIOECONOMIC
DIFFERENCES IN YOUNG PEOPLE'S HEALTH AND WELL-BEING
ANNEX. METHODOLOGY AND SUPPLEMENTARY DATA TABLES

A

RISK BEHAVIOURS
DRINKING WINE AT LEAST ONCE A WEEK

11-year-olds (%)				13-year-olds (%)				15-year-olds (%)			
Country/region	Boys	Girls	Total	Country/region	Boys	Girls	Total	Country/region	Boys	Girls	Total
Israel	9	4	7	Croatia	8	4	6	Croatia	17	7	12
Armenia	8	3	5	Israel	8	4	6	Malta	12	9	10
Slovenia	5	3	4	Albania	7	4	5	Hungary	12	8	10
Croatia	3	2	3	Slovenia	6	3	4	Israel	11	6	9
Lithuania	3	2	3	Greece	6	2	4	Italy	11	4	8
Austria	2	3	2	Hungary	5	3	4	Greece	10	5	7
Republic of Moldova	3	2	2	Italy	5	2	4	Albania	8	5	7
Romania	3	1	2	Romania	5	2	4	Romania	12	2	7
Hungary	3	2	2	Armenia	5	2	3	Slovenia	8	5	6
Albania	3	2	2	Bulgaria	4	2	3	Armenia	10	3	6
Bulgaria	3	1	2	Russian Federation	3	3	3	Bulgaria	6	3	4
Portugal	2	2	2	Malta	3	2	3	MKD[a]	5	3	4
Luxembourg	3	1	2	Austria	3	2	2	Netherlands	2	6	4
Canada	2	1	2	Portugal	3	2	2	Republic of Moldova	6	2	4
Malta	2	1	2	Republic of Moldova	4	1	2	Ukraine	5	2	3
Poland	2	1	1	Lithuania	3	1	2	Slovakia	4	3	3
Greece	2	0	1	Luxembourg	3	2	2	Austria	3	3	3
Italy	2	1	1	Canada	3	1	2	Belgium (Flemish)	3	3	3
MKD[a]	2	0	1	Switzerland	2	1	2	Canada	4	3	3
Czech Republic	1	1	1	Poland	3	1	2	Wales	2	4	3
Wales	1	0	1	MKD[a]	2	1	2	Czech Republic	2	3	3
Iceland	1	1	1	Finland	2	1	2	Poland	4	3	3
Latvia	1	1	1	Belgium (French)	2	1	1	Luxembourg	3	2	3
Russian Federation	1	1	1	England	2	1	1	Scotland	3	2	3
Belgium (French)	1	0	1	Czech Republic	2	1	1	Belgium (French)	3	2	3
Sweden	1	1	1	Wales	2	1	1	England	2	3	2
England	1	1	1	Slovakia	2	1	1	Russian Federation	3	1	2
Switzerland	1	1	1	Sweden	2	1	1	Germany	2	2	2
Scotland	1	1	1	Latvia	1	1	1	Switzerland	3	2	2
Germany	1	0	1	France	1	0	1	Lithuania	3	1	2
Slovakia	1	0	1	Germany	1	1	1	Denmark	2	2	2
Belgium (Flemish)	1	0	0	Denmark	1	0	1	France	3	1	2
Estonia	0	0	0	Scotland	1	0	1	Spain	2	2	2
Norway	1	0	0	Iceland	1	0	1	Latvia	3	1	2
Denmark	0	0	0	Estonia	1	0	1	Sweden	2	1	1
France	0	0	0	Ireland	1	0	1	Portugal	2	0	1
Ireland	0	0	0	Belgium (Flemish)	1	0	1	Iceland	2	1	1
Spain	0	0	0	Spain	1	0	1	Finland	2	1	1
Greenland	0	0	0	Norway	1	0	0	Norway	1	0	1
Netherlands	0	0	0	Greenland	0	1	0	Estonia	1	0	1
Finland	–	–	–	Netherlands	0	0	0	Greenland	1	0	1
Ukraine	–	–	–	Ukraine	–	–	–	Ireland	1	0	1
HBSC average	**2**	**1**	**1**	**HBSC average**	**3**	**1**	**2**	**HBSC average**	**4**	**3**	**3**

Note: no data were received from Finland (11-year-olds) and Ukraine (11- and 13-year-olds).

MEASURE Young people were asked how often they drink any alcoholic beverage and were given a list of drinks: beer, wine, spirits, alcopops or any other drink that contains alcohol. Response options ranged from never to every day. Findings presented here show the proportions who reported drinking wine at least every week.

[a] The former Yugoslav Republic of Macedonia.

RISK BEHAVIOURS
DRINKING SPIRITS AT LEAST ONCE A WEEK

11-year-olds (%)				13-year-olds (%)				15-year-olds (%)			
Country/region	Boys	Girls	Total	Country/region	Boys	Girls	Total	Country/region	Boys	Girls	Total
Israel	8	3	5	Israel	8	4	6	Malta	19	18	18
Slovenia	5	3	4	Croatia	6	4	5	Hungary	15	8	11
Austria	2	3	2	Albania	6	3	4	Israel	13	6	9
Lithuania	3	2	2	Bulgaria	5	2	4	Croatia	11	6	8
Croatia	3	2	2	Slovenia	5	2	3	Italy	10	5	7
Albania	3	1	2	Portugal	4	2	3	Denmark	9	5	7
Armenia	4	1	2	Hungary	4	2	3	Austria	8	6	7
Portugal	2	2	2	Austria	3	2	2	Greece	9	4	7
Luxembourg	3	1	2	Lithuania	4	1	2	Scotland	5	7	6
Bulgaria	3	1	2	Greece	3	2	2	Bulgaria	8	4	6
Poland	2	1	2	Russian Federation	3	2	2	Slovenia	7	6	6
Canada	2	1	1	Romania	3	1	2	Canada	6	5	6
Hungary	1	1	1	Luxembourg	3	2	2	MKD[a]	6	5	6
Romania	2	1	1	Malta	2	2	2	Wales	4	6	5
Italy	2	0	1	Poland	3	2	2	Slovakia	6	4	5
Latvia	1	1	1	Canada	2	2	2	England	3	5	4
Republic of Moldova	1	0	1	Armenia	3	1	2	Portugal	5	3	4
Switzerland	1	1	1	Scotland	2	2	2	Albania	5	3	4
Iceland	1	1	1	Wales	2	1	2	Spain	4	4	4
Russian Federation	1	1	1	Finland	3	1	2	Romania	7	1	4
Sweden	1	1	1	Slovakia	2	1	2	Czech Republic	5	3	4
MKD[a]	1	0	1	Italy	2	2	2	Luxembourg	5	3	4
Czech Republic	1	0	1	Switzerland	2	1	2	Lithuania	6	1	4
Estonia	1	0	1	MKD[a]	2	1	1	Belgium (French)	5	3	4
Wales	1	0	1	Belgium (French)	2	1	1	Germany	4	2	3
France	1	0	1	Republic of Moldova	2	1	1	France	4	3	3
Scotland	1	0	1	Sweden	2	0	1	Poland	5	2	3
Belgium (French)	1	0	1	Estonia	2	1	1	Belgium (Flemish)	3	3	3
Malta	0	1	1	Germany	1	1	1	Switzerland	4	2	3
Germany	1	0	0	Czech Republic	1	1	1	Russian Federation	5	2	3
Slovakia	1	0	0	England	1	1	1	Ukraine	5	1	3
England	1	0	0	Latvia	1	1	1	Estonia	3	2	3
Ireland	0	0	0	Spain	1	1	1	Armenia	4	1	3
Belgium (Flemish)	0	0	0	Ireland	1	1	1	Republic of Moldova	3	2	2
Norway	1	0	0	Iceland	1	1	1	Latvia	4	1	2
Spain	0	0	0	France	1	1	1	Ireland	3	2	2
Greece	0	0	0	Denmark	1	1	1	Greenland	4	1	2
Denmark	0	0	0	Belgium (Flemish)	1	0	1	Sweden	3	2	2
Greenland	0	0	0	Norway	1	0	0	Iceland	3	2	2
Netherlands	0	0	0	Greenland	0	1	0	Finland	3	1	2
Finland	–	–	–	Netherlands	0	0	0	Norway	2	2	2
Ukraine	–	–	–	Ukraine	–	–	–	Netherlands	2	2	2
HBSC average	**2**	**1**	**1**	**HBSC average**	**2**	**1**	**2**	**HBSC average**	**5**	**3**	**4**

Note: no data were received from Finland (11-year-olds) and Ukraine (11- and 13-year-olds).

MEASURE Young people were asked how often they drink any alcoholic beverage and were given a list of drinks: beer, wine, spirits, alcopops or any other drink that contains alcohol. Response options ranged from never to every day. Findings presented here show the proportions who reported drinking spirits at least every week.

[a] The former Yugoslav Republic of Macedonia.

GROWING UP UNEQUAL: GENDER AND SOCIOECONOMIC
DIFFERENCES IN YOUNG PEOPLE'S HEALTH AND WELL-BEING
ANNEX. METHODOLOGY AND SUPPLEMENTARY DATA TABLES

A

RISK BEHAVIOURS
FIRST ALCOHOL USE AT AGE 13 OR YOUNGER

Country/region	15-year-olds (%)		
	Boys	Girls	Total
Estonia	50	47	49
Lithuania	44	41	43
Greece	47	38	43
Hungary	46	37	41
Croatia	46	33	40
Slovenia	44	35	39
Austria	41	37	39
Portugal	38	37	38
Armenia	43	33	37
Germany	36	37	37
Bulgaria	38	30	34
Denmark	35	32	33
Poland	32	32	32
France	37	25	31
Ukraine	36	26	31
Luxembourg	32	27	29
England	31	27	29
Romania	40	20	29
Latvia	28	29	29
Albania	39	18	28
Scotland	29	27	28
Republic of Moldova	34	22	28
Netherlands	29	23	27
Spain	25	27	26
Belgium (Flemish)	29	22	26
Switzerland	29	22	26
Slovakia	28	22	25
Wales	25	25	25
Malta	25	25	25
Czech Republic	28	22	25
MKD[a]	30	17	24
Canada	25	22	23
Belgium (French)	25	18	21
Finland	22	20	21
Italy	26	12	19
Ireland	19	15	17
Russian Federation	18	15	16
Sweden	15	13	14
Norway	16	13	14
Israel	17	4	10
Iceland	6	5	5
HBSC average	**30**	**24**	**27**

Note: no data were received from Greenland.

MEASURE Young people were asked at what age they had their first alcoholic drink. Findings presented here show the proportions who reported first drinking alcohol at age 13 or younger.

[a] The former Yugoslav Republic of Macedonia.

RISK BEHAVIOURS
EVER SMOKED TOBACCO

11-year-olds (%)				13-year-olds (%)				15-year-olds (%)			
Country/region	Boys	Girls	Total	Country/region	Boys	Girls	Total	Country/region	Boys	Girls	Total
Lithuania	21	11	16	Lithuania	54	32	43	Lithuania	70	55	63
Latvia	15	8	12	Latvia	42	33	37	Latvia	61	60	61
Estonia	13	6	10	Estonia	37	31	34	Estonia	61	55	58
Poland	10	6	8	Slovakia	27	28	28	Czech Republic	51	56	54
Slovakia	10	6	8	Czech Republic	29	24	27	Slovakia	50	51	50
Czech Republic	9	6	7	Poland	25	23	24	Croatia	49	48	49
Ukraine	11	4	7	Finland	26	19	23	Poland	49	48	49
Russian Federation	9	5	7	France	22	21	22	France	47	48	48
France	8	3	6	Croatia	23	20	22	Finland	51	43	47
Israel	9	3	6	Hungary	23	18	20	Hungary	45	48	47
Croatia	9	2	5	Italy	16	21	18	Italy	43	48	46
Hungary	5	4	5	Bulgaria	17	17	17	Bulgaria	37	51	43
Armenia	9	1	5	Russian Federation	21	14	17	Slovenia	40	40	40
Romania	7	2	5	Switzerland	19	15	17	Austria	40	40	40
Finland	7	2	4	Romania	17	16	17	Luxembourg	32	42	38
Republic of Moldova	7	1	4	Germany	14	16	15	Romania	40	35	37
Bulgaria	5	3	4	Ukraine	19	11	15	Switzerland	40	35	37
Switzerland	4	4	4	Greece	17	12	15	Greece	37	37	37
Germany	5	3	4	Slovenia	17	12	14	Ukraine	41	33	36
Italy	4	3	3	Belgium (French)	15	12	13	Russian Federation	40	31	35
Slovenia	4	2	3	Republic of Moldova	19	6	13	Germany	32	38	35
Luxembourg	3	2	3	Luxembourg	13	12	12	Republic of Moldova	49	19	35
Wales	3	2	3	Austria	15	9	12	Netherlands	32	36	34
Sweden	3	1	2	Portugal	10	14	12	Portugal	30	35	33
MKD[a]	3	1	2	Netherlands	11	11	11	Belgium (French)	30	35	33
Albania	3	1	2	Wales	9	12	11	Denmark	31	33	32
Netherlands	3	1	2	Sweden	10	11	10	Sweden	29	33	31
Canada	3	1	2	Belgium (Flemish)	11	9	10	Spain	27	34	31
Austria	2	2	2	Spain	9	10	10	Belgium (Flemish)	30	26	28
Denmark	3	1	2	Israel	12	7	9	Scotland	26	30	28
Spain	2	1	2	Denmark	9	8	9	Malta	27	28	28
Portugal	2	1	2	Scotland	6	11	8	Wales	22	29	26
Ireland	3	0	2	Albania	10	6	8	MKD[a]	27	23	25
Greece	2	1	2	England	6	9	8	England	19	29	24
Iceland	2	1	1	Armenia	14	1	7	Norway	23	19	21
Belgium (Flemish)	2	1	1	Malta	7	6	6	Ireland	21	20	21
England	2	0	1	Canada	6	6	6	Israel	31	10	19
Malta	1	1	1	Ireland	7	6	6	Canada	18	19	19
Scotland	1	1	1	Norway	7	5	6	Albania	25	9	17
Norway	1	0	1	MKD[a]	8	4	6	Iceland	13	12	12
Belgium (French)	–	–	–	Iceland	5	4	4	Armenia	18	4	10
HBSC average	**6**	**3**	**4**	**HBSC average**	**16**	**14**	**15**	**HBSC average**	**35**	**34**	**34**

Note: no data were received from Belgium (French) (11-year-olds) and Greenland.

MEASURE Young people were asked on how many days (if any) they had smoked cigarettes. Response options were never, 1–2 days, 3–5 days, 6–9 days, 10–19 days, 20–29 days and 30 days (or more). Findings presented here show the proportions who answered that they had smoked on 1–2 days or more in their lifetime.

[a] The former Yugoslav Republic of Macedonia.

GROWING UP UNEQUAL: GENDER AND SOCIOECONOMIC
DIFFERENCES IN YOUNG PEOPLE'S HEALTH AND WELL-BEING
ANNEX. METHODOLOGY AND SUPPLEMENTARY DATA TABLES

A

RISK BEHAVIOURS
DAILY SMOKING

11-year-olds (%)				13-year-olds (%)				15-year-olds (%)			
Country/region	Boys	Girls	Total	Country/region	Boys	Girls	Total	Country/region	Boys	Girls	Total
Israel	5	2	4	Greenland	10	18	14	Greenland	43	46	44
Russian Federation	3	4	3	Russian Federation	7	6	6	Bulgaria	17	25	21
Denmark	2	1	2	Romania	6	4	5	Croatia	19	17	18
Greenland	2	1	2	Poland	4	5	5	Hungary	15	15	15
Bulgaria	2	1	2	Bulgaria	4	4	4	Romania	14	13	14
Poland	2	1	1	Lithuania	6	2	4	Italy	12	14	13
Ireland	2	1	1	Slovakia	5	3	4	Luxembourg	10	13	12
Romania	2	1	1	Croatia	4	2	3	Slovakia	11	12	12
Albania	1	1	1	Hungary	3	2	3	Greece	13	10	11
Ukraine	1	1	1	Israel	3	2	2	France	11	12	11
Republic of Moldova	1	1	1	Scotland	2	3	2	Lithuania	14	7	11
Armenia	2	0	1	Italy	2	2	2	Poland	10	10	10
Luxembourg	1	1	1	Wales	2	2	2	Latvia	12	8	10
Hungary	1	0	1	Ireland	3	1	2	Germany	9	10	10
Malta	1	1	1	Finland	3	2	2	Austria	10	9	10
Lithuania	1	0	1	Czech Republic	3	2	2	Russian Federation	13	7	10
MKD[a]	1	0	1	Ukraine	3	1	2	Czech Republic	8	10	9
Croatia	1	0	0	Latvia	2	2	2	Slovenia	9	8	9
Austria	1	0	0	Luxembourg	2	2	2	Finland	10	7	8
Portugal	1	0	0	Greece	2	2	2	Ukraine	11	6	8
Estonia	1	0	0	Germany	1	2	2	Scotland	8	7	8
Belgium (Flemish)	0	0	0	Denmark	2	1	2	Israel	12	4	8
Latvia	1	0	0	France	2	1	2	Estonia	9	7	8
Czech Republic	0	0	0	Republic of Moldova	2	1	2	Netherlands	8	7	7
Wales	0	0	0	Estonia	2	1	2	Belgium (French)	8	7	7
Greece	0	0	0	Belgium (French)	1	2	1	Belgium (Flemish)	7	7	7
England	0	0	0	Slovenia	2	0	1	MKD[a]	8	6	7
Slovakia	0	0	0	Albania	2	1	1	Malta	7	6	6
Canada	0	0	0	Armenia	2	0	1	Ireland	7	6	6
Norway	1	0	0	Spain	1	1	1	Switzerland	6	6	6
Italy	0	0	0	Belgium (Flemish)	1	1	1	Portugal	6	6	6
Germany	0	0	0	Portugal	1	1	1	Wales	5	5	5
Iceland	0	0	0	MKD[a]	1	1	1	Spain	4	5	5
Belgium (French)	0	0	0	Netherlands	1	1	1	Republic of Moldova	5	5	5
France	0	0	0	England	1	1	1	Denmark	5	4	5
Slovenia	0	0	0	Malta	1	1	1	Sweden	4	5	4
Scotland	0	0	0	Switzerland	1	1	1	England	4	5	4
Switzerland	0	0	0	Austria	1	1	1	Canada	3	3	3
Spain	0	0	0	Norway	2	0	1	Albania	5	1	3
Finland	0	0	0	Canada	1	1	1	Iceland	2	2	2
Sweden	0	0	0	Iceland	1	0	1	Armenia	4	1	2
Netherlands	0	0	0	Sweden	1	0	1	Norway	2	1	1
HBSC average	**1**	**0**	**1**	**HBSC average**	**2**	**2**	**2**	**HBSC average**	**8**	**7**	**8**

MEASURE Young people were asked how often they smoke tobacco. Response options ranged from never to every day. Findings presented here show the proportions who reported smoking every day.

[a] The former Yugoslav Republic of Macedonia.

RISK BEHAVIOURS
INVOLVED IN A PHYSICAL FIGHT AT LEAST ONCE IN THE PAST 12 MONTHS

11-year-olds (%)				13-year-olds (%)				15-year-olds (%)			
Country/region	Boys	Girls	Total	Country/region	Boys	Girls	Total	Country/region	Boys	Girls	Total
Belgium (French)	69	33	51	Czech Republic	65	25	44	Slovakia	51	22	37
Czech Republic	66	29	46	Belgium (French)	57	31	44	Greece	53	22	37
Armenia	70	16	43	Armenia	71	15	43	Albania	56	17	36
Hungary	62	24	42	Republic of Moldova	60	24	42	Armenia	69	12	36
Scotland	57	25	41	Greece	55	27	41	Czech Republic	50	21	35
Republic of Moldova	63	18	41	Romania	54	28	41	Republic of Moldova	52	17	34
Romania	61	21	40	Hungary	54	27	41	Belgium (French)	44	25	34
Latvia	62	20	40	Slovenia	58	21	39	Malta	44	24	34
Israel	62	20	40	Slovakia	55	24	39	Romania	49	22	34
Slovenia	57	22	40	Croatia	54	23	39	Bulgaria	45	19	33
Lithuania	61	19	40	Malta	51	25	38	Netherlands	39	24	31
Spain	52	27	39	Latvia	57	20	38	Lithuania	44	17	31
Ukraine	61	20	39	Bulgaria	51	23	38	Ukraine	48	17	31
Malta	54	22	39	Lithuania	55	20	37	France	41	20	31
Austria	59	20	39	Albania	54	21	36	Hungary	40	21	30
France	54	21	38	Austria	58	15	36	Croatia	41	14	28
Denmark	55	22	37	France	46	23	35	Latvia	43	14	27
Slovakia	58	17	37	Israel	53	18	35	Austria	44	14	27
Germany	53	20	37	Poland	50	19	35	Norway	41	13	26
Bulgaria	51	22	36	Ukraine	51	19	34	Russian Federation	39	16	26
Greece	51	20	36	Italy	49	19	34	England	35	17	26
England	51	17	35	Wales	43	25	34	Ireland	41	17	26
Russian Federation	54	20	34	Canada	44	22	33	Luxembourg	34	20	26
Luxembourg	51	19	34	Germany	50	14	33	Belgium (Flemish)	33	16	26
Estonia	54	14	34	Denmark	47	18	31	Poland	38	14	26
Netherlands	47	20	34	Netherlands	42	20	31	MKD[a]	36	15	26
Poland	51	15	33	Spain	41	22	31	Scotland	36	15	26
Switzerland	48	18	33	Scotland	41	21	31	Italy	38	13	25
Italy	46	20	33	Russian Federation	45	19	31	Denmark	38	14	25
Wales	45	20	32	England	40	21	30	Germany	36	14	25
Croatia	50	15	32	Luxembourg	41	18	28	Canada	32	17	25
Canada	48	18	32	Estonia	42	13	28	Wales	30	18	24
Norway	46	17	31	MKD[a]	38	18	28	Slovenia	36	14	24
Iceland	48	15	31	Switzerland	43	12	28	Israel	39	11	24
Sweden	47	14	30	Belgium (Flemish)	37	16	27	Spain	30	16	23
Albania	46	13	30	Norway	43	13	27	Estonia	31	10	21
Belgium (Flemish)	45	12	28	Ireland	44	17	27	Portugal	25	13	19
Greenland	47	9	28	Iceland	39	13	26	Switzerland	28	9	18
Ireland	40	16	26	Sweden	36	14	25	Finland	26	9	17
Finland	41	10	25	Finland	35	12	23	Sweden	24	11	17
MKD[a]	35	11	23	Portugal	33	11	22	Greenland	25	10	17
Portugal	35	10	22	Greenland	35	10	22	Iceland	22	9	15
HBSC average	**53**	**19**	**35**	**HBSC average**	**48**	**20**	**33**	**HBSC average**	**38**	**16**	**27**

MEASURE Young people were asked how many times during the past 12 months they had been involved in a physical fight. Response options ranged from none to four times or more. Findings presented here show the proportions who reported fighting at least once in the past 12 months.

[a] The former Yugoslav Republic of Macedonia.

GROWING UP UNEQUAL: GENDER AND SOCIOECONOMIC
DIFFERENCES IN YOUNG PEOPLE'S HEALTH AND WELL-BEING
ANNEX. METHODOLOGY AND SUPPLEMENTARY DATA TABLES

A

RISK BEHAVIOURS
BEEN BULLIED AT SCHOOL AT LEAST ONCE IN THE PAST COUPLE OF MONTHS

11-year-olds (%)				13-year-olds (%)				15-year-olds (%)			
Country/region	Boys	Girls	Total	Country/region	Boys	Girls	Total	Country/region	Boys	Girls	Total
Lithuania	59	56	57	Lithuania	53	56	54	Lithuania	51	48	49
Latvia	52	53	53	Latvia	53	56	54	Latvia	40	42	41
Belgium (French)	60	43	52	Belgium (French)	54	42	48	Belgium (French)	47	34	40
Russian Federation	53	49	51	Austria	46	39	42	Russian Federation	36	35	35
Estonia	48	49	48	Russian Federation	47	38	42	Portugal	36	33	34
Ukraine	44	42	43	Portugal	44	38	41	Wales	28	36	32
Portugal	47	36	41	Wales	36	44	40	Republic of Moldova	29	35	32
Switzerland	42	37	40	Romania	39	39	39	Ukraine	33	32	32
Canada	38	39	39	Ukraine	40	38	39	Canada	29	32	31
Scotland	35	42	39	Canada	33	43	38	Romania	33	28	30
Hungary	40	37	38	Estonia	42	34	38	Bulgaria	31	28	30
Bulgaria	41	36	38	Republic of Moldova	37	39	38	England	30	29	29
Luxembourg	38	38	38	Greenland	39	35	37	Austria	30	27	29
Austria	42	33	37	Scotland	32	41	37	Estonia	27	27	27
Wales	37	37	37	Bulgaria	36	34	35	Switzerland	26	27	27
Greenland	38	34	36	Switzerland	34	34	34	Greenland	27	25	26
Republic of Moldova	35	32	34	England	30	38	34	Ireland	25	27	26
Poland	36	31	34	Hungary	32	33	32	Poland	27	25	26
England	33	35	34	Poland	33	29	31	Scotland	24	28	26
Finland	37	29	33	France	30	31	30	France	26	26	26
Romania	39	27	33	Luxembourg	28	32	30	Luxembourg	21	26	24
Malta	36	24	30	Ireland	27	30	29	Slovakia	24	23	23
France	32	27	30	Finland	33	25	29	Finland	23	19	21
Slovakia	33	25	29	Malta	30	26	28	MKD[a]	22	18	20
Israel	39	20	29	Slovakia	28	26	27	Hungary	18	22	20
Ireland	25	29	28	MKD[a]	30	23	27	Germany	18	20	19
Denmark	28	26	27	Israel	34	18	26	Norway	18	18	18
Netherlands	24	29	26	Germany	25	27	26	Netherlands	18	17	17
Germany	27	24	25	Slovenia	28	23	25	Slovenia	17	17	17
Belgium (Flemish)	25	24	25	Netherlands	24	23	24	Malta	21	12	17
Norway	25	24	24	Greece	23	23	23	Greece	18	15	16
Slovenia	31	16	24	Belgium (Flemish)	24	20	22	Albania	18	14	16
Albania	29	19	24	Norway	22	19	21	Israel	23	10	16
Iceland	25	21	23	Croatia	21	20	20	Czech Republic	15	16	16
Italy	28	18	23	Albania	21	20	20	Belgium (Flemish)	14	16	15
MKD[a]	28	17	23	Denmark	18	21	20	Croatia	14	15	15
Spain	23	16	19	Czech Republic	20	18	19	Denmark	14	14	14
Czech Republic	21	17	19	Iceland	17	20	19	Spain	12	10	11
Croatia	19	14	16	Spain	20	13	17	Sweden	7	10	9
Sweden	14	16	15	Italy	15	15	15	Italy	10	7	8
Greece	16	14	15	Sweden	12	16	14	Iceland	12	4	8
Armenia	13	8	11	Armenia	11	6	8	Armenia	8	5	6
HBSC average	**34**	**30**	**32**	**HBSC average**	**31**	**30**	**30**	**HBSC average**	**24**	**23**	**23**

MEASURE Young people were asked how often they had been bullied at school in the past couple of months. Response options ranged from zero to several times a week. Findings presented here show the proportions who reported being bullied at least once or twice at school in the past couple of months.

[a] The former Yugoslav Republic of Macedonia.

RISK BEHAVIOURS
BULLYING OTHERS AT SCHOOL AT LEAST ONCE IN THE PAST COUPLE OF MONTHS

11-year-olds (%)				13-year-olds (%)				15-year-olds (%)			
Country/region	Boys	Girls	Total	Country/region	Boys	Girls	Total	Country/region	Boys	Girls	Total
Latvia	61	47	54	Latvia	70	59	64	Latvia	63	49	55
Lithuania	55	40	47	Lithuania	60	49	54	Lithuania	60	43	52
Russian Federation	52	43	47	Russian Federation	56	41	47	Ukraine	51	40	45
Estonia	51	30	40	Romania	51	41	46	Russian Federation	52	37	44
Belgium (French)	44	27	36	Republic of Moldova	46	41	44	Romania	53	37	44
Ukraine	41	29	35	Austria	58	30	43	Republic of Moldova	48	38	43
Switzerland	42	27	35	Ukraine	48	37	42	Austria	48	33	39
Republic of Moldova	39	29	34	Slovakia	41	36	39	Slovakia	42	36	39
Slovakia	41	27	34	Estonia	48	26	37	Switzerland	47	27	37
Luxembourg	38	30	34	Bulgaria	43	30	37	Bulgaria	43	26	35
Romania	40	26	33	Belgium (French)	40	33	37	Poland	43	28	35
Portugal	40	22	30	Switzerland	45	28	36	France	39	29	34
Austria	36	25	30	Luxembourg	39	30	34	Belgium (French)	37	27	32
Slovenia	38	18	28	Portugal	39	29	34	Luxembourg	40	25	32
Bulgaria	35	21	28	Poland	40	27	34	Germany	37	22	30
Hungary	35	20	27	France	36	31	34	Greece	38	20	28
France	29	22	26	Germany	39	23	31	Estonia	37	19	28
Poland	33	18	25	Slovenia	38	21	30	Canada	33	22	27
Albania	32	17	25	Greece	35	21	29	Portugal	32	21	26
Israel	34	12	23	Albania	31	22	27	Slovenia	32	20	26
Canada	24	18	21	Canada	28	25	26	Albania	28	21	24
Denmark	26	17	21	Hungary	34	18	26	Hungary	29	19	23
MKD[a]	25	16	21	MKD[a]	33	19	26	Netherlands	29	16	23
Finland	28	12	20	Netherlands	27	19	24	MKD[a]	27	17	22
Greece	27	12	19	Israel	34	13	23	England	25	14	19
Germany	23	15	19	Finland	32	14	23	Finland	26	12	19
Netherlands	22	14	18	England	25	19	22	Denmark	25	13	19
Belgium (Flemish)	23	10	16	Denmark	26	17	21	Belgium (Flemish)	22	13	18
Scotland	21	12	16	Belgium (Flemish)	27	14	21	Malta	24	10	17
Italy	21	12	16	Croatia	25	13	19	Wales	22	12	17
Spain	19	13	16	Wales	22	16	19	Spain	21	14	17
Wales	18	13	15	Spain	22	15	19	Croatia	22	11	17
Armenia	22	7	15	Scotland	21	14	18	Scotland	26	8	17
England	19	9	15	Malta	26	9	17	Ireland	24	11	16
Norway	19	9	14	Italy	21	13	17	Israel	27	7	16
Czech Republic	17	8	12	Armenia	24	8	16	Italy	18	12	15
Ireland	15	8	11	Czech Republic	21	11	15	Czech Republic	20	11	15
Iceland	16	6	11	Norway	19	9	13	Norway	20	10	15
Croatia	14	8	11	Ireland	15	9	12	Iceland	9	13	11
Malta	13	6	9	Iceland	14	7	11	Armenia	15	6	10
Sweden	9	4	7	Sweden	11	6	8	Sweden	12	5	8
HBSC average	**30**	**18**	**24**	**HBSC average**	**34**	**23**	**28**	**HBSC average**	**32**	**21**	**26**

Note: no data were received from Greenland.

MEASURE Young people were asked how often they had taken part in bullying (an)other student(s) at school in the past couple of months. Response options ranged from zero to several times a week. Findings presented here show the proportions who reported bullying others at school at least once in the past couple of months.

[a] The former Yugoslav Republic of Macedonia.

GROWING UP UNEQUAL: GENDER AND SOCIOECONOMIC
DIFFERENCES IN YOUNG PEOPLE'S HEALTH AND WELL-BEING
ANNEX. METHODOLOGY AND SUPPLEMENTARY DATA TABLES

A

RISK BEHAVIOURS
BEEN CYBERBULLIED BY MESSAGES AT LEAST ONCE

11-year-olds (%)				13-year-olds (%)				15-year-olds (%)			
Country/region	Boys	Girls	Total	Country/region	Boys	Girls	Total	Country/region	Boys	Girls	Total
Greenland	24	32	28	Greenland	23	39	32	Greenland	22	31	26
Russian Federation	20	27	24	Lithuania	21	24	23	Lithuania	22	26	24
Lithuania	21	20	20	Bulgaria	19	20	19	Hungary	17	22	20
Scotland	13	22	18	Romania	15	20	17	Ireland	9	23	18
Latvia	18	17	17	Hungary	15	20	17	Republic of Moldova	16	19	17
Romania	18	16	17	Scotland	12	23	17	Bulgaria	16	18	17
Ukraine	18	15	16	Russian Federation	18	17	17	Malta	16	17	16
Republic of Moldova	16	15	16	Wales	10	22	16	Scotland	12	19	16
Bulgaria	17	14	16	Latvia	14	18	16	England	11	20	16
Hungary	13	13	13	Malta	11	20	15	Russian Federation	15	16	15
Estonia	12	14	13	England	8	19	14	Romania	11	18	15
Wales	10	13	11	Republic of Moldova	13	15	14	Latvia	14	16	15
Slovenia	13	8	10	Ireland	10	16	14	Wales	10	19	15
Slovakia	10	10	10	Ukraine	11	16	13	Poland	11	15	13
Israel	14	6	10	Croatia	13	14	13	Slovenia	10	14	12
Ireland	8	11	10	Poland	12	14	13	Croatia	10	14	12
Malta	9	10	10	Slovenia	12	13	12	Ukraine	12	11	12
Croatia	10	9	9	Netherlands	9	15	12	Canada	8	15	11
Finland	7	12	9	Slovakia	11	13	12	Belgium (French)	9	12	11
Belgium (French)	10	8	9	Belgium (French)	9	14	12	Slovakia	10	12	11
Albania	12	6	9	Finland	9	13	11	Portugal	8	13	11
England	7	12	9	Estonia	10	12	11	MKD[a]	12	8	10
Poland	9	9	9	Canada	6	15	10	Luxembourg	7	12	10
Italy	9	9	9	Belgium (Flemish)	6	15	10	Belgium (Flemish)	6	15	10
Austria	9	9	9	Israel	13	7	10	Netherlands	8	11	10
Switzerland	8	10	9	Switzerland	7	12	9	Czech Republic	6	13	9
MKD[a]	10	7	9	Italy	6	12	9	Switzerland	8	10	9
Canada	8	9	8	Portugal	8	11	9	Israel	13	5	9
Netherlands	6	11	8	Sweden	5	13	9	Estonia	8	9	9
Luxembourg	7	9	8	Denmark	6	11	9	Finland	7	10	9
Denmark	6	10	8	Luxembourg	7	10	8	Spain	9	6	7
Portugal	6	9	8	MKD[a]	8	8	8	Austria	7	8	7
Norway	5	10	7	Spain	9	7	8	Norway	4	10	7
Spain	9	6	7	Czech Republic	6	10	8	France	4	10	7
Armenia	8	6	7	Austria	8	8	8	Denmark	7	6	6
Czech Republic	7	6	7	Germany	5	10	7	Sweden	4	9	6
Belgium (Flemish)	6	7	6	Norway	6	8	7	Albania	7	5	6
Germany	5	6	6	Albania	8	6	7	Italy	4	8	6
France	4	6	5	France	5	9	7	Germany	3	8	6
Sweden	4	6	5	Iceland	6	7	7	Armenia	5	6	6
Iceland	5	4	5	Greece	6	7	6	Iceland	4	5	5
Greece	4	2	3	Armenia	5	4	5	Greece	4	4	4
HBSC average	**10**	**10**	**10**	**HBSC average**	**9**	**13**	**11**	**HBSC average**	**9**	**12**	**11**

MEASURE Young people were asked whether they had experienced anyone sending mean instant messages, wall-postings, emails and text messages. The results presented here show the proportions who had experienced such messages at least once.

[a] The former Yugoslav Republic of Macedonia.

RISK BEHAVIOURS
BEEN CYBERBULLIED BY PICTURES AT LEAST ONCE

11-year-olds (%)				13-year-olds (%)				15-year-olds (%)			
Country/region	Boys	Girls	Total	Country/region	Boys	Girls	Total	Country/region	Boys	Girls	Total
Russian Federation	19	19	19	Latvia	16	19	18	Ireland	11	26	20
Lithuania	16	12	14	Russian Federation	17	17	17	Lithuania	18	13	15
Bulgaria	17	10	14	Bulgaria	18	15	17	Estonia	13	18	15
Latvia	13	13	13	Estonia	14	19	16	Denmark	13	18	15
Estonia	11	13	12	Greenland	12	20	16	Latvia	15	15	15
Greenland	10	11	10	Ireland	12	19	16	Greenland	14	15	14
Israel	15	5	10	Lithuania	17	14	16	Malta	14	14	14
Ukraine	9	10	9	Denmark	10	18	14	Russian Federation	15	12	14
Republic of Moldova	10	8	9	Scotland	10	18	14	England	9	18	13
Scotland	5	12	9	Ukraine	11	12	12	Bulgaria	15	10	13
Romania	9	7	8	England	7	16	12	Scotland	8	15	12
Denmark	7	8	8	Israel	15	7	11	Poland	10	13	12
Ireland	6	9	8	Finland	9	12	11	Hungary	11	13	12
Albania	11	4	8	Poland	10	11	11	Slovakia	10	10	10
Wales	5	9	7	Slovakia	8	12	11	Canada	8	12	10
Slovakia	7	6	6	Netherlands	8	13	10	Wales	8	12	10
Croatia	9	4	6	Wales	8	12	10	Netherlands	9	11	10
Spain	7	5	6	Croatia	10	9	10	Croatia	11	8	10
Hungary	7	6	6	Romania	9	10	10	Israel	13	6	9
Belgium (French)	9	3	6	Hungary	9	10	9	Republic of Moldova	9	9	9
Armenia	7	5	6	Republic of Moldova	9	8	9	Finland	9	9	9
MKD[a]	8	4	6	Iceland	7	10	9	MKD[a]	12	5	8
Iceland	6	6	6	Norway	7	10	8	Ukraine	10	7	8
England	4	7	6	Slovenia	9	7	8	Spain	10	6	8
Finland	5	6	5	Spain	10	6	8	Slovenia	8	7	8
Netherlands	5	5	5	Canada	5	10	8	Norway	6	9	7
Norway	3	8	5	Albania	8	7	8	Portugal	8	6	7
Slovenia	7	4	5	Italy	6	9	8	Belgium (French)	7	7	7
Czech Republic	6	4	5	Malta	4	11	8	Italy	8	5	7
Canada	5	5	5	Belgium (French)	8	6	7	Sweden	6	7	6
Italy	6	5	5	Czech Republic	7	7	7	Luxembourg	8	5	6
Malta	6	4	5	MKD[a]	8	5	7	Czech Republic	5	7	6
Switzerland	5	4	5	Sweden	4	8	6	Belgium (Flemish)	5	8	6
Poland	5	4	4	Armenia	6	5	6	Romania	6	6	6
Portugal	6	3	4	Austria	6	5	6	Albania	7	4	5
Austria	6	3	4	Portugal	7	4	5	Iceland	4	6	5
Luxembourg	4	4	4	Luxembourg	5	5	5	Switzerland	6	4	5
Germany	4	4	4	Belgium (Flemish)	4	7	5	Germany	4	6	5
Belgium (Flemish)	3	3	3	Switzerland	6	4	5	Austria	5	3	4
France	3	2	3	Germany	4	5	4	France	3	5	4
Sweden	2	2	2	France	3	4	3	Armenia	3	3	3
Greece	3	1	2	Greece	3	1	2	Greece	3	1	2
HBSC average	**7**	**6**	**7**	**HBSC average**	**9**	**10**	**9**	**HBSC average**	**9**	**9**	**9**

MEASURE Young people were asked whether they had experienced anyone posting unflattering or inappropriate pictures online without permission. Findings presented here show the proportions who had experienced such pictures at least once.

[a] The former Yugoslav Republic of Macedonia.

GROWING UP UNEQUAL: GENDER AND SOCIOECONOMIC
DIFFERENCES IN YOUNG PEOPLE'S HEALTH AND WELL-BEING
ANNEX. METHODOLOGY AND SUPPLEMENTARY DATA TABLES

A

RISK BEHAVIOURS
BEEN CYBERBULLIED BY PICTURES AT LEAST 2–3 TIMES A MONTH

11-year-olds (%)				13-year-olds (%)				15-year-olds (%)			
Country/region	Boys	Girls	Total	Country/region	Boys	Girls	Total	Country/region	Boys	Girls	Total
Russian Federation	7	8	8	Bulgaria	7	6	6	Russian Federation	7	4	5
Lithuania	7	5	6	Greenland	8	5	6	Israel	8	2	5
Bulgaria	9	4	6	Russian Federation	8	4	6	Bulgaria	7	1	4
Israel	10	2	6	Lithuania	7	4	5	Malta	5	3	4
Latvia	5	4	4	Israel	7	3	5	Ireland	2	5	4
Ukraine	5	3	4	Estonia	5	4	4	Lithuania	6	2	4
Estonia	5	3	4	Ireland	3	5	4	Scotland	4	4	4
Spain	4	3	3	Spain	5	3	4	Spain	6	2	4
Albania	4	2	3	Scotland	2	6	4	England	2	4	3
Croatia	4	2	3	Latvia	4	4	4	Canada	3	3	3
MKD[a]	4	2	3	Croatia	5	3	4	Greenland	5	1	3
Republic of Moldova	2	2	2	Denmark	3	4	4	Luxembourg	4	2	3
Slovakia	3	1	2	Ukraine	3	4	3	Latvia	4	3	3
Iceland	3	2	2	Poland	3	2	3	Denmark	3	3	3
Belgium (French)	3	1	2	Albania	3	2	3	Croatia	4	2	3
Romania	3	1	2	Iceland	4	2	3	Wales	3	3	3
Austria	2	1	2	Finland	2	3	2	Slovakia	3	2	3
Ireland	2	2	2	Norway	2	3	2	Ukraine	4	1	3
Armenia	2	1	2	MKD[a]	3	2	2	Norway	2	3	3
Greenland	3	0	2	Malta	1	4	2	Estonia	3	2	2
Scotland	1	2	2	Wales	2	3	2	MKD[a]	4	1	2
Czech Republic	3	1	2	Slovenia	3	2	2	Portugal	3	2	2
Canada	2	1	2	Canada	1	3	2	Poland	3	2	2
Denmark	2	1	2	England	2	2	2	Republic of Moldova	3	1	2
Luxembourg	2	2	2	Portugal	3	1	2	Finland	3	1	2
Portugal	2	1	1	Slovakia	2	1	2	Belgium (French)	2	2	2
Slovenia	2	1	1	Belgium (French)	2	2	2	Albania	3	1	2
Switzerland	1	1	1	Italy	2	2	2	Iceland	2	2	2
Poland	1	1	1	Austria	2	1	2	Netherlands	2	1	2
Wales	1	1	1	Luxembourg	2	1	2	Czech Republic	1	1	1
England	1	2	1	Armenia	2	1	2	Sweden	1	1	1
Malta	2	0	1	Republic of Moldova	2	1	2	Hungary	2	1	1
Germany	1	1	1	Netherlands	1	2	2	Slovenia	1	1	1
Belgium (Flemish)	1	1	1	Romania	2	2	2	Switzerland	1	1	1
Norway	0	1	1	Sweden	1	2	1	Belgium (Flemish)	1	1	1
Finland	1	1	1	Belgium (Flemish)	2	1	1	Italy	2	0	1
Hungary	1	0	1	Czech Republic	2	1	1	Armenia	1	1	1
Italy	1	1	1	Hungary	1	1	1	Austria	1	1	1
France	1	0	1	Germany	1	1	1	Romania	1	1	1
Greece	1	0	1	France	1	1	1	Greece	2	0	1
Sweden	0	0	0	Switzerland	1	1	1	France	0	1	1
Netherlands	0	0	0	Greece	1	0	1	Germany	0	1	1
HBSC average	**3**	**2**	**2**	**HBSC average**	**3**	**2**	**3**	**HBSC average**	**3**	**2**	**2**

MEASURE Young people were asked whether they had experienced anyone posting unflattering or inappropriate pictures online without permission. Findings presented here show the proportions who had experienced such pictures 2–3 times or more often per month.

[a] The former Yugoslav Republic of Macedonia.

REFERENCES

1. Currie C, Inchley J, Molcho M, Lenzi M, Veselska Z, Wild F, editors. Health Behaviour in School-Aged Children (HBSC) study protocol: background, methodology and mandatory items for the 2013/14 survey. St Andrews: Child and Adolescent Health Research Unit, University of St Andrews; 2014 (http://www.hbsc.org/news/index.aspx?ni=2418, accessed 17 November 2015).

2. Schnohr CW, Molcho M, Rasmussen M, Samdal O, de Looze M, Levin K et al. Trend analyses in the Health Behaviour in School-Aged Children study: methodological considerations and recommendations. Eur J Public Health 2015;25(Suppl. 2):7–12.

3. HBSC [website]. St Andrews: Child and Adolescent Health Research Unit, University of St Andrews; 2015 (http://www.hbsc.org/, accessed 17 November 2015).